REMAKING THE *American Patient*

STUDIES IN SOCIAL MEDICINE
Allan M. Brandt, Larry R. Churchill, and
Jonathan Oberlander, editors

This series publishes books at the intersection of medicine, health, and society that further our understanding of how medicine and society shape one another historically, politically, and ethically. The series is grounded in the convictions that medicine is a social science, that medicine is humanistic and cultural as well as biological, and that it should be studied as a social, political, ethical, and economic force.

REMAKING THE

American Patient

How Madison Avenue and Modern Medicine
Turned Patients into Consumers

NANCY TOMES

The University of North Carolina Press *Chapel Hill*

This book was published with the assistance of the Lilian R. Furst Fund of the University of North Carolina Press.

The paper in this book meets the guidelines for permanence and durability of the Committee on Production Guidelines for Book Longevity of the Council on Library Resources. The University of North Carolina Press has been a member of the Green Press Initiative since 2003.

Cover illustration: Candettes cough-jel advertisement, 1958. Courtesy of Medicine and Madison Avenue Digital Collection—MMA0406, J. Walter Thompson Company, Competitive Advertisements Collection, 1955–97, John W. Hartman Center for Sales, Advertising, and Marketing History, David M. Rubenstein Rare Book and Manuscript Library, Duke University. Candettes trademark is no longer in use.

Library of Congress Cataloging-in-Publication Data
Tomes, Nancy, 1952– , author.
Remaking the American patient : how Madison Avenue and modern medicine turned patients into consumers / Nancy Tomes.
p. ; cm. — (Studies in social medicine)
Includes bibliographical references and index.
ISBN 978-1-4696-2277-4 (cloth : alk. paper)
ISBN 978-1-4696-2278-1 (ebook)
I. Title. II. Series: Studies in social medicine.
[DNLM: 1. Delivery of Health Care—history—United States. 2. Consumer Participation—history—United States. 3. History, 20th Century—United States. 4. Marketing of Health Services—history—United States. W 84 AA1]
RA412.3
368.38′200973—dc23
2015029217

For BRITTANY, *who would have made*
a wonderful doctor,

for PHIL, *who helped me remember why*
medicine is a noble profession,

and for ANNIE *and* CHRIS, *who gave me*
the best reason to finish.

CONTENTS

A Tale of Two Medicine Bottles

A few years ago, while cleaning out the bathroom closet of my childhood home, I found an old prescription bottle. Its label carried simply the date, March 6, 1965, the name and telephone number of the drugstore, my name (misspelled), my home address (correct), my doctor's name, and these cryptic directions: "One every four hours until relieved." Unlike a prescription I recently filled at my supermarket pharmacy, there was no drug name with its generic equivalent, no number of allotted refills, no patient information leaflet explaining the conditions that the drug might remedy and the list of side effects I might expect.

Through the long labor of writing this book, I have kept that old bottle in front of me as a reminder of the past landscape of patienthood that I have tried to capture. My 1965 prescription came from Dr. William J. Moore, a Norman Rockwell–style general practitioner who still made house calls and had my family's worshipful respect. The medication was prepared at Frankel-Klapheke's, a tiny, dark drugstore that sold almost nothing except medicine. At that time, patients were to be seen and not heard, and no one—in my family at least—thought to second-guess the doctor's recommendations. At my local public library, the *Physicians' Desk Reference*—that Bible of all things prescription-drug-related—was likely kept behind the librarians' desk, along with the sex books, safe from inquisitive patient eyes. I saw plenty of drug ads on TV, but only for over-the-counter remedies; my generation grew up hearing about the plop, plop, fizz, fizz of Alka Seltzer and the fast, fast pain relief of Excedrin. But in my youth, ads did not invoke the magic of the lifesaving operation and miracle drug. Those seemed to be sacred goods, set apart from the commercial frenzy associated with hula hoops, cars with fins, and avocado green refrigerators. In those days, medicine seemed more protected from the unsavory aspects of modern capitalism.

As I have learned in writing this book, that image of separateness was in many ways illusory: already by the 1960s, the changes were under way that would turn my doctor's office and Frankel-Klapheke's drugstore into relics of a bygone age. But like most Americans, my awareness of that sweeping change came only later, in the 1970s and after. Now, looking back on my child-hood, the extent of the change through which I have lived seems breathtaking. In the early twenty-first century, Americans are expected to be in charge of their medical fates, always in possession of the latest and best information and ready to choose wisely among the many health choices now available to them—at least if they have the right kind of insurance. The family doctor has been replaced by a platoon of specialists tending to different parts of our bodies with an ever-changing array of high-technology and pharmaceutical remedies. From every media—television, radio, Internet, even the billboard at the baseball game—stream advertisements for every type of health service, from the mundane to the miraculous. Prescription drug ads urge us to "ask our doctors about" the latest, best medicine for erectile dysfunction, high cholesterol, and irritable bladder. Local medical centers offer to laser our eyes, staple our stomachs, or treat our cancer with more care and success than their competitor down the street. "It matters where you are treated first," the announcer intones against a backdrop of tasteful classical music. (God forbid that we be taken anywhere else, we think—at least until we hear the competitor's commercial.) At the local library, the *Physicians' Desk Reference* is shelved in a whole alcove of "consumer health information," including all the many guides to the best and worst of everything—drugs, doctors, diagnostic tests, and surgical procedures—required to counteract all the advertising.

In critically important ways, this new medical world is an improvement over the old: today's patients feel more entitled to information, choice, and voice in their health affairs. Few of us older folk (me included) are likely to hanker for an olden days when patients who wanted to learn about their ailments, to ask questions about their care, or otherwise to be treated as rational adults faced being called neurotics or closet communists. At the same time, there is no denying that for all its efforts to be more patient-directed and consumer-friendly, American medicine seems even more dysfunctional today than it did in 1965. This book reflects my curiosity about why that should be the case. Why has the "consumer revolution" in health care fallen so short of its goals?

That question first occurred to me in the course of writing *The Gospel of Germs*, a history of the popularization of the germ theory of disease. Study-ing the commercial invocation of the "germ menace" by the makers of toilets, paper cups, and mouthwash, I became fascinated by the way scientific claims were translated into advertising slogans. How ironic, I thought, that as phy-sicians defined scientific "truth" as the antithesis of advertising, advertising professionals became all the more effective at invoking modern bacteriology to sell a dazzling array of products. The idea for this book started with what I mistakenly thought were some simple questions: What difference did it make that modern medicine and modern advertising both came of age in the early twentieth century? How did patients and doctors respond to a host of commercial "strangers at the bedside" who used increasingly sophisticated sales techniques to sell various "new and improved" brands of medicine?

Tracking the parallel worlds of modern medicine and modern advertising, I spent many entertaining hours looking at old advertisements for products such as Listerine and Fleischmann's yeast. But as I began giving talks with titles such as "Medicine and 'Madison Avenue,'" using the nickname for the advertising industry, my audience's responses began to push me in additional directions. I wanted to analyze old Listerine ads; they wanted to talk about managed care and the health care crisis. In formal question-and-answer periods as well as private chats, people spoke with great passion about their frustrations with being a modern health consumer: about health care fragmented among many specialists, about sleazy junk mail promoting dubious medicines, about time-consuming hassles with insurance companies.

My initial reaction was to insist all the more loudly that the book I was writing would be "just about the advertising." I had no wish to engage with all that anger and anxiety. But my avoidance strategy eventually failed me when my dearly loved eleven-year-old niece (to whom this book is dedicated) developed lymphoma. My family's brutal introduction to "ped onc," or pediatric oncology, broadened my sense of what this book had to discuss. So next to my old prescription bottle came to sit Brittany's picture, to remind me what I learned from her while spending New Year's Eve in the pediatric ICU to keep her company as she lay dying and from my family's efforts to make sense of our ped-onc nightmare. As we sat in a corridor while she underwent yet one more MRI in a desperate and ultimately unsuccessful effort to save her, a relative voiced a worry that has haunted me ever since: "I hope they aren't torturing her just because we have good health insurance."

I did not believe then, nor do I believe now, that my niece was "tortured" to make money. But after writing this book, I better understand why so many Americans share a corrosive fear that the quality of their medical care depends too much on the size of their pocketbooks. Although the vast majority of individual physicians put their patients' lives above all else, the larger *culture* of medicine, including the expectations that both patients and doctors are encouraged to have, has been shaped in the context of modern consumer capitalism: we cannot help but think that healing consists of finding just the "right" combination of products and services and that "new and improved" medicine is better than its older—and usually cheaper—counterpart.

In fact, I believe that definition of healing is deeply flawed. Staying healthy or recovering from a serious disease usually involves far more than a magic pill or procedure. Some old remedies are better (and cheaper) than new ones. While often treated as the Cinderella of modern medicine, preventive medicine and public health repeatedly show that an ounce of prevention is indeed worth a pound of cure. But for reasons this book explores, we find it hard to give up the assumption that "new and improved" medicine is better and that expense equals quality. This book turns to the history of medicine's relations with consumer culture and consumerism as a way to help us better understand where those ideas originated. In so doing, I try to capture both Americans' great admiration for physicians and medical science as well as their persistent worries about the cost and value of their health care expenditures. I have also tried to describe the long efforts of many physicians to defend their profession's values against the corrosion of commercialism.

Like any historian, my point of view is inevitably bounded by my personal experiences and convictions. The reader should know in advance that although I am critical of some aspects of medicine, I am no medical Luddite. Blessed with reasonably good health and, more important, an excellent health insurance plan, I do not come to this subject with a personal sense of grievance against the medical profession. I am grateful for innovations such as antibiotics, Prozac, and an epidural during childbirth, three milestones of modern medicine that I have been privileged to enjoy. While I aspire to be an "intelligent buyer" and "constructively critical" of medical expertise, as my historical subjects termed it, I believe in finding a good doctor and putting my trust in her. Although there were no physicians in my family of origin, I married into a family of physicians who have taught me a great deal about what it means to be a good physician. My father-in-law, Phil, to whom this book is also dedicated, has helped remind me that when done right, medicine is indeed a noble profession.

Some readers will no doubt be disappointed because I do not hold one particular villain accountable—irrational patients, greedy doctors, evil pharmaceutical companies, or heartless insurance companies. But I have a different goal here: I want to understand why, despite a growing commitment to more consumer-friendly health care, American medicine still seems caught in such a dysfunctional set of institutions. In my view, no single-bad-actor explanation suffices to do this. In the absence of quick or easy solutions, we need to describe our problems as fully and accurately as we can. If, as many knowledgeable commentators suggest, we have a health care system "designed to fail,"[1] fixing it will require profound attitude adjustments on everyone's part; for needed change to occur, the values, expectations, and behaviors of patients and physicians, political and business leaders, all have to be transformed. I hope that this history contributes in some small way to that transformation.

ACKNOWLEDGMENTS

In the many years it has taken me to complete this book, I have accumulated more debts than can be properly acknowledged in a few paragraphs. Four scholarly communities have been particularly important in its writing. The first is the National Humanities Center in Research Triangle Park, North Carolina, where I spent two significant blocks of time. The first stint came during my tenure as the Burroughs Wellcome Fund Fellow in the History of Modern Medicine, a yearlong stay during which I benefited enormously from long conversations with my fellow Fellows, among them Jodi Bilinkoff, Susan Langdon, Louise McReynolds, Joanne Meyerowitz, Sherry Ortner, and Marjorie Woods, as well as the extraordinary assistance of librarians Jean Houston and Eliza Robertson. While at the Center, I also received an Ahmanson Foundation Grant that brought about a long and happy collaboration with Duke University's Hartman Center and the exceptional group of archivists there (chief among them Ellen Gartrell) who helped me create the website *Medicine and Madison Avenue*. More than a decade later, I was fortunate to have a chance to return to the National Humanities Center to teach a Jessie Ball DuPont Fellowship Program seminar, "Worried Sick, Worried Well." Through our weeks of reading and conversation, the participants in that seminar helped me better articulate what the book was about. So a big thanks goes to the "Worrieds"—Cole Barton, Steven Benko, Craig Bythewood, Katherine Goff, Victor Greto, Deborah Hawkins, Emily Mieras, Mickey Pellillo, Hilary Smith, and Jack Trammell—as well as my colleagues Carl Elliot and Andrea Tone, who came to visit our group.

The second community that helped shape this book was created by the Robert Wood Johnson Foundation. I was fortunate to participate in its Investigator Awards Program, which gave me the opportunity to join working groups on history and health policy, the future of public health, medical professionalism in the Internet age, and patients as policy actors. Attending the Investigator Awards' annual meetings was the best kind of interdisciplinary education I could ask for: a chance to listen to and learn from some of the country's best health economists, historians, political scientists, sociologists, and psychologists. I owe a special debt of gratitude to David Mechanic, who has been a wonderful mentor and friend for many years, and to his able assistants Lynn Rogut and Cynthia Church. Among the many scholars' work I got to know through the Robert Wood Johnson Foundation, that of Lori Andrews, David Blumenthal, Steven Epstein, Timothy Jost, James Morone, Marc Rodwin, and Deborah Stone has been especially useful to me. Above all, I benefited from the knowledge and support of my fellow collaborators on the Patients as Policy Actors project—Rachel Grob, Beatrix Hoffman, and Mark Schlesinger. They helped me make this book so much better.

The third scholarly community whose support made this book possible is at Stony Brook University. I am very lucky to be part of a history department filled with exceptionally smart and generous colleagues who have taken a big interest in this project from start to finish. They have provided excellent advice about shaping my arguments as well as bucked me up when I felt overwhelmed at the thought of getting the book done. I have also enjoyed the support of colleagues in other departments, chief among them Lisa Diedrich, who has been a treasured fellow traveler along the path of questions this study addresses. Stony Brook has also brought me some wonderful graduate students/research assistants: Amanda Bruce, Cynthia Dianne Creagh, Dennis Doyle, Amy Gangloff, and Kelly Hacker Jones. Kelly played an especially important role in helping me through the final ordeal of preparing the manuscript for copyediting. I am grateful to the College of Arts and Sciences Excellence Fund for helping to defray the cost of the illustrations.

Finally, I could not have written this book without the assistance of my fellow historians of medicine. For all the research I have done on my own, I could not have written a synthesis of this scope without building on the foundation provided by their work. I have been fortunate to have had as a first mentor and faithful friend the incomparable Charles E. Rosenberg. I have subsequently been mentored and befriended by other extraordinary scholars, among them John Burnham, Gerald Grob, Judith Walzer Leavitt, and Rosemary Stevens. Judy deserves special thanks for the personal as well as scholarly support she has given me over the years. Of my own generation, Joan Jacobs Brumberg and Susan Reverby get the same thanks for long service rendered. In addition, I have benefited from the research of a host of talented scholars, many of them also good friends, whose work has enlightened me: Emily Abel, Ava Alkon, Allan Brandt, James Cosgrove, Christopher Crenner, Jacalyn Duffin, Amy Fairchild, Daniel M. Fox, Joseph Gabriel, Janet Golden, Jeremy Greene, Burt Hansen, David Herzberg, Margaret Humphreys, Carla Keirns, Wendy Kline, Susan Lederer, Barron Lerner, Kenneth Ludmerer, Howard Markel, Gerald Markowitz, Gerald Oppenheimer, Martin S. Pernick, Nicholas Rasmussen, Leslie Reagan, Naomi Rogers, David Rosner, David Rothman, Sheila Rothman, James A. Schafer, Karen Cruse Thomas, Dominique Tobbell, Andrea Tone, Elizabeth Toon, Elizabeth Watkins, Keith Wailoo, John Harley Warner, and George Weisz. Two of the historians whose work most inspired me, Roy Porter and Harry Marks, died before I finished the project, but I want to remember them as well. One of my best memories of writing this book remains the long afternoon I spent with Harry, only months before he died, sharing ideas and chapter drafts. And I am beholden to Audra Wolfe for the insightful comments she provided on a very early version of the manuscript as well as the invaluable advice that she gave me about writing in general.

As every historian knows, we would get nowhere in our work without the aid of our archivist and librarian colleagues, and I am beholden to many of them. That debt started with the exceptional help I got at the National Humanities Center and at the Hartman Center and has continued with the years of assistance I have gotten from Stony Brook's Interlibrary Loan Office, where Donna Sammis and her staff have run down many a strange document for me. I am also appreciative for the help I got during shorter but still very fruitful visits to the Library of Congress, UCLA, the Hagley Museum and Library, and the Huntington Library. For personal as well as academic reasons, Arlene Shaner of the New York Academy of Medicine and Christine Ruggere of the Welch Medical Library at Johns Hopkins remain especially dear to me. I have benefited as well from the kindness of strangers such as Jim Armistead at the Truman Presidential Library and Museum, who copied and sent me Oscar Ewing's file on the American Patients Association.

As this book has reached its final stages, I have been fortunate in my choice of a publisher. Little did I know back during my first stay at the National Humanities Center that the article I did for the center's magazine, *Ideas*, would have such long-term significance. Many years later, it led Joe Parsons of the University of North Carolina Press to inquire about what had happened to that book manuscript I was working on. Joe has done a great job helping me get "the monster" done. I am also deeply grateful to Allan Brandt for his support of the project as part of the Studies in Social Medicine series he helps to edit. I owe much to Chris Crenner and Jonathan Oberlander for their excellent suggestions about how to revise and strengthen the book's argument. And Alison Shay, Stephanie Wenzel, and Ellen Goldlust have helped me through the complicated process of turning an untidy manuscript into a finished book.

Last but not least, I thank my friends and family for their support. Among my friends, Mandy Friskin, Brooke Larson, and Sara Lipton have been steadfast in their encouragement over the many years it has taken to get this project done. From her own experience of creative travail, my filmmaker friend, Lucy Winer, gave me some great advice about dealing with what was in my basement. Barbara Kos has helped me keep from driving myself and my family crazy. My Bethany "family" has done the same. My Sellers in-laws have spent many holidays and vacations listening to me maunder on about the modern patient. So thank you to Phil and Julia, Jeff and Laura, Randy and Laura, Pat and Kathryn, and my glorious niece and nephews for putting up with me. The Tomeses have done their share of supporting and listening, too, so thanks are owed to Linda, Wendy, Bob, and Lee. Russell, Angela, and Scott escaped the beginning of the book saga but are now with me at the end. I hope they will enjoy seeing their auntie's door-stopper in print. I owe a special debt to my sister-cousin, Regina Tomes Johnson, who showed up to support me when I most needed it.

As for Chris and Annie, I am truly a blessed woman, having the best of husbands and the best of daughters. Next to me, no one has had to suffer more than Chris to get this book done. He has become a master at talking me through the unfortunately frequent moments/days/months of despair when I thought I would never get done. Annie has helped in all kinds of ways: making copies, checking notes, giving me advice about the book cover, and introducing me to distracting entertainment fare such as *Orange Is the New Black* and *How to Train Your Dragon*. Chris and Annie, thank you for putting up with me. Our dogs, Lily and Wilson, can't read, but they will be glad I am done, too. More walks all around!

ABBREVIATIONS AND ACRONYMS

AARP   American Association for Retired Persons

ACA   Patient Protection and Affordable Care Act

AHA   American Hospital Association

AMA   American Medical Association

CCMC   Committee on the Costs of Medical Care

DRG   diagnostic related groups

DTCA   direct-to-consumer advertising

FDA   Food and Drug Administration

FTC   Federal Trade Commission

HCA   Hospital Corporation of America

HCFA   Health Care Finance Administration

HMO   health maintenance organization

IOM   Institute of Medicine

NIH   National Institutes of Health

NCPIE   National Council on Patient Information and Education

PDR   *Physicians' Desk Reference*

PSRO   professional service review organization

USP   United States Pharmacopeia

INTRODUCTION
This Isn't Your Father's Patient

In 2006, the trade periodical *Hospitals and Health Networks* carried a special supplement, "Patient Satisfaction and the New Consumer," prepared by Press Ganey Associates, a health marketing firm. The American patient, the supplement explained, was "more discerning and demanding" than in the past, a "savvy internet user" who valued "customer service, convenience and easy access to information." At a time when it was easier to "shop around with their health care dollars," Americans looked for "better amenities," chief among them doctors who treated them "with courtesy and respect," presented facts "in a way that patients can understand," and made pain control a top priority. In other words, "today's patient shouldn't be thought of as a patient, but as a consumer" whose expectations needed to be met in an increasingly competitive medical world. Rephrasing a line made famous by a 1988 Oldsmobile commercial, Press Ganey concluded, "This isn't your father's patient."[1]

The phrase "not your father's patient" captures a widely held assumption about our times: that Americans have become an enthusiastic nation of "doctor-shoppers," able and determined to get the best medical care possible by making savvy choices. By the term "shopping," I mean a set of behaviors that many Americans now regard as essential to their health: searching for the latest scientific information, reading labels carefully, asking lots of questions, and last but not least, feeling emboldened to challenge both medical opinion and bureaucratic decision making. Being a "good" patient now requires transferring habits initially developed to evaluate our automobiles and home appliances to the choice of our doctors and medical treatments. Pick up a trade publication from any health-related field today, and you are likely to see this new medical consumerism celebrated. According to optimists, we now live in a patient's Eden where empowered consumers have been liberated to make more choices for themselves and receive better care as a result.

But just as frequently, especially during the fierce debates over Obamacare, we hear far more pessimistic messages: the American health care system is broken and that the new breed of patient shoppers helped to break it. Americans, we are told, have completely unrealistic expectations about their medical care. We assume that doctors can fix every illness, including those we have brought on ourselves by our own bad habits, and then we shirk paying the cost of our cure. In this tale of entitlements gone wild, medical consumerism figures more as problem than as progress.

Consider, for example, the assessment rendered by Dr. Otis Webb Brawley, then head of the American Cancer Society, in a 2012 interview for the *New York Times*. While holding hospitals, doctors, and insurance companies accountable for the nation's problems, he also blamed patients for buying into "the notion that more care—more treatment, more screening, more scans, more drugs—is better care." At the same time the U.S. system failed to offer basic care to the poor and uninsured, "many Americans, particularly wealthier ones, are . . . gluttonous in their consumption of health care resources and often use them unwisely." As an illustration, Brawley described a patient with early colon cancer who had three doctors tell her that chemotherapy was unnecessary in her case; "she decided she wanted it, and she went doctor-shopping until she found a doctor who would give it to her." At the same time that this woman felt entitled to unnecessary chemotherapy, poor patients with more advanced cancer were receiving too little care. "Our health care system is messed up," Brawley concluded, and in order to fix it, everybody, including patients, had to learn to be more rational in their use of its resources.[2]

This is a very common assessment of today's health care troubles. But while I share Brawley's concerns about the overtreatment of some and undertreatment of others, his diagnosis neglects the problem that interests me as a historian: Where do those expectations come from? Why has shopping for particular diagnostic tests or treatments come to be likened to the hunt for the best automobile or flat-screen TV? In short, why have patients come to be thought of and to think of themselves as consumers?

Until now, explanations for when and how this consumer mind-set came to the American health care scene have focused on the recent past. The most common story line has consumerism first arriving in the 1970s, largely as a by-product of the women's health movement, and then exploding with the coming of the Internet in the late 1990s. In this accounting, the 1970s represented a radical break with a past in which patients were docile and medical authority reigned supreme, a break that cleared the way for the emergence of today's e-patients and medical Googlers. The coming of the Internet, so this argument goes, has ushered in a new era of patient empowerment that at long last will truly reshape the health care system.[3]

Remaking the American Patient makes a very different argument: today's patient-consumers, far from being the historical equivalent of something new under the sun, have a much older pedigree. While the 1970s women's health movement and the rise of the Internet are indeed very important developments, they are better understood as the end rather than the beginning of the story. As I see it, the birth of the patient as consumer lies not in the late *twentieth* century but rather a full century earlier. While they are completely unaware of it, twenty-first-century medical Googlers and their kin are indebted to several generations of Americans who sought to become more "educated" or "intelligent" patients, as they described themselves. Long before the 1970s, they began to seek out information, ask questions, and challenge medical authority; in the process, they started to reshape the culture of American medicine.

My version of consumerism challenges some widely held assumptions about medical history. The first of these is that a "golden age" of placid doctor-patient relationships existed in the United States from the 1910s to the 1960s. In the traditional textbook telling, the profession took a great leap forward in the early 1900s as a more scientific medicine emerged from a network of research laboratories, high-caliber medical schools, and technologically sophisticated hospitals. As the Harvard biochemist Lawrence H. Henderson liked to tell his medical students in the 1930s, "Somewhere between 1910 and 1912 in this country, a random patient with a random disease consulting a doctor chosen at random had for the first time in the history of mankind a better than 50–50 chance of profiting from the encounter." The American people, so the traditional narrative suggests, could not help but be awed into obedience by this superior type of medicine.[4]

Yet a deeper look soon demonstrates that these supposedly golden years were hardly so quiet. Presented with care that was more expensive but not necessarily more satisfactory, some laypeople expressed disappointment in its cost and quality. Although frequently told that only physicians could differentiate good and bad care, a discontented minority persisted in pointing out the gaps between the promise and the reality of medical progress. In articulating their concerns, these contrarians began in the late 1920s to use the term "consumer" as a synonym for "patient."

Of course, patients had been complaining about doctors (and vice versa) long before the 1920s. As medical historians well know, the United States has a long and rollicking history of questioning medical authority. From the nineteenth century onward, a long line of herbal doctors, homeopaths, Christian Scientists, chiropractors, osteopaths, and other healers have lambasted mainstream or "regular" medicine as ineffectual and despotic. What made the strand of discontent expressed in the 1920s different was its starting point;

these were lay critics who by and large accepted the legitimacy of modern science and the values of professionalism. Their complaints reflected a disappointment that doctors were not being scientific or professional *enough*, that their standards were being compromised by weak internal discipline and too close an embrace of commercial values.[5]

Along with the idea of a golden age of deferential patients, *Remaking the American Patient* challenges the assumption that prior to the 1970s, medicine existed completely separate from modern business. Contrary to the nostalgic view that money mattered little in the olden days, contemporaries already recognized by the 1930s that medical care had become "one of the largest industries of the country," in the words of physician-educator Ray Lyman Wilbur. On the eve of the Great Depression, medical care ranked sixth among leading American industries; measured by the size of its workforce, the value of the services and products it delivered, and investments in it, medicine stood ahead of automobile, iron, steel, oil, and coal production. As this history shows, the rapid growth in the medical economy between 1900 and 1940 created intense conflicts among doctors over how to reconcile the demands of being both scientific and businesslike. Long before the advent of third-party health insurance or for-profit health care corporations, the dual nature of medicine as profession and business had become a cause for concern among both doctors and patients. Indeed, medical consumerism appeared in the interwar period precisely because of fears that medicine was becoming businesslike in all the wrong ways.[6]

These concerns reflected the fact that medicine's great leap forward coincided with a broad shift in the economy toward greater dependence on consumer spending. Economic growth became increasingly driven by the decisions of millions of Americans to buy all kinds of goods, from expensive but rarely bought consumer "durables" such as automobiles and refrigerators to inexpensive and frequently consumed "nondurables" such as candy and cigarettes. An integral part of this expanded consumer economy was the role of advertising and marketing in getting people to buy more such goods. Starting in the early 1900s, the advertising industry, colloquially known as Madison Avenue as a consequence of its initial association with that New York City address, came to play an increasingly prominent role in the shaping of American wants and needs.

The intersection of these two broad trends—the changes in the medical economy and the expansion of a consumer-oriented culture—led to the debates that *Remaking the American Patient* explores. Despite efforts to shield physicians' services and medicinal drugs from the worst traits of marketplace competition, the provision of both inevitably got bound up with and measured against larger changes in consumption and consumer goods. Medicine's maturation during the expansion of twentieth-century consumer culture—in particular, its robust development of advertising, marketing, and public relations—blurred distinctions between professionalism and commercialism and thus complicated what it meant to be a "good" patient or a "good" doctor.

In examining those debates, I focus primarily on the influence of what I term critical medical consumerism in two key arenas, the doctor's office and the drugstore. By critical consumerism, I mean "the movement seeking to protect and inform consumers by requiring such practices as honest packaging and advertising, product guarantees, and improved safety standards," as the *American Heritage Dictionary* defines it. More specifically, my interest lies in the medical versions of the consumer rights articulated in 1962 by President John F. Kennedy: the rights to be safe, to be informed, to make choices, and to be heard. This medical consumerism is the direct ancestor of what in today's policy world is known as patient engagement and shared decision making. With those themes and locations as its moorings, *Remaking the American Patient* describes three distinct eras of consumerist agitation: a first peak occurring during the Progressive era, a second during the 1930s, and a third in the late 1960s and early 1970s. Medical consumerism gradually evolved from an orientation associated with cranks and communists to an approach endorsed by powerful political and business interests, albeit with their own aims in mind.[7]

To trace this evolution, the book starts with a description of the nineteenth-century version of "free-market" medicine and the concerns that brought it to an end in the late 1800s. For a variety of reasons, older traditions of "every man his own doctor" and the rule of caveat emptor (let the buyer beware) gave way to stronger forms of medical professionalism and drug regulation. In their wake, both medical innovation and health commercialism grew dramatically in the 1920s and 1930s, creating a raft of what economists would later describe as "shopping problems."[8] In the doctor's office and the drugstore, patient-consumers wrestled with rising prices, multiplying choices, and a host of misleading advertising claims. In response, some Americans, particularly affluent middle-class urbanites, started to adapt skills learned in making choices among other goods (food, clothing, appliances) and apply them to medical care. While recognizing that doctors and medicinal drugs constituted unique kinds of commodity, they nonetheless began to approach their purchase with a mind-set developed to deal with an expanding world of consumer goods and services.

Most physicians regarded consumerist aspirations as unwarranted and indeed downright foolish. In their view, the profession was doing a superlative job of caring for patients—or at least those willing to follow doctors' advice. But a large and influential minority of doctors shared consumerists' concerns that an excess of commercialism endangered medicine's scientific and ethical standards. They were joined by social scientists and welfare reformers troubled about the rising cost and uneven quality of medical care, particularly as the Great Depression worsened. Although neither physician reformers nor social scientists necessarily approved of the medical consumerists' tone, they agreed that Americans had good reason to be unhappy about the state of medical affairs. And as Chapter 4 reveals, far from being nonexistent or invisible, the complaining class of patients played a significant role in reshaping the interwar medical order—most notably, in strengthening drug and advertising laws in 1938 and softening physician opposition to private medical insurance.

As the middle third of the book shows, the changes adopted in the 1930s and 1940s did not solve patient-consumers' shopping problems. During the Cold War years, the cost of medical goods and services dramatically outpaced increases in other kinds of consumer goods, leading to renewed economic and political concerns. Physicians had many new and impressive services to offer their patients, both in their offices and in newly expanded hospitals, but they still faced troubling questions about the quality and pricing of those services. Unnecessary surgery and the cost and side effects of prescription drugs became particular focal points of popular anxiety. By 1960, both politicians and journalists declared that the United States was in the midst of a full-blown health care "crisis."

During the late 1960s, that sense of crisis escalated as a far more radical critique of medicine's failings gave rise to an even more sweeping "revolt of the patients." Out of that tumult came a new era of patients' rights, signified by such landmarks as the 1970 writing of *Our Bodies, Ourselves*, now in its ninth edition; the 1971 founding of Public Citizen's Health Research Group, which remains a major voice in policy debates to this day; and the 1973 patients' bill of rights, one of the founding documents of patient-centered medicine. In this time period, the consumerist concept of patient as watchdog gained enormous traction as both an organizing tactic and a policy principle. Advocates of empowerment argued that by teaching all Americans to be more active, informed patients, they could be turned into a powerful grassroots force for better medical care.

Physicians initially found the "new breed" of 1970s patient no more palatable than earlier versions of the "intelligent" patient. But as the last third of the book shows, a much-toned-down version of medical consumerism found growing favor with politicians and policymakers as a weapon to use in bringing a too-independent medical profession to heel. With medical costs now perceived as a serious drag on the national economy, both liberals and conservatives embraced the idea of increasing patients' role as market actors as a means to foster more competition among doctors and hospitals. In this context, critical medical consumerism became not just acceptable but admirable. Suddenly not just patient activists but politicians, government officials, and policy experts began to urge Americans to become better "doctor-shoppers," to use their powers of choice to improve the health care system. Once derided as a threat to the "American way" of medicine, discriminating patients became its salvation: by conscious choosing and wise consumption, they could redirect American medicine toward higher standards, in both therapeutic and economic realms.

As the political climate turned more conservative in the late 1970s and early 1980s, medical consumerism grew increasingly entangled—or perhaps more accurately strangled—by third-party payers' efforts to cut costs and limit physician autonomy. In the name of patient-consumers, both public and private health insurers began to manage doctors' fees and treatment decisions in dramatic new ways. At the same time, doctors had to contend with new for-profit health corporations and venture capitalist interest in the medical marketplace, including the rise of retail medical clinics, colloquially referred to as "docs in a box." Meanwhile, drugstores were losing their exclusive right to sell prescription drugs, so that now Walgreens had to compete with Kroger and Walmart for sales while pharmaceutical companies had to contend with the growing availability of generic medicines.

Thus the 1980s brought a new era of shopping mall medicine and medicine-chest roulette that has remained with us ever since. Paradoxically, while many of the changes of the past decades were justified in the name of patients' welfare, they led to frustrating new restrictions that left both patients and physicians unhappy. The side effects have included a relaxation of long-standing prohibitions on the advertising of prescription drugs and physicians' services, creating a deluge of claims about the "new and improved" virtues of medical care. In another grand irony, a medical consumerism founded on an intense dislike of modern advertising helped to justify the latter's expansion as a legitimate form of consumer health information. These new forms of advertising, along with managed care and its backlash, have helped create the very different perceptions of patient as consumer described at the outset of this introduction: the happy patient-shopper in a medical wonderland versus the overentitled abuser of a broken health care system.

For its true believers, medical consumerism holds out the hope not only that individual patients can avoid bad outcomes by being vigilant but also that their collective actions can become a force for reform throughout the whole system. This influence has been conceived in terms both of therapeutic quality (patients should reward doctors who offer the best care) and of cost control (patients should help hold down rising costs by shopping for good prices). Thus medical consumerism rests on a faith that well-informed patients can help curb our dysfunctional medical culture, with its tendencies to undertreat, overtreat, misuse, and overcharge for medical services. But in practice, the power of the patient as watchdog has been a weak corrective to the problems presented by a changing medical economy.

The weakness of critical consumerism in part reflects the difficulty of separating it from its uncritical counterparts. In addition to its association with "the movement seeking to protect and inform consumers," the term "consumerism" has other meanings that are also important to the history told here: according to the *American Heritage Dictionary*, these other meanings include the belief that a "progressively greater consumption of goods is economically beneficial" and the assumption that a deep "attachment to materialistic values or possessions" marks modern life. As this history amply demonstrates, those three strands are as hard to separate in medicine as in the rest of American life.[9]

In 1965, Jack Straus, the chair of Macy's board of trustees, described the nature of American consumerism: "The consumer is the key to our economy. Our ability to consume is endless. The luxuries of today are the necessities of tomorrow."[10] Insert the word "medical" before "economy," "luxury," and "necessity," and you have a good approximation of why the culture of "new and improved" medicine poses such a challenge to its patients. In the medical realm, critical consumerism has emerged in tandem with the emergence of the medical-industrial complex and a medicalized version of keeping up with the Joneses. The evolution of "good" consumerism has been articulated in opposition to its "bad" counterparts, such as the doctor-shopper in search of Oxycodone or the patient insistent on getting tests or procedures that may not be needed.

This historical perspective helps to clarify why American physicians have found the tenets of medical consumerism so off-putting even as they have endorsed the ideals of patient-centered medicine. While agreeing that patients need to be treated with respect and care, doctors do not necessarily see consumerism, with its emphasis on comparison shopping and second-guessing of medical advice, as the best way to reach that goal. As one doctor complained back in 1986, describing patients as consumers lends "a super-market touch" to the practice of a noble profession. Having devoted decades learning how to practice medicine, physicians understandably have balked at the idea of being "shopped for" by laypeople who may have spent an hour or two reading up on their symptoms. Many doctors share Brawley's worry that emphasizing consumerism has encouraged the wrong kind of choices; tellingly, physicians have long used "doctor-shopper" as slang for drug addicts looking for illegal prescriptions. Last but certainly not least, physicians today quite rightly associate the rhetoric of consumerism with the late-twentieth-century advent of managed care and the growing limits placed on medical autonomy by third-party payers. It is no wonder, then, that as one physician quipped to columnist Ellen Goodman, "every time a patient is referred to as a health care consumer, another angel dies."[11]

Yet ironically, as *Remaking the American Patient* shows, the medical profession has played a huge if inadvertent role in producing the modern doctor-shopper. For most of the twentieth century, its members passionately championed the principle of physician autonomy and successfully resisted centralized forms of professional control. The medical embrace of what came to be known as "free enterprise" medicine or the "American way" of health care contributed to the genesis of medical consumerism in two ways. First, it elevated the personal relationship between doctor and patient as the hallmark of good medicine, making it all the more likely that Americans would expect more of the service being rendered. Second, physician individualism allowed for the flourishing of an "anything goes" mentality that produced uneven standards of care and forms of medical entrepreneurship that seemed more commercial than professional in spirit. These conditions provided fertile soil for the rise of medical consumerism. Far from being an alien creed, imposed on doctors by misguided third parties, the patient-as-watchdog concept grew Frankenstein-like from the expectations that the medical profession had itself encouraged.

While physicians in other countries have also venerated innovation and progress, the culture of American medicine has nurtured a very product- and procedure-oriented style of practice since the early 1900s. This credo of "new and improved" medicine has promoted the idea that new treatments are invariably better than the old ones they replace and that if one new treatment is good, multiple treatments are even better. That credo has flourished in the United States thanks to the profession's comparatively decentralized status, its unusual insurance system, and most of all, the promotional culture of advertising and marketing that surrounds it. In short, it is a professional culture likely to increase the "doctor's dilemma," as George Bernard Shaw dubbed it in 1906: the temptation to overtreat and overcharge patients to make more money. Medical consumerism emerged so early and so strongly in the United States as a result.

Remaking the American Patient also reveals the growing tensions between two seemingly irreconcilable trends of modern culture: the elevation of individualism and personal autonomy on the one hand, and deference to scientific expertise and authority on the other. Here again, while other times and cultures have generated similar tensions, they became particularly intense in the United States as a consequence of the strong synergism that developed between modern science and modern consumer culture. As analysts of twentieth-century consumer culture have noted, it encouraged the search for a unique self, to be cultivated not only through education and self-discipline but also through participating in new kinds of consumption. This quest has been encouraged by neoliberal economic thinking that celebrates the power of free agents to act in free markets on their own behalf. At the same time, the rapid specialization of medical knowledge over the past century has required a growing deference to the doctor's expertise. Modern medicine has increasingly become identified with a scientific and technological complexity that even the most "educated" layperson finds difficult to comprehend. Perhaps more than any other area of economic thinking, medicine exposes the disconnect between market logics of personal choice and the need to trust and defer to experts.

The connection between the credo of "new and improved" medicine and medical consumerism also helps explain the latter's persistent weaknesses. It is hard to overcome the flaws of consumer economics and consumer culture by employing the same tools and values it promotes. Medical consumerism has proven a weak counterweight to medical commercialism in large part because its strengths and weaknesses mirror those of the larger medical culture. More suited to a focus on the trees instead of the forest, consumerist approaches tend to succeed better at directing attention to specific products (prescription drugs, hip replacements) and procedures (mammograms, coronary bypass surgeries) than they do to intangibles such as time, trust, and motivation that are essential to health promotion.[12]

These problems have become all the more obvious as policymakers have tried to scale up and universalize the ideal of the empowered patient-consumer. As this history shows, medical consumerism originated with what sociologist C. Wright Mills has termed the "new middle classes"—white, college-educated professionals who were far from "average" Americans. Inevitably, their conception of the "intelligent buyer" of medical care reflected their class, gender, and race privileges. When extolling the wise patient-consumer, consumerists initially pictured people like themselves: literate, well educated, white, and native born. While willing to allow that women of their own class could be educated to be better doctor-shoppers, male consumerists tended to assume, as did male physicians, that the "fairer sex" was a prolific source of medical error and confusion. They also believed that their poorer, darker, and less-educated fellow citizens were even less likely to know how to function as educated patients.

But while medical consumerism was closely associated with urban middle-class professionals, it had a wider resonance, in large part as a result of the growing emphasis on medical care as a symbol of the "American way of life" over the course of the twentieth century. The post–World War II perception of a transition from a "class society" where only a few enjoyed the best medical care to a "mass society" where all Americans had access to lifesaving goods lent the ideals of medical consumerism new force. Many Americans wanted to believe what Miriam Bredow wrote in her 1943 handbook for medical secretaries: "In a doctor's office people are perhaps more nearly equal than anywhere else in the world. For a physician there are only sick people and well people."[13]

In the 1960s, this aspiration to medical democracy opened up opportunities for groups outside the new middle classes, most notably in the labor and civil rights movements, to lodge their own complaints about the inequities of the health care system. As it turned out, people other than white middle-class urbanites also had strong feelings about the definition of a "good" doctor or a "good" patient. As Chapter 8 argues, the cross-fertilization of medical consumerism and other empowerment movements was a major reason that the former enjoyed so much success in the 1970s. In other words, the "shopping problems" that consumerists identified bothered quite a few Americans, including many who were not college educated or white.

Yet in the end, scaling up the patient-as-watchdog ideal proved difficult. While in theory a democratic approach to reform, its practice favored those possessed of more education, disposable income, and time to spend shopping for medical care. Although consumerism has certainly helped in advocating better care of everyone, including low-income, nonwhite, and foreign-born Americans, it has remained limited by its middle-class, college-educated origins. If making sense of prescription drug leaflets or hospital report cards constitutes a challenge for white Anglo-Saxon Protestant Americans with advanced degrees, it poses an even greater burden on people who have not finished high school, work two jobs, or do not speak English as their native tongue.

These failures do not necessarily reflect the breadth of consumerists' goals; consumerists have often been among the most articulate voices in identifying the systemic problems that work against all patients' interests. Rather, their frustrations stem from "upstream" problems over which they have little control. First, they are outnumbered in size and political influence by more powerful stakeholders. For all the increase in the number and visibility of patient advocacy groups since the 1970s, they tend, quite understandably, to promote specific issues and concerns: the safety of prescription drugs; the deficiencies of health insurance; the needs of vulnerable groups such as the poor, the elderly, and immigrants; and the challenges faced by people with specific diseases. While often in agreement on basic patient rights to safety, information, choice, and respect, each organization usually focuses on changes that benefit its particular constituency. On a practical basis, patient advocates often compete with one another for scarce funds and policy attention. Thus for all the greater visibility of patient activism, the political reality first noted in the 1930s—that patients are the least organized and weakest of health care stakeholders—remains just as true in 2015. The idea of an American Patients Association, proposed in 1954 by Oscar Ewing, former head of the Federal Security Administration, then again in 1970 by Theodore Cron, a colleague of Ralph Nader's, has never come to pass.[14]

Second, the language and aspirations associated with medical consumerism have proven all too easy for more powerful stakeholders to adopt as part of an effort to dilute or deflect change. Thus consumer requests for more information about their doctors or their prescription drugs have become rationales for more commercial advertising and marketing. Consumer interest in preventive health has become the justification for ordering expensive tests and scans. Meanwhile, stakeholders with diametrically opposed policy positions present themselves as the patients' best friend: the pharmaceutical company justifying its use of direct-to-consumer advertisements and the consumer groups calling for their elimination; the insurance companies imposing benefit limitations and the doctors and patients who challenge them; the policy camp arguing for insurance exchanges and the policy camp opposing them. Grassroots patients' efforts now compete with "astroturf" groups created and funded by corporate lobbyists. Given that all the actors in current policy debates now justify their positions in the language of patient empowerment, sorting the faux from the real benefit has become that much harder.[15]

For all these reasons, the increase in medical consumerism's respectability over the past fifty years has not resulted in a magical transformation of the American health care system. While expanding the recognition of patients' rights to be safe, to be informed, to make choices, and to be heard has been all to the good, it has not proven a magic bullet for all that ails our medical care. In some ways, what has been done in the name of the patient-consumer has only amplified some of the system's worst flaws. Much like the homeopathic "law of similars," the consumerist cure has become a diluted form of the disease. But as this history also helps to explain, we continue to return to this solution, in large part because it is the best lever for change within the limits of the American political system.

In tackling this big and sprawling set of issues, I have inevitably had to make some difficult decisions about what to include and emphasize. To start with, while the book's title refers to the remaking of *patients*, this history does not focus primarily on very sick people treated in hospitals or otherwise in the midst of life-threatening medical crises. Rather, my interest lies in what I think of as "potential patients," to borrow a useful phrase I found in a 1935 book, *The Patient's Dilemma*. As S. A. Tannenbaum and Paul Branden wrote, "The time for the potential patient to stop, look, and listen, is while he is still in full possession of his faculties and his bank account."[16] The kinds of deliberation involved when we look for a doctor to visit, ponder a visit to the drugstore instead, and wonder about insurance coverage are an important part of how adults are expected to interact with the world of modern medicine, yet they rarely get much attention. Therefore, I have chosen to start with the doctor's office and the drugstore rather than the hospital and the chemotherapy unit, while also keeping in mind how all of these places are connected.

For similar reasons, I do not focus primarily on the patient experiences or activist traditions that have grown up around specific diseases, such as polio, tuberculosis, HIV/AIDS, or breast cancer. Here again, I recognize that medical consumerism has been intimately linked to the rise of "expert patients"—that is, people with chronic illnesses who both participate in and shape the therapeutic regimens that keep them alive. But as with my decision to focus on the doctor's office rather than the hospital, I have chosen a more diffuse angle of vision: the perspective of laypeople who still dwell in the "kingdom of the well" rather than the "kingdom of the sick," to use Susan Sontag's famous dichotomy. This choice does not mean that I ignore the "kingdom of the sick"; on the contrary, the requirement that very sick people undergo intense and possibly risky treatments has been a powerful driver of laypeople's demands for rights and information. But while I take that dynamic into account, my focus ultimately remains on the slightly sick and the worried well rather than the seriously ill.[17]

As I will be the first to acknowledge, the kind of deliberative thinking associated with the patient-as-watchdog mode often gets dramatically revised or even cast aside when a person moves from the kingdom of the well to the kingdom of the sick. Critics of medical consumerism have often pointed out this phenomenon as one of its fundamental flaws. In line with the adage that there are no atheists in foxholes, we might say there are no medical consumerists in the emergency room. Yet acknowledging the limits of deliberation does not detract from the reality that in many situations, people were and are expected to exercise their due diligence regarding important medical choices. Moreover, to a greater degree than any other developed nation, the United States has constructed a health care system that requires people to make skillful choices to get good care, giving us all the more reason to try to understand the reasons why.

In exploring the evolving definition of the prospective patient, I have chosen here to concentrate primarily on *medical* consumerism as distinct from a broader *health* consumerism. Many consumption choices have health consequences, from buying a package of cigarettes to visiting a tanning salon. I acknowledge the general ways that commentators linked changing disease patterns to changing consumption habits, among them a more stressful, sedentary lifestyle; a richer diet; and increased use of alcohol and tobacco. The rise of medical consumerism must be set within the context of a larger set of debates about whether the "American way of life" may itself be "hazardous to your health," as one 1978 commentator put it. But I concentrate here primarily on consumerist perspectives as they concern the more specialized goods and services we associate with doctors' offices and drugstores.[18]

Although I am mindful of other perspectives, this book remains primarily a chronicle of a version of medical consumerism closely associated with educated middle-class professionals. I focus on that version not only because its proponents left behind such a rich paper trail but also because their complaints got such a visible reaction from the medical and political powers that be. But I do so in full awareness that theirs was not the only consequential vision of change existing at any particular time. I assume that whatever their income or education level, people had (and have) their own senses of what it means to be well treated by their doctors and that those expectations mattered (and still matter) to the shaping of medical institutions. As future studies open up the history of medicine to include a more diverse array of actors, I anticipate that the story line I present here will be greatly expanded and corrected, and I welcome that prospect.

The same caveat applies to the book's focus on the twentieth-century United States. Rising concerns about medical costs, quality of care, and physician accountability are by no means unique to this country. Other affluent countries whose health care systems differ substantially from our own face similar challenges in accommodating the fast pace of scientific and technological change and the growing expense of providing it. Nor is the idea of patient engagement a modern American invention; as recent studies of early modern medicine have shown, the practice of doctor-shopping is a very old one. Still, I think it is fair to say that the particular version of doctor-shopping that emerged in the twentieth-century United States is both influential and interesting. By putting its evolution in historical perspective, I hope to contribute to the transnational history of patients' rights and consumer movements.[19]

Finally, in exploring the history of the patient as watchdog, I have remained acutely aware of the story's relevance to present-day controversies. Questions about how much market thinking should be encouraged in American medicine and how much protection and guidance patient-consumers need in making medical choices are central to the highly polarized and partisan debate currently raging in the United States. The book's conclusion lays out some historical insights that might be useful to today's patients, physicians, and patient advocates.

Although this book is not written as a brief for any particular fix to the current health care system, my argument inevitably reflects my own predilections. I do not worship in what some have called the "church of the free market." I strongly favor empowering patients, but I do not long to return to the "good old days" before the federal government or other third parties got involved in medicine's affairs. After learning more about what doctor-patient relations were like back in the not-so-good old days, readers will better appreciate why I hold that view. But I hope that those who disagree with my viewpoints will still find this book useful.

It may come as cold comfort to find out that the problems we face today did not start with the Internet or the Affordable Care Act, and that patients and physicians have long struggled over issues of money and trust. But there is value in realizing that our problems are *not* entirely new. Knowing more about the origins of the concept of patient as consumer, why many people resisted that idea for so long, and why it finally "triumphed" in the late twentieth century provides much-needed insight into why, despite striking changes that seemingly empower patients, so many Americans still feel unhappy and confused about their medical choices.

A 2009 cartoon, "Everybody! Let's Play Health Care," portrayed that sense of confusion as a medical version of Candyland, the classic board game introduced in 1949. In the original version, players move through a landscape of sweet adventures in which a common fate is to move a few steps forward and then fall as many steps backward. As reimagined by cartoonists Robert and Donna Trussell, the patient-consumer's journey is far from sweet and simple; he or she must evade many pitfalls—"depression and isolation," "claims denial, bankruptcy, death," Koko the clown visiting the chemo ward, and erectile dysfunction ads that cause impotence—to arrive at the happy ending of an old age of canasta playing and senile dementia.[20]

In negotiating our medical Candyland, much of the advice and commentary written in the 1930s remains surprisingly relevant. I hope that this history will prove useful to today's young people, including my twenty-one-year-old daughter and the young people I teach, some of whom want to become doctors—and all of whom inevitably become patients. They have no memory, as I do, of the world before managed care and prescription drug ads on television or of the circumstances that led to the remaking of patients into consumers. Widening our memories of past patients and their complaints may increase the odds that we can improve our future.

PART ONE

The Hazards of New Choices
The 1920s to the 1940s

{ONE}

Farewell to the Free Trade in Doctoring

When today we lament the loss of a "golden age" when the goods of medicine, both real and symbolic, were untouched by the entrepreneurial spirit of modern consumer culture, we mourn a past of our own imagination. The remaking of patients into consumers started not with managed care or the Internet but with the nineteenth-century market revolution and the rise of modern consumer capitalism, which dramatically changed the way Americans received both their doctor's care and their medicinal drugs. During the first half of the 1800s, the United States saw the closest approximation of free-market medical care to ever exist. For both practical and ideological reasons, nineteenth-century Americans embraced a freewheeling approach to health care, characterized by enthusiastic self-medication and unapologetic questioning of medical authority. As one contemporary wrote of the national mood in 1848, "We go for free trade in doctoring."[1]

That "free trade in doctoring" began to be curtailed in the late 1800s on the grounds that the patient public needed to be protected from bad and unscrupulous purveyors of medical goods and services. Physicians convinced state legislatures to pass laws tightening the requirements to get a license to practice. City and state governments created new boards of pharmacy that oversaw how and by whom drugs were sold. With the 1906 passage of the Pure Food and Drugs Act, the federal government got involved in the work of consumer protection. Invoking the advance of scientific knowledge, new groups of experts successfully pressed for an end to the "free trade in doctoring."[2]

Underlying this restriction was a clear logic: patient-consumers would surrender the freedom to make certain kinds of choices in exchange for the guarantee of better goods and services. That logic met with fierce resistance from both providers and patients, neither of whom wanted their choices restricted. Progressive-era reformers eventually convinced enough voters and politicians to get legislation passed by emphasizing the promise of protection: seek out the licensed physician, use the drug as directed, and all will be well.

But from the outset, the guarantees implied by licensing and labeling reforms raised expectations that they could not fulfill. Manufacturers, physicians, pharmacists, and government officials had different notions of what constituted quality control and full disclosure. The pressure to soften standards to preserve economic interests was strong and unrelenting. As consumer-oriented capitalism accelerated, insulating medicine from the robust influences of commercialism turned out to be very difficult. The resulting tensions in the doctor's office and the drugstore created the forcing ground for the emergence of a more assertive kind of medical consumerism.

The Free Trade in Doctoring

To appreciate the end of the "free trade" in doctoring in the late 1800s, we need first to understand how it operated. The Progressive-era turn to patient-consumer protection followed decades of great turbulence in medicine brought about by the twin forces of democratization and industrialization. The result was intense battles over the proper balance between self-care and deference to medical authority as well as the necessary distinctions between professionalism and commercialism.

Dating back to the colonial period, the scarcity of formally trained doctors in many parts of the United States had inspired a strong tradition of "Every man his own doctor," the title of the first domestic medical manual published in the British colonies, which appeared in 1734. The American Revolution fostered a distrust of what its leaders deemed "aristocratic" traditions of law, while the rapid growth of commercial capitalism after the War of 1812 encouraged new forms of economic entrepreneurship. In this climate grew a spirit of medical democracy that bred do-it-yourself approaches to medical care and a questioning of doctors' skills and ethics that would persist into the twentieth century.[3]

The democratic mind-set rested on a foundation of confidence in what historians term domestic medicine—that is, home remedies and nursing routines overseen by laypeople, mostly women but also some men. Calling for a professional physician usually came not at the start of an illness but only after other measures had failed. It was a habit reinforced by the fact that in many parts of the rapidly growing nation, trained doctors were few and far between. Early histories of life on the American frontier often included harrowing tales of settlers driven to desperate acts because no doctor was available, as in the case of an Illinois man who amputated his own toe to escape death from gangrene, an event recorded by a local historian as the community's "first surgical operation by white people."[4]

While such dramatic episodes of do-it-yourself medicine earned a place in communal folklore, domestic medicine was more often associated with the nineteenth-century equivalent of "Dr. Mom." Learning how to treat symptoms and nurse the sick formed part of what American mothers taught their daughters about how to run a home. In dooryard gardens, women cultivated plants prized for their healing qualities, mixing Old World standbys such as angelica, chamomile, feverfew, and foxglove with New World additions such as bee balm, goldenseal, and American pennyroyal. They shared favorite recipes for homemade pain relievers, fever reducers, wound cleansers, and bowel openers and traded advice about managing specific illnesses as well as the dangers of childbirth. This trading of information expanded to include Native American and African American cures along with those from a variety of European immigrant groups.[5]

Within the broad tradition of domestic medicine, laypeople who showed a special talent for managing illness became sought after by their neighbors; such was the case with midwife Martha Ballard in Maine, housewife Mrs. Gardner Randolph in Illinois, and African slave Binah in South Carolina. In the first half of the nineteenth century, trained physicians and lay healers usually cooperated rather than competed with each other. For example, when Ballard faced a difficult delivery, she called in the local doctor for assistance; he in turn let her care for uncomplicated cases and concentrated instead on the more difficult births.[6]

Trained physicians represented the very narrow tip of the medical-care pyramid, to be consulted only when the domestic store of solutions had been exhausted. Most people regarded seeking out the doctor as a serious step, one not to be entered into lightly, an attitude that would persist well into the twentieth century. Moreover, they did so with the expectation of getting specialized services that domestic healers could not provide, such as bone setting and bloodletting. Physicians also had a broader armamentarium of drugs. They could prescribe plant-based drugs in much higher concentrations than could be achieved in homemade brews, among them aconite (from monkshood), digitalis (from foxglove), and opium (from poppies), and a wide array of strong-acting metals, minerals, and salts such as mercury, borax, and alum.[7]

Until the mid-1800s, most doctors learned their specialized skills by apprenticing to other doctors; only the most ambitious attended medical school as well. They delivered their medical services almost exclusively in patients' homes. While practitioners in cities and towns began to maintain offices, usually located in their homes, they treated only a tiny percentage of cases there— chiefly those involving single men.[8] Hospitals existed only in very large cities and then primarily served the "poor and friendless"; even wealthy people had surgery or delivered children at home. For all but a very few doctors, making a living was not easy. At a time when cash was still scarce, patients often paid with cords of wood or bushels of fruit.

Although some aspects of this medical system, including the preference for self-medication and the reluctance to go to the doctor, would long persist, the dynamics of medicine began to change in the 1810s and 1820s.[9] High rates of literacy, especially in the North and the Midwest, coupled with technological breakthroughs in paper and printing, enabled a rising tide of health advice and advertising to enter American homes. The print revolution cheapened the cost of almanacs and home health manuals, adding to the store of domestic medical knowledge. Many American households came to possess not only a copy of the Bible but also family medical guides such as William Buchan's or John Gunn's *Domestic Medicine*, the latter evocatively subtitled *Poor Man's Friend, in the Hours of Affliction, Pain, and Sickness*. More drugs and drug advertising also began to enter the American home as changing methods of making glass and paper containers brought down the price of store-bought remedies, such as Thomas Dyott's line of Dr. Robertson's remedies. Taking advantage of the very favorable postal rates set by the U.S. Congress, which wanted to encourage an informed citizenry, newspapers became a major vehicle for promoting proprietary medicine products. The bundles of reading matter arriving in the American backwoods that so impressed French observer Alexis de Tocqueville in the early 1830s included an abundance of drug advertisements.[10]

As the possibilities for self-education and self-dosing expanded, so too did the number and types of trained doctors available for consultation. In the new republic, the ranks of regular physicians expanded rapidly, as did their efforts to upgrade their educational standards. By the 1830s, nearly every state in the Union had a medical society in operation, and state legislatures had granted most of them authority to issue medical licenses. But regular physicians found themselves challenged by new medical sects that disdained the prevailing "purge and puke" methods, including homeopathic, Thomsonian, botanic, and eclectic practitioners. These alternative doctors created their own medical schools, professional societies, and journals. Faced with warring groups of physicians, state legislatures proved reluctant to favor one over the other. In some states, alternative practitioners were permitted to set up their own societies and licensure systems; in others, the main licensing body was required to include representatives of different sects; in still others, licensing laws were eliminated altogether.[11]

To fend off these challenges, regular practitioners banded together in 1847 to form the American Medical Association (AMA), a national organization dedicated to professional uplift. In 1848, the AMA issued a code of ethics designed to clarify what made its members superior to both sectarian physicians and the makers of proprietary nostrums. A good physician, the code specified, did not openly criticize his fellow doctors, steal patients from his colleagues, claim to have secret remedies that cured deadly diseases, or advertise his own services. But the AMA's efforts were all too often undercut by the behavior of their fellow regulars, who in the entrepreneurial spirit of the era rushed to found for-profit medical schools that churned out poorly trained doctors and started up proprietary medicine companies that offered cheap alternatives to visiting a doctor.[12]

By the eve of the Civil War, then, the American medical marketplace was deeply fragmented and relatively unregulated. Medical training and medical licenses did not provide a very reliable guide to a doctor's skill or trustworthiness. Physicians were divided into rival camps that attacked each other ferociously. Coupled with the growing profusion of health advice and drug advertising, the free trade in doctoring meant that potential patients confronted a very rich and confusing set of choices. The burden of that confusion was likely lightened by the fact that all this competition made for relatively affordable doctors' fees—from as little as fifty cents to a dollar for a consultation early in the nineteenth century to an average of two to five dollars by its end. Doctors used what today we would call a "sliding scale," charging more for wealthier patients than for the poor. Since doctors delivered the great majority of care in patients' homes, they had ample opportunity to assess the family's circumstances before deciding on fees.[13]

Looking back from a twentieth-century perspective, many commentators would characterize this free trade in doctoring as an abundance of care, none of it any good. At worst, patients had the freedom to be defrauded by outright quacks and charlatans; at best, they had the option of being cared for by well-intentioned but ineffectual doctors. But that perspective requires serious qualification. Patients' notions of what worked did not reflect a modern sense of the scientific method—as yet nonexistent in 1850—but rather a personal sense of relief. According to this standard, laypeople valued home remedies to soothe sore throat or sour stomach and respected the midwife's experience in delivering a great many babies. When people decided to seek out trained physicians, they did so out of conviction that such practitioners had valuable knowledge and skills—for example, how to manage a difficult birth, set a compound fracture, reduce a dislocation, prescribe a stronger drug, and perhaps most important, relieve pain. In short, nineteenth-century physicians by no means approached their patients empty-handed. As the distinguished dermatologist William Allen Pusey wrote of his physician father, "For 90 per cent of the ills of life, he gave them useful service," and the high regard he enjoyed in the community reflected that value.[14]

Nineteenth-century patients respected the specialized skills that trained physicians offered but do not appear to have approached them with extreme deference or passivity. As the letters and diaries they left behind suggest, many patients felt entitled to patronize a wide variety of healers. If they encountered a doctor whose treatment they found unsatisfying, they had no compunction about moving on to another one more to their liking and letting all their friends and relations know why. As physician Arthur Hertzler recalled of old-time country practice, the older women in the community could make or break a doctor's reputation: "The doctors of that day were tried at the quilting bees of the community, not in courts of law."[15]

Yet even at its most lightly regulated, the free trade in doctoring operated according to rules designed to protect patients against the special harms posed by bad doctoring or dangerous drugs. In fact, nineteenth-century medicine produced some of the clearest exceptions to the principle known as caveat emptor (Latin for "let the buyer beware"). First recorded in a 1534 English case concerning a horse trade, "caveat emptor" came into widespread use in the late eighteenth century, as the free-market principles championed by Adam Smith and others became dominant. As Kent's commentaries on American law observed in 1840, caveat emptor "very reasonably requires the purchaser to attend, when he makes his contract, to the quality of the article he buys." Should the product prove to be defective—as was the case with the sixteenth-century horse—buyers had no legal claim against the seller. Hence the buyer had to exercise great care when making a purchase.[16]

But American courts also recognized that in contracting for medical care or buying medicinal drugs, patients needed some degree of protection from the incompetent and the fraudulent. As free-market principles gained favor in the 1800s, American jurists began to recast the old common-law concept of medical malpractice, redefining the doctor-patient relationship as a contract in which the doctor promised the patient a specific service. Medical malpractice cases began to increase rapidly in the 1840s, largely as a result of cases involving surgeons charged with badly setting broken bones, a concrete procedure whose outcome was comparatively easy to assess. In deciding such cases, American courts held that patients had the right to expect an "ordinary standard of care, skill, and diligence" from their physicians and turned to physician experts to establish what constituted this "ordinary standard" of care. Although malpractice represented neither an easy nor a cost-effective way to resolve disputes, it reinforced the contractual view of medical practice as an agreement entered into by doctor and patient as well as the existence of an "ordinary standard of care" to which the former could be held.[17]

Departures from the traditional rule of caveat emptor likewise applied to the sale of potentially dangerous drugs. Dating back to medieval times, the handling of substances that could kill or maim humans and animals had been subject to special care. Even with the legal embrace of free trade, special precautions continued to govern the sale of poisons, especially after several high-profile murders were committed using arsenic and other poisons freely available from grocers and druggists. After the British Parliament passed the 1851 Arsenic Act to regulate its sale, many American states followed suit, passing statutes instituting special precautions for the sale of poisons. In an influential 1852 decision, *Thomas v. Winchester*, the New York State Court of Appeals decided in favor of the patient-consumer suing over the mislabeling of the powerful drug belladonna as dandelion oil, setting the precedent that those who traded in poisons needed to observe special care in labeling their products.[18]

So as of the 1870s, the medical marketplace had what today we would consider remarkably light limits. States allowed medical societies to issue licenses using standards that fell far short of the AMA's goals. A medical practitioner who did an exceptionally bad job of treating a patient could be sued for malpractice; manufacturers could not sell poisons as harmless medicines. Within these bounds, American patients could choose among a wide array of medical advice givers and self-treatment regimens.

Even at its most open, this medical marketplace did not operate fairly or equitably for all. Very poor people, then as now, faced enormous disadvantages. They had to rely on charitable people and institutions for care, and such aid was denied to those thought unworthy of it for moral reasons. Both before and after slavery's abolition, a white-dominated culture worked on racist assumptions that imposed additional burdens on African Americans, who had good reason to fear mistreatment at the hands of white doctors. New immigrant groups faced discrimination as well and often preferred to care for their own rather than depend on native-born Americans for help. Poor women of all races faced legal and economic constraints on their autonomy. In medicine and in other areas of life, patients who were free, white, and affluent had clear advantages in the quest for good outcomes.

The freewheeling medical marketplace did not meet its demise primarily because of widespread public discontent with its terms. In fact, the growing limitations on the choice of doctor and medicine proved very unpopular with many patient-consumers. While we have no opinion polls or survey data to gauge the overall state of opinion, medical reformers acknowledged that their efforts to restrict the free trade in doctoring ran against the majority public opinion. The preference for do-it-yourself care, the desire to mix and match healing services, and the general distrust of authority meant that patients preferred to pick their physicians and direct their care. The impetus to change those habits and thereby to close down the free trade came from a determined minority of physicians and laypeople who convinced state and federal legislatures that some bad choices needed to be eliminated for the public's own good.

During the Progressive era, this refashioning of the medical marketplace occurred along two distinct but related pathways. The first was the strengthening of medical education and licensure, which helped the regular profession gain a competitive edge over its sectarian competition; the other was the emergence of stronger drug regulations designed to protect consumers against the excesses of the proprietary medicine industry. In the long run, both developments would have important consequences for the rise of medical consumerism. But at the time, those consequences emerged with much more fanfare in the drugstore than they did the doctor's office.

Building the Regular Brand:
Late-Nineteenth-Century Medical Reform

Institutional reforms implemented gradually after the American Civil War laid the foundation for a much more confident medical professionalism. The spectacular successes of late-nineteenth-century laboratory science—in particular, physiology and bacteriology—greatly strengthened the regulars' efforts to upgrade their professional position. Starting in the 1870s, elite medical schools began to strengthen their curriculum, replacing a two-year, undifferentiated round of lectures with a three-year graded curriculum and requiring more hospital experience at every stage of teaching. By linking medical degrees to licensure, medical leaders used this more demanding medical school curriculum to improve professional standards in general.

With support from the AMA, state medical societies convinced state legislatures to create physician-run medical boards to oversee a more rigorous system of medical licensure. By 1900, every state had such a body to license physicians. Six state boards simply issued licenses to any doctor with a diploma, while eleven required either a diploma from an "approved school" or passage of an examination, a mechanism they hoped would weed out graduates of diploma mills and other inferior schools. Twenty-two states required both diplomas from approved schools and passage of an examination. By virtue of their licensure authority, these state boards became an increasingly powerful force within the profession.[19]

While presented as negotiations on behalf of the patient public, these new medical practice acts were essentially deals brokered in state legislatures among physician groups. As regular medical leaders admitted, laypeople were at best ignorant or indifferent and at worst suspicious or antagonistic to efforts to restrict their choice of a doctor. A case in point was the continued public support for alternative medicine. Much as members of the regular profession hoped to deny the competition license to practice medicine, they found that many state legislators were reluctant to grant them a monopoly on the term "doctor." First homeopaths and later osteopaths and chiropractors persuaded state legislatures to safeguard patients' right to select their own brand of care. The success of these efforts depended heavily on the support of patients, whose willingness to sign petitions and provide funds fueled both the institutions of alternative medicine and their legislative defense. This strategy triumphed because the right to choose one's doctor was presented as an economic prerogative in a free-market economy: consumers should be allowed to purchase desired goods and services unless they were unsafe.[20]

But this range of choices remained limited to groups such as homeopaths, chiropractors, and osteopaths who followed the AMA strategy of limiting membership predominantly to white men and linking credentialing to formal medical training. It did not extend to more traditional modes of domestic healing, such as herbalism and midwifery, that were now defined as "foolish" choices that a modern system of licensure could not tolerate. Although many state boards continued to allow midwives to practice among rural and poor families, the new specialty of obstetrics denounced them as ignorant, unskilled, and unsanitary.

By tying licensure to the completion of a medical degree, American reformers made the upgrading of medical school facilities the key to professional uplift. This process culminated in the publishing of the 1910 Flexner Report, which created a new benchmark for medical education. The report advocated requiring medical students to have college degrees before entering medical school and made hospital training an integral part of a medical education. Taking the elite Johns Hopkins Medical School as its gold standard, the Flexner Report created an ABCD ranking system that consigned the majority of American medical schools to the lowest ranks. This ranking disadvantaged schools that accepted women and black physicians: barred from admission to "approved" schools, they found it increasingly hard to get licensed. Thus, the new licensing laws tended to equate "good" choices with white men educated at recognized medical schools.[21]

The growth of professionalism represented an important modification of the informal philosophy of medical caveat emptor. Although initially focused on regulating doctors' behavior with regard to other doctors, professional ethics imposed new burdens on patients as well. As the doctor-patient relationship came to be perceived as a contract for care, the latter bore greater responsibility to vet the former in advance. By highlighting the importance of credentials, professionalism encouraged patients to verify those credentials before placing themselves in someone's care. The implied social promise held that anyone who chose a doctor in good standing with a medical society would be safe from bad treatment. Thus the "right" to choose one's own doctor was modified through a closing down of choices deemed acceptable to earlier generations of patients.

As part of this new and improved professionalism, physicians implicitly pledged to adopt a higher code of conduct shaped by both scientific and ethical rigor. Professionalism would be the antithesis of commercialism; patients would have no need to fear that doctors would be corrupted by the businesslike spirit of the day. As a sign of their higher calling, members of the regular medical profession deliberately rejected the kinds of self-promotion becoming so common in business culture. In his widely read advice book for physicians, first published in 1873 and reprinted well into the 1920s, D. W. Cathell explained that the refusal to advertise was the bedrock of professionalism: "*Merchants and tradesmen* attract customers by *handbills and newspapers*, and yet, even though these do exaggerate, and make claims that are worse than untrue; yet such methods are not considered dishonest, because all *customers are supposed to know* something of the price and quality of the articles offered; besides, they can go from one place to another to examine and compare before buying." In contrast, "the unthinking public and the stranger" had no such "safeguard" against the false claims of the medical quack. Thus, Cathell concluded, "*advertising is not resorted to by honorable, upright, and self-respecting members of our profession,*" and he warned against departing from this "established custom."[22]

By the 1910s, then, the regular profession had undergone a major renovation that put its members at great advantage over their medical rivals. In upgrading medical education and licensure standards, its leaders set a premium on aligning their standards with the values of the new laboratory-based science. They also promoted a style of professional behavior designed to reassure the lay public of their trustworthiness. In many respects, it was a very effective makeover: many of the principles hammered out in the second half of the nineteenth century remain the bedrock of modern medical professionalism. At the turn of the twentieth century, the worst threats that rampant commercialism posed to the public health appeared to emanate from outside the medical profession: from untrained quacks and deceitful snake-oil salesmen.

But this state of relative quiet did not last forever. For all their rigor, these medical reforms could not and did not assure patients a consistent level of medical expertise. The seemingly simple advice to look for a doctor with a new-style license did not guarantee much in the way of knowledge or ethics. Having promised that stronger licensing laws would resolve patient difficulties in finding well-trained doctors, the medical profession would find these raised expectations hard to meet.

Pioneers of Novelties

In the second half of the nineteenth century, the dangers of medical commercialism in the drug trade sparked a far more public sense of unease than did the state of the "doctoring" business. For the latter, strengthening the hand of the regular medical profession would bring order to the doctor's office. Far harder was the challenge of reining in the extraordinary growth of the proprietary medicine companies and the changes they brought to the drug trade. Their extraordinary success as entrepreneurs made them the focal point for turn-of-the-century efforts to impose new rules on the selling of medicine. Out of the battles over pure food and drugs would emerge the principles of a new kind of medical consumerism.

Renowned as "pioneers of novelties," proprietary drugmakers epitomized the American business dream in that an enterprising individual with an appealing product and a clever advertising plan could get very rich very quickly. The business required little in the way of capital investment or product development. Many of the "toadstool millionaires," as Oliver Wendell Holmes nicknamed the proprietary manufacturers, were physicians, but a medical background was by no means a necessity. To embark on a career in the medicine trade, a person need only mix together a number of ingredients (the more the better, preferably combined with a substantial amount of alcohol), design a distinctive bottle and trademark, and compose some imaginative advertising copy.[23]

The proprietary drug industry also illustrated the potential of a new kind of medical consumption based on frequent repeat purchases of relatively inexpensive manufactured goods. Unlike what economists refer to as consumer durables, such as household furnishings or appliances, these nondurable goods were designed to be used up and replaced frequently. Demand for them was more elastic, as economists would later term it, because people could be more easily persuaded to consume more tonics or gargles than to buy another piece of furniture. The key to success lay in expanding sales to a broader swath of the population and getting those sales to repeat, which in turn depended on the marketing and advertising of the product. The more widely and effectively a medicine was advertised, the more likely it was to sell well.

Investing heavily in marketing and advertising worked only if companies could protect their products' distinctive identities, which they did through the use of copyright and trademark law. Although remedies were often referred to as patent medicines, very few companies in fact had patents because getting one required manufacturers to disclose the remedy's contents, which meant that competitors could reproduce the formula. Manufacturers instead relied on the expanding reach of copyright and trademark law to protect a drug's brand name and distinctive packaging. That strategy allowed them to keep the ingredients a secret while building and protecting brand-name recognition for the product itself.[24]

For all the scorn that reformers would later heap on them, the "novelties" introduced by the proprietary medicine companies represented a range of new consumer-friendly measures that would ultimately transform the entire pharmaceutical business. To wean Americans away from remedies such as homemade pennyroyal tea and old-fashioned calomel pills, drug manufacturers sought to make their mixtures easier and more pleasant to take. For example, drugmakers rolled medicines into pills that could be coated with a sugar shell to disguise their bitter taste, added cinnamon and other flavored extracts to make syrups more palatable, and put menthol into salves to make them smell better. This impetus also led to the liberal addition of alcohol, an excellent solvent for other drugs (and still used in many medicines today), and of narcotics that relieved pain and anxiety. The generous use of alcohol and narcotics eventually would help bring down the wrath of reformers on the industry's head. But proprietary manufacturers' efforts to make medicines more palatable ultimately forced regular pharmacists and physicians to do the same to compete.[25]

Proprietary medicines appealed to the eye as well as the heart. Their attractive packages and appealing advertising drew on new printing techniques such as rotogravure to provide buyers with a dazzling array of images that still beguile the modern viewer. The proprietary medicine industry also addressed a growing need for advice and reassurance. As economic change forced people to move more frequently, their access to old family remedies and neighborly advice diminished. In their place, drug manufacturers and their advertising agents created comforting icons of reassurance assumed to have vast experience in caring for others' ills. The native healer became the inspiration for Sagwa, an Indian tonic marketed by the Kickapoo company; the housewife skilled in herbal medicine gave rise to Lydia Pinkham's vegetable compound; and the wise old family doctor stood behind Dr. Winslow's Soothing Syrups and a host of other remedies carrying physicians' names. Similarly, user testimonials mimicked the old-time community knowledge of a remedy by providing personal authentication for the new packaged medicines. The testimony of fellow patients was offered for its own convincing power, the late-nineteenth-century version of what today's marketers refer to as peer-to-peer influence.[26]

Perhaps more than any other industry of the day, proprietary medicine helped turn advertising into an essential part of modern business. While critics found much to dislike in its methods, the proprietary medicine industry fomented a revolution in providing product information via labeling, packaging, and advertising. It was the first industry to use national advertising campaigns, direct-mail advertising, personal testimonials, outdoor advertising (including sandwich boards), promotional giveaways (almanacs, trading cards), product placement (having vaudeville comics mention specific nostrums in their performances), and infomercials (the medicine show).

No domain of American commerce better illustrated the power of new manufacturing and marketing methods to penetrate every nook and cranny of even so vast a nation as the United States, epitomized by stories told half ruefully, half admiringly, about travelers venturing into a seemingly pristine wilderness only to be greeted by advertisements for patent medicines painted on rocks. The proprietary industry continued to make good use of the favorable discounts offered by the U.S. Postal Service as well. With the inauguration of rural free delivery in the 1890s, this information network could reach into every part of the United States. In effect, the 1900 Sears Catalog offered the equivalent of a drugstore in its pages, including both name-brand proprietaries and store brands of ague pills, cod liver oil, and tonics.[27]

These innovations changed the marketing not only of medicines in general but also of other consumer goods by demonstrating the dramatic impact that marketing and advertising could have on sales. As advertising pioneer Charles Hopkins noted in his memoirs, "The greatest advertising men of my day were schooled in the medicine field." Writing ad copy for proprietary remedies was "the supreme test" of a writer's ability, he explained, because such "medicines were worthless merchandise until a demand was created." The tactics used to sell them were easily adaptable to other commodities such as processed foods and hygiene products.[28]

The Pure Food and Drug Crusade

Both reviled and emulated as an economic marvel, the proprietary drug trade set the pace for a new kind of consumer-oriented capitalism in the late nineteenth century. It grew so fast and so audaciously between 1865 and 1900 that it became a lightning rod for many different kinds of anxieties about the growing commercialization of American culture. Far more than medical reform, it aroused those anxieties because of its connection with larger transformations in the economy—the growing distance between the makers and the users of manufactured goods. As Americans consumed more products made in factories far from their homes, they became more vulnerable to lapses in quality. Of the modern goods being consumed in growing quantities, none seemed more prone to both dangerous adulteration and fraudulent advertising than those actually ingested in the body—foods and drugs. Buyers of these industrial goods, who were increasingly referred to as "consumers," needed protection from those who made them, now termed "producers."[29]

In confronting those challenges, Americans were greatly influenced by British developments. In 1872 and 1875, Parliament passed laws strengthening safeguards against food and drug adulteration, inspiring American reformers to introduce similar legislation in the U.S. Congress. While that effort failed at the national level, it did much better at the city and state levels, where many localities passed laws setting standards for food and drug manufacture and sale in the late 1800s. The setting of standards was bolstered by major advances in analytic chemistry that made adulteration easier to detect. In evaluating the purity of drugs, for example, state boards could rely on the standards laid out in successive editions of the United States Pharmacopeia (USP) and the American Pharmaceutical Association's National Formulary.[30]

The power of new analytical methods was evident in the career of Harvey Wiley, who would go on to become the chief architect of the 1906 federal food and drug law. Hired as chief chemist of the U.S. Department of Agriculture in 1882, he began to study the extent and impact of food adulteration, a topic much on the minds of agricultural producers. Under his direction, the Bureau of Chemistry (later renamed the Food and Drug Administration, or FDA) increasingly focused on the dangers of food adulteration. In 1902, Wiley embarked on a landmark study in which he fed human volunteers large quantities of the most common food preservatives, including borax, salicylic acid, and sulfites. Thanks to extensive press coverage, this "poison squad," described as having "Been Eating Doctored Food Five Months and Don't Like It," in a 1904 *New York Times* headline, helped to popularize the idea that food adulteration was both common and potentially hazardous.[31]

None of Wiley's poison squad experiments involved medicinal drugs, which interested him far less than food products. But he shrewdly realized that linking food and drug dangers could win him much-needed support from powerful groups such as the Woman's Christian Temperance Union and the General Federation of Women's Clubs. For women reformers, the alcohol and narcotics in proprietary drugs represented a much greater danger than food preservatives because their deceptive advertising led the unwary to take the first dose and become lifelong addicts. In addition, Wiley gained the support of a small group of journalist reformers concerned by what they saw as the proprietary industry's subversion of the democratic traditions of a free press. Led by Edward Bok, the editor of the *Ladies' Home Journal*, they objected in particular to the "red clause," which threatened newspapers with the loss of advertising revenue if they reported on laws unfavorable to the industry, and the duplicitous writing of testimonials, such as those supposedly penned by Lydia Pinkham long after her death.[32]

Especially important was the muckraking work done by journalist Samuel Hopkins Adams, who arranged to have samples of proprietary remedies analyzed by an independent chemical laboratory and then published the results in *Collier's* along with a detailed critique of the remedies' marketing and promotional claims. Later published as a book, *The Great American Fraud*, Adams's work in essence constituted the first handbook of critical consumerism: a layperson's guide to learning to detect fraud and deception in the medical marketplace. People interested in protecting themselves against quackery, he explained, could do so by observing "a few very simple rules": never trust a doctor who advertised and never believe a medical claim that appeared in the popular press. "Shut your eyes to the medical columns of the newspapers," he wrote, "and you will save yourself many forebodings and symptoms."[33]

Yet for all the negative publicity generated by Wiley's poison squad, the muckrakers' revelations about the red clause, and Adams's list of dangerous drugs, the revelations about meatpacking contained in Upton Sinclair's 1906 novel *The Jungle* finally led to passage of reform legislation. One convert to the cause was President Theodore Roosevelt, who threw his support behind the idea of a federal law regulating food and drug safety after investigators confirmed that Sinclair had not exaggerated.[34]

The debates regarding the 1906 law revealed very different representations of the consumers' situation. The bill's supporters emphasized the grave disadvantages that Americans faced because they could not count on the safety and purity of the products they were buying. As Adams wrote, "Our national quality of commercial shrewdness fails us when we go into the open market to purchase relief from suffering." Setting out to "buy a horse, or a house, or a box of cigars," the average American "is a model of caution," but that prudence deserted him when it came to medicinal goods. He thus needed standards to govern the claims appearing on labels and advertising, without which he might accidentally be lured into consuming alcohol and narcotics.[35]

The bill's detractors dismissed these fears as hysterical. Not surprisingly, proprietary drugmakers insisted that their products were perfectly safe and that consumers did not need a government agency to make choices for them. In this view, drug regulation was a violation of Americans' right to self-medicate as they saw fit. Some politicians agreed: as Representative William Adamson of Georgia put it, the proposed pure food act was in fact "pure foolishness." Invoking fears of what a later generation would call the nanny state, Adamson fumed that "the Federal Government was not created for the purpose of cutting your toe nails or corns"—or by implication, inserting itself into the buying and selling of medicines. In an era of widespread concern over the growing power of business combinations, some critics also portrayed the law as the work of a "doctors' trust" determined to discourage self-medication and thus increase their fees.[36]

Perhaps because of that perception, the AMA did not campaign hard on behalf of the 1906 law. To be sure, the recently reorganized group encouraged members to write letters and generate petitions supporting the measure and helped to finance the publication of *The Great American Fraud*. In its own publications, the AMA made a case for disclosing the contents of patent medicines: asserted an editorial in the *Journal of the American Medical Association*, "The public had the right to know what it is taking when it prescribes for itself." It also set up the Council on Pharmacy and Chemistry to help physicians distinguish between the many good and bad remedies coming on the market. At the same time, physicians were wary of giving the federal government authority over any aspect of medical care, a sentiment that would grow even stronger during the controversy soon to come over Prohibition.[37]

Congress eventually passed the Pure Food and Drugs Act, the first great piece of national consumer legislation in American history, and President Roosevelt signed it into law on June 30, 1906. Its provisions were by no means as strict as reformers had hoped or manufacturers had feared. Both proponents and opponents of drug regulation portrayed the measure as a victory for their side. Rather than dwell on the act's limitations, reformers celebrated the principles of transparency in terms of labeling that had been established and that they hoped would be strengthened in the future. Drug industry leaders claimed they had gotten a bill that they could work around, leaving them free to do much of what they had done before. As the law took effect, both proved to be correct.

Like much Progressive-era regulation, the Pure Food and Drugs Act turned out to be a boon for manufacturers. With key terms such as "adulterated" and "false or misleading" only vaguely defined, intense battles over their meaning occurred between government officials and drug manufacturers, with the drugmakers usually winning. Whereas the Meat Inspection Act passed the same year set up a preventive apparatus of inspection, the Pure Food and Drugs Act did not. It merely gave consumers more information—of a very limited sort—through federal oversight of drug labeling.

Whereas reformers had originally asked that labels be required to list all of a product's ingredients, business objections led to a congressional compromise in which manufacturers had only to disclose the presence of ten drugs deemed especially hazardous: alcohol, morphine, cocaine, heroin, opium, eucaine, chloroform, cannabis indica, chloral hydrate, and acetanilide. Should manufacturers choose to list other ingredients on the label, those ingredients needed actually to be in the preparation and, if listed in either the USP or the National Formulary, at the strength and purity specified by those authorities. Finally, the law stated that the label could not contain "any statement, design, or device" regarding the product that was "false or misleading in any particular." Manufacturers that complied with these guidelines were entitled to include on product labels the statement that they had been "guaranteed under" the terms of the 1906 law.[38]

As a result of the extensive publicity surrounding the law's passage, the public thought its provisions were far more sweeping than they actually were. Charged with implementing the new law, the Bureau of Chemistry staff quickly realized that consumers interpreted the phrase "guaranteed under" to constitute a disinterested vote of confidence from the federal government that the product was a good one. To clarify the matter, the bureau modified the statement in 1908 so that "guaranteed by" was followed by the name of the manufacturer. Even that change did not suffice, so in May 1914, the bureau asked manufacturers to stop invoking the law on their labels in any way.[39]

Federal regulators' attempts to enforce the ban on false or misleading claims immediately produced legal challenges. After the government seized shipments of Dr. Johnson's Mild Combination Treatment for Cancer on these grounds, lawyers for Johnson, an eclectic physician from Kansas City, Missouri, filed suit in March 1907, claiming that the new law did not include such sweeping powers. In a 1911 decision, the U.S. Supreme Court decided in Johnson's favor; the majority opinion, written by Justice Oliver Wendell Holmes, agreed with the defense's argument that medical views of what constituted a cure were so divided that the government had no grounds for "establishing criteria in regions where opinions are far apart." The court echoed an old common-law distinction that had long allowed for advertising claims to be asserted as opinion rather than fact. The minority opinion insisted that despite the current "conflict between the schools of medicine," "there still remains a field in which statements as to curative properties are downright falsehoods and in no sense expressions of judgment," and Congress had intended to outlaw those "downright falsehoods."[40]

With the backing of the new president, William Howard Taft, Congress passed the Sherley Amendment (named after the representative from Kentucky who proposed it) to clarify that it had indeed intended to prevent labels from offering false or misleading claims about a product's therapeutic value. The amendment was immediately challenged in the courts, but this time the judiciary sided with the government. Thereafter drug manufacturers who wanted to sell drugs across state lines had to abide by the Bureau of Chemistry's definition of what was false and misleading. But out of this legal wrangling emerged a ruling that would shape the future direction of medical consumerism in the United States: the courts held that the Sherley Amendment applied only to statements on the bottle and its packaging, not to claims made elsewhere. Thus, companies could and did make claims in their advertising that they could not make on the bottles themselves. Off-label claims did not come under federal review until the 1920s, when the Federal Trade Commission (FTC), set up in 1914, assumed responsibility for policing misleading drug advertising not as a health issue but as a form of unfair business competition.[41]

Still, for all its weaknesses, the 1906 law changed the drug industry in important ways. In the first ten years after its passage, the agency used its authority to seize hundreds of improperly labeled products. For every company that took the federal government to court over the new drug laws, many others changed their curative claims to avoid the negative publicity and costly legal fees that accompanied a Bureau of Chemistry citation. The bureau also collected and published information designed to offset the 1906 law's limits. For example, in 1910 it published a bulletin listing specific products, among them Mrs. Winslow's Soothing Syrup and Dr. Miller's Anodyne for Babies, that contained drugs such as morphine and chloral hydrate but were not required to list them on their labels because "they are not sold as remedies for any disease." Citizens could obtain this "directory of habit-forming drugs" simply by writing to the bureau and asking for a copy.[42]

Concerns about addiction fueled further restrictions on the drug trade in the 1910s. In 1914, Congress passed the Harrison Narcotics Act, which imposed stricter marketing procedures on the sale of all opium and coca products and made it illegal for any but physicians to prescribe drugs containing these substances. The act required that all medications containing controlled substances be clearly labeled with the statement, "Under the Harrison Law, effective March 1, 1915, this prescription can be refilled only by obtaining a new prescription from your physician." Ironically, while the Harrison Act increased scrutiny of doctors' prescription practices regarding opiates and cocaine derivatives, it allowed the continued use of small amounts of these drugs in proprietary medicines. Similarly, the 1918 Volstead Act, which went into effect in 1920, forbade the manufacture and sale of alcohol as a beverage but allowed its use as a medicine as long as it was procured with a physician's prescription. The act also permitted alcohol to be used in proprietary medicines as long as it was listed on the label. While failing to put an end to addiction, both laws significantly complicated the practice of pharmacy and medicine.[43]

As all three acts showed, federal regulation of medicinal drugs hardly constituted a magic wand that suddenly made consumers safe or rational. Drug reform proceeded in bits and pieces, as new laws were passed, implemented in the face of fierce resistance, and challenged in the courts. The resulting web of regulation proved difficult for drug manufacturers, pharmacists, and physicians—much less patients—to untangle. So despite the new regulation, choosing safe and effective drugs remained difficult for all concerned. The end of Wiley's career at the Bureau of Chemistry illustrates the pitfalls that plagued those determined to draw a clearer dividing line between good and bad products. Faced with growing complaints that Wiley had too much independence, the secretary of agriculture created a board of scientific experts to review his decisions. After conflicts with the new board, Wiley resigned in protest in 1912, becoming only the first of many government regulators to learn firsthand how hard the business of consumer protection could be.[44]

The Hazards of New Choices

By the early 1920s, both of the chief threats to good medicine, the untrained quack and the "wily patent medicine man," had been brought under more control. The combined forces of medical professionalism and government regulation meant that patient-consumers could now depend on stronger licensing laws and federal oversight of drug labels to make safer, wiser choices about their medical care. For their own protection, their rights to pick an unlicensed healer or to self-medicate at will had been narrowed; in exchange, they could assume that the doctors hanging up their shingles were better prepared to treat them and that the drugs available were more accurately labeled.

But many problems remained as the Progressive era came to an end. While educational and licensing standards had been upgraded, the medical profession still possessed relatively little authority to discipline individual physicians who departed from those standards. Likewise, the new system for regulating medicinal drugs left considerable scope for commercial influences to flourish. Establishing and enforcing scientific guidelines for what constituted quality, in terms of either medical procedures or medicinal drugs, was no easy matter. As prosperity returned after World War I, the sense of having tamed medical commercialism proved very short-lived.

During the 1920s, the United States entered a period of rapid economic growth characterized by rising rates of consumer spending. As more companies adopted methods of mass production, the need to stimulate consumption through national marketing and advertising campaigns grew as well. Both manufacturers and retailers competed fiercely for shares of consumer spending, resulting in an avalanche of new goods, including both comparatively expensive purchases meant to last indefinitely (automobiles, radios, and electrical appliances) and inexpensive items meant to be used up quickly and repurchased (cigarettes, shampoo, and movie tickets). As the Great Depression would soon demonstrate, this new consumer-dependent economy proved fragile because important economic sectors, including agriculture and textiles, never recovered from the postwar recession. Many workers remained too poor to participate in the new consumption patterns. But for those who fared well, such as middle-class white-collar workers and the upper echelon of industrial workers, the benefits of modern prosperity seemed evident in the abundance of available consumer goods.

The postwar consumer culture was closely identified with the expansion of American cities. By 1920, half of all Americans lived in urban areas, defined by the Census Bureau as having a population of 2,500 or more; a quarter of them resided in the country's sixty-eight cities of 100,000 or more. Big cities were by their nature consumption oriented in that urban households depended on others to supply food and other necessities on a cash basis. The larger the city, the greater the variety of its retail establishments and leisure-time activities. The combination of growing population and better mass transit fostered a growing segmentation of cities into specialized commercial areas. The main downtown commercial districts were anchored by huge department stores and large movie theaters, with smaller satellite areas featuring groceries and variety stores aimed at the "shawl" trade (thrifty shoppers from immigrant families) as well as the growing number of southern blacks moving north. Within this urban culture, going out to spend money became a major pastime. While women remained the chief purchasers of household goods, men also became deeply involved in interwar consumption, buying tickets to sporting events and movies as well as choosing their own reading matter and tobacco products. Wherever they went, men and women encountered a sea of advertising pitches. Newspapers, then avidly read by all classes of society, carried many pages of display advertising pitches. Subways and buses carried "car cards"; buildings were plastered with posters and billboards; theater marquees lit the night with electric bulbs.[45]

Although the contrast between the city slicker and the country cousin remained a staple of early twentieth-century comedy routines, the spread of print culture, mail order, and later radio meant that these trends reached rural areas as well. Affluent farm families subscribed to newspapers and magazines that carried the same advertising pitches as their urban counterparts. They used the Montgomery Ward and Sears Catalogs, colloquially known as "dream books," to order the goods advertised there. When they went into town to shop, billboards along rural roadsides sought their attention. With the advent of the movies and commercial radio, the messages of commercial culture would reach even deeper into rural America.

These changing consumption patterns generated heated debates over the kinds of values they promoted. Interwar opinion leaders disagreed over whether the "democratization" of luxury indicated by factory girls wearing silk stockings and midlevel office managers sporting handmade suits was a good development. Some saw a positive prod to work hard in the growing effort to "keep up with the Joneses" (a phrase that came into use in the 1920s) by buying nicer houses, stylish clothes, or fancier cars, while others felt that pressure to consume bred discontent and materialism. Parallel debates surrounded the emergence of a new hierarchy of highbrow, middlebrow, and lowbrow culture that threatened to dilute American intellectual life.[46]

These concerns showed up in discussions of how medicine figured in the postwar consumption economy. Unlike previous eras, when reports of scientific innovation spread very slowly, new forms of mass media spread awareness of medical advances much more quickly. The "medical breakthrough" story entered modern journalism in the 1880s with coverage of Louis Pasteur's development of a rabies vaccine. By the 1920s, reporting on the latest discoveries had become a staple of newspaper and magazine coverage. The advertising that bankrolled the expansion of the print media and later radio also featured its own version of scientific progress, populated by images of microscopes, laboratories, and white-coated doctors with nurses at their sides.[47]

Even more dramatically, the films that Americans flocked to see starting in the 1910s circulated images of medical innovation, among them emergency rooms (*The Gentleman from Indiana*, 1915), childbirth in a hospital (*Sowers and Reapers*, 1917), blood donations (*The Gift Supreme*, 1920), and incubators (*Oh, Doctor*, 1925). While these films featured many heroic moments, not all the portrayals of medicine were flattering: the plot of *The Penalty*, a 1920 film that launched the career of actor Lon Chaney, revolved around an incompetent surgeon who unnecessarily amputated both of his character's legs. As the commercial film industry added sound to its product, portrayals of physicians, hospitals, and medical miracles became even more effective. Films about the modern *Men in White*, as a 1935 hit starring Clark Gable was titled, became a staple of Hollywood cinema, starting a still-ongoing tradition in which physicians' medical skills were juxtaposed with their romantic and moral dilemmas. Hollywood introduced viewers who had never set foot inside a hospital not only to the medical miracles that could occur there but also to the conflicts between idealism and moneymaking that came with them. Movie plots familiarized audiences with both doctor heroes and their opposites—in particular, the money-hungry and social-climbing physician.[48]

In sum, the spread of popular media helped ensure that anyone who could afford a newspaper or a movie ticket was likely at some point to get the message that medicine had much to offer in the way of new products and services, but that its costs could be prohibitive. Medical miracles did not come cheap, and this fact raised troublesome questions about access to them. In trying to make sense of the new medical economy, both physicians and laypeople frequently compared medical care to other forms of consumer goods and services, using terms such as "fashion," "taste," "luxury," and "necessity" to mark both its similarities and differences. Unlike other areas of consumer spending, where the play of personal preferences and circumstances seemed appropriate, modern medicine operated more clearly on a hierarchical model: experts declared its goods and services to be valuable, and the patient public was to accept those judgments without question. To doubt expert judgment was the mark of the ignorant. Moreover, unlike ladies' hemlines or automobile styling, medicine presumably changed in response to scientific advances that left little room for taste or preference in their valuation.

But in practice, this deference to scientific judgment presented its own set of problems in that it made doctors far more responsible for guiding their patients' choice of treatment. A car salesman or a department store clerk could promote a particular model or style as just the thing; the customer presumably had sufficient knowledge of the product to satisfy his or her preferences. If afflicted with a case of buyer's remorse, the consumer could return the product and try another style. But medicine operated by a different set of rules in that patients could neither easily judge the quality of the goods and services they received nor easily return them if they did not "work." Patients were also expected to understand that sometimes doctors could do nothing to help them yet still be entitled to present a big bill. Medical care consequently involved a degree of deference to expert judgment virtually unique within the dynamics of interwar consumer culture.

Medical care also diverged from that larger consumer culture because barriers to its access seemed especially reprehensible. Whereas class stratification might be tolerated in the possession of expensive jewelry or luxury cars, it appeared repugnant with regard to medicine. Cheap reproductions of luxury goods might suffice in which the rhinestone substituted for the diamond and the ready-made suit for the tailor-made. But the medical equivalent of the bargain basement or knockoff item was inherently suspect: there could be no substitute for a lifesaving drug or operation. Whereas the aspirations of working-class families to acquire fur coats or fancy cars could be derided as inappropriate, their desire to experience the kind of medical miracles portrayed in advertisements and the movies was far harder to dismiss. The prospect of a scientific medicine affordable only by the top half of American society seemed fundamentally unfair. Hence, the more valuable the doctors' services became, the more troublesome loomed income-related limits on their availability.

Concerns about medicine's affordability converged with growing awareness of another corollary of rising prosperity, namely a longer life span. Improved collection of vital statistics confirmed what public health authorities had begun to note even before World War I: death rates from infectious diseases, especially among infants and children, were in steep decline. As a result, the average American life span grew dramatically from barely forty years at birth in 1850 to sixty years in 1930. As further proof that science was improving the human condition, the decline in infectious diseases seemed cause for celebration. It helped inspire postwar enthusiasm for what health educators termed "positive health," a state of being not simply free of disease but also physically and mentally fit. Thanks to new scientific certainties as well as economic progress, the task of "taking care of yourself," as one guidebook termed it, took on new importance. How individuals cared for their bodies and their minds became an integral part of tending what sociologist Charles Cooley termed the modern "looking-glass" self: a sense of individual worth formed in relation to others' judgments.[49]

In both not-for-profit health education and commercial advertising, "taking care of yourself" became increasingly defined in terms of making better product choices. Positive health required a medicine cabinet stocked with tooth powder to preserve teeth, a reliable laxative to open the bowels, and an antacid to calm the stomach, all of which the interwar drugstore was happy to provide. To be sure, people could still make homemade versions of such products, using baking soda for brushing teeth and prunes as a laxative. Home economists and other experts often urged Americans to free themselves of the fetish of the store-bought. But the disposition to equate good health habits with the frequent purchase of modern hygiene products was hard to fight. As home economist Marion Harland observed, "In case of indisposition, the first question in this country is: 'What shall I take?' 'What shall I do?' is left unasked."[50]

While those Americans blessed with prosperity aspired to positive health, they also wrestled with the fact that modern comforts and conveniences constituted their own kind of health menace. A sedentary lifestyle weakened the body, especially the heart, while the accelerated pace of everyday life encouraged the consumption of "too many highballs and too much food," as one commentator observed. The factories and office buildings in which modern workers labored presented all manner of unhealthy conditions, including long commutes, stale air, and overbearing bosses. To compensate for a hard day's work hunched over a desk or a machine, urban dwellers flocked to commercial entertainments, such as amusement parks, movies, and nightclubs, which left them tired and unsettled the next day. Indulging in cigarettes, candy, and alcohol (still widely available despite Prohibition) gave immediate pleasure but had long-term drawbacks: smoker's cough, added pounds, and extended hangovers. At the same time, the constant excitement of work and leisure activities produced health-robbing mental pressure, tension, and anxiety.[51]

Worries about what medical educator Iago Galdston termed the "pathogenicity of progress" intensified as newspaper and magazine articles began to acknowledge another disturbing health fact: as infectious diseases declined, they were being replaced by equally frightening ailments. In 1921, heart disease replaced tuberculosis as the leading cause of death in the United States, followed closely by cancer, another disease associated with longer life. Experts disagreed over what these trends meant. Some suggested that they were an artifact of better record keeping and diagnosis, while others argued that they reflected a real change in disease patterns. Whatever the case, physicians and patients now faced the "ironic paradox," as one commentator put it, that "prolonging the span of life" meant increasing the risk of cancer and other diseases of mid- and late life.[52]

Moreover, despite all its advances, the new medical science did not offer much insight into the causes of degenerative heart disease and cancer other than equating them with a "civilized" lifestyle. Articles on heart disease listed many possible causes, including heredity, diet, lack of exercise, smoking, and stress—what eminent cardiologist Paul Dudley White referred to as "the speed of life and its evil accompaniments." The best recourse, he concluded, was to "try to stem the tide by preaching better habits, such as exercise in moderation, food in moderation, and work in moderation," especially for those with a family history of the disease. The causation of cancer was even murkier: as physician Harry Saltzstein acknowledged in a 1934 article, "Cancer—Its Status Today," experts knew little about the causes of cancer except that it "most frequently starts in body regions or spots that have been mildly irritated for a long time."[53]

The recognition that "we die differently now," as the Literary Digest declared in 1932, made decisions about how to live and what to consume all the more momentous. Urges to overeat and avoid exercise seemed far harder to evade than external foes such as microbes. Noted the Literary Digest, "We have been able to fight the germ diseases with success, but ourselves we cannot control." In other words, the new disease order created a constant battle between self-gratification and self-discipline that many people seemed destined to lose. The advent of what a later generation would term "lifestyle diseases" or "diseases of affluence" placed a high premium both on learning to consume more carefully and on monitoring the body's early warning signs of trouble. Articles in popular magazines emphasized the fact that early recognition followed by prompt treatment could make the difference between life and death.[54]

For heart disease, preventive messages focused on watching for the danger signs of high blood pressure (headaches and dizziness) and heart attacks (indigestion, shortness of breath, and chest pains following exertion). Similarly, messages about cancer prevention enumerated a long list of changes to watch for, including mouth ulcers, hoarseness, persistent cough, lumps in the breast and other parts of the body, and recurrent indigestion. Health educators urged people with these symptoms to see a doctor without delay, noting that those who "waited too long" to do so often died unnecessarily. Yet as commentators acknowledged, early warning signs of serious disease were easy to confuse with the minor health problems of everyday living. Ob-gyn specialist George Gray Ward observed in 1936, "As the early symptoms seem so unimportant it is not strange that the average person fails to appreciate their possible significance."[55]

Learning to negotiate the challenges of interwar consumer culture was no easy task. Somehow one had to remain healthy, well rested, good looking, and calm in the face of a modern lifestyle that seemed designed to undermine every one of those goals. Some people appear to have responded by ignoring the warnings and embracing the "eat, drink, and be merry" path. But for others, the new disease order and its uncertainties inspired another reaction: cultivating useful knowledge and protective behaviors as a way to lessen the risk of a long, slow decline from heart disease or cancer.

In the new interwar disease order, health information itself became a valuable commodity to be traded for profit as well as public benefit. Similar to the advent of the Internet almost a century later, the early twentieth-century information revolution made facts and opinions into commodities to be judged by their freshness, accuracy, and utility. As ad man Wallace Boren wrote in 1930, people needed the informational equivalent of the sandwich shops and soda fountains: "a mental lunch counter" that "serves various stimulating and nourishing bits of information to prospects who scurry in—who turn the leaves of a magazine while the radio is selling socks and savings accounts and tooth paste all over the dial."[56]

As "nourishing bits of information," medical breakthroughs and preventive advice featured prominently in both newspapers and magazines, which peaked in number and importance in the pre-1940 period. Newspaper syndicates developed medical columns in which physicians, among them William Brady, Royal Copeland, and Logan Clendenning, offered expert advice about how to negotiate the health hazards of modern life. After his departure from the federal government, Wiley found a successful second career as head of the Good Housekeeping Institute, overseeing its "seal of approval" program, which was designed to guide women readers' choice of better products. Film created more new possibilities for health education, among them newsreels, a 1930s innovation that carried a variety of health and medical news. Most powerful of all, radio became an important source of health information, sponsored by both nonprofit and for-profit groups.[57]

This new informational worldview elevated the importance of scientific change as a touchstone of modern life. As Morrill Goddard, the editor of *American Weekly* (the prototype of the Sunday newspaper magazines) told the creative staff at the J. Walter Thompson ad agency, "The public mind has come to feel that science is a wonderful thing—that science can do almost anything." In the new information order, journalism's task as well as that of advertising consisted of "telling [people] what the trouble is—that what they have been doing is futile and telling them the right way to do it as science finds." Much of that process involved "upsetting the things that grandma used to do and told mother and mother told us" and convincing people to say "now, I am going to do that" instead.[58]

The worship of modern science meshed nicely with the "cult of the new" so central to modern consumer culture, promoting the assumption that old was bad and new was good in medicine as elsewhere. Modern science progressed by a constant process of questioning received wisdom; each generation sought to test and if necessary overturn its predecessors' truths. As Mayo Clinic internist and health columnist Walter Alvarez noted, many leading scientists made their reputations by questioning "textbook statements." Newspapers and magazines hoped to attract readers by keeping them up-to-date on those shifts in scientific thinking. Yet intensifying media exposure also tended to undermine scientific authority. The more extensively and intensively the press covered medical and health issues, the more apparent it became that scientists disagreed over many aspects of many issues. A case in point was the great diversity of advice about what constituted a healthy diet. As Alvarez lamented in a 1928 letter discussing indigestion, "Here I am—a trained observer and intensely interested in the problem—and I am not really sure what I should avoid."[59]

The advertising industry's invocation of scientific progress only compounded the confusion. For all their seeming incompatibility, the dynamics of modern science actually served the purposes of advertising quite well. Ad agencies tasked with having to come up with new selling propositions year after year found plenty of inspiration in medical science. As a Thompson agency executive noted at a 1930 staff meeting, "The discovering of new merchandising angles and of themes for advertising campaigns which wish to be sound as well as novel, is leading more and more into territories formerly populated solely by chemists, biochemists, dieticians, doctors, specialists in all the several branches of science." More sarcastically, the humor magazine *Ballyhoo* opined in 1932 that an ad agency's definition of "Great Scientist" was "any doctor who will sign an endorsement." While attracting considerable scorn, advertising nonetheless promoted the idea that "science is a wonderful thing," in Goddard's words.[60]

The "march of science" and the "cult of the new" dovetailed to create a constant churning of news, information, and advertising in which "debunking," or exposing unscientific opinions, became a common sport. With the textbook opinion thrown aside, debate flourished over which of the latest theories was correct. While physicians were used to having such debates among themselves, they were less enthusiastic about journalists attempting to do their own debunking. As medical experts would increasingly warn the American public, not all this health-related information was equally good. Becoming a skilled information consumer required becoming an astute judge of what one public health leader termed "grade A Facts."[61] The savvy American had to sift valuable knowledge out of the deluge of messages, assessing the reliability of the source and the currency of the information. In the process, patient-consumers trying to follow health debates might easily conclude that none of these so-called experts knew what they were talking about. Once that process of doubting began—for example, in the aisles of the drugstore—it would not necessarily stop when the skeptical layperson moved on to the doctor's office.

All these developments—the new health dangers posed by prosperity, the lack of scientific certainty over many health matters, the increasingly rich variety of information and advertising surrounding every aspect of health—fed into the growing expectation that ordinary Americans become more skilled at making medical choices. The modern citizen had to become a better shopper in terms not only of products and services but also of information. Given the conflicting messages bombarding the public, the skills required to remain healthy, wealthy, and wise were by no means easy to master, even for the highly educated.

The Progressive-era upgrading of licensing and labeling laid the foundation for a vibrant and often confusing medical marketplace in the post–World War I period. The advent of a new disease landscape, a rapidly changing information environment, and new forms of consumption contributed to a growing profusion of choices. Long before they entered the doctor's office or the drugstore, patients were likely to have been exposed to a great many messages about how to manage their health affairs. Those messages included not only the prompts offered by commercial advertising but also the rising volume of often contradictory expert advice. In many ways, these messages reinforced the new medicine's idea that more and better knowledge was the essence of progress. Yet perversely, the rising tide of health advice also helped create an "informed" patient-consumer who would be more difficult to manage.

Thus during the interwar period, a new standard of what it meant to be a good versus a bad consumer slowly emerged in the doctor's office and the drugstore. "Good" consumers knew to distrust any whiff of ballyhoo and to regard modern advertising with automatic skepticism. They distrusted experts' and entrepreneurs' claims of having their best interests to heart. Conversely, "bad" consumers believed everything that they heard on the radio. They naively believed that modern science and modern medicine were as magical as the advertisers made out. Being an easy mark, in the language of the time, identified a person as a "rube," a "hayseed," or a "greenhorn"—that is, an unsophisticated soul who did not know how the world worked and could easily be taken advantage of.

In health matters as well as other areas of life, a growing number of people, blue collar as well as white collar, assumed that the growing commercialism surrounding medicine required them to think more, not less, for themselves. The crowning sign of that modern maturity was a sardonic disregard for advertising. As the humor magazine *Ballyhoo* summed it up in a parody of Rudyard Kipling's famous poem "If," "If you can tune in on the programs nightly, and yet not buy a single tube of [tooth]paste . . . you'll be a man, my son."[62] As the next two chapters show, the changes taking place in the interwar doctor's office and drugstore soon provided many opportunities for such skepticism. The closing down of the comparatively open market for medical goods and services by no means eliminated the hazards of patient choice. On the contrary, the shopping problems of the modern medical consumer were only just beginning.

{TWO}

The High Cost of Keeping Alive

In 1926, the *Saturday Evening Post* ran an article, "The High Cost of Keeping Alive," that described the replacement of the old-style family doctor with a new and better kind of medical man. As physician-author Stanley M. Rinehart explained, "It takes more time, more money and more education to be a doctor now than it did, say, forty years ago." In the post-Flexner era, a good medical degree cost anywhere from $10,000 to $25,000, while setting up a properly equipped office could add as much as $15,000. To pay off those expenses, the modern doctor had to tend to "the business side of medicine" more than his country predecessor had. Modern patients had to get used to coming to the office rather than receiving house calls and to getting regular itemized bills rather than a slapdash accounting every six months or so with "the total amount guessed at or reckoned according to sentiment." But, Rinehart insisted, while "the family-friend phase is gone," the doctor's new businesslike attitude "in no way interferes with or lowers the high ideals of a great profession." The new physician's services now cost more because they were *worth* more.[1]

Yet for many patients, the transformation that Rinehart described was far from satisfying. As another doctor writing in the late 1920s observed with dismay, "Many folk seem to regard the modern medical man as a deteriorated pigmy of the idolized old-time country doctor." The former might have more effective treatments to offer, but the new style of practice was not necessarily so easy to appreciate. Patients had to pay more for increasingly sophisticated, technologically advanced services, the need for which they could not easily judge for themselves. Perhaps the new medicine cost more because it was worth more, but how were patients to know for sure? And at a time when medical insurance did not yet exist, the "high cost of keeping alive" came straight from the patient's pocket.[2]

Doctors attributed grumblings about rising fees to the fact that "any medical bill is too much, at least from the patient's viewpoint," as one doctor wrote in 1928. "That is only human nature," he concluded. Doctors likewise dismissed as nonsense the idea that medical care varied in relation to the size of the patient's pocketbook rather than the number and quality of treatments rendered. Not surprisingly, many patients saw the situation differently. They perceived the reordering of doctors' offices as the imposition of a colder, harsher medical regime dictated by doctors' convenience rather than patients' needs. Despite medical reassurances to the contrary, they worried that the more businesslike doctor was becoming too mercenary in his approach. Anxieties already evident during the relative prosperity of the 1920s only deepened as the Great Depression set in. Thus rather than constituting an era of easy good feelings between doctor and patient, the interwar period marked the start of a lively public debate about the new style of doctoring. And out of this debate emerged the beginnings of medical consumerism in the doctor's office.[3]

A Better Class of Doctors

Paradoxically, these debates flourished at a time when the American profession was celebrating dramatic advances on many fronts: higher educational standards, tougher licensing laws, and a closer link to the technological marvels represented by the modern hospital. After a half century of hard-fought reforms, medical leaders had good reason to think they had at long last put their profession on a solid foundation. But all too soon new problems arose, creating discord both within the profession and between physicians and the patient public.

As the Flexner reforms took hold, medical schools began to attract a more elite type of student. By the mid-1930s, more than half of all schools required applicants to have completed at least three years of college work. Once admitted, medical students took a demanding curriculum that included bacteriology, physiology, and pharmacology and received intensive training in hospital wards and outpatient clinics. By the 1930s, most states required medical students not only to complete medical degrees at "approved" schools but also to pass licensing exams. Starting in 1915, medical graduates could also choose to take another round of "severe and searching" exams administered by the National Board of Medical Examiners. By the early 1930s, approximately 200 students each year, or about 9 percent of all medical school graduates, passed the National Boards. As hospital experience became increasingly integral to medical training, many students began to spend a fifth year training as hospital interns before entering private practice. Gradually many states, starting with Pennsylvania in 1914, required the internship as a requirement for licensure. By 1940, virtually all young doctors had completed internships before beginning practice.[4]

These higher educational and credentialing standards produced a medical profession that was far less diverse than it had been in the late nineteenth century. The Flexner reforms led to the closure of many medical schools willing to accept women and blacks, leaving a profession that was 95 percent white and male by the 1930s. Quotas that limited Jewish applicants added another layer of discrimination. The more elite the medical school, the more likely its students were to be what Nicholas Butler referred to as the "country club type"—white college graduates from wealthy backgrounds. The rising cost of obtaining a medical education and setting up a practice made it harder for applicants from less privileged backgrounds to become physicians. So while the range of Americans needing medical care remained very diverse after 1920, the physicians available to care for them became more uniform in terms of class, race, and gender.[5]

Perhaps because of the profession's greater homogeneity, medical groups became far better organized and effective political agents in the post–World War I period. In the wake of its thorough reorganization in 1901, the AMA oversaw the integration of county and state medical societies into a more effective vehicle for protecting the profession's interests. While not all doctors agreed with its positions, the AMA spoke often and powerfully as the voice of the American physician.

In the AMA's optimistic view, the profession had honored its social contract with the patient public. Having surrendered the old traditions associated with "every man his own doctor," the American people were reaping the rewards: well-trained physicians were now both easily identifiable and affordable.[6] Yet beneath that comforting message lay a more complex reality. Having promised a generation of physicians who were uniformly excellent in their training and demeanor, interwar medical leaders found that promise hard to deliver on. Not only was the upgrading of standards more slow and uneven than they admitted, but the profession was also unsettled by the rapid advance of specialization. In the words of physician Arthur Hertzler, the public had been promised a more "standardized profession" than could actually be delivered.[7]

The trend toward specialization was a natural consequence of the growing importance of hospital-based medicine. By the late 1920s, the United States had some 7,000 hospitals with a capacity of around 900,000 beds and representing some $5 billion in investment, much of it in surgical suites, laboratory facilities, and radiology departments. This increasingly complicated array of medical technology became a seedbed for ever-more-complex procedures for testing and treating an expanding range of illnesses. Combining these technological assets with a growing supply of patients as clinical material, hospitals nurtured the trend toward medical specialization, allowing doctors to deepen their understanding of particular organs and ailments.[8]

Whereas in 1900 relatively few doctors limited their practice to a single area such as surgery or neurology, by the early 1930s many had come to think of themselves as full or partial specialists. A 1931 survey found that 23 percent of doctors described their practices as entirely limited to one specialty, another 21 percent combined general practice with some specialty work, and only 56 percent considered themselves to be general practitioners. The most common area of specialization was surgery; other popular areas were ear, nose, and throat; obstetrics and gynecology; and ophthalmology. Although specialization was most prevalent in cities, its impact was felt in smaller towns as well. For example, a study of rural San Joaquin County, California, found that in its largest town, Stockton, nearly 40 percent of its seventy-nine physicians were full or partial specialists.[9]

The trend toward specialization represented not only a response to expanding medical knowledge but also a pursuit of economic incentives. By 1929, specialists' net income was more than twice that of the general practitioners—an average of $10,000 versus $3,900. In rural areas, general practitioners made far less, with 50 percent making under $2,500 a year. Moreover, standards for entering specialty practice remained very loose. In contrast to Europe, where physician organizations maintained more centralized control over specialist practice, voluntary national societies set standards for specialist training in the United States. Elite surgeons, for example, formed the American College of Surgeons in 1913; thereafter patients in search of good surgeons were advised to seek out a member of that group. By 1940, sixteen such specialty boards were in existence, but all their standards remained voluntary, and they had no legal authority to stop doctors who did not meet them from representing themselves to patients as having a specialist level of knowledge and experience.[10]

While in theory a testimony to medicine's growing scientific prowess, the rapid growth of specialization in general and surgery in particular became a recurrent source of conflict within the profession. General practitioners complained that specialists were stealing patients who could be treated just as effectively—and at less expense—by nonspecialists. Although medical societies routinely advised against doing so, many patients bypassed general practitioners' referrals and went straight to specialists, who welcomed them without reservation. General practitioners also complained about the rapid proliferation of outpatient clinics and dispensaries, where interns and residents provided free or very low cost care as part of their training. One solution, much decried on ethical grounds, was the system of fee splitting, in which general practitioners referring patients to a surgeon received a portion of the fee.[11]

Thus, while medicine appeared to be making marked scientific and professional gains, its economic evolution in the interwar decades produced very uneven patterns of growth. On the one hand, medical incomes rose overall: compared to other middle-class occupations, doctors fared relatively well, receiving better pay than teachers and only slightly less than engineers. On the other hand, studies of physician incomes in the late 1920s showed a larger minority of poorly paid members than was present in other fields: urban specialists earned handsome incomes, while doctors in rural and poor areas were barely making ends meet.[12]

These uneven patterns of growth not only created conflict among physicians but also posed problems for patients trying to find medical care. The services offered by licensed physicians remained anything but uniform in terms of quantity, quality, and cost. For all the rhetoric of first-class medical schools and hospitals as the doctor's workshop, the variety of medical providers and the goods and services that flowed through their hands remained highly variable. In a still highly individualistic profession, physicians practiced in dramatically different ways; as a consequence, laypeople intent on getting good care needed to learn more about how the new medical order worked.

Setting Up the Doctor's Showroom

While interwar commentators often highlighted the hospital as the exemplar of medical progress, patients rarely ended up in one without having first been seen by a physician in private practice. For all the importance of the hospital, both to medical training and to treatment innovations, doctors continued to provide more than 80 percent of their services outside its walls. Whether specialists or generalists, doctors needed to attract private patients in order to make a living. As part of that process, managing office-based practices became increasingly important to practitioners' success. The doctor's waiting room, as one advice manual put it, was "the 'show window' of his profession."[13]

Creating a "practice-building office," as *Medical Economics* styled it, was all the more important because many Americans still assumed that they should "not go to the doctor for every little thing," as one commentator observed.[14] The proliferation of drugstores encouraged long-standing habits of self-medication among town dwellers, while the sale of proprietary medicines through mail-order catalogs did the same for rural folk. At the same time, alternative healers such as chiropractors, osteopaths, and Christian Science practitioners continued to offer their services. So in country and city alike, doctors had to promote their new brand of scientific medicine to a patient public also being courted by drugstores, proprietary medicine ads, and other healers.

Positioning the doctor's services as superior to these options was all the more challenging because of the restrictions that medicine's professional codes placed on self-promotion. Despite the new pressures on doctors to be more businesslike, they were still expressly forbidden to advertise their services. As Rinehart noted in the *Saturday Evening Post*, the modern physician "must keep up appearances" because his office constituted "his only means of advertising, except that which is done by the G.P.s"—"grateful patients."[15] Even as physicians complained about the commercialism rampant in American culture and particularly that associated with drugstores and drug advertising, they could not afford to ignore the rising standards of service that consumers were starting to expect. Succeeding in medicine required a delicate balancing act: appearing businesslike but not commercial, prosperous without being ostentatious, and welcoming yet dignified. As a result, the interwar renovation of the doctor's office reflected a curious mix of features that said "come hither" yet "obey me," an apt characterization of the doctor-patient relationship.

The stakes involved in this balancing act were heightened by what was perhaps the most significant change in medicine from the patients' point of view, namely doctors' efforts to shift the locus of care from the patient's home to the doctor's office. In the nineteenth century, doctors had provided the great majority of their services as house calls. The doctor's office typically was a room in his own home, used only a few hours a week for walk-in patients, with his wife often serving as receptionist. This arrangement began to shift as medicine became more instrument- and technology-dependent and local transportation became easier. While doctors continued to make house calls, they sought to shift the bulk of routine medical care into their offices, now increasingly set up separately from their homes.[16]

By the 1920s, with this shift well under way, one hallmark of the "new doctor" was his expectation that the patient should come to him for care rather than the other way around. Not surprisingly, many people disliked this change, and much medical advice literature consequently focused on the best ways to wean patients off the house-call habit. To that end, rehabilitating the doctor's office into a more welcoming space had obvious merits. In the words of H. Sheridan Baketel, the editor of *Medical Economics*, investing in a "pleasing arrangement of furniture need not be expensive" and could go a long way toward reconciling patients to the necessity of the office visit. Whether one's patients lived on Park Avenue or Main Street, such efforts "spell courtesy, and courtesy isn't expensive."[17]

Baketel made setting up a "practice-building office" sound easy, but in fact it posed a challenge for young physicians. Success involved a number of important decisions: choosing a good location, investing in the right equipment and staff, and last but not least, deciding what kind of services would attract a loyal clientele. Medical school training did little to prepare its graduates for making these decisions. As economist Maurice Leven noted in 1932, "After years of purely professional preparation, [the doctor] is turned loose in a commercial world to compete for business as well as professional success." For all his specialized training, "his first and primary concern after graduation must, of necessity, be that of a small-scale business man."[18] In a highly individualistic profession, young doctors had to find their own way, relying on informal networks of friends and colleagues to guide their choices.

One consequence of this decision making was a growing mismatch of doctors to patient populations. As of 1932, the United States had approximately 156,000 physicians, or one physician for every 780 people, theoretically the most favorable ratio of any developed nation. But those numbers were not evenly distributed. In search of patients, doctors followed the post–World War I flow of population into large cities and their suburbs. By the late 1920s, rural areas had 48 percent of the population but only 31 percent of the physicians. Commentators explained that trend by noting that rural areas were far poorer than urban areas, making it hard for doctors to make a living, and lacked the hospital and laboratory facilities needed to practice up-to-date medicine. As economist Harry H. Moore noted in 1927, the doctors who left country practice tended to be the "younger, more enterprising men," leaving behind the older men "now in quite a different class from those who in recent years have graduated from Class A schools." At the same time, rural doctors faced pressure to update their style of practice, as affluent families took advantage of improved transportation to go to nearby towns for care. Because of the greater ease of travel, Hertzler noted in 1938, "the modern country doctor's office is as carefully kept as the city doctor's."[19]

Within cities, similar pressures led to a clustering of doctors' offices in areas deemed most likely to present a favorable mix of potential patients. Urban doctors' offices tended to be concentrated either in the central business district or the city's more prosperous suburbs. Office location varied depending on the doctor's background and aspirations: someone seeking to be a general practitioner or a pediatrician might seek out a family-oriented suburb, while the aspiring specialist would locate downtown in the so-called doctors' districts, where purpose-built "professional buildings" just for doctors and dentists began to spring up, for example, around Rittenhouse Square in Philadelphia and on Park Avenue in Manhattan. Doctors might change locations as their careers prospered, starting out in modest offices in modest neighborhoods and then moving to "better" locations in the central business district or the suburbs after their practices became successful. Such moves often coincided with growing commitments to specialty practice; after some years in general practice, doctors would relocate to be closer to the hospitals providing referrals. Over time, the range of doctors' offices that a patient might encounter in a single city grew very diverse.[20]

Already by the 1930s, social scientists were beginning to note how these currents of change affected patients differently depending on their class and race. For patients who could afford the costs of mass transit, the clustering of doctors' offices in commercial districts had some advantages. As social scientists I. S. Falk, C. Rufus Rorem, and Martha D. Ring noted in 1933, "Even in towns of 5,000 to 10,000 population, most physicians are located on 'Main Street' rather than in residential sections," so that "the patient may call during a temporary absence from employment or during a shopping expedition." These authors also noted that having doctors' offices located in the same area encouraged "the public to 'shop around' for a physician" rather than stick to just one practitioner.[21]

At the same time, fewer and fewer doctors chose to locate in very poor neighborhoods, forcing residents of those areas to make long, expensive trips to other parts of the city for care. Entrenched racism compounded this problem in predominantly black neighborhoods. In districts where few private practices remained, doctors felt less pressure to modernize. Low fees, long hours, and forgiving collection practices mattered more to their clientele than did the appearance of their waiting room. In poor neighborhoods, doctors continued to work out of offices that differed little from the late-nineteenth-century version that Hertzler described: a single room with a row of books over the desk, "an old couch, three chairs," and "a small table" for instruments.[22]

In contrast, practitioners who moved to doctor-rich areas of the city, particularly the young ones just going into practice, had to invest more heavily in the appearance and conduct of their "showroom." Simply put, the more choices that patients had for comparison shopping among physicians, the more consequential became their first impressions of a medical practice. When presented a choice of doctors to patronize, patients took into account factors such as the cleanliness and attractiveness of the office space and the friendliness of the doctor and his staff. In order to compete effectively for "good" patients—that is, those who could pay their bills on time—interwar doctors had to invest more time and thought into practice management. As an unnamed "Doctor's Wife" explained in *Harper's Monthly*, professional success required that a doctor "must, in the common phrase, 'sell himself,' or 'put himself over,' with his patients." That subtle art of self-promotion started with the look and feel of his private office.[23]

To instruct physicians in that subtle art, *Medical Economics*, a journal aimed at private practitioners, carried regular articles about office decor and management. The makeover of the interwar doctor's office began with the reception room. As a 1927 article warned, "Too many physicians . . . take it for granted that a patient's impressions begin and end in the consultation room" when in fact "they are in the making long before that." Indeed, the author suggested, "one of the best possible advertising campaigns that the medical profession could put on" would be "a general uplifting of the reception room." To that end, articles presented tips on how to make a waiting room appealing, among them displaying fresh flowers, providing cigarettes and ashtrays, and installing a "neat little telephone box" for use of "the businessman who drops in a few minutes too early for his appointment." To keep nervous patients occupied, the physician should supply magazines for them to read; one favorite was *Hygeia*, the AMA's popular health magazine started in 1923. The goal was to create a light and pleasant environment: as another *Medical Economics* article counseled, the waiting room's furnishings should have "nothing about them to suggest pain and suffering."[24]

The same theme of convenience and comfort applied to the next stage of the office visit, when the patient entered the doctor's inner sanctum and prepared for the examination. In "Some Dressing Rooms I've Seen," a "veteran patient" reported that "most up-to-date doctors are now arranging their offices" so that they had a space dedicated for use as a dressing room where patients might disrobe in privacy and hang their clothing neatly prior to being seen. Such a space need not be big or fancy as long as it sufficed to "give privacy, be convenient and immaculate." Providing such an amenity, the author concluded, is "one of the best practice-builders I know of speaking from a patient's viewpoint."[25]

Efforts to make patients feel at home prepared them for the most important phase of the office visit: the clinical encounter itself. Here again, physicians looking to build their practices were advised to invest in the right kind of furniture and equipment. As a combination advertisement for office furnishings in a 1927 issue of *Medical Economics* explained, "Modern equipment is one means of bringing a physician and his patients together with a feeling of complete confidence on both sides." Another ad in the same issue began, "Do You Value Your Patients' Opinion?" and then followed with the observation that "Allison's matched office suites are looked upon as Builders of Good Will and as an ethical way of advertising." In similar fashion, interwar companies promoted examining tables, instrument tables, instrument cabinets, and arc lighting as necessities for the properly furnished office.[26]

When examining patients, the new doctor had many more forms of medical technology at his command than his old-fashioned predecessor. As the "Doctor's Wife" explained in 1932, only thirty years earlier, the best doctor reached a diagnosis primarily by "whatever he could find out by his eye and ear, unaided by any instrument except the stethoscope" and only rarely by a urinalysis. In contrast, the modern physician's "diagnosis and opinion are backed by the facts recorded by a blood count, a blood chemical examination, a tracing of the heart showing its contours, an electrocardiogram showing how it acts, chemical analysis if indicated, giving all the current gastrointestinal news, and other accurate laboratory facts for which the subjective symptoms or the history have indicated the necessity."[27]

At a bare minimum, patients seeing a doctor for an office visit might anticipate that he would use the same tools he carried in his black bag: stethoscope, clinical thermometer, otoscope, scalpels, and forceps. In addition, many doctors' offices had heavier, more complex instruments that could not be easily transported: microscopes and slide-making equipment, autoclaves to sterilize instruments, scales for weighing the patient, and devices to read blood pressure. Beyond those basics, patients might see many more devices, depending on the doctor's personal taste and specialty. Late-1920s medical journals carried advertisements for X-ray units, ultraviolet lights, diathermy devices, and physiotherapy equipment along with the latest versions of more familiar tools such as office scales, clinical thermometers, steel needles, surgical knives, and syringes.[28]

These advertisements often mentioned the equipment's value not only in making the doctor's practice more effective and efficient but also in impressing patients. Thus in 1925, the W. A. Baum Company advertised the Baumanometer, a blood-pressure-monitoring device, by declaring, "It's confidence that counts—your patient's confidence in you—your confidence in your instrument." The ad featured an imagined conversation between a doctor and a patient in which the latter, identified as "a consulting engineer," commented, "That seems to be a much more accurate instrument than some doctors use for blood pressure." Similarly, a 1926 advertisement for the Castle sterilizer pictured a mother and child visiting the physician and announced, "Everyone has faith in Castle Sterilization": having such a device made it "a simple matter to visually demonstrate your thoughtful care."[29]

How much of all this equipment a patient might see in use during an office visit remained highly variable. While all interwar physicians were in theory trained to provide a standard physical examination, in practice they did not follow the same protocols. But a patient might reasonably expect that during a first visit, the doctor would take a medical history, focusing on whatever problem had brought the patient there, and then conduct a physical exam, taking the pulse, temperature, and blood pressure; listening to heart and lung sounds; and palpating parts of the body. Depending on the symptoms presented, the doctor would then decide on additional tests, such as an X-ray, throat culture, or blood analysis. In some cases, those tests might be done in the doctor's office; in others, the patient would be referred to a nearby clinic or laboratory.[30]

Once the exam and follow-up tests were completed, doctor and patient met again to discuss treatment. Here again, the comparison with the old-fashioned doctor seemed very much in the new doctor's favor. As commentators frequently noted, physicians no longer had to rely so heavily on a reassuring bedside manner to serve their patients well: now they had much more concrete and effective goods to offer in exchange for patients' loyalty. As social scientist Michael Marks Davis noted, to get a sense of how much medicine had changed, one need only compare the Chicago Medical Society's listing of common procedures: in 1892, that list took up only half a printed page, whereas by 1940, it consisted of "six times the space in fine print."[31]

As accounts of medical progress emphasized, the interwar physician not only could do a better job of diagnosis but had many more treatment options at his command, including new drugs, specialized diets, and office-based treatments. In addition to the big breakthrough "magic bullets" of the era, such as insulin to treat type 1 diabetes or neosalvarsan to treat syphilis, surgical advances placed a new premium on early diagnosis of conditions that if left untreated might result in chronic debility or even death. For example, prior to the 1890s, appendicitis had been treated by bed rest and painkillers. As surgery became safer, some surgeons urged quick removal of the organ rather than a "watch and wait" approach. By the 1920s, early surgical treatment of the disease had become widely accepted in the American profession.[32]

Not surprisingly, given the fulsome accounts of medical progress circulating in newspapers and magazines, patients came to doctors expecting to receive one or more of these new and improved treatments. Having made the decision to visit the doctor's showroom, they did not intend to leave empty-handed. One of the most prized of such treatments was a prescription for a drug not available over the counter. As economist Allon Peebles noted in a study of Indiana, in the late 1920s when patients went to the doctor, they "want medicine, expect it, and as one physician reported, if the doctor does not give it to them, even though he may have given them far more valuable service in the way of advice, they feel dissatisfied and in some measure cheated." Thanks to the expanding array of medications listed in the pages of the USP, the National Formulary, and the AMA's New and Nonofficial Remedies, doctors had little reason to deprive patients of this satisfaction. Along with the advertisements for office furnishings and equipment, medical journals carried many promotions for new products designed to appeal to patients. As an ad for Gray's Glycerine Tonic in the October 1927 issue of *Medical Economics* explained, "The Patient Estimates the Value of His Treatment by Immediate Rather Than Ultimate Results."[33]

In addition to the prescription pad, interwar physicians had a rapidly growing array of other measures they could recommend. For patients bothered by poor digestion or weight issues, a variety of special diets had been developed. For those suffering from fatigue or nervousness, a glandular extract or treatment with a sunlamp might be prescribed. Treatments with ultraviolet and infrared rays, quartz light, and electric heat were especially popular between the two world wars. Last but not least, doctors could perform a wide range of surgical procedures in their offices. As a survey conducted in the late 1920s revealed, 30 percent of all surgery took place in the office, including operations on the sinus and nasal cavities, lancing of boils, and removal of hemorrhoids.[34]

The types of treatments offered reflected the growing influence of medical specialism. Although full-time specialists still comprised only a minority of doctors, they helped to promote an activist style of medical practice throughout the profession. Whether full time or part time, specialists led the way in promoting new theories of treatment, such as the dangers of "focal infection" used to justify the removal of infected teeth, tonsils, and appendixes, operations that could easily be performed by physicians in general practice. Specialists were also early adopters of new laboratory tests and improvements in X-ray and other imaging devices that soon became common in more general practice. As one contemporary described them, specialists constituted the "go getters of the scalpel and stethoscope," and other doctors had to copy their ways to compete.[35]

Becoming a Better Doctor-Shopper

The great reorganization of American medicine that took place in the first three decades of the twentieth century created a host of what economists would later describe as "shopping problems" for patients. To be sure, the nineteenth-century "free trade" in doctoring had required patients to make complicated decisions about which doctors to patronize. But the interwar medical scene became even more confusing as the distance between scientific and lay understandings of disease widened. While being reassured that the new doctors were better than the old, patients did not find their services easy to understand or evaluate. Precisely the changes that supposedly made the new doctors better made their performance harder for patients to judge. These problems were evident in the popular advice offered about how to pick a "good" doctor.

At one level, picking a good doctor seemed a simple process. By taking proper care with the initial selection, patients could easily avoid any danger of poor treatment. Writing in *Hygeia*, the AMA's lay magazine, in 1927, physician William Everett Musgrave emphasized the importance of that selection. As he noted, "Among our remaining personal liberties is the right to select our dogs, our marital mates and our doctors." To exercise that right wisely, Musgrave outlined the markers that patient-consumers should use to judge the physician's "merits." A good doctor was known by his professional credentials: possession of a medical degree from "some worthy institution of learning"; membership in local, state, and national medical societies; and possession of a valid medical license (although Musgrave noted that licenses meant little in states that issued licenses to irregulars). Further, according to Musgrave, a good doctor should consider "the patient rather than the disease," be willing to provide preventive advice, be aware of his own limitations, and be amenable to collaborations with other doctors. He should also possess a high moral code that included charging only what patients could afford to pay and a strong interest in keeping up-to-date on current medicine. Totally opposed to "personal puffery," "he relies for the growth of his own clientele on the influence of the ever-widening circle of those friends whom he has served."[36]

On the face of it, Musgrave's advice seemed quite straightforward: do this and all will be well. Yet the realities of choice turned out to be more complicated. Patients' first task was determining whether a physician was trustworthy, which required that they become more knowledgeable about medical standards. But the more patients interacted with the real world of doctors' offices, the more likely they were to encounter disparities between ideal and practice that inspired confusion and disappointment, leading some to become less trusting of medical authority.

In the first place, doctors' training turned out to vary far more than scientific professionalism would seem to allow. For example, the practice of grandfathering in older practitioners meant that many practicing physicians had received their education and licensing under late-nineteenth-century standards far below those associated with the Flexner reforms. In the days before continuing medical education requirements, doctors had no motives other than personal curiosity or sense of professionalism to follow the latest medical developments.[37]

Moreover, even recent graduates of medical schools remained unevenly trained. Although the original Flexner ABCD grading system was replaced by a simple dichotomy between "approved" and "unapproved" schools, a substantial distance remained between the elite schools and their less rigorous counterparts. Licensure requirements also varied greatly from state to state. Therefore, discriminating patients came to understand that physicians could be distinguished by the quality of the medical schools they had attended; by the standards of the states where they had initially been licensed; by other professional certifications, such as passage of the National Boards or board certification in specific specialties; and by their overall degree of specialization.

Finding the "good" doctor was further complicated by the profession's bans on self-promotion, which made finding out this kind of information difficult. In theory, patients were supposed to be able to find a doctor simply by relying on local medical authorities. According to the "Doctor's Wife," those who could not find good doctors clearly lacked "the forethought enough to acquire a regular physician by looking up the local doctors in the medical directory or calling up the county medical society or a recognized hospital and getting the name and address of a good doctor near their home."[38] Yet in practice, the limits on physician publicity left patients with little concrete information about the doctors' ability, personality, or affordability. In the effort to distinguish themselves from "quacks," doctors deliberately made their professional listings very uninformative. Directories gave only the most basic information, such as the address and office hours of the practitioner. As Ruth Evelyn Henderson lamented in 1928, people very much wanted an "alert, personal, friendly" doctor, and she had no doubt that doctors "with the 'home town spirit'" could be found even in the biggest metropolis. But as she noted wryly, doctors were not classified as such "in the directories of large, strange cities."[39]

In light of these limitations, the first office visit became all the more important as a supplement to prospective patients' knowledge about a physician. In magazine articles and advice books, a range of commentators proffered tips about how to "read" the appearance of the office and the demeanor of the doctor as a predictor of good care. Yet here again, the advice proved confusing and contradictory. On the one hand, patients were told that they could tell a great deal about a style of practice from the comfort and cleanliness of the doctor's waiting room as well as the organization and equipment of his examining room. But they were also warned against assuming that a finely furnished office alone constituted evidence of quality. An excellent doctor might practice effectively in a very small office if he had access to local laboratory and hospital resources; conversely, a very bad doctor might well work in what appeared to be a medical palace.

As Falk, Rorem, and Ring wrote in 1933, "One physician may conduct an independent practice in a single room or at most with a waiting room and an adjoining examining room," while another "may maintain a suite of offices with several examining rooms, a telephone clerk and admission girl in the waiting room, a laboratory technician, and a roentgenologist in separate quarters, and several nurses and possibly an attendant to assist him in the conduct of minor operations."[40] The variance in doctors' fees clearly reflected the different costs of running such an office. Presumably "good" doctors could be found at both extremes, but the question remained: How was the patient to understand and interpret such striking differences in their office spaces? The discerning patient needed to learn to look carefully at both the doctor and his office.

Medical and lay advice givers alike warned against being taken in by the lavish offices kept by "society doctors" who offered the medical equivalent of "the rental of a Park Avenue apartment or a parterre box at the opera." Rinehart warned his readers, "There are fads in doctors as in dress, dogs, and restaurants," and while the fashionable doctor "may deliver, medically speaking, sterling and not pewter," he noted, "you pay extra for the frills." Echoing that sentiment, a 1925 article by Ida Albright described the sense of buyer's remorse experienced during a visit to a specialist's office. At first, the beautiful surroundings gave her a "happy glow of appreciation—until I cast an appraising eye at the appointments of the room" and started to think: "These Oriental rugs—they looked frightfully expensive." "Had the diagnostician paid for them, or would he put them on my bill?" She concluded, "The thought terrified me." The same suspicion extended to treatments ordered. "Mammon, M.D.," as Lloyd Morris dubbed him, followed the precept to "get yourself a practice among wealthy, fashionable people" by offering the latest in fashionable treatments, among which Morris classified appendectomies, electrical treatments, and sunlamp bathing.[41]

By this same logic, patients should not assume that a successful doctor was necessarily a good doctor. Disputing the conventional wisdom that doctors never promoted themselves, Cleon Mason warned that many of his fellow physicians prospered only because they were talented at the art of self-promotion: "The public still likes its bally hoo, not only in the side-show but in the doctor's office, and far too often the public runs to clever medical salesmanship while it completely ignores medical competency and scientific efficiency." He concluded that patients who felt taken in by physicians charging high prices for ineffective treatment had only themselves to blame: "You cannot sell a brand of medical treatment which the public does not like, no matter how right it may be."[42] Equally confusing was the advice about what to look for in terms of the doctor's bedside manner—that is, how he handled the personal and emotional dimensions of patient care. Here again, physicians provided scorching criticism of their brethren, complaining that doctors with little scientific skill established flourishing practices on the strength of personal charm and affability. "Medical knowledge and personal charm often go together, but not necessarily," noted the "Doctor's Wife."[43] A savvy patient had to learn to judge a doctor not on superficial traits of personality but on reliable signs of ability.

As a way out of all these difficulties, advice givers fell back on the reassurance that the real secret to getting good medical care was "to find a good family doctor—and hold on to him after you find him," as Hugh Grant Rowell wrote in a 1931 article, "How to Get Your Money's Worth from Your Doctor."[44] Patients should find competent and trustworthy general practitioners and allow them to provide guidance through the increasingly dense thicket of conflicting claims about what constituted good doctoring. Yet that advice became increasingly difficult to follow as the ratio of generalists to specialists steadily declined, making the family doctor with that "home town spirit" even more of a rarity.

Not surprisingly, the problems posed by specialization figured prominently in discussions of what was amiss in the doctor's office, as battles within the profession spilled over into the popular literature. Positioning themselves as the conservators of the old country doctor's virtues, general practitioners presented themselves as superior to specialists in that they looked after the whole patient, refused to follow mere therapeutic "fashion," and still took time to listen to patients. But as the generalists well recognized, specialists effectively portrayed themselves as scientific trendsetters, due to their continually changing arrays of complicated tests and procedures. The rise of specialism, as one doctor complained in *Harper's* in 1928, had encouraged patients "to diagnose their own cases rather than go to their family physician . . . and let him decide what special work is needed."[45] Given the long-standing emphasis on patients' right to choose their personal physician, little could be done to stop this behavior other than to keep advising patients to seek out the dwindling population of general practitioners.

Meanwhile, patient complaints about negotiating the confusing and expensive landscape of medical specialism became commonplace. Many symptoms, such as headaches, backaches, fatigue, heartburn, and indigestion, could have any number of origins, so the person seeking relief might well visit a number of specialists before finding one who could help. A 1925 article in the *Independent* joked about the process: a patient afflicted with mysterious pains goes to Dr. Hocus, who fails to find the cause and sends him on to Dr. Pocus, a process that continues through Drs. Hodge, Podge, Namby, and Pamby, who finally refers him back to Dr. Hocus. But the search for Dr. Right could have disastrous economic as well as therapeutic consequences. An unlucky choice of physician meant not only physical suffering but also "a heavy financial penalty for every doctor whose theory is mistaken," as one commentator noted. Nor was this a problem solely found among wealthy patients. Studying low-income families in New York City, social worker Gladys V. Swackhamer found that many reported disappointment with medical specialists, including an Italian baker's wife whose family came to financial ruin after treatment by the real-life equivalents of Drs. Namby, Pamby, and Podge.[46]

Some advisers characterized such tragedies as functions of individual ignorance: unfortunate patients allowed themselves to be taken in by "salesmanship." Lamented Albright, "The specialist, without fanfare of trumpets, or blare of advertising, has sold himself with complete success to the public."

Other commentators suggested that patients did not deserve all the blame for these problems. Even people who confined their choices to doctors in good standing with local medical societies might well have problems. As insurance executive Donald Armstrong noted, not all criticisms of the medical profession came from those "too ignorant or stupid to know the difference between a supposedly well-qualified physician and a so-called 'doctor' of chiropractic." Legitimate complaints also came from "those who recognize that still in the practice of medicine today there is a great deal that is chaotic, unintelligent, and irresponsible."[47]

Ironically, the medical profession's emphasis on personal choice increased patient-consumers' incentives to put more time and effort into selecting their physicians and treatments, in other words, to become informed consumers of medical care. To tell "good" doctoring from "bad," patients had to exercise some degree of medical judgment. To avoid being taken advantage of by quacks, patients needed to learn what distinguished a proper doctor. In this spirit, the AMA worked hard to "educate" patient-consumers to be watchdogs against the kind of quackery presented by the likes of Norman Baker, who promised cancer cures over his own radio station. Yet in the end, keeping this watchdog outlook trained only on unlicensed practitioners proved impossible, and AMA members found it turned on themselves as well.[48]

The Bill Comes In

Deciding who bore the blame for the patients' shopping problems took on an even more bitter edge when the bill came in. Among the features of the "new" doctoring that patients found unappealing, perhaps the most painful was its more businesslike approach to billing. Modern doctors not only had more care to offer but also charged more for its provision. While hospital care remained the most expensive, the rise in costs spread to the doctor's office as well, as the whole medical economy seemed caught in a perpetual cycle of rising prices.

The rise in cost coincided with the medical profession's embrace of a more businesslike approach to practice. For decades, its leaders had cultivated an image of medicine as a higher calling that practitioners entered for altruistic rather than economic reasons. They took pride in doctors' reputation for being "bad" businessmen. That image may well have been exaggerated: as a study of rural Indiana in the late 1920s observed, "the financial records of the physicians are superior to their medical records." But the conviction that the old-time doctor had been an indifferent businessman remained a commonplace of interwar commentaries on medicine. As Rinehart wrote in "The High Cost of Keeping Alive," his knowledge was based on long familiarity with his patients and their families rather than scrutiny of X-rays or lab tests. He did not need to keep track of individual visits and sent out his medical bills once or twice a year "because he was too busy doing things to reckon the charges." But the new doctor could not afford to be so casual because he had to pay off the costs of his expensive education and office equipment.[49]

One practical factor contributing to the rise of the more business-conscious doctor was the 1914 institution of the federal income tax. Form 1040 not only required physicians to declare their practice income but also allowed them to deduct professional expenses, including the costs of running an office and maintaining an automobile, from their taxable earnings. Physicians consequently had an important incentive to keep better track of both income and expenses. The advent of the income tax, suggested accountant E. S. Woolley, convinced "the up-to-date physician" that "it is just as necessary for him to know the business end of his profession, as it was for him to study the profession in the first place."[50]

In other ways, the business-friendly climate of the 1920s encouraged more attention to the economic side of medical practice. That trend was evident in the 1923 founding of *Medical Economics*, a journal explicitly intended to address the business aspects of professional life. As its editor H. Sheridan Baketel noted, until very recently "the business side of medicine was simply taboo." But the profession had started to recognize that "scientific progress in medicine is not so very far removed from economic progress," ushering in "a new era of medicine" in which "the physician is becoming efficient." The old-time doctor's casual approach to sending bills, collecting debts, and accepting barter in exchange for care seemed woefully out of step with modern economic principles.[51]

In explaining why doctors had to change, physician commentators frequently drew parallels between medicine and modern businesses such as department stores or automobile showrooms. Explained Miles Brewer in "The Basis of the Doctor's Charges," "a physician works on a margin of profit quite as directly as a merchant." Just like an automobile salesman, the doctor's "overhead must be considered in fixing fees." Similarly, Mason explained that in raising their fees, doctors were simply acting in accord with modern market principles: "A doctor has only one thing to sell, his time, which of course comprehends his talent or abilities"; he "quickly finds that the article he has to sell is subject to economic laws, just as any other commodity, and the law of supply and demand soon begins to operate." While patients found higher fees unpleasant, these laws were a fact of life "in the commercial world, and will continue to exist in the medical world until some radical changes come to pass."[52]

The monetarization of medical practice inevitably facilitated comparisons between medicine and other commodities and services that did not necessarily favor the doctor. While industrialization drove down the cost of many goods thereby making them more affordable, the economics of the doctor's office were going in the opposite direction: physicians were offering more goods but only at much higher prices. Woolley suggested that doctors needed to reeducate their patients to realize that they had to pay their doctor bills just like they did their department store charges because "in coming to the Doctor for professional services, a contractual obligation has been assumed." But in the process, assessing whether those services had been necessary or valuable was likely to become a sticking point. Asking patients to pay bigger bills inevitably provoked them to take a closer look at what they were being charged for.[53]

In fact, how doctors decided on the size of their fees remained puzzling not only to patients but also to economists. Not only did great regional variations exist in what physicians charged, but fees varied dramatically even within a locality, and for reasons doctors themselves had difficulty articulating. As Brewer noted, "Hard and fast rules for fee fixing are more often broken than kept." Of two doctors practicing in the same neighborhood, one would charge $5 and the other $25 for the same service. A public health laboratory would charge fifty cents to perform the Wassermann blood test for syphilis, while a private lab charged $5. Even more dramatic differences showed up in the pricing of surgical procedures. For example, the cost of a simple tonsillectomy might be $5 when performed by a hospital resident or $300 when performed by a specialist.[54]

To explain these variations, physicians noted that many doctors adjusted their fees according to the patient's ability to pay, charging wealthy patients more and discounting their services to the poor. According to physician Linsly Williams, "Some of [a doctor's] work is done for nothing, some is done at what might be called bargain rates, and some is done at what might be called the list price." William Allen Pusey argued that doctors were simply following the practices common in other fields: "The banker, the real estate man or the lawyer will charge in proportion to the size of the transaction he undertakes." Since a lawyer might charge a man $25,000 for handling a half-million-dollar matter, why, Pusey asked, "should the doctor not get fully as good a fee for performing an important operation on the same man?" He concluded, "We are entitled to base our charges, to a considerable extent, on what the services are worth to the individual."[55]

But open acknowledgment of the "sliding scale" brought with it a host of problems. First, the business of guessing what patients could afford to pay was fraught with difficulty. As critics noted, doctors were not trained as social workers, so their ability to assess what their patients could afford to pay seemed limited. Commentators frequently related stories about doctors fooled by duplicitous patients. For example, Rinehart repeated the tale of a colleague who gave a deep discount to a shabbily dressed woman, only to discover that she was fabulously wealthy. Conversely, well-groomed, educated, middle-class patients trying to keep up appearances were being charged far more than they could actually afford. Second, the huge disparities between the fees charged different classes of patients undercut the idea that doctors were delivering a standardized service priced solely in terms of the time and skill required. The fact that in New York City, the same doctor might charge patients of "small means" $125 for an appendectomy while billing those of "large means" for $1,135 suggested a "what the market will bear" strategy rather than a rational calculation of the technical skill or overhead costs involved.[56]

Differential fees inevitably raised the question of whether the services were really equivalent. For his higher fee, did the wealthy man get better care than his poor neighbor? Physicians might insist that such was not the case, that the $125 operation was every bit as skillful as its $1,135 counterpart. But for patients familiar with the way other aspects of consumer culture worked, this assertion seemed hard to credit. Moreover, the variation in fees suggested the emergence of class segmentation in medical care that made some observers profoundly uncomfortable.

Physicians tended to dismiss complaints about rising fees as predictable if unwarranted grousing. In their experience, patients had a long tradition of "paying the doctor last." A 1927 cartoon in *Medical Economics* depicted patients' good reasons not to pay for each month, starting in January ("Didn't get that raise") to December ("Getting Christmas Presents"). The doctor's bill was unique, Williams noted, in that it was neither regular nor predictable and offered little opportunity for the "bargaining instinct." Thus, its arrival usually evoked "a certain amount of melancholy, surprise and perhaps even resentment." Now that those bills were starting to come in more frequently and for higher amounts, it was no surprise that "kicking about the high price" of doctoring had become a popular pastime.[57]

Such grumblings came from male as well as female patients. Physicians customarily established medical accounts in the name of the male head of household, so the monthly bill for everyone's care was sent to him. As a consequence, family medical bills often became the focus of joint decision making—and worrying—between husband and wife. This was the case even in affluent households: while living in the White House, First Lady Eleanor Roosevelt forwarded their son's medical bill to her president-husband for payment, along with the warning that he would "have a fit" when he saw the size of it. (He replied, "Pay it. Have had the fit.")[58] While these fits likely occurred in households of all income levels, the sense of grievance seemed especially intense among those in the middle: families who were neither too poor to qualify for free care at teaching hospitals or clinics nor rich enough to pay big doctors' bills without great sacrifice. Middle-class couples whose expectations of medical care were rising faster than their ability to pay for it led the way in complaining about the "high cost of keeping alive."

When responding to patients nearer their own social class, physicians found it harder to fall back on an uncomplicated assertion of paternalistic authority. As a California doctor noted rather wistfully of his farmer patients, they regarded him as their "boss," and "once the confidence of these people is placed in you, it is almost impossible to make them think you can make a mistake." For this class of patients, "your position in their family is next to the priest in affection and trust." But increasingly physicians, especially those practicing in large cities, faced a more consumer-savvy clientele, accustomed to being bombarded by ads filled with medical "information" and courted by drugstores. Grumbling about fees became all the harder for doctors to ignore when it came from their social equals—business and professional men who had enough experience with fees and bills in their own lines of work to feel entitled to "kick" about the doctors' business practices. Presented with very large doctors' bills, they not unreasonably expected a clear accounting for the price and quality of the goods they were paying for, an accounting that doctors found it hard to deliver. Selling such patients on the "doctor knows best" philosophy of medical practice was no easy task.[59]

Luxury or Necessity?

In discussing their concerns about cost, both doctors and laypeople frequently compared doctors' bills to other kinds of consumer spending, such as grocers' bills and department store charges. They did so with a clear understanding that medicine was an unusual commodity in that patient-consumers had to rely on doctors to select it. As Falk and his economist colleagues put it in 1933, "The patient does not know whether he should purchase a particular type of medical service and is frequently unable to determine whether or not the medical service has been satisfactory after its receipt."[60] Thus paying bills often prompted a kind of buyer's remorse in which purchasers wondered if the new treatments were really worth their higher prices, using the language of retail—bargain and value, fad and fashion, luxury and necessity—to express their concerns.

With regard to bargain and value, there was widespread agreement that price alone was not a good guide to picking a doctor. The concept of bargain-basement medical care held very little appeal for potential patients. Working- and middle-class families had negative opinions of the charity care delivered in public hospitals, which they assumed, often with good reason, to be of poor quality. At the same time, they also understood that medical goods could be wildly overpriced. In interwar popular culture, the high-priced but incompetent Mammon, MD was a stock character, familiar from works such as Sinclair Lewis's novel *Arrowsmith* and Sidney Kingsley's play *Men in White* as well as the Hollywood films based on them. Price alone clearly was not a reliable guide to medical quality.

Nor could patient-consumers assume that the newest treatment was necessarily the best treatment. For all its advances in scientific rigor, medicine still seemed far too prone to indulge in what physician and lay commentators decried as medical "fashions." Just as women's hemlines or hat styles changed, doctors' enthusiasm for particular treatments waxed and waned. As they competed with one another, doctors faced the temptation to adopt the latest therapeutic fad as a means to attract affluent patients. Warnings about medical faddism often appeared as part of a larger critique of specialism and its influence on the profession. Given that many doctors questioned theories such as autointoxication or focal infection, it was all the harder for patients to determine if a new treatment was in fact groundbreaking or simply an expensive fad.

Doctors who were "not keeping up" with the latest scientific information and thus offered their patients out-of-date advice posed a different sort of problem. Consumer advocate Arthur Kallet reported having a throat specialist "at high fees" recommend he use Listerine as a gargle, evidently unaware that the *Journal of the American Medical Association* had published several exposés of its ineffectiveness as an oral antiseptic. Likewise, insurance executive Donald Armstrong lamented that people who heeded experts' good advice to get an annual preventive health check often found that their general practitioners had no idea how to conduct such exams.[61]

In theory, the strict oversight of medical professionalism was supposed to correct such problems. But in practice, patient-consumers looking to find clear distinctions between treatments that did and did not work were bound to be disappointed. Reputable doctors offered treatments that seemed perilously similar to the kind of quackery that the AMA vigorously opposed. Thus while the association railed against Henry Gaylord, inventor of the ionizing I-ON-A-CO device; William J. Bailey, maker of Radithor, a water infused with radium; and John R. Brinkley, patron of goat gland treatments to preserve youthfulness, many regular physicians in good standing with the AMA enthusiastically employed similar electrical devices, radium treatments, and glandular products. A reasonable patient might well wonder what made Brinkley's goat gland treatment a "bad" remedy while an AMA member's prescription for an estrogen extract was not.[62]

Warnings about the dangers of medical fashion cropped up frequently in discussions of surgery, which had long been the exemplar of a more activist approach to treatment. As early as 1896, one physician complained that "surgery has run wild and there has been a great deal more of operative work than was needed." Surgery was the inspiration for playwright George Bernard Shaw's 1906 articulation of the "doctor's dilemma"—that is, the temptation to order more treatment to profit from it. As rates of surgery rose in the interwar period, so too did worries that medicine's tilt toward commercialism was evident in the too hasty use of the surgeon's knife. In 1929, popular science writer T. Swann Harding observed that "exploratory abdominal operations are performed with considerable abandon and thoughtlessness." Surgery also revealed the profession's difficulties in enforcing the AMA's code of ethics, which prohibited the practice of fee splitting. While medical leaders insisted that only a few bad apples engaged in the practice, its persistence created doubt about how effectively medical discipline was working to offset the temptations of profit.[63]

The question of what was medical fad and what was medical value inevitably led to an even more vexed discussion of what medical services were "necessities" as opposed to "luxuries" and how the average family might be helped to save for the rising expense of the former. In differentiating between medical necessity and luxury, physician and lay commentators often invoked very different sorts of goods such as automobiles, furs, and jewels. The automobile analogy was a particular favorite, given the growing rates of car ownership among both middle- and working-class families. The car analogy was used to argue for going to the doctor sooner rather than later: paying for a tune-up to forestall a major repair. It also served more crudely to express patients' fear of being overcharged, as in the case of a man who responded to his doctor's advice to get an immediate operation by saying, "I guess he needs a new car. . . . Well, he's not going to buy it at my expense."[64]

Similarly, car comparisons were used to articulate concern about class distinctions in treatment. If "Cadillac" care was the best, how were patients who could only afford a Ford going to purchase it? Albright reported that when she complained to a New York City doctor about the unaffordability of specialist care for the middle classes, he responded, "You do not realize that you are reaching for something beyond your grasp. It is just as if you were riding down Fifth Avenue in a Ford, and suddenly decided that you were entitled to a Rolls-Royce" or becoming "dissatisfied with your string of beads when you saw a woman in a box at the opera wearing pearls. It is the middle-class woman reaching out for what only the rich woman can have." The middle classes, he concluded, needed to invest in prevention and the care of a good general practitioner (both of which might be hard to find). Countered Albright, "My child, no less than the child of the woman with the limousine or the string of pearls, is heir to and flower of the ages," and she demanded "the best for him as passionately as" wealthier women demanded the best for their own. She concluded, "Why should the splendid and thrilling results of specialization in modern medicine be employed for the benefit of two minority groups—those who are rich enough to pay enormous prices, and those who are poor enough to go to the clinic?"[65]

The development of the medical equivalent of the luxury trade clearly made some interwar commentators uncomfortable. To be sure, they realized that class distinctions were nothing new. Physician Joseph Collins recalled that one of his mentors, "an admirable business man" rather than a compassionate one, had two entrances to his office: "When one went to consult him, with five dollars, one rang the stoop door bell; but if one had only a dollar, the basement bell admitted." But the widespread perception that when done well, the new medicine was far superior to the old made these class distinctions far more problematic. The choice of Cadillac, mink coat, and pearls fell into the realm of show; the choice of a lifesaving operation meant something far different.[66]

In his 1927 study, *American Medicine and the People's Health*, Moore suggested that while Americans accepted class stratification in services such as higher education (Ivy League colleges versus public universities) and railroad accommodations (first-class versus second-class fares), it was not clear that they would tolerate the same trends in medicine. The fact that in large cities, physicians catering to wealthy patients now welcomed them into lavishly decorated offices with uniformed doormen while many families went without any treatment at all clearly bothered some observers, among them Moore. Distinguishing between a luxury and a necessity mattered more in the realm of health care than it did in other arenas of consumer economics.[67]

Our Medical Muddle

By the eve of the Great Depression, the shopping problems presented by the new doctor's office had already become the subject of anxious discussion among physicians and patients. Patients were expected to pay for increasingly expensive services whose necessity could not be evaluated by even the most intelligent layperson. Middle-class patients feared being priced out of the new medical marketplace, while troubling questions about waste and efficiency loomed over the whole medical economy. While the word "crisis" had yet to be applied to medicine's problems, there was a growing sense of distress over what one commentator styled "our medical muddle."[68]

Well before the stock market crashed in 1929, an increasingly vocal minority of doctors and social scientists had begun to argue that the problems with the new medicine required serious study and redress. In 1927, proponents of that view convinced eight private philanthropic foundations, including the Carnegie Foundation for the Advancement of Teaching, the Milbank Memorial Fund, the Russell Sage Foundation, and the Twentieth Century Fund, to fund a study of "the economic factors affecting the organization of medicine." Commanding what was at the time a huge budget of more than $1 million, the Committee on the Costs of Medical Care (CCMC) recruited a distinguished advisory board of physicians and laypeople and hired a thirty-person staff to collect and analyze information about medical care and its costs.[69]

In line with the best social science of the time, the CCMC staff started with what today would be termed metanalysis of existing statistics on illness and treatment. Quickly realizing the limits of the available data, its researchers decided to conduct their own survey of a nationwide sample of 9,000 families to see what ailments they developed and what medical services they obtained in the course of a year. In addition, the CCMC conducted more focused studies on medical care in different parts of the country. Over the next five years, its staff compiled all this information into twenty-eight reports and two summary volumes: *Medical Care for the American People* (1932), which briefly stated the group's overall findings and recommendations, and the much heftier *Costs of Medical Care* (1933), which reported its results in great detail.

The CCMC's approach was heavily influenced by the work of economist

Wesley C. Mitchell, who studied the nature of recessions, and sociologist William F. Ogburn, who developed the concept of the "cultural lag" to describe mismatches between societal reality and cultural beliefs. Through applying these concepts, committee staff hoped better to understand the dynamics that made medicine so different from other sectors of the consumer economy, which followed the so-called Fordist model, named in homage to Henry Ford and his Model T. In the Fordist model, a growing population, increased demand for goods, and innovations in technology and labor management led to more and better products at cheaper prices. As Ray Lyman Wilbur, the CCMC's chair, noted in the foreword to the 1933 summary volume, science's impact was having the opposite effect in medicine: as care became more efficacious, it also became more expensive. "We may anticipate that the costs of personal *services* will increase while the costs of machine-made *things* will decline," he wrote, so that "increasingly for many people the choice is to live with disease or to suffer with debts."[70]

In that same volume, authors Falk, Rorem, and Ring stressed the economic peculiarities of medicine: "Medical care is not merely an economic commodity, it is also a personal service involving individual relationships between a medical practitioner and a patient." To ignore that personal element, they warned, "would be as absurd as to overlook the laws of mechanics in the construction of a bridge." The physician "is judge both of the patient's need for the service which he has to offer, as well as of the time and conditions under which it shall be purchased." As Falk and his colleagues concluded, "The conditions surrounding the delivery of medical care are therefore unique and unlike those which characterize ordinary economic phenomena, because there is but one buyer and one seller and because the commodity itself is of priceless value if received."[71]

The CCMC's thousands of pages, statistics, charts, and the like identified many misalignments between patient needs and medical services. Some regions of the United States had too few doctors and hospital beds to meet their burden of illness and disability, while other parts had ample doctors and institutional facilities but families could not afford to use them. Perhaps most damningly, the study showed that the utilization of medical care varied in direct relation to a family's income level rather than the extent of illness; 1 percent of all families consumed 13 percent of the services provided, while 70 percent of families received only 24 percent of the total. Observed Falk, Rorem, and Ring, "Just as some people go hungry though the country produces more food than people can consume; many are inadequately clothed though we manufacture more clothing than we can use; even so millions are sick, hundreds of thousands suffer pain and anguish, and tens of thousands die prematurely for lack of medical care which available personnel and facilities could supply."[72]

While committee members agreed on the seriousness of these problems, they could not reach a consensus about how to solve them. Their final report, *Medical Care for the American People*, included competing sets of recommendations. The majority report, signed by most of the social scientists and a few of the physicians, advocated having more medical care provided by groups of physicians and using group insurance plans to finance the costs of medical care. The majority also called for financing health care in ways that would reward the prevention rather than treatment of disease. One minority report, supported by most of the physician members, disagreed with the group principle, in terms of both medical practice and prepaid insurance plans, and argued that the maldistribution of care could be rectified within the traditional fee-for-service system. Yet another minority report, submitted by two of the academic experts, argued that the majority report did not go far enough and called for more radical change.[73]

Read eight decades later, the CCMC's studies seem remarkably mild in tone. At the time, however, they provoked a violent reaction from the AMA. Under the leadership of editor Morris Fishbein, the organization used the editorial pages of the *Journal of the American Medical Association* and affiliated publications to attack the report as dangerous radicalism. According to Fishbein, the uniquely personal nature of medical service doomed economists' attempts to apply Fordist logic to medicine: "Until we become a nation of robots with interlocking, replaceable, and standardized parts, there will be little need for completely standardized doctors." He denounced any program of medical insurance as representing "state medicine" or "socialized medicine"—"encroachment of the State on private medical practice."[74]

In retrospect, Fishbein's ability to portray the CCMC's work as medical radicalism is hard to fathom. In its emphasis on eliminating waste and rationalizing production, the summary report seems far more heavily indebted to corporate managerial methods than to the Communist Manifesto. But in 1932, invoking the "bugbear" of socialism, as economist Isaac M. Rubinow termed it, turned out to be a highly effective way to undercut the authority of social scientists and other nonphysicians to question how physicians ran their own affairs. In essence, Fishbein implied, the CCMC's approach was Bolshevik at heart, as would be any deviation from completely private practice.[75]

But the CCMC's work would not be so easy to dismiss, for it captured a clear sense of interwar patients' paradox. While careful never to attribute base motives to the medical profession, the summary volumes suggested in no uncertain terms that the new medical order was failing to meet the needs of the average American patient. By refusing to abandon an outmoded faith in fee-for-service medicine, physicians were failing in their professional obligation to act in patients' best economic interests. Patients were being simultaneously asked to spend more on medical services and told that they could not possibly appreciate their real value. While many households were struggling to pay their bills, the new medical economy had particularly dire implications for the poorer families. As Michael Marks Davis concluded in 1931, between 25 and 30 percent of people with "relatively serious" illnesses did not receive any medical care at all.[76]

Two very different explanations emerged to account for why the new medical economy was not working as anticipated. One line of argument, preferred by many physicians, laid the blame squarely on patients. They could easily afford good medical care if they stopped patronizing quacks, found good doctors, and obeyed their instructions. If the public gave up wasteful spending on useless drugstore items and unhealthy items such as cigarettes and candy, they would have no problem paying their bills on time. The other line of argument suggested that the medical profession bore a significant amount of responsibility for the "medical muddle." The profession's economic organization was not keeping pace with its scientific prowess. While not excusing patients from the need to behave more prudently, this line of argument held doctors even more accountable precisely because they were the more scientific party. With some important modifications, those two lines of argument would persist for decades. For all their disagreements, they fostered similar emphases on educating patients to make better choices. Thus, the growing sense of being in a "medical muddle" became a prime impetus for the pursuit of medical consumerism.

Starting in the mid-1920s, in realms as diverse as popular magazines and academic journals, critical voices began to articulate the problems that Americans faced at the doctor's office. As the next chapter shows, these concerns often intersected with worries about the appearance of a new kind of drugstore. The same currents of change remaking the doctor's office were simultaneously transforming the old-fashioned pharmacy into the "new corner store." For critics of the new medical order, the deficits of good doctoring were exacerbated by the often-dubious wares available in these establishment, which proved even more fertile ground for medical consumerism than doctors' offices.

{THREE}

The New Corner Store

In 1925, writing in the *American Mercury*, essayist Thomas LeBlanc reflected on the demise of the traveling medicine show. As a boy in rural Michigan, he had looked forward to the annual visit of the Professor and his sidekick, Sambo, to promote Tono Tonic, their "secret compound of roots, herbs, barks, leaves, berries, buds and balsams." The local physician joined in the fun, LeBlanc recalled, because he knew that the Professor's song and dance routines posed no real competition. But now, LeBlanc noted sadly, a new kind of drugstore was driving the old medicine shows out of business. "Instead of the gasoline torches, the reassuring Professor and the tinkle of a banjo," he wrote, "there are nitrogen bulbs, a busy but efficient salesman, a clanging cash register and profit sharing coupons," all designed to sell an "avalanche of tonics, oils, pills, pastes, creams, ointments and muds." Whereas the old-time doctor had little to fear from the charms of the snake-oil salesman, LeBlanc concluded, today's physician had good reason to beware the slickly advertised "flood of nostrums" now on offer in the modern drugstore.[1]

LeBlanc's sentiment that "the medicine show is dead, long live the medicine show" was frequently voiced in the 1920s. During the same decades that physicians were struggling to justify the "high cost of keeping alive," they faced increased pressure to compete with the new "toothpaste temples" appearing on American urban street corners.[2] Entrepreneurs such as Charles Walgreen and Louis Liggett blended modern science and salesmanship into a commercial health culture that offered a cheaper, friendlier alternative to the doctor's office. Yet neither physicians nor even professional pharmacists considered the new-style drugstore a force for medical progress. In their view, this new retail innovation brought nothing but trouble.

That hostility reflected the role of these stores, the modern ancestors of today's Walgreens and CVS chains, in preserving and extending the great American tradition of self-medication. While continuing prominently to feature their prescription departments, promotional drugstores also marked out an easier path to care. In the place of a long wait in the doctor's office followed by a big bill, they held out an appealing alternative: relatively inexpensive medical goods able to promote good health and relieve minor illnesses. In an era when roughly two-thirds of the medicines purchased were over-the-counter rather than prescription items, drugstores offered a tempting prospect, particularly because those medical goods nestled side by side with a host of other appealing commodities not available in the doctor's office—cosmetics, tobacco, and ice cream sundaes from the lunch counters.[3]

Behind the drugstore's rise lay another development with profound implications for both physicians and patients—the growing reach and sophistication of product advertising. While professional ethics limited how physicians could promote themselves, the makers and sellers of over-the-counter medicines faced few such constraints. With their profit margins heavily dependent on selling more products to more people, drugmakers and drugstore owners invested heavily in the latest advertising and marketing techniques. First in print and later in radio as well, advertising campaigns enthusiastically invoked the wonders of modern medicine to sell goods. By 1930, the drug industry was spending approximately $70 million annually on advertising. As a result of those herculean efforts, patients often arrived in physicians' offices with expectations that their doctor could not necessarily meet.[4]

Those who profited from the drugstore's success—proprietary drugmakers, store owners, and their advertising agents—saw its innovations in a far more favorable light than did doctors. Where physicians perceived dishonesty and hype, the drugstore's advocates beheld a wonderful innovation: a "new corner store" catering to the comfort and convenience of busy, hardworking Americans. Far more flamboyantly than the doctor's office, the new corner store celebrated the medical credo of "new and improved": the belief that new products were always better than old ones and that buying more was always better than making do with less. In addition, the goods for sale in the drugstore were labeled and packaged more like other familiar commodities, making them seem easier to select and evaluate than the more mysterious services encountered in the doctor's office.

But for its growing legion of critics, the exuberant advertising and selective truths associated with the new-style drugstore seemed little to celebrate. Interwar medical consumerism cut its critical teeth on denunciations of the updated "medicine show" taking place in its aisles. Many modern skills now deemed essential to being a more "educated" patient, from careful reading of product labels to decoding of drug advertisements, first emerged in response to the drugstore's alleged excesses. Becoming an "educated" medical consumer involved learning not only how to find a good doctor but also how to resist the commercial appeals associated with the modern drugstore.

What consumerists perceived as the medical profession's failure adequately to police the drug industry's influence on its members contributed to their unwillingness to place blind trust in medical authority.

From Pharmacy to Drugstore

The new-style drugstore of the 1920s was the end product of changes that began in the late nineteenth century, when a handful of entrepreneurial pharmacists began to imitate what they saw happening in other retail sectors. In this regard, they were heavily influenced by chain groceries such as the Great Atlantic and Pacific Tea Company (A&P), which used bulk buying and efficient distribution systems to cut prices, and department stores such as Macy's and Filene's, which enticed shoppers with glass-topped counters, elaborate window displays, elevators, and escalators. In comparison, turn-of-the-century pharmacies had a reputation for being "small and musty" establishments focused primarily on the compounding of drugs, with a small side trade in packaged remedies and penny candies.[5]

Although the retail revolution came relatively late to pharmacies, once it arrived it moved very fast, as Charles Walgreen's career demonstrates. The Chicago store where the young pharmacist first went to work in the late 1890s was only twenty by fifty feet in size. Dimly lit by gaslight, it had narrow aisles, a cracked dirty floor, and shelves laden with products that had been there for years. By the 1910s, Walgreen had transformed the old-style pharmacy into a new kind of medical department store. His "promotional" drugstores, as they were referred to in trade publications, boosted profits by increasing sales volume through a combination of strategies: acquiring multiple stores in heavily trafficked locations, carrying a wide variety of goods, and most important, investing lavishly in aggressive advertising.[6]

While Walgreen became famous for his retail methods, his success also reflected advances in the science and practice of pharmacy in the late 1800s. The pharmacy profession, like medicine, upgraded its training, transitioning from an apprenticeship system to a program initially requiring two years and later four to get a license to practice. The upgraded pharmacy degree emphasized the hospital and the laboratory as the lodestones of scientific progress. As a licensed pharmacist in good standing, albeit one of the last generation trained solely through apprenticeship, Walgreen thought of himself as helping to distribute the goods associated with this more scientific pharmacy.[7]

His fellow pharmacists did not necessarily share this opinion. The retail side occupied a very low place in pharmacy's professional hierarchy, in part due to its association with the proprietary medicine companies, which many pharmacists disliked almost as much as physicians did. Charles Walgreen won the hand of his wife, Myrtle, only after her pharmacist brother had dismissed a previous suitor whose father sold patent medicine from the back of a wagon. Ultimately, however, some professional pharmacists would come to regard Myrtle's husband an even worse sort of turncoat because of the promotional techniques he introduced to the field.[8]

Walgreens stores attracted customers using bold signage promising "Drugs and Surgical Dressings." Company policy required that every customer be greeted as he or she walked through the door. Although still tiny by modern standards—the first Walgreens store, on Cottage Avenue in Chicago, would have fit comfortably in the space later devoted just to the cosmetics department—its look was dramatically different, with glass countertops to showcase their wares, displays rotated frequently so goods always appeared fresh, bright electric fixtures to illuminate the whole interior, and a durable, easily cleaned floor to project an air of neatness. The prescription department was strategically placed at the store's back, requiring customers to walk past all the attractively displayed goods on the way to pick up their orders.[9]

Using this formula, Walgreen enjoyed extraordinary success. By 1934, when Walgreens stock was first publicly traded on the New York Stock Exchange, the company owned 483 stores and had around 12,000 employees. The company's success naturally inspired other drugstore owners to copy its methods. Promotional stores, as Herman C. Nolen and Harold H. Maynard described them in their 1941 textbook on drugstore management, made "an aggressive and competitive type of selling as the cornerstone of . . . operations" and surrounded the customer "with a carnival atmosphere of pennants, posters, and compelling displays of merchandise."[10]

This promotional style was closely associated with the chain store—that is, a single business that operated multiple stores using the same distribution system, management structure, and advertising budget. The years from 1900 to 1930 marked the golden age of chain stores, which expanded beyond groceries and department stores to include shoe stores and variety stores, also known as five-and-dimes. Largely a big-city innovation, twenty-four drug chains operated in the United States by 1932, with Walgreens the largest. By the early 1940s, chain stores accounted for about 7 percent of all drugstores but 25 percent of all drugstore sales. Disadvantaged by the chains' aggressive cost-cutting and advertising practices, independent store owners sought legislative protection: during the 1930s, almost thirty states passed chain store taxes in an attempt to slow their spread. But these efforts eventually lost momentum because consumers liked what they were getting—more goods at lower prices.[11]

To survive, many independent store owners adopted elements of the chain store's approach. For example, Louis Liggett's Rexall Company became highly successful by providing independent franchisees the advantages of bulk buying, store brands, and national advertising that chain stores enjoyed. Other pharmacies succeeded by doing the opposite, catering primarily to physicians and doing a high volume of prescription business; such establishments were referred to as "professional" or "ethical" stores to distinguish them from their promotional counterparts. Still others sought to cultivate loyal client bases by offering good soda fountain service or stocking the remedies preferred by various local ethnic groups. In an era of rampant segregation, black-owned drugstores became a retail anchor in many black neighborhoods.[12]

Americans flocked to drugstores in all their varied guises; by the 1930s, they ranked second only to grocery stores in the number of shoppers they attracted. According to a 1941 estimate, 21 million people, or one in seven Americans, visited a drugstore each day. Drugstores also earned a reputation as immune to the boom-and-bust cycles that plagued other retailers; even during the Great Depression, in which at least a quarter of all Americans lost their jobs, the number of drugstores remained relatively steady at around 58,000—roughly one store for every 2,200 people. While considerably less than food or clothing, the amount spent on medicinal drugs still constituted a significant part of the average family's budget. In the late 1920s, the CCMC estimated that between 15 and 20 percent of the annual spending on medical care went for drugs—a total of $715,000 per year. By 1939, the total sales volume for drugstores had risen to about $1.5 billion.[13]

In achieving their retail dominance, interwar drugstores benefited from their relationship to state boards of pharmacy. Modeled on their medical counterparts, these boards had been founded in the late 1800s both to grant pharmacists license to practice and to protect the public against unsafe drugs. Most states required that prescriptions requiring compounding of any sort could only be dispensed by a pharmacist or a doctor; thus for a drugstore to sell drugs, it had to have a licensed pharmacist in charge. States also recognized some form of what was known as the "proprietary exemption," which allowed general merchants to sell packaged remedies, a necessity for people who lived far from a drugstore. But by and large, interwar drugstores retained dominance in sales of not only prescription drugs but also over-the-counter remedies.[14]

In part, this dominance stemmed from the growing web of state and federal laws covering pharmacy practice. Interwar pharmacy textbooks devoted hefty chapters to the laws governing drugstores' operation, including not only the rules of commerce that applied to all stores but also the highly specialized laws that applied only to them. State pharmacy laws varied enormously in their scope, so staff had to be well versed in what applied to their locale. Federal law added yet more complexity. The 1914 Harrison Act required that pharmacists keep detailed records of all the narcotic prescriptions they filled, while national Prohibition, in effect from 1920 to 1933, forced pharmacists to contend with its confusing and frequently changing requirements concerning the prescription sale of alcohol. Unlike proprietors of five-and-dimes, drugstore owners faced huge fines and jail terms for violating the laws surrounding the sale of narcotics, alcohol, and poisons. Moreover, pharmacists had to contend with the popular image of drugstores as hotbeds of illegal activity. In F. Scott Fitzgerald's 1925 novel, *The Great Gatsby*, the central character, Jay Gatsby, owed his great wealth to illegal drugstore sales of alcohol, while the plot of A. L. Furman and Harold Hadley's 1935 novel, *Drugstore*, revolved around a small-town store that became the hub of a national illegal drug network.[15]

While imposing special burdens, these regulatory concerns had advantages as well in that they helped cement the drugstore's control over the prescription counter. With the exception of large department stores, which hired pharmacists to offer prescription services to shoppers, drugstores maintained a virtual monopoly on this part of the drug marketplace, which gave them an immense advantage over their retail competitors. Consumers might buy cosmetics or ice cream sodas elsewhere, but if they wanted a prescription filled or a good selection of proprietary products, to the drugstore they went.[16] Paradoxically, this advantage was not necessarily reflected in the store's bottom line. Prescription drugs accounted for only 27 percent of the medicines sold. While professional pharmacies might fill as many as 100 prescriptions per day, most drugstores averaged only 8 to 10, approximately 10 to 12 percent of the total volume of sales. Yet drugstore owners still considered prescription services essential to success because they brought customers into the store. Prescription sales constituted the "heart" of the drugstore, as Nolen and Maynard put it, and thus had "to be shown considerably more attention than the volume of prescription business might appear to warrant."[17]

In essence, the prescription department functioned as a lure that promoted more profitable lines of packaged medical goods. In addition to their location at the back of the store, pharmacies were positioned adjacent to large selections of over-the-counter products. By the 1930s, the standard merchandise categories included cough and cold relief, laxatives and other "elimination aids," antacids, internal analgesics, external analgesics, external antiseptics, tonics and "alteratives," oral hygiene products (toothpastes, toothbrushes, and mouthwashes), and miscellaneous remedies for hemorrhoids, burns, poison ivy, acne, and athlete's foot. In addition, drugstores carried extensive lines of first aid and sickroom supplies such as packaged bandages, adhesive tape, and fever thermometers; surgical elastic goods such as stockings and trusses; home rubber goods such as hot water bottles and syringes; feminine hygiene products; and baby supplies. Also nearby was the widening variety of goods associated with personal cleanliness, such as bath soap, which thanks to several generations of hygiene education had acquired a strong association with healthiness. As Nolen and Maynard wrote, "Modern hygiene as publicized over the radio, in magazines, and in newspapers has made the American public more health conscious than ever before, and as a result the per capita sales possibilities on this type of merchandise are far greater than ever before." Keeping the teeth and mouth clean was touted as a crucial safeguard against both infectious disease and social rejection. Sales of toothpaste, mouthwash, and toothbrushes—cheap to make and comparatively easy to sell—consequently boomed.[18]

Not only did drugstores offer a widening array of medicines and health-related goods, but they also offered a choice of many different brands within each category. A customer coming in search of a particular remedy would find it available from multiple companies. By 1935, for example, Walgreens stores carried five different brands of aspirin, "all of the same standard strength and purity," twenty-two kinds of toothpaste, four varieties of liver pills, and eighteen antiseptic mouthwashes. Extensive advertising campaigns meant that consumers tended to ask for medicinal items and toiletries by brand name, giving stores incentives both to stock the most heavily advertised brands and to offer cheaper house brands that were presented as just as good as the national ones. Thus while selling a tin of 12 name-brand aspirin for a dime, Walgreens offered its own bottle of 100 aspirin for thirty-nine cents.[19]

Besides stocking products useful in avoiding an expensive visit to the physician, new-style drugstores exemplified the virtues of convenience by offering goods and services that had little to do with health. As the trade journal *Printers' Ink* noted in 1920, "The modern drugstore will sell you a soda or an umbrella as conscientiously as it will a dose of medicine." Along with their medical departments, promotional drugstores offered a huge array of other goods, including cosmetics, candies, tobacco products, camera supplies, stationery, and what were termed sundries—board games, playing cards, and picture frames. Some stores even stocked small appliances, such as toasters, radios, and clocks—anything that was small and easy to sell.[20]

In other ways, drugstores recognized that busy Americans wanted convenience and worked hard to oblige them. Roughly 70 percent of them offered fountain service, so a shopping trip could be combined with the 1920s version of fast food: sandwiches, griddle dishes, ice cream, pastries, and coffee. To capture sales, drugstores also developed the policy of opening earlier and closing later than other stores. A 1927 article in the trade periodical *Advertising and Selling* praised this policy as a sign of American progress: "If you want the contrast, try to buy a tube of toothpaste late in the evening in London or Paris." Success would be elusive in those major cities, "but in any fair-sized town in America you may alight from a train, note that you are minus a hairbrush or a toothbrush and stop at almost any corner and be served promptly."[21]

The new corner store flourished by offering one-stop shopping for the care and maintenance of the looking-glass self. "Your druggist takes the light cream from the trade of every merchant," explained a 1935 *Fortune* article, leaving competitors with "the cumbrous, slow-moving residue." Drugstores concentrated on products that came neatly packaged, were easy to display, sold quickly, and posted nice profit margins. Even with its many sidelines, Walgreens estimated in 1935 that medicinal products accounted for more than 55 percent of its total sales. Thus even as other retailers tried to chip away at their retail advantage, drugstore owners fought fiercely and successfully to hold onto the edge derived from the sale of medicines.[22]

The Business of Medicine Making

For all the toasters and umbrellas to be found there, drugstores derived their selling advantage from the sale of medicines. Their success, therefore, was intimately linked to the companies that made those remedies. Like other sectors of the American economy, pharmaceutical firms experienced dramatic changes in the early twentieth century. As LeBlanc noted in 1925, the drug "business has been turned into an industry with all the trappings of capital, quantity production, distribution, service and advertising." But just as the more businesslike doctor's office did not always please, so too this more businesslike approach to drug development and marketing presented a host of complications.[23]

Like the doctor's office, the interwar drugstore's aura benefited from the perception that after decades of false starts, modern laboratory science had finally begun to discover "magic bullets"—that is, powerful remedies effective against specific disorders. In the late 1800s, new laboratory methods produced the rabies vaccine and the diphtheria antitoxin. In 1897, German chemist Felix Hoffman, who was working for the Bayer Company, developed aspirin, a drug with remarkable properties to control fever and pain. A few years later, his countryman Paul Ehrlich developed an arsenical compound effective against the microorganism responsible for syphilis. In the 1920s, Canadian researchers Frederick Banting and Charles Best achieved a dramatic success in isolating the hormone insulin, which resulted in a lifesaving treatment for juvenile (type 1) diabetes. Other hormones such as thyroxin and progesterone soon followed, adding other powerful drugs to physicians' therapeutic repertoire.[24]

These successes inspired scientists around the world. In the United States, the Rockefeller Institute for Medical Research oversaw an extensive research program designed to develop new serums and vaccines. Following the lead of American expatriate Henry Wellcome, founder of the British Burroughs Wellcome Company, American firms such as Parke, Davis began to invest in research facilities, hoping to find new drugs that would not only save lives but also be profitable. When World War I halted the flow of German pharmaceutical goods, American companies quickly stepped in to pick up the slack.[25]

While these developments gave physicians some very powerful new remedies, the vast majority of medicines sold in the interwar drugstore were far from wonder drugs. Outside of a few notable exceptions, many of the drugs being combined, packaged, and promoted for sale, both by prescription and over the counter, did not represent dramatic improvements over their 1900 counterparts. Much interwar drug "development" consisted of making drugs more palatable by altering their taste or increasing their ease of use. Firms such as United Drugs made a show of setting up drug laboratories in homage to the Rockefeller Institute, but what they produced were actually new combinations of old drugs. Especially sought after were "ethical specialties"—packaged drugs sold by prescription. As C. Rufus Rorem and Robert F. Fischelis noted in their 1932 overview of the drug industry, a growing number of prescriptions were being written for "the manufacturer's brand of some well-known combination of drugs" that would have cost less if compounded by the pharmacist.[26]

While the drug trade had long been competitive, the 1920s marked a period of particular uncertainty and change. The industry was increasingly dominated by a group of big firms that competed fiercely with each other to sell similar product lines; their profit margins depended heavily on their ability to use sophisticated marketing and advertising campaigns to induce both doctors and patients to ask for goods by brand name. Drug companies also benefited from the public perception that drugs were safer and more reliable than they had been before passage of the 1906 federal drug legislation. Most drug companies had little difficulty in meeting state and federal standards for drug safety and advertising, while the new laws helped suppress the most extreme forms of quackery that had made the whole industry look bad. Convinced that the marketplace was now safe, Americans eagerly bought more medicine than ever before. But the reality was considerably more complex, as consumerists would soon begin to warn American shoppers.[27]

In the competitive 1920s, the dividing line between proprietary and ethical firms began to blur as doctors began to prescribe the former's goods and the latter advertised product lines directly to patients. Large proprietary companies such as Sterling Products, Bristol-Myers, and United Drugs became increasingly dominant actors, battling for national (and sometimes international) sales of packaged medicines and health-related goods. At the same time, the ethical firms, which had traditionally kept their distance from the proprietary trade, began to adopt some of the latter's tactics. As Arthur Cramp, director of the Bureau of Investigation of the AMA, noted, Parke, Davis's 1887 catalog had boasted, "We rely for the reputation of our products on their superior excellence. We protect none of them by patent, copyright or trade-mark," but by the mid-1920s, the company sold "dozens of preparations that are protected by trade-mark," advertising them directly to consumers. Perhaps to mitigate any resentment spurred by its move into the over-the-counter trade, Parke, Davis became a leader in goodwill advertising extolling the virtues of the medical profession.[28]

This blurring of categories reflected the fact that drug companies boosted their bottom lines not via new treatments but via innovations in marketing and advertising directed not only at consumers but also at the trusted intermediaries—pharmacists and doctors—who helped them choose their medicines. More than any other feature of the interwar drugstore, this growing dependence on new forms of advertising sparked criticism from both physicians and patients. While persuasions directed at the public initially attracted the most attention, the increasing sway of drug companies over physicians also came under criticism.

Whoever Shouts the Loudest Sells the Most

A deepening investment in advertising and marketing meant that long before patient-consumers set foot in a drugstore—or the doctor's office—they had been exposed to an avalanche of commercial messages about what goods were necessary to "take care of yourself," to use Jerome Ephraim's phrase. Of course, lavish advertising centered on medicine and health was by no means new; the late-nineteenth-century expansion of the proprietary medicine industry had helped create the field of modern advertising. But like the products it promoted, post–World War I advertising claimed to be "new and improved": more informational and psychologically sophisticated than its predecessors.

Health-related advertising expanded as part of national corporations' effort to take advantage of post–World War I prosperity. Improved printing technologies, the advent of radio, and the development of popular psychology produced an extraordinarily creative period in American advertising. By 1932, the United States had approximately 2,000 national and local advertising agencies, and companies were spending almost $2 billion on advertising messages. Promotions for over-the-counter medicines and health and beauty aids figured prominently in the interwar advertising boom. Through print and electronic sales pitches, companies paid for agencies to develop the "come hither" blandishments that brought customers to the drugstore. As one pharmacist explained the spirit of the day, "Whoever shouts the loudest . . . sells the most."[29]

Although print advertising remained extensive, the new medium of radio attracted the most attention. In contrast to other countries, where the airwaves were kept under tight government control, the United States allowed the rapid and unregulated expansion of commercial radio in the late 1920s, creating fierce competition for corporate sponsorship of popular shows. By 1935, companies were spending $87 million on radio advertising, of which roughly 12 percent was dedicated to medicinal drugs and another 13 percent to personal hygiene products; the only larger expenditure was on food products, which constituted 19 percent of the total spending.[30]

Radio's ability to project drug advertising into millions of American homes made it a powerful tool for familiarizing patient-consumers with new products. That reach extended even into the farthest, most remote reaches of the country: as a Longtown, North Carolina, woman proudly told an interviewer in 1938, her family owned a battery-powered set and sometimes bought the medicines advertised "like you hear on the radio." Radio ads were all the more powerful because of their novelty. As Cramp testified before the Federal Communications Commission in 1935, years of print advertising had left the American consumer with "a defense mechanism against the printed word, and . . . much less likely to be carried away by false or fraudulent claims made in cold type" than "when similar claims are made verbally by a plausible announcer." Able to ignore drug ads when reading newspapers or magazines, people could hardly "avoid listening to the patent-medicine ballyhoo that comes in to their homes over the radio."[31]

Commercial radio essentially etherized the ballyhoo traditions of both the medicine show and vaudeville, its more sophisticated urban counterpart. Many early radio stars, among them George Burns, Gracie Allen, and Red Skelton, were veterans of the medicine-show circuit and knew its style well. In the radio version of the medicine show, the announcer assumed the role of the barker, delivering the sales pitch between the songs, jokes, and skits. Radio listeners grew accustomed to the now familiar alternation of entertainment and advertising. As the comedian Skelton once quipped, "and now a word from our sponsors" was "the single longest word in the English language." Radio shows also practiced what today is known as "product placement" by working the sponsors' products into plots. For example, in the show *Real Folks*, sponsored by the makers of Vaseline, the script called for someone to cut his finger, call for Vaseline, and have someone "rush up and put it on," as the ad executive in charge proudly reported.[32]

These tactics were so heavy-handed that radio celebrities routinely mocked them, inviting listeners to do the same. Advertising professionals had a low opinion of radio as well. Noted one ad executive of a Chicago radio personality sponsored by Dr. Strasska's toothpaste, "His program is just terrible, awful. None of us would like to listen to it, but the people who buy toothpaste like it." Meanwhile, ethical drug companies' attempts to do more refined advertising, such as sponsoring informative talks by doctors, did nothing for sales. Radio advertising, however bad, was effective, meaning that enjoying free entertainment over the airwaves required putting up with "ballyhoo for medicines of one kind or another," as a commentator wrote in 1935. To "have the privilege of listening," he lamented, "we must swallow the insult to our intelligence together with some of the medicine."[33]

Whether on the radio or in print, advertising for medicines and health goods remained only lightly regulated in the 1920s and 1930s. Its regulation fell to the FTC as part of its responsibility to deter unfair business practices: making false claims in an advertisement allowed a company to lure customers away from its more honest competitors. Investigating complaints about advertising made by one company against another became such a big part of the agency's work that in 1929 it set up the Special Board of Investigation just to deal with such matters. In deciding what medical and health claims to go after, the FTC consulted closely with the FDA and the AMA's fraud division. Those companies deemed to be violating fair trade standards were issued cease-and-desist orders specifying which claims needed to be removed from their advertisements.[34]

By 1930, policing proprietary medicine claims had become a substantial part of the Special Board's workload. In 1930–31, the FTC acted on 119 false advertising claims, the vast majority of which concerned health-related products. It put a stop to companies that used the word "laboratories" in their name or advertising copy "when neither owning nor operating laboratories" and that claimed a product cured asthma "when in fact it only alleviates the inconveniences occasioned by the disease." But the FTC's advertising work suffered a major setback in 1931 when the U.S. Supreme Court ruled in the *Raladam* case that its enabling legislation gave the agency authority only to act against claims that limited business competition, not those that purposefully misled consumers. Dismay over this ruling eventually led to the 1938 Wheeler-Lea Act, which explicitly gave the FTC powers to prosecute misleading advertising on consumers' behalf.[35]

Many national corporations voluntarily moderated their product claims to avoid negative attention from either the FTC or the AMA's fraud division. In part, this softening reflected the advertising profession's desire to distance itself from its proprietary medicine past. As William Legler of the J. Walter Thompson agency, one of the era's leading advertising firms, noted in a 1923 talk to his fellow executives, the company had made its name as "the greatest patent medicine advertising agency in the country," a fact that some viewed as "a skeleton in the closet." But, he insisted, professionally done, modern health advertising had become a very different force in American life: "Ours are excellent products of the highest quality . . . while the majority of the old patent medicines were practically worthless."[36]

The change in strategy also reflected advertisers' recognition that consumers were becoming too sophisticated to be taken in by the kind of extravagant promises that had worked in the past. As J. Walter Thompson's *News Bulletin* noted in 1923, "Competition has become too keen, housewives have become too critical and too well-informed, to make it possible for dishonest advertising to pay." The new advertising sought to win over the educated consumer with a more informative kind of ad. Whereas the old snake-oil sales message had been entirely spurious, product claims now were "based on actual facts which are subject to the censorship and the constant scrutiny of competent people," Legler asserted.[37]

A new reverence for modern science was essential to this more informative kind of advertising. As Thompson's president, Stanley Resor, wrote in a 1927 essay on "Advertising as a Career," "Advertising is helping to turn the light of science on the path not only of the housewife but of the average consumer." In addition to alerting people to "new devices for their comfort," advertising helped to popularize the latest scientific discoveries concerning health. Advertising agencies now subscribed to scientific journals so that they could "constantly consult medical, chemical, and physical authorities in the preparation of their copy" and make only such "inferences . . . as are warranted by available clinical and laboratory experience."[38]

While presenting ads as a useful addition to the consumers' "mental lunch counter," advertising professionals acknowledged that their claims often involved the "puffing" or exaggeration of scientific truths. However, they believed that puffing caused no harm because unlike the quack's product, the national brands they promoted were perfectly safe. Magnifying their effectiveness might even contribute to the desired relief by inducing what a later generation of psychologists would christen the placebo effect: the ads helped the patient believe the medicine would work and thus increased the likelihood that they would find relief. And thanks to the virtues of the free enterprise system, if the drugs proved unsatisfactory, consumers could simply stop buying them.[39]

A 1931 article in *Hygeia*, the AMA's magazine for the public, declared that advertising had become "a much more subtle affair than it was twenty years ago." Respectable companies now knew better than to promise to cure specific, life-threatening diseases but instead focused on "ill-defined conditions" and an "evasive appeal to the health desires of the public."[40] But while claiming to adopt a more truthful tone, interwar advertising's medical messages often relied on heavy-handed approaches that in retrospect seem anything but subtle.

A case in point was the 1930s vogue for so-called scare copy or fear copy to promote sales. Legler explained the logic behind the fear sell: while "nobody likes to be reminded of unpleasant possibilities," it remained the case that "fear is a vital human characteristic—one that we simply cannot ignore in this business." He pointed out that people commonly ignored the advice that exercise was good for them until "a doctor tells us that our blood pressure is dangerously high, that we need some form of exercise"; then "we hasten to the handball court or the golf links." He concluded, "If the strongest way to sell a product (legitimately, of course) is with scare headlines and scare illustrations—then that's the way it should be done, even if we do it with our tongue in our cheek."[41]

Following this strategy, advertisers evoked fears of serious illness to promote a wide variety of goods. A seemingly minor ailment left untreated could be the first step on a fatal slide toward some terrible end. Concerns about infection and contagion topped the list of fear copy appeals. Dating back to the 1870s, American advertisers had found that making consumers more germ conscious was the royal route to selling a whole multitude of products. Even as death rates from infectious diseases declined, the persistence of life-threatening diseases such as tuberculosis and influenza kept this type of promotion alive. At the same time, health educators' efforts to make Americans more "heart conscious" and "cancer aware" opened up additional avenues for scare copy. As long as advertisers were careful to avoid claims that a product could cure a specific disease, advertisers could and did make good use of the sense that "we die differently now."[42]

Ads thus cleverly mirrored the lists of warning signals so common to educators' discussions of cancer and heart disease. A 1928 Sal Hepatica advertisement provided a checklist of the "7 common ailments" of modern living that its use could alleviate, including constipation, headaches, auto-intoxication, bad complexion, rheumatism, indigestion, and colds. Ad copy frequently emphasized how modern society encouraged overeating, smoking, nervous anxiety, and lack of exercise, leading to ill health. As another Sal Hepatica advertisement noted, "Radio and motors, restaurants and clubs have changed the complexion of life," bringing with them "too much food— too little sleep—too much nervous excitement," and *"nature doesn't like it a bit."* So when the first symptoms appeared, the ad urged, the modern health consumer should *"do something about it."* In this fashion, ads encouraged consumers to use drugstore purchases as "bodyguards," in the words of a 1933 Phillips' Milk of Magnesia ad.[43]

Counter Prescribing

At a time when competition among doctors was fierce and patients were "kicking" over the size of their bills, the medical profession regarded the new-style drugstore and its advertising methods with enormous suspicion. While drug manufacturers and store owners went out of their way to appear respectful to physicians, the new medicine show occurring in the drugstore nonetheless appeared threatening; a trip to the corner store could all too easily be substituted for a more expensive visit to the doctor's office. Physicians became increasingly worried over the prospect of "counter prescribing"—that is, pharmacists practicing medicine at the doctor's expense.

From the medical profession's standpoint, the transformation from the old-time pharmacy to the new-style drugstore represented not progress but regress. Like LeBlanc, they saw a strong resemblance between medicine-show ballyhoo and the new corner store's commercialism. As Walter Alvarez, an internist and medical writer, noted scornfully in 1928, "Nowadays drugstores sell writing paper, cameras, [and] cosmetics and have practically nothing to do with physicians or legitimate medicine." In the doctors' eyes, only the ethical pharmacy retained the ideals of professionalism. In its 1935 article on Walgreens, *Fortune* reported that "most doctors take care to send you to those few 'ethical' drugstores that specialize in prescriptions [and] soft-pedal the patent-medicine trade."[44]

While they disliked the promotional side of the drugstore business, physicians were becoming increasingly dependent on its prescription-filling services. As part of the era's changing medical culture, town-based doctors stopped compounding their own medicines (though rural physicians continued to so). Instead, pharmacists in towns and cities took on that task along with responsibility for making sure that patients understood how to take their medications.[45] For all that doctors tried to steer patients to pharmacies that rejected the promotional stores' ballyhoo, their enthusiastic embrace of medical "liberty" meant that they could not hope to control where patients took their trade.

In the context of patient complaints about the "high cost of keeping alive," physicians frequently pointed out that money "wasted" on useless drugstore remedies would have been far more wisely spent on doctors' fees. Studies of household budgets confirmed that families spent substantial amounts on drugstore products. Rorem and Fischelis estimated that Americans spent around $665 million on medicines and home remedies in 1929. Many patients regarded modest expenditures on products available at the drugstore as the first line of defense when indigestion or headache struck. Although some people still swore by homemade preparations, many now preferred the convenience of packaged medicines. The poorer the family, Rorem and Fischelis noted, the higher the percentage of their medical dollar spent on drugstore goods. As journalist James Rorty summarized in 1939, "The patent medicine maker is the 'poor man's doctor.'"[46]

The interwar drugstore's convenience reflected the continued strength of the self-help tradition. As K. E. Miller, medical director of the U.S. Public Health Service and medical adviser to the FTC, conceded in 1940, self-medication had a secure place in "our social order" by virtue of the fact "that many of the simpler ailments are too trivial to justify a requisition upon the time of a skilled physician who has more serious duties to occupy his attention." In a medical economy where patients paid directly for care, the high cost of medical care compared to a home remedy "may decide the issue as to whether the patient is to receive some degree of relief from his ills or none at all." In sum, he concluded, "regardless of its limitations, self-medication is the inalienable right of Americans."[47]

At best, the medical profession could try to educate the patient public about the dangers of inappropriate self-medication. To this end, the AMA sponsored consumer education programs promoting caution in the use of drugstore remedies. The most ambitious of these efforts was its seal of approval program. Taking as its model the Good Housekeeping Institute set up by Harvey Wiley after he left the FDA, the AMA introduced the program in 1930 to help consumers cope with the increasingly aggressive use of the health sell. As *Hygeia* explained, "One way of distinguishing between reliable statements and nonsensical advertising puffery is to look for some sign of actual consideration by a scientific group, an indication of this being the appearance on the package or in advertising matter of a 'seal' such as those of the Councils of the American Medical Association and of the American Dental Association." Manufacturers submitted products and advertising material to the appropriate AMA council, and if the health claims were found "unobjectionable," they received permission to feature the AMA seal in their advertising. Only products bearing the seal might purchase advertising space in *Hygeia* and the many other AMA publications, so manufacturers interested in cultivating medical goodwill had considerable incentive to comply.[48]

The AMA's consumer efforts concentrated primarily on the same flamboyantly fraudulent remedies that concerned the FTC and FDA, such as Norman Baker's cancer cure and John R. Brinkley's goat gland treatment. Less often, the association took national manufacturers to task for advertising claims that the FTC had allowed to pass, with limited success. Listerine, for example, ran ads implying that its germ-killing ingredients met scientific standards for disinfection; a 1930 ad proclaimed, "We could not make this statement unless prepared to prove it to the entire satisfaction of the U.S. Government and the medical profession." The following year, the AMA's Chemical Laboratory issued a report disputing the product's germicidal powers, but Listerine ads continued to tout its germ-fighting powers.[49]

The AMA also tried to keep physicians from doing paid product promotions, vigorously protesting the use of medical authority to promote the sales of Fleischmann's yeast, among other products. In 1928, faced with flagging sales, the J. Walter Thompson Company started to use testimonials from physicians to promote eating yeast as a "natural" way to tone the intestinal tract, stop constipation, clear the skin, and restore vigor. To get around the AMA's ban on medical testimonials, Thompson chose to feature distinguished European doctors, hoping to trade on their international cachet. The AMA responded by reaching out to its counterparts in Austria and other countries, asking them to resist the advertising agency's overtures. Here again their efforts brought mixed results, as doctors from one country were easily replaced by physicians from other locales.[50]

Although the AMA had some success in making its own members wary of giving product testimonials, it had limited power to discipline those who were not. Those limits were made very clear when a former AMA president, distinguished dermatologist William Allen Pusey, provided endorsements for the Woodbury Company's Camay soap, a lapse in professional discipline that lay critics of advertising noted with some glee.[51] Likewise, for all its efforts to discourage testimonials, the AMA had no way to stop individual physicians from exercising their own consumer choices in ways that advertisers could exploit. Perhaps the most embarrassing example of this freedom was the enthusiasm with which doctors took advantage of the free cartons of cigarettes offered by Lucky Strike, which became the foundation for its ad campaign featuring lines such as "20,679 physicians say 'Luckies' are less irritating."

Advertisers also played up prevention as a medical blind spot. As one Thompson executive noted while working on a promotional campaign aimed at mothers, doctors "are so busy treating specific illnesses that they often overlook things that should be considered when the baby is well." Laypeople, even those who disliked commercial ballyhoo, tended to hear medical protestations against the drugstore as a self-interested defense of their economic interests. As journalist Richard Lee Strout noted, "possibly the medical profession's jealousy of its prerogatives played a part" in shaping doctors' opinions. For their part, drug manufacturers worked hard to keep alive the long American tradition of medical self-help by portraying any and all regulation of drug markets as a threat to the "sacred right" to self-medication.[52]

Establishing doctors as a trustworthy source of consumer advice about drugstore products was not as easy as the AMA had hoped. That goal was further complicated by another troubling theme that began to emerge in the interwar decades: the fear that both doctors and pharmacists were succumbing to the evils of commercialism and thus becoming unreliable allies for the "intelligent" consumer. The threat of ballyhoo seemed to be spreading from over-the-counter preparations to the prescription department. As a result, some laypeople began to wonder if the prescribing habits of physicians were as scientific as the profession claimed.

A major reason that patient-consumers decided to visit doctors was the desire to get medicines stronger than those available over the counter. As economist Allon Peebles noted in 1929, "Their faith in the efficacy of bottles of brightly-colored medicine is strong."[53] Patients tended to assume, with doctors' encouragement, that what the doctor ordered via prescription was in fact different from—and better than—medicines that could be bought over the counter. In this regard, narcotics remained the prototype of the "doctors' drugs"—that is, medicines so potentially dangerous that they could only be given under medical supervision. But as those familiar with the pharmaceutical industry pointed out, more and more doctors were writing prescriptions for drugs available over the counter, adding to the medication's cost to the patient-consumer. The growing percentage of prescriptions written for proprietary remedies reflected the breaking down of distinctions between the way ethical and proprietary drug companies behaved due to increasing competition. At the same time that ethical firms began to develop their own lines of consumer goods, proprietary firms moved in the opposite direction: they began to direct more advertising at physicians, adopting practices long in use by ethical firms to shape physicians' prescribing habits. As awareness of this trend spread, so, too, did troubling questions about the corrosive effect of commerce on medicine's scientific standards.

Advertising directed at physicians had long been a small but well-defined specialty within the advertising field. In his authoritative 1897 encyclopedia, Nathaniel Fowler praised the medical trade press for the high quality of its advertising, which he described as "the very cream of printed integrity." Doctors read the ads as well as the articles, he suggested, because there they could find "news and information of benefit to [them] financially and to the health and happiness of all humankind." But in the aftermath of the 1906 Pure Food and Drugs Act, that view of professional advertising as the antithesis of rank commercialism and the doctor as impervious to persuasion began to change.[54]

As Daniel Hoyt noted in his 1914 pharmacy textbook, drug manufacturers increasingly competed to market "old remedies under unusual names" and attempted to capture doctors' loyalty "by numerous small presents." As long as the new drug worked better than the old, Hoyt saw no problem in this trend: "A patented medicine . . . is a perfectly legitimate remedy for a physician to use if he is convinced that it is of definite value in a given case." Convenience often determined the choice of the packaged good over its USP counterpart. Hoyt used Phillips' Milk of Magnesia as an example. "It is an excellent preparation," he wrote, "but in no way superior to magnesia magma . . . if the latter be properly made." Of course, the doctor might worry about whether the "corner druggist can properly make up the product," which Hoyt considered "a very practical objection." If physician and pharmacist "will take the trouble," they need not rely on the packaged good, Hoyt concluded. But in fact, most medical professionals no longer had the time or inclination to do the work necessary to ensure quality and thus became a promising audience for commercial cultivation.[55]

The bulk of this new promotion came via direct-mail advertising: starting in the 1920s, doctors began to receive a heavy volume of circulars touting the merits of various proprietary drugs, with free samples offered for many of the products. As ethical firms had done for decades, proprietary firms also began to send drug salesmen, known as "detail men," to visit physicians and pharmacists in order to promote their product lines. By the late 1920s, detail men were a common fixture in not only urban areas but rural counties as well. In Shelby County, Indiana, a doctor reported seeing agents representing fifteen different companies, "each of whom visits him about every six weeks." The goal was simple: convince physicians to prescribe products by brand name; for example, instead of prescribing milk of magnesia, the physician would order the more expensive Phillips' Milk of Magnesia. If the doctor failed to specify a brand, companies hoped to persuade the pharmacist to choose their particular label when making up the prescription.[56]

In the early 1900s, an industry observer had predicted that "the proprietary medicine of the future will be advertised through 'medical' channels,' and physicians and drug companies alike would reap the benefits." By the 1930s, that prediction seemed to have been fulfilled. When the editors of the National Formulary undertook a comprehensive analysis of prescriptions written between 1885 and 1931, they found that the number of proprietary products appearing as an ingredient in prescriptions rose from 7 percent to 41 percent of the total over that span. To be sure, they remained only 16 percent of the total drugs prescribed, far less than the 65 percent of prescribed drugs listed in the USP. As the National Formulary analysis noted, much of what was being sold by proprietary firms were drugs listed in the USP and National Formulary that had been turned into tablets, capsules, and ampules, products that were not only easier to dispense but also easier for patients to take. According to the report, "Manufactured medicines, ready for prompt and rapid dispensing, have increased greatly in recent years." In other words, instead of preparing drugs, pharmacists opened products that had been prepared at factories and repackaged them for patient-consumers.[57]

Physicians committed to the cause of "rational prescribing" were concerned that the "weak sisters" in the medical profession were succumbing to the wiles of the "pharmaceutical Barnums," in the words of the AMA's Arthur Cramp. Particularly troubling to physician experts was the increasing number of prescriptions that physicians were writing for products that did not appear in any of the recognized bibles of scientific therapeutics, the USP, the National Formulary, or the AMA's list of new and unofficial remedies. Cramp estimated that by the mid-1930s, two-thirds of all drugs dispensed by prescription were medicines that patients could buy more cheaply over the counter. In this respect, the volume of advertising addressed to the "professional trade" of physicians and pharmacists seemed to be working all too well.[58]

In a 1929 article, "How Scientific Are Our Doctors?," popular science writer T. Swann Harding presented a cynical view of this process: "Suppose you consult a physician [who] looks at you wisely and writes a prescription for 'Blank's Compound No. 17.'" The patient dutifully takes the prescription to the pharmacist, and he "soaks the original label off the bottle, sticks on his own, compels you to wait an hour for purposes of prestige and financial gain, gives you the tonic, and you get well," but having paid more than if you had purchased the same tonic off the druggist's shelves. As Harding suggested, the growing evidence that some physicians were failing the test of being rational prescribers called into question their ability to act as the patient's trusted intermediary. The ease of dispensing and taking drugs came at a price: patient-consumers paid more for packaged goods than for their base ingredients. Once they became familiar with this fact, consumers might well choose to dispense with the middleman and buy the same ingredients themselves, a solution that consumerists such as Harding would soon begin to promote.[59]

The growing sensitivity to these issues was reflected in the redesign of prescription departments according to a "semi-open" plan. As the name suggests, the new layout left most of the compounding area open, so that consumers could watch pharmacists make up prescriptions and hence appreciate the care and labor that went into doing so. At the same time, the design provided a sheltered space where druggists could perform tasks they did not want consumers to see, such as repackaging proprietary remedies as prescription goods for resale at a higher price. (The semi-open plan had the added virtue of deterring other indiscretions: Charles Walgreen supposedly adopted it during Prohibition after discovering a pharmacist entertaining two girls with a bottle of whiskey.)[60]

Unlike fee splitting, which received more popular-press attention during the 1930s, the ethical questions surrounding the prescribing of over-the-counter medications remained a matter of debate only among insiders in the medical and drug industry. Patients had little chance of figuring out that they were being prescribed goods that they could buy over the counter thanks to the tradition of writing prescriptions using Latin terms and arcane symbols. As pharmacists acknowledged, this system was adopted not only for the sake of precision but also to ensure that patients did not know what their doctors were ordering.

Frederick Gerrish explained in his popular late-nineteenth-century guide to prescription writing that Latin was "often desirable to keep the patient in ignorance of what he is taking." Gerrish justified this ignorance as a kindness meant to keep patients from unnecessary worries. Writing in the tradition of medical paternalism, he noted that in the same way that it would be unnecessarily "cruel" to give a patient a detailed pathological description and prognosis, "so it is generally unwise to permit him to know just what he is taking for a remedy." If people knew, for example, that their doctor had ordered a medicine that might be addictive or otherwise dangerous, they might be afraid to take it. But the system also kept the patient from understanding exactly what the doctor was ordering and buying the medicine directly.[61]

Remington's textbook, which was widely used in pharmacy colleges, justified the use of Latin in similar terms. Not only was Latin "the language of science," understood "throughout the civilized world," but also "it is frequently necessary, and always advisable, to withhold from a patient the names and properties of the medicinal agents administered," a requirement that "can usually be effected by the use of the Latin technical terms." The Latin stood out all the more because other parts of the prescription, such as the *signa* (the instructions for taking the medicine), had to be written in English. Thus the prescription drug's label presented an uneasy linguistic mix of the mysterious and the familiar.[62]

For precisely these reasons, some interwar consumers began to complain about the use of Latin and ask for more understandable descriptions of what was in their prescriptions. As Samuel O. L. Potter and R. J. E. Scott noted reproachfully in their 1931 pharmacy text, "The use of the Latin language in writing prescriptions is criticized by a certain class of patients who like to know what they are taking, or wish to exercise their judgment upon the prescription of a physician whose learning and skill they professed to have confidence in when they consulted him." The textbook continued, "This feeling frequently crops out in our State legislatures, where bills are frequently introduced making it a crime for a physician to write a prescription in any other than the vernacular tongue."[63]

But perhaps because the cost of prescription drugs remained comparatively small—on average only a few dollars—the economic sleights of hand going on in the prescription department attracted less hostile commentary than did the changes in doctors' billing practices. Since so many drugs were more or less equivalent, no single seller could raise prices very high without losing trade, and the cost differential between prescription and over-the-counter drugs remained relatively small. Moreover, prices for prescription medications did not vary as dramatically as did physicians' fees. Pharmacists relied on standardized systems for calculating drug costs, such as the Evans Rule, used by the National Association of Retail Druggists and named in honor of its pharmacist inventor. In essence, these systems doubled the cost of the ingredients to cover containers and overhead and added a set rate for the labor of compounding the prescription, with an ultimate goal of achieving a profit of between 10 and 20 percent.[64]

At a time when patients could repeatedly get the same prescription filled, so long as it was for non-habit-forming drugs, pharmacists also had to be careful not to vary prices, lest the refill cost be higher than the original. Instead of putting the price right on the label, pharmacists substituted ciphers: in the early 1900s, the phrase "COME AND BUY" stood for the numbers one through zero, so a dollar would be written "C.Y.Y." In the late 1930s, the National Association of Retail Druggists had replaced the overt commercialism of the earlier code with a more neutral cipher, "PHARMOCIST," in which a dollar would be written "P.T.T." In another indication of price sensitivity, physicians and pharmacists developed codes to recognize very poor patients for whom the customary pricing should be waived. Explained Remington's, "It frequently happens that physicians desire to indicate that a patient is poor and is a proper subject for charity"; in such cases, doctors would write the letter P in the lower corner of the prescription, "or if very poor PP." Continued the text, "It is customary and humane to regard these marks if assured of their genuineness."[65]

Yet another factor that helped to keep the cost of both prescription and proprietary medicines low was the intensification of price competition among retail outlets. The big chain drugstores featured one-cent sales and specials to bring in customers; the independents had to counter with their own price cuts and sales promotions. During the Great Depression, some entrepreneurs opened so-called pine board stores, where packaged drugs were piled on rough boards in a space devoid of retail niceties. To limit cutthroat price competition, states began to pass "fair trade" laws in the mid-1930s, allowing manufacturers to set minimum retail prices below which their products could not be sold. In 1937, the U.S. Congress passed the Miller-Tydings Act, which made fair trade principles national policy. While these laws would be tested in the 1950s, they essentially remained in place until the 1970s. But compared to doctors' bills, a trip to the drugstore still seemed to promise a bargain.[66]

In the fierce competition for customers, pharmacists introduced other innovations designed to appeal to discriminating shoppers. Aware that a more discerning class of patients was patronizing the drugstore, pharmacists took more care with preparing prescription medications. The gaudy labels common in the late nineteenth century gave way to a more refined, serious look. Pharmacists expanded the use of accessory labels to help patients quickly distinguish their medications: some stores used red stickers (sometimes with a skull and crossbones) to denote potentially poisonous substances and blue labels for habit-forming drugs. Others added messages such as "Shake well before using" or "For external use only." The use of symbols and stickers not only pleased the educated consumer but also helped the less literate patient.[67]

Pharmacists also had an advantage over physicians in that their professionalism was more easily adapted to a retail setting. Even the most welcoming doctor's office could not compare with the kind of "come hither" atmosphere that characterized the drugstore, where prompt and friendly service was a key way to beat out the competition. As Charles Walgreen liked to enjoin his employees, "Do not talk about service; let it speak for itself." To underline this point, Walgreens developed a routine known as the two-minute drill: when a patient called to put in an order for nonprescription items, the pharmacist would write it down, give it to the clerk, and then keep the person on the line talking about baseball or the weather. After rapidly assembling the order, the clerk would run to deliver it while the customer was still on the phone. Walgreens promised the same prompt and courteous service to customers who came into the store. Before the advent of self-service in the 1950s, buying "over-the-counter" goods meant literally that: patients asked for the medicines they wanted, and clerks fetched them. Advertising campaigns and in-store displays and promotions sought to get a customer to point to a product on a shelf and say, "I'll have one of those."[68]

Pharmacists thus tried to build their custom by providing superior personal service. Unlike physicians, they were easily available to patients—no appointment was needed for a consultation—and the cost of their service was folded into the price of the product. Not surprisingly, these consumer-friendly features of the new drugstore created tensions between pharmacists and physicians. Physicians not unreasonably worried that a well-liked pharmacist could easily steer consumers complaining of indigestion or headaches toward over-the-counter remedies rather than urge them to see a doctor. As drug retailing texts warned, the pharmacist had to steer a fine line between engaging in the salesmanship essential to retail success and practicing medicine without a license, a charge that could bring the local medical society down on his head. Nolen and Maynard warned the pharmacist had to avoid "aggressive personal selling" lest he be accused of "counter prescribing." He might "describe the product, explain its uses, and in other ways make it easier for the consumer to buy, but under no conditions must he be insistent or offer 'medical' advice."[69] The suspicions of "counter servicing" were particularly directed at the chain stores: physicians worried that the same zeal used to sell pinochle sets carried over into the prescription department.

Even as the main note of caution sounded about drugstores remained directed at foolish patient-consumers taken in by foolish advertising, another set of worries emerged regarding doctors and pharmacists as patients' trusted intermediaries. The new commercialism not only threatened to make patients more irrational but also had a corrosive effect on the professionalism of those helping to guide their choices. In the drugstore as in the doctor's office, the interplay between modern science and modern capitalism seemed to be blurring rather than sharpening the markers of real quality. As some consumer advocates were beginning to realize, physicians were coming under the same blandishments as the lay public and, despite their superior scientific training, were not sufficiently resistant to the spirit of ballyhoo. In time, these revelations about what was going on behind the prescription counter would further erode trust in the doctor's judgment.

Consumer Wonderland or Rotting Miasmal Swamp?

While these troubles were brewing behind the prescription counter, commentaries about the new drugstore remained primarily focused on its relationship with patient-consumers, not physicians. Its boosters suggested that the drugstore gave Americans just what they wanted: more goods at lower prices. With its eye-catching displays and soda fountain treats, the new corner store seemed like an institution made to order for modern living: a welcoming place stocking all the essential goods that patient-consumers needed to take care of themselves. But an increasingly vocal cadre of critics warned against being taken in by that image. The business of making and selling drugs had become incredibly complicated, they argued, and consumers who got distracted by the colorful balloons and ice cream sundaes were likely not only to waste their hard-earned money but also potentially to harm their health.

In "Consumers in Wonderland," first an article and later a chapter in their best-selling 1927 book, *Your Money's Worth*, economist Stuart Chase and engineer Frederick Schlink stressed the dangers that lurked in the new-style drugstore. "In buying soap and shoes and sealing wax, the consumer has at least trial and error to help him," they observed, but such was not the case where drugstore medicines were concerned. Most minor illnesses were self-limiting: people recovered regardless of the treatment they did or did not receive. The crafty drug manufacturer and retailer relied on the fact that "you are sick; you drink a few bottles of Pepso-sene, and pretty soon you are well" to cultivate devoted users of worthless remedies.[70]

Americans wrongly assumed that since passage of the Pure Food and Drugs Act, nothing in those bottles could hurt them. Yet as Chase and Schlink noted, that legislation's weaknesses had become glaringly apparent. The law required that only a very few dangerous drugs be listed on labels, applied only to goods traded across state lines, and did not cover cosmetics and weight-loss remedies. Moreover, its ability to command truth-telling covered only what was written on the label and the box, not what was claimed in off-label advertising. Hence even though the courts agreed that Doan's Kidney Pills could not cure kidney disease, the government had no authority to stop the company from advertising such benefits. Pretending to be a consumer "wonderland," the drugstore might better be described as a "rotting miasmal swamp" presided over by proprietary drugmakers, the "vultures of modern civilization."[71]

While some critics simply dismissed Americans' penchant for over-the-counter medicine as proof of their ignorance, other observers pointed out the special difficulty involved in assessing the worth of such goods. "In the barter, sale or exchange of practically every line of merchandise save one, the purchaser has a chance of learning, eventually, whether or not he has been swindled," explained Cramp. If someone bought "an automobile, a piano, or a suit of clothes" that turned out to be inferior in quality, "it is but a matter of time before the purchaser learns the fact, and so acquires knowledge which, if he has brains, may prevent him making the same error the next time." But when purchasing one group of goods, "the public never does and never can get an even break: products or services that are sold for the alleged alleviation or cure of human ills." "The healing power of nature" or "vis medicatrix naturae" ensured that roughly 80 percent of all illnesses improved on their own, leaving consumers to mistakenly believe that their latest drugstore purchases deserved the credit.[72]

Curiously, while most commentators worried about American consumers being routinely misled by crafty advertising, marketing surveys and public opinion polls suggested the opposite: most Americans did not like the new advertising any more than the old and regarded its claims with intense skepticism. Studies done in the early 1930s by the U.S. Office of Education and the National Committee on Education by Radio uncovered deep dissatisfaction with the new broadcast commercialism. Although audiences enjoyed the entertainment that radio presented, they felt that advertising "interrupts the programs so often as to destroy the pleasure of even the good features" and was of "questionable honesty." Of the many products advertised, listeners expressed a special distrust regarding claims about proprietary medicines.[73]

Perhaps the most telling evidence of advertising's low reputation was its central place in interwar humor. Radio comedians and other humorists frequently made advertising the butt of their jokes. For nearly a decade, *Ballyhoo*, a humor magazine founded in 1931 by George T. Delacrote Jr. and Norman Anthony, made spoofing advertising a central theme, beginning a tradition of poking fun at Madison Avenue that remains a staple of American humor. Health-related promotions featured prominently as an object of mirth. The first item on *Ballyhoo*'s list of the Advertisers' Ten Commandments was, "Thou shalt not have for thyself any unpleasant breath, any cough, any film on thy teeth, any athlete's foot, or the likeness of any disease that is in Heaven above or on the earth beneath or in the waters under the earth." A full-page ad for the fictional Ballyhoo Institute and Medical Center detailed the many ways that modern science was helping "all those suffering from advertising diseases," including pink toothbrush, dandruff, body odor, and throat irritation.[74]

But while such advertising was easy to ridicule, it still seemed to influence many people's attitudes and behavior. As Rorty wrote in his 1934 book on advertising, *Our Master's Voice*, "True, the saps laugh, but they also buy!"[75] Questions about how wisely Americans used the drugstore were closely related to the debate over how they were handling the tidal wave of advertising directed at them. By one reckoning, the American people had learned to tune out advertising hype and sort through its messages for the kernels of truth they valued—lower prices and desirable products. In this view, common sense triumphed: Americans could work around the drugstore's blandishments to get what they wanted. From another perspective, however, they remained easily duped "saps who buy," helpless to resist the promise of a miracle. Their ignorance was a fundamental cause of the problems with American medicine. The unrealistic expectations with which modern drugstores and their advertising schemes filled patient-consumers' heads led to wasteful spending and neglect of the real expertise offered by modern doctors.

With the image of the sap who buys, interwar commentators suggested the many contradictions wrapped up in the new corner store. On the one hand, a trip to the drugstore represented a far more enticing prospect than a visit to the doctor's office. It appealed to the long-standing American love of self-medication with new and improved products that reflected the wonders of modern science and the vigilance of the FDA. The drugstore offered an attractive mix of opportunities for constructive self-improvement and reclamation from modern sins, with some pampering thrown in. On the other hand, the drugstore was an enabler, conveniently assembling together an array of goods associated with the unhealthy pace of modern life, an unholy alliance of the cosmetics, shaving products, and cigarettes needed to complement a night out on the town and the headache tablets, cough drops, and indigestion aids necessary to recover from those excesses.

The rise of the modern drugstore and its association with an aggressive health commercialism contributed to growing confusion over the question of whose claims were worth heeding. Drug manufacturers, advertising agents, drugstore owners, health educators, and physicians claimed to be devoted to telling the truth and serving the public yet offered remedies that were often at odds with each other. Both staying well and spending one's money wisely required that patient-consumers become more inquisitive about the story "that lies back of the bottles on drugstore shelves," as Chase and Schlink put it.[76] As a consequence, drugstore aisles became an important arena in which medical consumers developed their skills.

In short, developments in the drugstore converged with those in the doctor's office to create a growing sense that patient-consumers needed to educate themselves about what was good medicine. To that end, a host of self-appointed consumer guardians began to step forward, working not only to educate the public about how to shop more wisely as individuals but also to bring collective pressure on the medical profession and the federal government to do a better job of protecting patient-consumers' interests. Against the backdrop of the Great Depression, their efforts would give rise to a burst of consumer politicking that permanently changed the American way of medicine.

{FOUR}

The Guinea Pigs' Revolt

In 1935, an article with the provocative title "Shopping for Medical Care" appeared in the *Confidential Bulletin*, published by Consumers' Research, a nonprofit organization set up in 1929 to advocate for consumer interests. "In shopping for medical care it is necessary to be even more skeptical and vigilant than in shopping for food and clothing," former nurse Katharine A. Kellock wrote. Prospective patients needed to learn how to negotiate the twin dangers of "medical ignorance" and "medical racketeering"—that is, poorly trained doctors and unethical practices such as fee splitting and unnecessary treatment. Although she admitted there was "always danger in advising patients to be critical of their doctor's work because on occasion it put unfair burdens on able, honest practitioners," Kellock urged those in search of "intelligent medical care," as she assumed the *Bulletin*'s readers to be, to become more assertive: to ask pointed questions about physicians' qualifications, to get copies of X-rays and lab reports, and to read medical journals to learn about the "consensus of opinion" regarding treatment of particular ailments. In essence, she outlined a playbook for the watchdog patient.[1]

Kellock concluded her piece with some reflections on the changing consumer mood: "There is a growing irritation and objection among consumers with the tendency of medical men to arrogate to themselves the prerogatives of the deity and to treat their patients as persons who should gratefully pay the high charges for medical services, and question those services and their value as little as possible." But expectations of patient docility were in vain, she suggested, for much as they might wish to be godlike, "medical men and medical ethics are in a notably unstable and hesitating state at the present time." With medical benefits being discussed as part of the new Social Security program under congressional consideration, "the increasing and sharpening threat of state and socialized medicine has put physicians in a mood to listen to, and even at times to heed, criticism by intelligent laymen." She confidently asserted that "medical care will improve mightily under intelligent consumer demand."[2]

Against the backdrop of the Great Depression, Kellock was among a growing chorus of voices urging Americans to become more "intelligent buyers" of medicine. This consumerist advice was formulated primarily by laypeople for laypeople, with heavy borrowings from a few physicians who shared similar concerns. At its core lay anxiety about what journalist James Rorty referred to as the "marriage of medicine and business" and its impact on both the doctor's office and the drugstore. For all its scientific achievements, the "new medicine" and the drugs and procedures associated with it were getting caught up in their own version of ballyhoo. Those authorities delegated to be the consumers' protectors—the FDA and the medical profession—were failing to stand up to the forces of commercialism. The result was a nation of unwitting "guinea pigs," as Arthur Kallet and Frederick Schlink described their fellow Americans in a 1933 best seller, *100,000,000 Guinea Pigs*, exposed to the dangers of deceptive advertising, unsafe drugs and cosmetics, unnecessary medical procedures, and unaffordable doctors' bills.[3]

To avoid those hazards, this generation of critics argued, Americans needed to become warier, smarter consumers. That goal required rejecting both the enthusiastic commercialism espoused by the business community (blind faith in the free market) and the professional paternalism advocated by medical leaders (blind faith in one's personal physician). Instead, these critics promoted a third path increasingly referred to by the term "consumerism," by which they meant a more systematic, critical approach to consumer decision making. Simply by educating themselves, informed patients would become a positive force for change. As Schlink, one of the founders of Consumers' Research, wrote in 1936, "We will get good medical service only insofar as those who need it are critically informed and as expert as laymen can be toward it."[4]

This new faith in the power of critical medical consumerism met with both ridicule and resistance. Most business and medical leaders rejected consumerist complaints as unfounded, insisting that Americans enjoyed better medical care and drugs than ever before. Physicians shared the consumerists' dislike of quackery but reacted with outrage to the suggestion that members of their profession ever succumbed to the "doctor's dilemma" and overtreated for profit. They portrayed consumerists as neurotic, irresponsible, perhaps even subversive gadflies who grossly overestimated the dangers lurking in the doctor's office and on the drugstore shelves. Consumerists did not help their own cause by frequently fighting with each other.

Yet while often disorganized and divided, advocates of a new kind of medical consumerism found considerable political traction in the New Deal era. Through books, magazine articles, and letter-writing campaigns, they drew attention to the shopping problems created by the changing economics of the doctor's office and the drugstore and promoted medical consumerism as the mark of a well-informed citizen. Their persistent complaining helped to bring about the New Deal's most significant health legislation: the 1938 laws strengthening the consumer protection powers of both the FDA and the FTC. In addition, their criticisms of the medical profession helped bring about changes within the AMA, chief among them endorsement of the concept of private health insurance. So while often derided, the guinea pigs' revolt of the 1930s had long-lasting if sometimes paradoxical results.[5]

Getting Their Money's Worth

The medical consumerism articulated in the 1930s reflected the culmination of several decades of growing academic interest in what surgeon Hugh Cabot referred to as the "problem of the consumer." The economic collapse following the end of World War I, marked by both an inflationary spiral and unprecedented political violence, motivated academic economists to devote new attention to the mechanisms of supply and demand. As consumer goods became more central to economic growth, old concepts of saving and spending had to be rethought. Some economists, chief among them Simon Patten at the University of Pennsylvania, argued that an "economics of scarcity" was giving way to an "economics of abundance" in which encouraging consumers to spend rather than save would foster economic growth.[6]

Likewise, the growing field of home economics sought to educate the nation's primary shoppers, namely its womenfolk, about how to spend wisely on their family's behalf. Home economists believed that by teaching women to shop more "scientifically," using objective measures of quality and value, they could help make consumer capitalism work better. An educated wife and mother could distinguish among different cuts of meat, types of cloth, and household cleansers and consequently get more value for her money. By the 1920s, courses in home economics had become part of the standard curriculum in the upper grades of public schools. Women's clubs and social workers took the same message to adult women, including not only middle-class ladies but also working-class mothers, many of whom were recent immigrants or rural-urban migrants.[7]

While it built on postwar interest in consumers, the critical consumerism of the 1930s took a more jaundiced view of their situation than either mainstream economics or home economics. In essence, depression-era consumerists thought that neither the federal government nor the medical profession was doing enough to keep patient-consumers safe. Moreover, they believed that consumer protection had to be far more than just "woman's work": the men of the new middle classes—engineers, lawyers, and accountants—needed to become more involved as well.

This more masculine version of consumerism debuted in a 1927 best seller, *Your Money's Worth*. Written by Stuart Chase, a certified public accountant and former staff member of the FTC, and Frederick J. Schlink, an engineer and former staff member of the National Bureau of Standards, the book provided an overview of the economic changes affecting the average consumer. As Chase and Schlink explained, industries now battled fiercely for "the largest possible share of the national purchasing power," primarily through advertising that was far from truthful. As a result, "we are all Alices in a Wonderland of conflicting claims, bright promises, fancy packages, soaring words, and almost impenetrable ignorance." The book presented more than 200 pages of disturbing evidence about how this consumers' wonderland worked, including long chapters on proprietary medicine and medical quackery. For those wanted to escape Wonderland, the authors urged that "there is a way out," and *Your Money's Worth* marked the path.[8]

Chase and Schlink argued that because "the market always responds to organized pressure," consumers needed to become more assertive in expressing their demands. "Pending the coming of organization," they wrote, "the individual can create no little nuisance value in the right direction, and inform himself besides," by learning more about what he was buying. To this end, they made a range of suggestions. Consumers should "ask advertisers to produce the scientific facts upon which their claims are based" and always read product labels carefully. They should write to the AMA for "information on the quality and character of advertised drugs and medical appliances" and share that information with "your druggist and your neighbors." Finally, consumers should "never believe advertisements" and make sure to "say so, loudly, clearly and on every possible occasion."[9]

Not only did *Your Money's Worth* become a Book-of-the-Month Club selection, but it also inspired readers to want more such advice. In 1929, after receiving hundreds of letters from readers, Chase and Schlink joined with Kallet, also an engineer, to form a nonprofit organization they christened Consumers' Research. Its goal was to provide the kind of objective information that more and more consumers seemed to want: scientific, substantive, and not beholden to advertising interests. In exchange for dues payments, subscribers received regular issues of the group's *Confidential Bulletin*, which contained detailed evaluations of a wide range of products, including appliances, antiseptics, and even doctors' services.[10]

Consumers' Research staff initially focused on digesting product information collected by government agencies, congressional subcommittees, and other groups; in later years, they also set up facilities to evaluate products as diverse as automobiles and underwear. Consumers' Research accepted no paid advertising or financial support from any group that might profit from their evaluations. They believed this no-advertising policy was critical to their credibility and gave them a big advantage over the "seal of approval" programs run by *Good Housekeeping* and the AMA, both of which depended greatly on advertising revenue. This strategy clearly had appeal: the organization's subscriber base increased from 565 in 1929 to 42,000 in 1933. Moreover, readers soon showed they not only valued the *Confidential Bulletin* but also were willing to join the leadership's appeals to participate in more collective efforts to exert political pressure.[11]

The Consumers' Research approach to "getting your money's worth" had particular appeal to urban middle-class Americans. Although enjoying rising levels of educational opportunity and prosperity, they still needed to spend wisely in order to enjoy a comfortable way of life. Whereas the Progressive-era consumers' leagues had linked activism to improving labor conditions, the interwar version focused more on consumer protection as an end in itself: consumers of all classes deserved to be offered quality goods at fair prices. And unlike the Progressive-era consumer leagues, Consumers' Research was headed by white male professionals. Although women held important positions in the organization and its later offshoot, Consumers Union, interwar consumerism was far more identified with men than had been the Progressive movement. Perhaps as a consequence, depression-era consumerists proved far more willing to challenge medical authority than had the previous generation of reformers.[12]

Although successful in galvanizing action, the acerbic tone of Consumers' Research earned it many detractors. These included not only the businesses they attacked, but also other groups vying to speak on consumers' behalf, including the AMA. Thus in 1935, when Consumers' Research became embroiled in an internal battle over unionizing its employees, its many critics rejoiced. The organization eventually split, and the pro-union faction led by Kallet founded a rival organization, Consumers Union. Although both groups survived the battle, Consumers Union went on to enjoy the greater long-term success.[13]

In spite of their difficulties, assertive advocacy first by Consumers' Research and then by Consumers Union garnered new visibility for consumerism in general and medical consumerism in particular. Their articulation of consumers' interests inspired other individuals and groups to advance versions of the same message: consumers needed to become educated and more organized as an interest group. Academic social scientists and home economists might have qualms about the "guinea piggers'" combative tone but shared their general concerns about commercialism and its hazards. The "problem of the consumer" also attracted attention from the Roosevelt administration, where New Deal reformers sought to cultivate consumer interests as a counterweight to business and labor groups.[14]

Against the backdrop of the Great Depression, efforts to articulate consumers' interests came from a variety of directions. Academics trained in the new fields of institutional economics and sociology sought to develop a more empirical, objective view of the problems consumers faced, an approach exemplified by the studies undertaken by the CCMC; many researchers associated with it, including Michael Davis and Isidore Falk, became widely recognized experts on the economics of medicine. Others writing about medical consumerism were journalists and popular science writers who sought to explain the workings of the new medical economy to a general audience, among them adman-turned-journalist James Rorty, part-time science writer T. Swann Harding, and Vassar-educated publicist Ruth deForest Lamb. Last but not least, lay writers were joined by a small group of dissident physicians, among them surgeons Hugh Cabot and Bertram Bernheim, who broke ranks with the AMA and offered their own critical perspectives on the problems of modern medicine.

A major force propelling the popularization of critical medical consumerism was its appeal to editors and publishers. The success of both *Your Money's Worth* and *100,000,000 Guinea Pigs* provided concrete evidence that an audience existed for the advice they offered. As Jerome W. Ephraim noted in his 1937 book, *Take Care of Yourself: A Practical Guide to Health and Beauty*, "countless books on diseases, drugs and cosmetics line library shelves throughout the land," and "unending streams of health articles fill columns of magazine and newspaper space." As much as readers seemed to like upbeat stories about medical innovations, they also apparently wanted to know more about the dark side of the drugstore and the surgical suite. Publishers and editors competed to find writers adept at writing about medical topics. Some authors addressed political and policy controversies directly, while others concentrated more on the "how tos" of smart shopping.[15]

Rank Flowers in the Garden of Rugged Individualism

Of the two strands of medical consumerism, the one directed at the drug-store developed earlier and more robustly, in part because it built on long-standing complaints about the proprietary drug industry and its advertising techniques. But after several decades of regulation under the 1906 act, the Great Depression generation had a much less optimistic view of what government and scientific expertise could deliver in the way of protection. Consumerists believed that the public had a right to know what they were buying via an accurate label, to be guaranteed that the product was safe when used as directed, and to be assured that the maker's claims for the product's value were reasonably truthful. On all three counts, they found the interwar drugstore sadly lacking.

The case against the drugstore was powerfully and persuasively summed up in Kallet and Schlink's widely read *100,000,000 Guinea Pigs*. It was among the five top-selling works of nonfiction in the United States for both 1933 and 1934 and appeared in the public libraries of small towns such as Osage, Iowa, and Sauk Centre, Minnesota. Like Chase and Schlink's earlier *Your Money's Worth*, Kallet and Schlink cast their book as an insiders' guide to the modern marketplace: an objective, hard-nosed look at current business practices and their consequences. The foreword explained, "This book is intended not only to report dangerous and largely unsuspected conditions affecting the health and safety of all consumers of foods, drugs, and cosmetics, but also, so far as possible, to give the consumer some measure of defense against such conditions." While concerned with a broad range of consumer issues, Kallet and Schlink devoted many pages to the hazards of choice presented by the new drugstore.[16]

In Kallet and Schlink's view, the combination of the American penchant for self-medication with the regulatory weakness of its watchdog agencies created a very dangerous situation. "Of all the rank flowers in the garden of rugged individualism," they wrote, "few have a more vile and pervasive stench than the huge $350,000,000 patent-medicine blossom." At best, the industry was "guilty of the economic fraud of selling necessary drugs under meaningless or fantastic claims, with absurd claims of special merit, at from five to a thousand times their ordinary value"; at its worst, the industry was committing murder by selling poisons capable of making people far sicker than the ailments they were trying to cure.[17]

Among the worst sins of the proprietary industry was its financing of the "little white lies" spread by modern advertising, which helped delude consumers into buying these dangerous products. As Kallet and Schlink noted, doctors spent six or seven years earning the right to prescribe drugs, while pharmacists devoted between two and four years to earning the right to dispense medicines. But "Dr. Copy-Writer" could "diagnose and prescribe for all known diseases and conditions, without benefit of even ten minutes of medical education." At the same time, the reliable product information needed to counter misleading advertising remained difficult to access because of copyright and trademark protection. Commercial law allowed the withholding of "vital information" about drug products on the grounds that they were "trade secrets" that had to be guarded from competitors.[18]

Nor should the public think that the goods sold in the prescription department were any better. Kallet and Schlink sought to puncture consumers' confidence that pharmacists and physicians were looking after their interests. Many pharmacists made no effort to ensure the freshness of their drug supplies, and a large percentage of the prescriptions they compounded were made of ingredients that did not appear in either the USP or the National Formulary. Few states did any kind of routine checking to make sure that the drugs being dispensed were those actually prescribed, and the few checks that were performed uncovered many discrepancies. These problems reflected the inevitable results of "a drug and prescription dispensing system which mixes a minor profession with a major business." Kallet and Schlink also blamed the medical profession for the drugstore muddle. Not only were physicians complicit in the writing of unsound prescriptions, but their rising fees were helping to drive patients into the arms of the proprietary drugmakers.[19]

The book levied even harsher judgment on the federal regulators who were failing to do their job to protect the public. Here again, Kallet and Schlink sought to puncture consumers' confidence in supposedly protective forces. Americans greatly overestimated the strength of the food and drug laws protecting them. The FDA had too few resources to do its job adequately, while the courts had undercut the FTC's authority to regulate deceptive advertising on consumers' behalf. The FDA came in for particularly tough criticism as being too easy on "the quacks and the crooks" in the medicine business. Food and drug officials had failed to deter "self-serving business men and politicians in the act of breaking down the regulatory system," forcing consumerists to undertake the work themselves.[20]

Kallet and Schlink concluded that consumers needed to "wake up" to the dangers they faced and mobilize as a political lobby. The last chapter of *100,000,000 Guinea Pigs* presented a list of actions that concerned citizens needed to take. Consumers should write to their political representatives to demand stronger food and drug laws. They should punish dishonest drug-makers by boycotting unsafe and misleadingly advertised goods. They should cultivate scientific and independent sources of information about medicinal products, such as signing up to receive notices of judgment rendered against specific companies for violating the law. "Above all," the authors concluded, "let your voice be heard loudly and often in protest against the indifference, ignorance, and avarice responsible for the uncontrolled adulteration and mis-representation of foods, drugs, and cosmetics," which constituted "a menace to your health that ought no longer be tolerated."[21]

In the wake of the book's publication, some readers did indeed act on its suggestions, writing to President Franklin D. Roosevelt, First Lady Eleanor Roosevelt, their congressmen, and FDA officials. New York pharmacist Edward Davis sent a copy of the book to the president, telling him, "If what Messrs. Kallet and Schlink have written is true, it deserves your undivided attention." Mrs. E. M. Winters of Altoona, Pennsylvania, wrote to Mrs. Roosevelt that if the FDA lacked the power to "prosecute the offenders," the law needed to be strengthened. "Everything is commercialized," Winters lamented, "money is the God of most of the manufacturers and they have little or no concern for our welfare so long as the money rolls into their pockets."[22]

Although some reviewers criticized the book for its tone, described by one writer as "too sensational and too deficient in detached judgment and scientific objectivity," few disagreed with its basic argument that the existing laws for consumer protection were deeply flawed and that the standards of quality and truthfulness adhered to by drug manufacturers, drugstore owners, and advertisers left much to be desired. Despite feeling unfairly vilified, FDA officials believed that the volume performed a useful service by pointing out the defects in the current law. As William G. Campbell, the FDA's director of regulatory work, wrote to a colleague in early 1933, "The book contains a vast amount of good material in the nature of incontrovertible facts to which we would unhesitatingly subscribe." Moreover, he had no quarrel with Kallet and Schlink's assertion "that the law is weak and that the facilities for its enforcement are woefully inadequate." Both the law and its enforcement needed to be strengthened, and, he believed, "if this muckraking publication furthers these aims it will not have been published in vain."[23]

At the very least, the response to *100,000,000 Guinea Pigs* created a widespread assumption among politicians and businesspeople that consumers were indeed riled up. The book went through thirteen printings in the first six months after publication and inspired follow-up books on the subjects of women's hygiene, food and nutrition, and children's health. In 1933, Con-

gress began to hold hearings concerning the need to strengthen the regulation of food, drugs, and cosmetics. Over the next couple of years, legislators
would hear extensive testimony regarding the problems involved in making
informed choices in the drugstore.[24]

One key theme in that testimony concerned the deficiencies in drug labeling. Home economists had for decades been telling consumers to read labels
as the royal route to product safety, but in the case of medicine, that advice left
much to be desired. Ruth deForest Lamb, a Vassar graduate hired as the FDA's
chief educational officer in 1933, emphasized exactly that point in the agency's
exhibits for Congress about the need for a stronger law, which she published
in 1936 as *American Chamber of Horrors*. The existing law required disclosure
of only ten drugs known to be "addictive or poisonous," leaving many other
dangerous substances, among them arsenic and strychnine, liable to be used
with no mention on the labels. Lamb also questioned the usefulness of simply
listing an ingredient without elaborating on why and at what dose it might
be harmful. As an example, she pointed to acetanilide, a coal tar derivative
with painkilling properties that taken at high doses could depress the heart
rate and destroy the blood's hemoglobin. "How many people who see the
declaration of acetanilid [*sic*] on a headache powder or cold remedy know
that it might kill them?" she asked. In the absence of sufficient information,
a patient might well die from taking two doses of headache powder in quick
succession, as had occurred in one case reported to the FDA.[25]

Advertisers' freedom to make fanciful claims for products so long as they
did not appear on the label only compounded the problem. When the law was
originally passed, Lamb wrote, "requiring labels to tell the truth was thought
to be ample protection against dishonest claims." In 1906, the law's architects
could hardly imagine the volume of "wildly extravagant advertising" that
would develop in the decades to come. Lamb, who had worked for a time at
an advertising agency, noted the irony that by limiting what could be put on
the label or package, the 1906 act "forced fraudulent selling appeals out into
the wide, open spaces of collateral advertising where they may romp without
restraint and, in their coursing, round up vast herds of victims who would
never have been snared by the label."[26]

Faced with growing grassroots pressure for change, Congress began to
debate the possibility of extending both the FDA's and the FTC's powers
of consumer protection. The first version of such legislation was drafted by
Rexford Tugwell, an economics professor brought into the Agriculture Department as part of Roosevelt's brain trust. Tugwell's measure required that
all ingredients be listed on the label, transferred oversight of drug advertising

from the FTC to the FDA, included penalties for publishers who printed false advertising, and provided manufacturers no way to appeal the FDA's decisions. The measure was widely considered too tough to pass, a fate that was assured after Tugwell made a two-week trip to the Soviet Union, making him an exemplar of the supposed Bolshevik influence within the New Deal. A more viable bill was drafted by Senator Royal Copeland of New York, a former homeopathic physician and health columnist for the Hearst newspaper syndicate. Having provided personal testimonials for various products, including Pluto mineral water and Fleischmann's yeast, Copeland had a far more relaxed approach to advertising. His version of the bill called for only limited disclosure of ingredients on the label, left drug advertising in the FTC's hands, dropped the punishments for publishers, and set up a mechanism for appeals.[27]

Even the more moderate Copeland bill aroused enormous opposition. Drug manufacturers insisted that changes to the law were not needed because the current system represented no threat to American consumers. Publishers dependent on drug advertising income objected to any expansion of the FTC's powers, protesting that it "should not be set up as a final authority on matters which relate to differences of opinion." Business leaders characterized the Copeland bill as an unnecessary and even dangerous assault on the American system of free enterprise. Despite the fact that the proposed law exempted medical journals and advertising to physicians from its regulatory provisions, the AMA also failed to lobby on its behalf. AMA conservatives saw Copeland's bill as yet another attempt to extend government control over medical practice that needed to be opposed on principle. The fact that its congressional sponsor was a homeopathic physician only reinforced medical suspicions. On the other side of the question, groups such as Consumers' Research and Consumers Union attacked the bill for making too many concessions to industry. Finally, its chances were not helped by the fact that Copeland, like Tugwell, fell out of favor with President Roosevelt.[28]

The legislative deadlock persisted until a tragedy occurred in 1937. In the early 1930s, the German pathologist Gerhard Domagk had discovered sulfonamides, a group of drugs that could cure potentially life-threatening infections. American physicians lagged behind in adopting the "sulfa drugs," until 1936, when a White House physician used one of them to treat twenty-two-year-old Franklin Roosevelt Jr., who was near death from a sinus infection. As the news media spread the story of Roosevelt's miraculous recovery, physicians began to prescribe the new sulfa drugs to treat strep throat among children and gonorrhea among adults.[29] In 1937, Tennessee drug manufacturer S. E. Massengill decided to develop a liquid solution of the drug as an alternative to tablets or injections. The company's chief chemist, Harold Watkins, made up the solution using diethylene glycol, a chemical closely related to automobile antifreeze, unaware of warnings published in medical journals that the solvent was poisonous to humans. Doctors began prescribing the new drug, Elixir Sulfanilamide, but rather than curing people, it sickened and killed them. After doctors reported the deaths to the FDA, the agency mounted a huge effort to alert the public and recover all shipments, but more than 100 people in fifteen states ultimately died as a result of taking the medicine.

In the tragedy's aftermath, the FDA could only prosecute Massengill on the relatively minor charge of "misbranding" the elixir: the label listed alcohol rather than diethylene glycol as the solvent. The incident clearly showed the limits of the existing law, which did not require that drugs be safe for human consumption but only that certain ingredients be listed accurately on the label. Concluded FDA commissioner Walter Campbell, unless the testing provisions of the law were strengthened, "these unfortunate occurrences may be expected to continue because new and relatively untried drug preparations are being manufactured almost daily at the whim of the individual manufacturer, and the damage to public health cannot accurately be estimated."[30]

Widely covered in newspapers and magazines, the Elixir Sulfanilamide deaths seemed to confirm that the guinea piggers' dire warnings were correct. One doctor wrote to the FDA of his "mental and spiritual agony": "Six human beings, all of them my patients, one of them my best friend, are dead because they took medicine that I prescribed for them innocently," believing that any product from such a "great and reputable pharmaceutical firm" must be safe. Similarly, the mother of one of the dead children wrote to President Roosevelt, "It is my plea that you will take steps to prevent such sales of drugs that will take little lives and leave such suffering behind and such a bleak outlook on the future as I have tonight." Aware that their son's more fortunate experience with the drug had inadvertently helped precipitate the tragedy, both Franklin and Eleanor Roosevelt were deeply affected by that letter, and the First Lady threw her considerable political resources behind passage of the new drug legislation.[31]

After years of political stalemate, the U.S. Congress finally passed the Food, Drug, and Cosmetic Act of 1938, which expanded the FDA's regulatory powers, and the Wheeler-Lea Act, which did the same for the FTC. Manufacturers now had to show that drugs introduced on the market were safe (although not necessarily effective). The law laid down new requirements for the labeling of drugs, requiring greater disclosure of ingredients, adequate directions for administration, and warnings against possible misuse. The Food, Drug, and Cosmetic Act also reinforced the principle that some drugs were so powerful that they had to be used only under a doctor's supervision, thus widening the regulatory distinction between prescription and over-the-counter drugs. At the same time, the law allowed manufacturers to appeal government rulings. In Copeland's words, "Procedurally, the law is written so as not to harass business." As conservatives had wanted, the regulation of advertising remained with the FTC, which lobbied hard to retain it. But the Wheeler-Lea Act gave the commission expanded powers to regulate advertising on behalf of consumers as well as businesses, thus closing the loophole opened by the Supreme Court's *Raladam* decision.[32]

The consumer groups that had lobbied for regulatory change had mixed feelings about the 1938 legislation. As Louise Baldwin and Florence Kirlin noted in a 1939 article, "Consumers Appraise the Food, Drug, and Cosmetic Act," most viewed it as "a long step forward" and an "imperfect but perfectible" law. In their view, a flawed bill was better than no bill at all. The extension of regulation to cosmetics, an area where women had suffered from particular harm, was definite cause for celebration. But consumerists were disappointed with the legislation's weaknesses, particularly in advertising oversight. The FTC's sanctions had far more limited force than those of the FDA. The Wheeler-Lea Act was not a criminal statute and thus did not provide for imprisonment. Businesses much preferred its "cease and desist" orders to the FDA's seizure powers. Investigating complaints took a long time and the manufacturer "can reap the profits of his misrepresentations until compelled to desist," wrote law professor Milton Handler, "and then by adopting new copy, continue his depredations of the public until again forced to stop." Handler concluded, "Unless buttressed by clarifying amendments broadening its prohibitions and implementing it with effective sanctions, it will not effect an abiding solution of the vexing problem of false and misleading advertising."[33]

So the guinea pigs' revolt produced only mixed results in the effort to change the drugstore and its promotional culture. A few battles had been won, but the war was far from over. The new laws gave consumers additional information and guarantees of safety but by no means eliminated the need for vigilance. Like the Progressive-era laws they replaced, the new food and drug legislation passed in 1938 would leave plenty of room for the continued growth of medical consumerism in decades to come.

Skeptics in the Doctor's Office

The same consumer skepticism carried over into the depression-era doctor's office. Medical consumerists acknowledged that the medical profession had higher standards than drug manufacturers or advertising agencies but still found much to criticize in doctors' service to their patients. To rectify those deficiencies, they sought to extend what Jerome Ephraim termed "a constructively critical attitude toward everything we see or hear" to the affairs of organized medicine.[34] That aspiration put them at odds with interwar physicians, who anticipated that the profession's new scientific prowess entitled them to more rather than less deference from patients. Despite strong medical disapproval, medical consumerists persisted in calling attention to the shopping problems that the new medicine presented to patients.

Of course, fierce criticism from laypeople was nothing new to American medicine. But prior to the 1930s, that criticism came primarily from adherents to what today we call alternative medicine, including homeopathy, chiropractic, and Christian Science. In contrast, this set of medical detractors accepted the legitimacy of modern science but contended that physicians were not being scientific enough and were allowing both their therapeutic standards and their professional discipline to be corrupted by the forces of commercialism. The 1930s generation took a much less respectful stance toward the medical profession than did their Progressive predecessors.

This new harshness in tone was evident in *100,000,000 Guinea Pigs*, which chided the profession for its complicity in prescribing worthless proprietary medicines as well as for doing too little to discipline the incompetent and unethical among their number. While taking a far less confrontational tone, academic social scientists affiliated with elite research universities and private foundations also suggested that the medical profession was failing to meet the nation's health needs, largely because of its commitment to an outmoded concept of fee-for-service practice. At a time when "no institution was being spared a critical and searching re-examination of its role in the American way of life," Morris Fishbein later recalled in his autobiography, "American medicine was no exception."[35]

In some ways, the application of critical consumerism to medical care was a logical progression: the same principles of intelligent buying useful in the drugstore came in handy at the doctor's office. The medical profession's own advice about how to pick a personal physician depended on teaching patients to "shop around" by checking doctors' credentials and distrusting those who advertised themselves too enthusiastically. At the same time, patient-consumers faced obvious disadvantages in judging the quality of their medical care. Economist Walton Hamilton summed the problem up in a comment on the CCMC's final report: "An old maxim, long known to every student of social philosophy, calls for a restriction of personal choice when 'the consumer is not a proper judge of the quality of the ware.'" Medicine was clearly such a case, for "in medicine, almost more certainly than anywhere else, the patient has not the knowledge requisite for judgment." Relying so heavily on "the personal choice of the physician" came at a cost of "the expense and suffering which attends wrong choice and 'shopping around,' [which] add greatly to the avoidable human costs of medicine."[36]

Although they acknowledged the special difficulties posed by medical choices, consumerists nonetheless concluded that laypeople could become more skillful in making such decisions. To that end, they focused on the kinds of problems previously described in Chapter 2: difficulties in finding good doctors, negotiating the new specialism, and above all, affording the "high cost of keeping alive." Those failings pointed to the limits of Progressive-era reforms to protect patients' best interests. States had granted the medical profession the right to govern itself on the condition that it used that power for the greater good. While emphasizing that most physicians were good, honest individuals, medical consumerists argued that professional organizations, in particular the AMA and local affiliates, were failing to control those who were not. Instead, the guardians of professionalism aimed first and foremost at protecting doctors' economic interests, often at patients' expense.

At the simplest level, medical consumerists pointed out how the current system of medical education and licensing failed to eliminate incompetent and unethical practitioners. While the Flexner reforms had raised standards at many schools, the overall quality of physician training remained highly uneven, and the profession hesitated to discipline members for incompetence or unethical behavior. As Kallet and Schlink wrote in *100,000,000 Guinea Pigs*, the AMA "has not seen fit to expose in any forthright manner the incompetence of physicians, except for those engaged in obvious quackery."[37]

Patients looking for good doctors had very little information with which to work. The AMA's prohibition on physicians' promoting themselves meant that they gave only the most minimal information—their addresses and office hours—to prospective patients. Local medical societies steadfastly refused to differentiate among licensed doctors, saying all were equally good. As a consequence, patients had no guarantee that the doctor whose name they found in the city directory or the medical society's roster was either properly trained or ethical in his behavior. Only by trial and error could the intelligent patient find a really good doctor and might well waste a great deal of money on incompetent healers in the process. As Harding concluded, "If a man gets sick in this country to-day there is no sure way for him to procure the services of a conscientious and competent medical doctor."[38]

Despite providing services of uneven quality and value, doctors still felt entitled to charge high fees. The rising cost of medical care figured prominently in consumerist complaints. As Kallet and Schlink argued, rapidly rising doctors' bills were driving many Americans into the arms of the proprietary drug industry. "It costs money to be sick, to go to doctors, to specialists and hospitals; it costs more money than most people have or can spare." A woman worrying about a lump in her breast "knows that if she goes to the doctor, it will mean visits to high priced, mysterious, and uncommunicative specialists, costing a year's income." It was far easier for her to believe in the advertising claims of a quack remedy costing seventy-five cents, especially given the business community's insistence that "advertising is essentially honest and in the public interest."[39]

Medical consumerists also turned a jaundiced eye toward the AMA's claims to be a guardian of the consumer's health interests in the drugstore. While praising the work of Arthur Cramp's fraud department, these critics had many more reservations about the AMA's Seal of Approval program and advertising policies. The organization held itself up as a scientific authority yet made profitable deals to get advertising revenue. As Schlink noted, although *Hygeia* did not accept cigarette advertising, the AMA's popular health magazine contained many other ads for products of dubious medical and nutritional value, among them mercurochrome and chocolate milk. In like spirit, Harding pointed out the often glaring contradictions between the medical journals' scientific content and their advertising pages. For example, during an outbreak of influenza in late 1929, an editorial in the *Journal of the American Medical Association* chastised a number of companies for advertising flu remedies when it was clear that the only way to treat the illness was rest, warm drinks, and nourishing food. Yet the same issue of the journal also carried ads for flu treatments including Syrup Thioral Roche, Calcreose, Neutral Acriflavine Throat Troches, and several types of electric vaporizers.[40]

Even worse than the hypocrisy apparent in its advertising policy was the AMA's inability or unwillingness to discourage the overtreating and overcharging of patients for doctors' economic gain. Even a cursory reading of the medical literature suggested an awareness of how commonly doctors practiced fee splitting; general practitioners who recommended patients to specialist colleagues for treatment, most often surgery, got a cut of the specialists' fees. This unethical custom could be eliminated, Harding noted, "if the profession really wished to get rid of it"; instead, it appeared to continue unchecked.[41]

By pointing out medicine's flaws, Harding aimed to awaken his readers to the need to abandon blind trust in medical authority. In his view, patient-consumers should no more passively defer to medical opinion than they did to the messages promoted by "Dr. Copy-Writer" and his radio ballyhoo. Instead, people needed to aspire to being intelligent buyers when it came to the doctor's services as well as the drugstore's nostrums. The same habits of skepticism would serve patient-consumers well in both places.

This approach was clearly laid out in Kellock's 1935 article. Although the *Bulletin* had previously featured articles on how to evaluate drugstore products, "Shopping for Medical Care" represented the publication's most ambitious attempt to apply consumerist skills to doctors' services. In explaining the necessity for this vigilance, Kellock showed considerable familiarity with the problems concerning medical standardization and medical ethics. Citing the Flexner Report and other studies of medical education, she noted that only 10 percent of practicing physicians had been adequately trained in scientific medicine. She also referred to the weakness of professional discipline that allowed some doctors to charge excessively high fees for unneeded treatments.[42]

Kellock's article outlined the duties of the watchdog patient in considerable detail. In some respects, her advice mirrored that given by William Everett Musgrave and other physicians: people should compile a list of "reliable" sources of care, including a general practitioner or internist, a surgeon, and a hospital, before illness struck. But Kellock went on to suggest far more assertive attempts to assess physician quality. Patients should ask pointed questions about qualifications before agreeing to treatment and treat any "evasions and excuses" in response to those requests as "signs of deficiencies." Patients should secure copies of their X-rays and lab reports so that they could easily get second opinions. Finally, Kellock advised reading up on the current state of medical knowledge: "A person suffering from a condition that defies diagnosis or treatment, or who is being given drugs and treatments of which he is doubtful, can go to the nearest medical library, and with the aid of the *Index Medicus*, check up on the points that trouble him." By reading the same medical literature as their doctors did, laypeople could determine the prevailing "consensus of opinion" about proper treatment and thus reject unproven or possibly dangerous measures.[43]

In addition to advocating the "patient as watchdog" approach, medical consumerists critiqued the way physicians organized their practices. Many 1930s reformers argued that the problems with American medicine stemmed largely from its horse-and-buggy style of delivery: a solo practitioner providing care on a fee-for-service basis. As alternatives, some advanced the idea of the prepaid group medical practice, in which a person paid a set amount monthly. Another option was a government-sponsored program modeled on Social Security, in which people paid into a medical fund that they could draw on for support when they became too sick to work.[44]

In expressing an interest in alternatives to fee-for-service medicine, medical consumerists were influenced by the burgeoning field of medical economics. Beginning with the CCMC reports and continuing with work supported by private foundations, academic researchers compiled evidence about the economics of medicine. With many charts and graphs, these studies documented the limitations of the traditional fee-for-service approach. As long as doctors were paid by office visit and procedure, they had no incentive to keep their patients well. In the context of a more commodified, procedure-based style of practice, fee for service offered too big a temptation to practice pocketbook medicine. The answer, reformers argued, was to rethink the fee-for-service system and to devise ways to make medical care more affordable.

The medical profession's response to both the medical consumerists and the academic social scientists was essentially the same: the criticisms were unwarranted and insulting. For example, Consumers' Research's physician subscribers responded to Kellock's piece with "vociferous and numerous" letters of complaint, violently objecting to the idea that patients should shop for a physician the same way they chose a toaster or a refrigerator. According to one Cleveland practitioner, Kellock's approach would only "make people suspicious and critical, an attitude which is directly against good results." A doctor from Wichita Falls, Texas, derided the "suggestion, which is nothing short of silliness, that the patient read up on his condition via the 'Index Medicus'" and declared himself "discouraged and dismayed to find such junk in our highly reveared [sic] CR." Nearly all of the forty letters sent by physicians were similarly hostile.[45]

The AMA took an equally hard line in responding to lay critics. While acknowledging that the depression had created problems for both doctors and patients, its leadership insisted that nothing was fundamentally wrong with the existing system and that doctors were the only ones qualified to fix whatever problems needed fixing. In his editorials in the *Journal of the American Medical Association*, Fishbein described the profession's critics as mentally unbalanced and politically subversive. In 1929, he observed that "the problems of medical practice and of the cost of medical care are today like a patient suffering with a superfluity of advisers, some scientific, some logical, some informed; others ignorant, biased or with the one sided perspective of the situation that a chiropractor has in studying the ailments of the human body." In the absence of competent and informed voices, "popular periodicals have accepted the contributions of the propagandists and loud-speakers," among which the "yawping, sneering, exaggerated and, indeed, comical lucubrations of T. Swann Harding" were the worst.[46]

A 1934 editorial in the *Journal of the Indiana State Medical Association* echoed Fishbein's disdain. It was time, the editor announced, to "blackball those mavericks whom we have reason to suspect of long-haired theories and pop-eyed reforms as regards goose-stepping the medical profession." (Goose stepping was a style of military marching associated with both fascist Germany and Soviet Russia.) Expressing contempt for the new breed of critics, the editor urged that they be sent back to the "farms and forges and ribbon-counters and trash-littered desks and dust-covered law books" from whence they came, or "otherwise, in their guinea-pig-o-mania, they will march our ideals and idealisms, one by one, single file, up that long, last hill for crucifixion."[47]

Physicians' zeal to punish lay critics was evident in the "Milk Bottle Wars." After the CCMC disbanded, two of its former staff members, Edward Sydenstricker and Isidore Falk, went to work at the Milbank Fund, a charitable foundation set up by Alfred Milbank, the head of the Borden milk company. With the blessing of the fund's executive director, John Kingsbury, Sydenstricker and Falk devoted some Milbank funds to studying the workings of voluntary health insurance plans, which they saw as a promising way to finance medical care. Considering any form of health insurance tantamount to what Fishbein termed "medical socialism," conservative physicians organized a 1935 boycott of Borden to protest the actions of Kingsbury and his staff. Borden had recently introduced a new line of so-called prescription products advertised chiefly to physicians, including Biolac, an evaporated baby food, and Beta Lactose, a modified milk sugar product. The boycotters urged their fellow physicians to stop using Borden products in their homes and recommending them to patients and to pressure hospitals to do the same. As Borden began to lose significant money, Milbank bowed to the pressure, fired Kingsbury, and recanted any support for the idea of health insurance.[48]

But while medical conservatives won the Milk Bottle Wars, that success came at a cost. The stridency of physician response to outside criticism reinforced consumerists' conviction that the medical profession was growing too arrogant. As Schlink summed up the response to Kellock's article, "Many physicians have vehemently criticized our drawing attention to defects in medical care in this article. All too many of them, I regret to say, are still holding to the old ground that physicians and organized medicine are pretty much above lay criticism." Likewise, when Rorty wrote about the Milk Bottle Wars in his 1939 book, *American Medicine Mobilizes*, he raised questions about the conflict between democratic values and a medical autocracy. As the debates over medical care continued into the mid- and late 1930s, the AMA's harsh response to any and all critics of medicine would become an increasingly fraught issue, not only in public discussions but within the profession as well.[49]

Medicine at the Crossroads

While lay critics and conservative physicians denounced each other, a broader sense of unease swept through the medical profession. While few doctors subscribed to the consumerist ideal of the skeptical patient, a growing number were willing to grant that all was not well in the doctor's office. In so doing, they were influenced not by reading *100,000,000 Guinea Pigs* or *Consumers' Research* but rather by what they saw in their own practices. These doctors believed that the rising cost of medical care, the uncoordinated spread of specialization, the unevenness of access to good care, and the overtreatment associated with fee splitting were serious problems that needed redress. An influential minority of physicians, including some very distinguished individuals, thus came not only to agree with some lay criticisms of medicine but also to challenge the AMA's refusal to admit the profession's flaws.

That sense of disaffection emerged in a major study of the medical profession funded by the American Foundation. Created in 1925 by Edward Bok, the editor of the *Ladies' Home Journal* who had so staunchly supported the 1906 Pure Food and Drugs Act, it was run after his death in 1930 by his lawyer son, Curtis Bok. As part of a broader "studies in government" series, the younger Bok hired Esther Everett Lape, a social worker with close ties to Eleanor Roosevelt, to conduct a study of medical opinion about the need for reform. To guide her work, Lape formed a medical advisory committee of thirteen prominent doctors, all members in good standing of the AMA, among them surgeon Hugh Cabot of the Harvard Medical School and nephrologist John P. Peters of the Yale Medical School.[50]

With their assistance, Lape chose a sample of more than 2,000 physicians, including both established clinicians and recent graduates of the best medical schools, and sent them a list of questions designed to elicit their thoughts about whether some "essential change" was needed in the medical system. By conducting what in today's parlance would be described as an open-ended survey, Lape aimed to "collect and summarize the experience and thought of medical leaders throughout the country." The result was almost 1,500 pages of testimony, published in 1937 in two massive volumes under the title *American Medicine: Expert Testimony Out of Court*.[51]

Lape's study confirmed that physicians were well aware that the shopping problems described by critical consumers did indeed exist. Their commentaries detailed the many ways that the convergence of modern science and commercialism had complicated the doctor-patient relationship. For example, a New York City specialist shared the sentiments of the medical economists, writing, "Of all things the public buys they are least able to judge the *quality* of the medical care they purchase." The chief surgeon at a West Virginia hospital questioned whether physicians were the best judges of their own worth. When a patient was sick, he wrote, "the medical man is king," and "his slightest word becomes a law; folks scurry at his command." He observed that the "frequent repetition" of this experience "causes him to have a superiority complex—which makes him entirely unfit to fix his place in the national economy."[52]

Many physicians confirmed the uneven qualifications and unscientific behavior about which consumer critics had complained. According to a member of the National Board of Medical Examiners, "The average physician ceases to learn when he is licensed to practice" and thereafter "derives most of his inspiration from the pharmaceutical detail men, who make good livings largely from his ignorance." A number of doctors commented on the sad state of physicians' prescribing habits thanks to the commercial power of the drug companies. They also noted the trend toward overtreatment. Observed an Iowa doctor, "We have in this county twenty doctors struggling to make a living," a situation that inevitably led to "commercialism—to the doing of unnecessary operations." Despite efforts to stop it, doctors reported that fee splitting was very common. And a midwestern physician wrote of the expense being generated by the multiplying number of X-ray machines and diagnostic laboratories in his community: "In my opinion, the layman has a perfect right to ask the question, 'Who is to pay for all this duplication of equipment and effort?'"[53]

In sum, the American Foundation report suggested that far from being the irrational ramblings of neurotic or subversive cranks, the problems patients reported having in the doctor's office were real; the ultimate expert—the physician—recognized problems with the quality, cost, and accessibility of the medical care available to the American public. As a professor of bacteriology and hygiene from a Grade A medical school put it, "The public is not receiving the quality of service to which it is entitled, considering the advances made in the medical sciences in the past century." Moreover, contrary to the AMA orthodoxy, the study correspondents seemed far more willing to consider changes to the traditional fee-for-service system that might improve the situation, from voluntary medical insurance to a national health insurance plan.[54]

The publication of the American Foundation report in the spring of 1937 attracted widespread media attention. When Lape and interviewee Samuel J. Kopetzky went to the June meeting of the AMA to discuss their findings, *Time* covered the trip in detail, including a cover portrait of Morris Fishbein. Given the political conservatism of the magazine's editor, Henry Luce, the reportage was remarkably evenhanded. On the one hand, Fishbein's objections were quoted at length, including his warning, "Shall medicine remain a profession or become a trade?" under his cover portrait. But the article also suggested that some of the reforms Fishbein opposed "embodied so much prudent common sense" that doctors should not dismiss them so quickly. If implemented, "patients would get the world's best medical care, because they would not fear to consult a doctor on account of his bill."[55]

In the wake of the report's publication, Lape's medical advisory committee, led by Cabot and Peters, reformed as a new group, the Committee of Physicians for the Improvement of Medical Care. The committee drafted a set of "Principles and Proposals" designed to counter the AMA's "ten points" or "ten commandments," written in response to the CCMC report. Committee members convinced 430 eminent physicians to sign a declaration that "the health of the people is a direct concern of the government" and calling for a more equitable and prevention-oriented health care policy. Peters's November 1937 release of the declaration and the list of signatories warranted a front-page story in the *New York Times* that opened with the line, "Many noted physicians join 'revolt' against American Medical Association." The press coverage emphasized the stature of the physicians involved, among them Nobel laureate George Minot of Harvard as well as the deans of the leading U.S. medical schools. The signers were described as "insurgents" issuing a "medical declaration of independence" from the conservative AMA leadership, an event hailed "in medical circles as the first open revolt against the hitherto unquestioned authority of the ruling body of America's organized medical profession."[56]

Fishbein struck back, suggesting in an editorial in the *Journal of the Ameri-*

can Medical Association that the signatories had been tricked into endorsing the declaration. Other medical commentators dismissed the American Foundation study as just another piece of "propaganda" and repeated their belief that "the restiveness of the public" was "due solely to the propaganda of foundations, eager to justify their existence, and to the machinations of social workers and lay 'meddlers,' eager to make jobs for themselves under the state medicine schemes they proposed." So intense was the pressure to recant that thirty-two of the original signers withdrew their names.[57]

But the willingness of over 400 prominent physicians in the United States to sign the Cabot-Peters declaration created a "panic in some parts of the medical profession," as Fishbein later recalled. AMA leaders regarded the American Foundation report as far more damaging than the CCMC studies because, as Fishbein put it, "the persons concerned were influential." In the wake of its publication, the thirty-two who recanted were soon replaced by several hundred physicians who asked to sign the petition retroactively. These medical "progressives," as journalists dubbed them, became more outspoken within the AMA; state delegations that had long chafed at Fishbein's politics, in particular those from New Jersey and California, began publicly to criticize him at annual meetings. The Michigan state delegation urged the AMA to create a separate public relations office to combat the negative press physicians were getting, while the progressives spearheaded the formation of the American Medical Students Association, hoping to organize medical students, who were generally more liberal than their elders, into a political lobby.[58]

The *New York Times* published a November 1937 editorial, "Medical Democracy," that suggests how much ground the AMA had lost since 1932, when that newspaper had uncritically endorsed Fishbein's view of the CCMC. The paper praised the proposals put forth by the Committee of 430 as a welcome break with the AMA's "opposition to social progress in medicine." That opposition fueled the "suspicion . . . that the economic status of the private practitioner must be defended against even the semblance of outside interference, though thousands die for lack of competent medical advice and care." The editorial described the insurgents as "enlightened practitioners who are imbued with a deep concern for the national health." Between the AMA's "aimless drifting" and the medical progressives' plan for reform, the editorial concluded, "the choice is easy."[59]

The unrest produced by the American Foundation study and the Committee of 430 Physicians was compounded by the release in late 1937 and early 1938 of the results of the National Health Survey conducted under the auspices of the U.S. Public Health Service. Initiated by Sydenstricker and Falk, the researchers at the center of the Milk Bottle Wars, the survey represented the most ambitious effort yet to document the extent of illness in the United States. Using funds from the Works Progress Administration, they hired unemployed workers to conduct interviews with a representative sample of Americans about the illnesses and treatments they had experienced over the previous year. The scope of the sample was unprecedented: during 1935 and 1936, surveyors interviewed almost 3 million people in nineteen different states. Initial analyses of the data confirmed with statistics what critics had been saying with anecdotes: one in six Americans had suffered a serious illness or physical defect in the previous year, for which almost 30 percent of families had been unable to afford treatment. In Rorty's words, the survey "revealed an appalling volume of unmet medical need, and striking correlations between low incomes and high incidence, duration, and severity of illness."[60]

Nor could the AMA take much comfort in the results of public opinion polls, which were becoming an increasingly popular feature of American political life. Magazines and newspapers not only reported the results of professional pollsters such as Elmo Roper and George Gallup but also conducted their own polls. In September 1938, the *Ladies' Home Journal*, one of the most popular women's magazines of the era, published a poll of its readers' views about the medical profession. The article was part of a yearlong series reporting women's opinions on "the subjects that most concern them," including birth control, war, religion, divorce, and alcohol consumption. By interwar standards, it was a very large sample: 37,000 respondents, chosen to get a wide cross-section of opinion by class, marital status, and "all races and creeds." The results, published in "What Do the Women of America Think about Medicine?" could not have made the AMA very happy.[61]

The results of the poll clearly showed, as author Henry F. Pringle wrote, that "the women of the country want something done—something done to ease the fearful burden that comes when ill health strikes their loved ones." While doctors and social workers debated the pros and cons of different systems of care, women lived with the practical results, "for illness to them is a fact not a theory." The poll suggested that women wanted a system of health insurance, free government-sponsored care for the poor, and free medical care for schoolchildren. The article's impact lay in linking numbers—52 percent of respondents said "doctors' bills are too high"—with personal testimonies, such as one in which a woman wrote, "Right now we are trying to raise $150 to pay the doctor. My husband had his appendix out, but how are we ever going to find the money to pay for it?"[62]

The survey revealed a high level of concern about "the high cost of illness, the fees charged by doctors and the degree to which hospital expenses can wreck any household budget." Not surprisingly, the more affluent the reader, the less likely she was to report being unable to afford medical care. "The woman who has watched her children suffer—possibly even die—because a doctor was beyond reach financially, has a different reaction to the subject of state medicine from that of her well-to-do sister who can afford general practitioners, and specialists as well when they are needed," Pringle noted. Many respondents liked the idea of a medical insurance plan that allowed families to pay three dollars a month toward hospital expenses. In the words of one nineteen-year-old Indiana girl, "I could stop worrying about breaking a leg." But some did worry that under such a plan the care might not be the best. Worried a woman married to a painter, "Doctors wouldn't take as much interest" in patients like her; another woman whose husband was a lawyer agreed, "You'd just get what you paid for. Cheap pay would bring cheap care." But all the women were united about the need to make medical care more affordable for children. According to a woman married to a druggist, "In many cases the children must go without because the parents can't pay," while an insurance executive's wife wrote, "A great deal of misery and anxiety could be prevented by early diagnosis and treatment."[63]

Despite the dryness of the technical debates involved, the drama inherent in the experts' battles over doctors' bills made for good copy in a highly competitive news environment. As a reviewer observed in 1939, "As everyone knows by this time, the medical profession has been taking a pretty thorough going over in the prize-ring of print." Both big-city newspapers and mass-circulation magazines ran stories about the "revolt" among the doctors. Articles about the controversy within the AMA appeared not only in the left-leaning magazines such as the *Nation* and the *New Republic* but also in more mainstream magazines such as the *Saturday Evening Post* and *Time*. And the coverage in the more conservative, business-oriented publications was not necessarily favorable to the AMA.[64]

That trend was evident in a lengthy article on medicine that appeared in *Fortune*, Time-Life's business magazine, in late 1938, only a few months after the *Ladies' Home Journal* story. "The American Medical Association Dissected" provided an overview of the current controversy in terms that male professionals and businessmen could understand. While hailing the AMA's success in transforming itself from a negligible operation into a powerful "trade association," the article provided a long account of the last decade of controversy, starting with the CCMC report, and suggested that the organization deserved much of the criticism it had received. "While Dr. Fishbein is a brilliant promoter he has not displayed much flexibility when faced with new medical and political realities," the article concluded. By refusing to admit any problems with the current practice of medicine, the AMA "has been in the backwash of social forces that are threatening to crumble it."[65]

Press coverage of the "war among the doctors" documented a growing tendency to present the AMA as the medical equivalent of a labor union. Over the course of the 1930s, the phrase "organized medicine" came into widespread use, suggesting that the profession operated as an economic interest group in the same way as "organized labor" or "organized business." Moreover, while the local general practitioner might credibly present himself as an independent entrepreneur, the more affluent sectors of the profession seemed increasingly connected to drug manufacturers and hospital facilities that operated in more corporate ways. As Bernheim wrote in *Medicine at the Crossroads*, "Medicine is Big Business; let there be no illusions about that."[66]

Medicine's arrival as a member of the big-business fraternity seemed confirmed by the Justice Department's 1938 decision to charge the AMA, several of its constituent state societies, and a number of individuals (including Fishbein) with conspiracy to violate antitrust law. The lawsuit grew out of charges that the Washington, D.C., medical society was punishing local doctors who worked with the Group Health Association, an experimental prepaid medical plan organized for employees of the Federal Home Owners Loan Corporation. Under the leadership of Thurman Arnold, an ambitious young assistant attorney general, the antitrust case threatened to become a much more sweeping examination of organized medicine and the state of American medical care.[67]

AMA leaders suspected with good reason that the antitrust suit was timed to soften up medical opposition to the new health insurance bill about to be presented to Congress. Disappointed with President Roosevelt's decision to leave medicine out of the 1935 Social Security Act, out of reluctance to take on AMA opposition, a powerful group of New Deal officials sought to undo what they regarded as a very bad mistake. In 1938, this group, the Interdepartmental Committee on Health and Welfare Activities, convened a National Health Congress in Washington, D.C., to collect testimony about the flaws in the traditional fee-for-service system of medical care.[68]

Addressing that group, Cabot predicted that American medicine was on the verge of a major transformation. One had only to look around, he observed, to see "evidence of a movement of tremendous power." Cabot acknowledged that his generation had been trained to think that doctors alone should dictate the terms of medical care. But now, that entitlement was being challenged. "The consumer, known to the profession as a patient," he said, "is beginning to wake up to the fact that he has a collateral interest in this problem, that he is the boy who is paying the bill or is going to pay it, and that he has a right to a very large word in what is done and in how it is done." In short, physicians could no longer make decisions without taking to heart "the problem of the consumer."[69]

In February 1939, Senator Robert F. Wagner of New York introduced a bill meant to take the first step in that transformation. Although impressively titled the "National Health Bill," it was a comparatively modest set of proposals to let states experiment with federal monies to finance public health services, maternal and infant care, hospital construction, and disability relief. Despite the measure's modest aims, the AMA was gearing up to oppose the plan when World War II broke out in Europe, creating a crisis that put an end to the immediate prospect of reform. As the United States was inexorably drawn into what became a worldwide war, the debates concerning the nation's "medical muddle" were suspended. They resumed in the mid-1940s, as soon as the prospects for victory in the war seemed assured, but on very different political terms.

Many medical progressives remained lukewarm to what today we term the "single-payer system." It was not just conservatives who found the prospect of a New Deal–controlled health care system unappealing. As one of Rorty's reviewers put it, "However efficient the government scientist and hygienist may be, the independent physician, human as he is, is better trained to exercise the priestly functions of the practitioner of medicine than is a government official." Confronted with a choice between an independent doctor and a bureaucratic functionary, many liberal physicians, including members of the Committee of 430, preferred the former.[70] Ultimately the idea of a national health program would fail again, paving the way for a different solution to the problems patients faced in the doctor's office.

Good Patient, Bad Patient

By the late 1930s, the shopping problems Americans faced in making medical choices had reached a higher level of definition but little resolution. A generation of "guinea pig books" had raised wide fears about the safety and effectiveness of many products considered essential to health and well-being. A generation of studies, from the CCMC through the American Foundation report and the National Health Survey, had documented the deficiencies of fee-for-service medicine. Americans had been introduced to a new cast of consumer advocates, medical experts, and journalistic interpreters, all claiming to provide the inside story on medicines and doctors' services. Extensive media coverage of the doctors' revolt meant that laypeople were more likely to know that physicians disagreed over fundamental economic issues and that the AMA functioned not only as a scientific organization but also as a trade association. According to Rorty, a widespread sense existed that "the marriage of medicine and business is a bad marriage" and that "the better half—the professional half—will be sick as long as that marriage lasts, and we, the patients, will in consequence be sick, too, sicker than we need be."[71]

Harold Aaron, medical consultant for Consumers Union, summed up the case for medical consumerism in his 1940 book, *Good Health and Bad Medicine*: "The new Food, Drug and Cosmetic Act is, in some respects, a marked improvement over the old Act, but there are still too many loopholes through which the artless consumer can be peppered by drug advertisers' dum-dum bullets." Given that advertising targeted at laypersons still consumed close to $4 million a year of drug companies' money, their "grip on the minds and pockets of the public is an important feature of American society, and any health book that fails to take this into account, fails to teach." Aaron consequently repeated the advice to cultivate a healthy sense of skepticism: "In health care, next to the ability to buy competent medical care, it is perhaps the most important quality that the consumer should possess." It "will save him much discomfort and disability, not to speak of hard coin."[72]

For medical consumerists like Aaron, the skeptical patient had become the model of the good patient. But the spread of the patient-as-watchdog attitude was by no means universally applauded. Critics of the new mood shared angry doctors' fear that Kellock's advice would undermine the necessary trust between doctor and patient. Many people likely shared the views of the lay reviewer who wrote of Bernheim's *Medicine at the Crossroads*, "Such fluoroscoping of medical failing might be terrifying to the casual reader," and concluded, "Nowhere could a little knowledge be more disturbing." After reading the book, a patient "may wonder if he is being rushed into unnecessary surgery." And "if we turn from scientific medicine, where can we go" for trustworthy advice?[73]

Apparent in these debates was a growing conflict over what it meant to be a "good" patient. One model conformed to what a later generation would term a compliant patient: one who knew just enough to make him or her willing to accept a physician's authority and to do whatever the doctor ordered. The other, newer model was closer to what we today would call an "engaged" or "empowered" patient: knowledgeable enough to differentiate good and bad practice. The skills of checking facts, asking questions, and second-guessing medical opinion had become desirable components of modern adulthood. Underlying the growing divergence between these models of the good patient were two unresolved issues of growing importance: the difficulty of agreeing on scientific truth, and the tensions between personal autonomy and the need to defer to expert knowledge.

The interwar debates over medical consumerism exposed the weaknesses of looking to scientific methods and standards to induce patient compliance. As both lay and medical critics were realizing, the ideal of a more scientific medicine had the potential to complicate rather than clarify the issue of trust between doctor and patient. If physicians disagreed over what really worked, how could laypeople know whom to trust? Observed the publisher George D. Eaton, "The medical profession has for a long time admitted that from 40 to 60 percent of [their] diagnoses are wrong."[74] So how could patients not start to ask questions? In the face of this dilemma, many physicians could only promise to try to achieve greater scientific certainty and better communicate that certainty to their patients.

But physicians who agreed that medical consumerists had some cause for complaint did not see their skepticism as helpful. Walter Alvarez expressed the common perception that laypeople's attempts to influence medicine had always been to the profession's detriment: "Every time we have tried to stop the doors against ignoramuses, the public has opened them again, and allowed more to get in under some subterfuge." He believed that it consti-tuted "a big mistake" to think "that the average layman will have higher ideals than we have," citing the new Nazi regime in Germany, where "quacks were boosted into high positions." And "average" or "ignorant" patients were not the only ones who held mistaken views; the highly educated did so as well: "If you want to find a lot of half cracked people who, when they are ill, are particularly fond of going to chiropractors, osteopaths and Christian science practitioners, go to a University town." In short, Alvarez did not believe that the "intelligent" public constituted a reliable support for a more scientific medicine.[75]

Understandably, physicians found it easier to accept criticism from other physicians than from laypeople. Debates over medical consumerism under-lined what publisher Eaton termed the "strategy of position": the reaction generated by an idea depended on who suggested it (lay critic or doctor), where it appeared (in a newspaper or a private letter), and who was reading it (layperson or doctor).[76] Doctors resented having their supposed defects dragged before the public by publishers and editors eager for sales. But for the same reasons, laypeople believed that fellow patient-consumers better understood their concerns about finding good doctors or paying medical bills than Morris Fishbein did. They appreciated a frank discussion of the "doctor's dilemma" more than the medical profession's tendency to deny that any economic conflict of interest existed.

Medical consumerism also exposed the growing sense of tension between professionalism and individualism. Doctors and patients had to grapple with two seemingly irreconcilable trends: the spread of education and democracy and the personal autonomy that went with it, and the growing deference to expertise and authority seemingly required by the advance of scientific knowledge. American culture stressed the importance of individual autonomy and the duty to cultivate a personal authenticity through reasoned choice and self-discipline. At the same time, the rapid expansion and specialization of knowledge constrained what the ordinary person could understand, thus increasing the need to defer to scientific expertise. Perhaps more than any other area of American life, the doctor-patient relationship raised fundamental questions about how modern consumer-citizens were supposed to both think for themselves and defer appropriately to expert authority.

At the same time, the interwar version of medical consumerism remained constrained by its own limitations. Its advocates positioned themselves as spokespeople for what Harding claimed were the 75 percent of Americans who were neither rich enough to afford whatever medical care they wanted nor poor enough to be eligible for charity care. In reality, the language of critical consumerism, with its frequent use of phrases such as "intelligent buyer" and "educated patient," reflected the anything-but-average background of its leading exponents. Not only academic types such as Davis and Falk but also more popular commentators such as Chase, Schlink, Kallet, Rorty, Harding, and Lamb were college graduates at a time when the average American had only an eighth-grade education and someone who had completed high school was considered well educated. A significant subset of these authors had not only college degrees but postgraduate or professional training as well. Put simply, they had a degree of education that made them feel able to understand the complexities of the modern world and that they deserved respect not only from business leaders but also from doctors. This preponderance of white, highly educated, and male voices made critical consumerism so hard to ignore.[77]

To stand toe to toe with the druggist and the doctor, critical consumerism emphasized the growing clout of the "intelligent" and "educated" patient-consumer. This kind of careful parsing of labels and advertising in the light of modern science and economics was likely to be difficult for people who lacked formal education. The ideology of critical consumerism projected a strategy for lifting all boats: the better-educated consumers would pave the way for improvements that would benefit everyone else. In fact, middle-class white families had no monopoly on the concept of "constructively critical" habits of mind: as the era's frequent food riots, store boycotts, and other consumer-themed protests suggested, immigrant and nonwhite families had their own conceptions of market fairness and their own strategies for trying to achieve it. But members of those groups could back their preferences with less financial and political clout than their better-educated contemporaries.

Last but not least, medical consumerism had an Achilles' heel that would become all too evident in the years to come: the potential to blame patient-consumers for their bad choices. As Jerome Ephraim concluded in his 1937 guide *Take Care of Yourself*, every American had to learn "what constituted truly sound practice in body care" as well as to resist the misleading claims of modern advertising. People could not wait for government or business to look out for their well-being but had to take responsibility for protecting themselves. "Deception and dishonesty and the accompanying wastefulness and dishonesty and threat to the public health would not be profitable or even possible if the consuming public were of a higher level of intelligence, and alertness." Concluded Ephraim, "My moral is this: Consumer, reform *yourself!*" But in the decades to come, the expectation that Americans should be more skillful in shopping for medical care would prove hard to fulfill.[78]

PART TWO

Free Enterprise Medicine
The 1940s to the 1960s

{FIVE}
The Fourth Necessity

In December 1944, with the end of World War II in sight, the business magazine *Fortune* carried a lengthy article on "U.S. Medicine in Transition." It opened with a sharp observation: "Nobody gives a hoot whether or not night clubs or even movies are made cheaply available to all, but people who cannot find or pay for proper medical care are resentful, as are those who see the effects of such deprivations upon neighbors, and in the long run, upon the community." Resentment was rife, the author suggested, because medical costs had outstripped the average American's ability to pay them. "The best medical care is bought by the rich and—in some large cities—obtained free by the very poor, but to get first-rate care the middle-income group must mortgage itself." Given that 29 percent of American men inspected for the draft were rejected for medical reasons, "the state of American health is nothing to cheer about." The AMA thus had only itself to blame, *Fortune* suggested, for the fact that 68 percent of respondents recently polled thought it was "a good idea" to expand the Social Security system to cover physician and hospital care. If the AMA wished to stave off the American equivalent of the British National Health Service, its standpatters needed to rethink their opposition to private medical insurance.[1]

The *Fortune* article heralded the fact that at war's end, debates about the nation's medical system would resume. If nothing else, the prewar battles had firmly established the importance of medical care as the "fourth necessity" of modern life, as one contemporary put it, on a par with food, clothing, and housing. Having fought long and hard for their democratic way of life, Americans wanted a postwar order that reflected those values, including more and better medical care. As U.S. assistant attorney general Wendell Berge told an audience of physicians in late 1944, "Millions of soldiers, returned from the front, are going to demand for themselves and their families the instruments of health to which they are entitled." Predicting that a "new medical order" was on the way, Berge advised doctors to heed the maxim "if you can't stop a movement, join it."[2]

While agreeing that change was inevitable, commentators differed sharply on what shape the postwar medical order would take. While a minority advocated for an American equivalent to Britain's National Health Service, the majority agreed that a more "free enterprise" system would better suit the nation. But that term had very different meanings in the mid-1940s. For many business leaders and their political allies, free enterprise required that the federal government step out of their way and allow wartime trends toward concentration of economic power to accelerate even if prices rose as a consequence. For New Dealers and consumer advocates, free enterprise meant that the government would promote competition in industry and moderate rapid hikes in prices. In the late 1940s, the business-backed model of free enterprise prevailed, creating a medical economy that moved in the opposite direction from what consumerists had hoped for.[3]

In the short run, these free enterprise modifications to the medical economy laid the foundation for an extraordinary expansion of the health care system. Through a complex process of regulatory compromise and voluntary action, government, business, and medical leaders brought American medicine into even closer alignment with the dynamics of postwar consumer capitalism. These dynamics brought a dramatic upsurge in the number of medical products and services available to American patients. But in the long run, free enterprise medicine not only failed to solve the underlying problems that produced the 1930s unrest but ultimately made them worse. The postwar triumph of the "American way" of medical care led inexorably to more consumer dissatisfaction, which would build to new heights in the 1950s and 1960s.

Free Enterprise Medicine

The new medical order that emerged in the late 1940s rested on a series of important political developments. While unwilling to pass any kind of national insurance program, the U.S. Congress strove to advance the cause of "medical democracy" by other means.[4] Instead of guaranteeing a right to medical care, legislators voted to spend public funds on hospital construction and basic medical research as a means to yield more and better treatment. To make that treatment affordable, the federal government looked to the private sector for help, using tax policy to encourage the growth of employee insurance plans. In this fashion, postwar political and business leaders hoped to create a free enterprise alternative to "socialized" medicine.

The first step toward expansion came in 1946 when Congress passed the

Hill-Burton Act, which funneled federal funds into hospital construction and expansion. Over the next two decades, Hill-Burton funds would be used on almost 5,000 projects, many of them in rural areas that previously had had no hospitals. The program proved very popular, giving local communities a new institution to be proud of while creating more "doctors' workshops" for medical education and private practice. At the same time, Congress vastly increased funding for medical research, from about $4 million in 1947 to $100 million by 1957. Postwar political leaders found appealing the idea of tackling cancer, mental illness, and other dread diseases through "a medical research program equal to the Manhattan Project," as the National Health Education Research Committee urged in 1958. Taxpayer dollars helped to build up the National Institutes of Health (NIH) in Bethesda, Maryland, as the hub of what a later generation would christen the "medical-industrial complex": a network of researchers located in American universities and scientific institutes whose careers depended on the generation of medical innovations.[5]

These investments paid off quickly, as laboratory-based researchers produced new drugs and vaccines and hospital-based clinicians developed more sophisticated forms of treatment for many ailments, including heart disease and cancer. But despite the public tax subsidies invested in research laboratories and hospitals, the new products and services associated still came with a potentially unaffordable price tag. If the United States was not going to develop a government-sponsored insurance program, what would it offer instead? As befit a free enterprise system, the preferred solution became the purchase of another new product, namely the private health insurance plan.[6]

The concept of private insurance originated as a means to cover hospital care, the largest and most unpredictable of patient-consumer expenses. In 1929, Baylor Hospital in Dallas introduced the first prepaid group hospital plan: by paying a small fee each month, participants were enrolled in what became known as the Baylor plan. Having people regularly set aside small sums for medical emergencies was an appealing extension of already established "insurance habits." According to one Baylor official, "We spend a dollar or so at a time for cosmetics and do not notice the high cost." By the same token, "the ribbon counter clerk can pay 50¢, 75¢, or $1 a month, yet if she endeavored to do this by herself it would take about twenty years to set aside a large hospital bill." With the Baylor plan, however, "a thousand ribbon counter clerks can go together and protect themselves over night."[7]

In response to Baylor's success, other hospitals began to develop similar plans. Fearing that competition to sign up subscribers might create disruptive price wars among local hospitals, a group of hospital administrators formed

Blue Cross, a nonprofit company that let participants pick the hospital of their choice for treatment. Blue Cross then paid the hospital directly rather than requiring the patient to do so, a "service benefit" that was very popular with subscribers. And since it did not have to provide returns to shareholders, Blue Cross promised to keep its premiums affordable while providing a steady, reliable stream of income to hospitals, a tremendous boon during the Great Depression. Blue Cross's success subsequently led to the development of Blue Shield, a parallel plan to cover physicians' fees for hospital services.[8]

While popular with employers and employees, these new-style insurance plans aroused concerns among doctors who fervently believed that "no third party must be permitted to come between the patient and his physician in any medical relation," as the AMA House of Delegates had voted in 1934. This opposition was especially intense regarding plans that provided for payment of physician fees, so enrollment in Blue Shield lagged far behind that in Blue Cross. In time, that resistance softened as individual physicians discovered the ease with which they got paid with Blue Shield plans. Meanwhile, voluntary plans continued to attract subscribers; on the eve of World War II, about 10 percent of Americans had insurance that covered hospital costs.[9]

Wartime policies facilitated the expansion of coverage as union leaders accepted wage limits in exchange for employer contributions to workers' medical insurance. That approach became particularly attractive after the Internal Revenue Service ruled in 1943 that insurance payments by both employer and employee were exempt from taxation, an exemption later made permanent with the 1954 revision of the Internal Revenue Code. While some labor leaders preferred more progressive alternatives, such as union-run medical clinics or prepaid medical plans of the type pioneered by Kaiser Permanente, they were often willing to settle for the Blues' more conservative approach.[10]

For its part, the AMA faced a series of political setbacks in the 1940s that softened its opposition to private health insurance. After years of litigation, the Supreme Court in 1944 finally decided the 1938 antitrust suit in favor of the Justice Department, agreeing that organized medicine's opposition to prepaid medical plans, in this case the Group Health Association of Washington, D.C., represented an illegal restraint of trade under the Sherman Antitrust Act. While modest in its legal reasoning, the 1944 decision represented a victory for a type of medical practice that the mainstream profession found anathema: doctors on a salary. The AMA tried to downplay the importance of the Court's decision, but as Morris Fishbein, the longtime editor of the *Journal of the American Medical Association* and a defendant in the case, admitted, the decision served "to convict the AMA in the eyes of the people as being a predatory, antisocial monopoly."[11]

At the same time, the AMA faced the return of an even more repugnant enemy—reformers bent on the passage of some kind of national health insurance. In 1943, even before the war's end, New York senator Robert F. Wagner had reintroduced the bill that had generated such intense battles in the late 1930s. After Franklin Roosevelt died in April 1945, Harry Truman assumed the presidency and soon made clear his determination to push for a Social Security–style government health insurance plan financed by payroll contributions. The decision of Great Britain, America's closest ally in the recent war, to set up its National Health Service in 1946 gave Truman reason to think he could succeed.[12]

These political setbacks further deepened the lines of division already apparent in the depression-era "war among the doctors." Concerned that an unholy alliance between liberal New Dealers and their journalist allies was softening public opinion toward the idea of national health insurance, a vocal and influential minority within the AMA urged its leadership to change political course. In response to those worries, the board of trustees in 1946 hired a public relations firm, Raymond Rich Associates, to assess the association's public standing and suggest how to improve it. The results were not reassuring: the Rich report found a widespread perception that the AMA put physicians' economic interests ahead of patients' well-being. To combat that impression, the firm urged the AMA to soften its opposition to voluntary health insurance and replace Fishbein with a more conciliatory public spokesman. The AMA board of trustees chose not to act on the report, trusting that a Republican would win the presidency in 1948 and put an end to discussions about national health insurance. When Harry Truman unexpectedly won reelection, the AMA leadership embraced a dramatic makeover of the group's public image.[13]

This makeover began with a national campaign on behalf of private health insurance developed by another public relations firm, Whitaker and Baxter. Invoking Cold War themes of democracy versus totalitarianism, the husband-and-wife team of Clem Whitaker and Lenore Baxter developed a patriotic brief on behalf of a distinctly American way of financing medical care. As Whitaker explained to a meeting of New England doctors, "Hitler and Stalin and the socialist government of Great Britain all have used the opiate of socialized medicine to deaden the pain of lost liberty and lull the people into non-resistance." Americans needed to reject this "Old World contagion of compulsory health insurance," which "if allowed to spread to our New World, will mark the beginning of the end of free institutions in America." As a more concrete example of what Americans were fighting to maintain, the campaign featured reproductions of Luke Fildes's painting *The Doctor*, which idealized the sacred tie between doctor and patient.[14]

In what would become a public relations legend, the Whitaker and Baxter campaign helped burnish the image of private insurance as the foundation of free enterprise medicine, keeping "politics out of medicine" and honoring patients' "sacred right" to choose their own physicians. After three years and almost $5 million worth of investment, financed by a special fee assessed against every member, the AMA scuttled Truman's legislation. Recognizing that its lobbying had proved far more effective than the president's efforts, Truman's adviser Oscar Ewing concluded that only an equally well funded "American Patients Association" could ever hope to match the AMA's influence.[15]

Now that it had the AMA's imprimatur, the private insurance idea became even more popular among political and business leaders. Its respectability was confirmed by the Eisenhower administration's willingness to allow the tax-exempt status of business spending on medical insurance to become part of the 1954 tax code. Medical insurance quickly became part of the fringe benefit packages offered to white-collar executives as well as elite union workers. Eager to compete with the private sector, city and state governments began to provide the same benefits for public employees.[16]

Moreover, the success of the nonprofit Blue Cross/Blue Shield plans inspired for-profit insurance companies, which had previously hesitated to write medical policies, to offer their own coverage. To compete with the Blues, which signed up everyone at the same rate, a practice known as community rating, commercial plans adopted experience rating, setting premiums according to the enrollee's health status and keeping costs low by signing up younger, healthier people. Commercial plans also kept costs down by setting high deductibles (amounts that patients had to pay before insurance coverage began) and by excluding maternity care, the kind of hospital utilization that young families were most likely to need. Because for-profit commercial plans offered superior cost-saving features, many employers came to prefer such plans to the Blues. To win them back, the Blues began to add cost-saving features such as deductibles.[17]

During the 1950s, private health insurance became "a booming competitive industry," as economists Herman Somers and Anne Somers wrote, with more than 700 companies offering a wide range of medical plans. By 1959, 128 million Americans had some level of coverage: around 72 percent had insurance for hospitalization expenses, 66 percent had coverage for surgical fees, and 47 percent had coverage for medical fees connected with hospital stays. The majority of those covered, 65 percent, were enrolled in group plans, usually sponsored by employers; individual plans remained far more expensive to purchase and limited in their coverage. While most insurance worked on the traditional fee-for-service model, prepaid group plans, such as Kaiser Permanente, Group Health of America, and Health Insurance Plan of New York, continued to grow thanks to their more comprehensive array of covered services.[18]

Support from mid- to large-sized American businesses helped drive the expansion of private insurance plans. While small businesses found their expense prohibitive, companies with large numbers of employees could cover their cost and saw many advantages in doing so, starting with the fact that such spending was tax-exempt. Medical insurance plans kept employees loyal to the company. As an advertisement in *Newsweek* for the Key Men Group Accident and Sickness Insurance Company promised, "This is the kind of security your key men need—the kind that ties their future to that of your company." At the same time, when employees left the company's payroll, the obligation to cover their hospital bills ceased. Employers also liked the personal responsibility built into the system of payroll deductions and deductibles.[19]

Advocates of free enterprise principles pointed to the rapid expansion of private insurance plans as proof that Americans did not want a government-sponsored program of health insurance. Insurance executives, businessmen, and medical leaders praised the private option as a better way of financing medical care than the "socialistic" plans of other countries. A generous insurance plan constituted a just reward for the most productive members of the workforce. By relying on employee contributions and using deductibles and copays to discourage unnecessary doctor's visits, it reinforced the principles of hard work and discipline that had made the United States a great nation. In short, private health insurance plans seemed like the ideal solution to the "problem of the consumer."[20]

But as quickly became apparent, the growing availability of private insurance hardly resolved the difficulties attendant to paying doctors' bills. With the exception of a few plans negotiated by very powerful labor unions, most insurance plans required workers to make substantial payroll contributions. Some companies matched their employees' contributions on a 50–50 basis, though others paid far less. Many plans also had high deductibles or required copays to discourage overuse of doctors' services. Even after the maximum reimbursements had been reached, many patients who contracted serious illnesses found themselves with onerous bills to pay.[21]

Moreover, most private plans covered only hospital-based care, following the reasoning that patient-consumers could and should finance more routine costs of care on their own. As medical costs rose, the burden of this out-of-pocket expense grew as well. Patient-consumers postponed seeing doctors to save money but then got sick and ended up with large hospital bills, for which they were still partly responsible. The logic common within the insurance industry (provide more care and patients will overuse it) conflicted with the logic associated with preventive medicine (intervene early in the disease process and circumvent a more expensive illness). On this count, the prepaid group plans covering routine care clearly seemed to have an advantage. As an alternative, insurance companies began to offer "major medical" plans that covered a wider range of services. Liberty Mutual became the first company to offer such a plan in 1949, and by 1960, about 12 percent of individual plans offered more comprehensive coverage—at a much higher cost. Correcting flaws in private insurance plans by expanding what they covered become a common strategy, but one that ultimately did little to hold down medical costs.[22]

The cost problem stemmed from the fact that while private insurers set up barriers to consumer overutilization of medical care, they provided no such measures to guard against a different kind of moral hazard—the temptation for providers to raise fees and offer more treatments for patients with insurance. By letting hospitals and physicians set their own rates of reimbursement, the new funding system set in motion a powerful inflationary force. Because more patients had coverage, providers felt entitled to raise their charges as well as to bill patients for additional services. Observed one indignant labor spokesman, the growing availability of insurance seemed to encourage some doctors and hospitals "to color professional ethics with the business ethics of charging all the traffic will bear."[23]

Insisting that doctors were too high-minded to take undue advantage of their patients, defenders of the medical profession claimed that the rising cost of medical care was a straightforward reflection of its higher quality and technological sophistication. Critics begged to differ: Anthony Remuglia, a researcher working for the California Congress of Industrial Organizations, told Truman's Health Commission in 1952, "Doctor control, like any one-sided control, leads to abuses sooner or later." Those fears seemed borne out by a scandal that same year involving the California Physicians' Services, a nonprofit insurance plan sponsored by the California Medical Association, in which almost 200 physicians were discovered to have billed for services that they had not provided.[24]

Meanwhile, the "American way" of private insurance was showing yet another very serious flaw. By tying insurance only to some kinds of employment, it left substantial numbers of citizens with no coverage at all. The ranks of the uninsured included the many workers whose employers did not offer benefits, as well as the self-employed unable to afford the high cost of individual plans. It also included retired people, a grave disadvantage given that the loss of insurance came at precisely the time when older Americans began to need more care than ever before. For all its "booming competitive" bustle, the insurance industry had little interest in developing plans for low-income workers and the elderly. To make matters worse, the price inflation brought about by private insurance plans raised the cost of care for the uninsured as well. Over the course of the 1950s, the plight of the uninsured, especially the elderly, became an increasingly important political issue.

Promoted with such patriotic fervor during the early Cold War years, private insurance plans could not deliver on their promises of anxiety-free medical care. While much of the criticism came from advocates of government-sponsored insurance, even supporters of the private solution began to worry about the growing gap between Americans with and without insurance as well as the lack of comprehensiveness in what conventional plans covered. As doubts grew about the rationality and fairness of the private insurance system, so too did questions about the medical profession's economic motivations in supporting that system. Having championed the American way, including the right to be reimbursed at their "usual and customary rates," doctors would soon find the defects of private insurance laid at their doorstep.

The Doctors' Drugs

During the same years that its fate grew more entangled with the economics of private insurance, the medical profession also became more dependent on another industry undergoing a profound transformation: pharmaceuticals. Following passage of the landmark Food, Drug, and Cosmetic Act of 1938, a combination of scientific innovation, corporate reorganization, and government intervention led to dramatic changes in the drug business. A generation of new wonder drugs came on the market and fundamentally transformed the practice of medicine. Ironically, the more exacting requirements for consumer-friendly labeling and directions for use contained in the 1938 law helped stimulate the redefinition of so-called doctors' drugs—those available by prescription only—as products to be delivered with a minimum of information for the patient-user. Along with their rising cost, the "black box" nature of postwar prescription drugs would become a focal point for consumer concern. And as with private medical insurance, the medical profession would find itself held responsible for the problems that developed in the new drug order.

Free enterprise principles played out very differently in pharmaceuticals than in the medical insurance marketplace. The insurance industry's postwar expansion involved growing competition among nonprofit and for-profit companies and attracted a host of new vendors; in contrast, the drug industry moved toward a greater concentration of economic power in the hands of fewer and larger companies. While those companies produced many new prescription products, the methods of promoting and pricing them became more uniform. Even more than with private insurance, the changing prescription drug marketplace provoked debates over how well free enterprise principles were working for patient-consumers' benefit.

Those debates reflected wartime changes that catapulted a small group of American companies to the forefront of the international drug industry. In 1942, the Office for Scientific Research and Development, a federal agency created to help the U.S. military, enlisted a select group of drug companies to boost production of penicillin. That program's success in engineering a massive output of high-quality product transformed the entire drug industry. Companies able and willing to invest in a more industrial model of research and development enjoyed unprecedented dominance over their smaller, more traditional counterparts. While their new drug products became a source of national pride, the changing configuration of the pharmaceutical industry also aroused concerns about its growing size and ability to minimize competition.[25]

In a 1944 article, "Science and Monopoly," Assistant Attorney General Wendell Berge tried to sound the alarm about those dangers. Wartime exigencies had led to the "concentration of productive facilities in the hands of a relatively small number of gigantic corporations." While Berge believed that large companies should be allowed to profit from their ability to concentrate talent and capital, he insisted that "it is not in the public interest to allow the small competitors to be killed off in the uneven fight." He warned that "when competition is absent the consumer suffers not only from exorbitant prices but from inferiority of products." In 1945 testimony to Congress, Berge took an even harder line: "Cartel domination of essential medical products has jeopardized the health and welfare of millions in this country and elsewhere." Reflecting that concern, under Berge's direction the Justice Department blocked the Wisconsin Alumni Research Foundation from patenting the process for synthesizing vitamin D on the grounds that vitamins needed to be manufactured as widely and cheaply as possible to promote the public's health.[26]

But as the postwar political climate grew more conservative, Berge's New Deal faith that antitrust regulation was essential to maintaining a free enterprise culture fell decidedly out of favor. In Congress, conservative southern Democrats joined Republicans to block any continuation of New Deal policies. What Truman nicknamed the Do-Nothing Congress was "not in the mood," as one journalist put it, for further antitrust action. In 1947, Berge departed from government service for private practice, an event widely noted as the end to the New Deal era of trust-busting. As a consequence, pharmaceutical companies were able to influence government regulation in ways that proved very beneficial to their interests.[27]

One very important set of changes involved patent law. Reflecting a nineteenth-century association of inventions with machinery and manufacturing, patent law initially forbade patenting the products of "nature," including medicines derived from organic sources. Thus penicillin, the 1940s wonder drug derived from mold, received no patent, even though major innovations had been required to turn it into a therapeutically usable substance. In the absence of a patent, many different companies began producing penicillin, causing the price to plummet from almost $4,000 a pound in 1945 to $282 a pound in 1950. While a boon to widespread use, the penicillin model gave companies little incentive to discover new antibiotics. Pharmaceutical companies consequently began to seek patent protection as a way to recover their investments in research and enhance their competitive positions relative to each other.[28]

In that quest, Merck won a key 1948 ruling from the U.S. Patent Office that allowed the company to patent the chemical process needed to synthesize its new antibiotic, streptomycin, derived from a soil bacterium. Merck received the patent on the grounds that streptomycin was a "new composition of matter" made valuable only through the process the company had developed. With concerns about cartelization and price gouging still intense, Merck agreed to a request from Selman Waksman, who headed the lab where the drug was discovered, not to exercise exclusive patent rights; instead, the company agreed to license the new drug for manufacture by other companies, a solution that had emerged in Great Britain as a pragmatic way to balance profitability with access to valuable new medicines. Other drug companies quickly took up the proffered opportunity; like penicillin, streptomycin was widely manufactured as a generic drug without a brand name, and its price fell accordingly.[29]

As wartime memories of price gouging faded, pharmaceutical companies grew far less willing to be so generous, preferring instead the "integrated" model of development: seeking to patent new drugs and regulate their supply to keep prices high during the patent's term, customarily seventeen years from its issuance. A 1952 revision to patent law formalizing the recognition of a medicinal drug as "a new composition of nature" encouraged the turn to the integrated model. Even more important, in defining what constituted a new composition, the Patent Office proved willing to patent drugs that differed only in very slight ways from existing products.[30]

The result was a wave of new medicines that differed relatively little from each other and remained more stable in price. A pattern first set with new antibiotics, it applied as well to subsequent "wonder drugs" such as cortisone and both major and minor tranquilizers. While the new patent system intensified competition among pharmaceutical companies, it did little to reduce the prices consumers paid for the drugs. Each company now developed its own lines of antibiotics, steroid preparations, and psychoactive drugs, priced essentially the same regardless of brand. A company's profits rested on its ability to persuade physicians to favor its brand over the competition through the intensive marketing system known as detailing.[31]

These developments helped to make prescription drugs far more expensive by the mid-1950s than they had been in the 1930s, a trend that increased critical scrutiny of the pharmaceutical industry. At the same time, the 1938 Food, Drug, and Cosmetic Act led to important changes in how drugs were sold that left patient-consumers not only with higher price tags but also with a lack of information about their prescription medications. Ironically, the law's provisions intended to meet popular demands for better labeling and instructions for use sharpened the distinction between over-the-counter and prescription drugs in ways that made the latter even more mysterious.

With the exception of medications covered by narcotic and poison laws, most drugs prior to 1938 could be sold either by prescription or over the counter. The 1938 law had little concern with sharpening the distinction between the two categories. In fact, the distinction was mentioned only in one place, section 502, which gave the FDA the right to exempt some drugs from the law's labeling requirements because they were deemed too dangerous for use without a physician's supervision. Such drugs or devices were to bear a label reading, "Caution: to be dispensed only by or on the prescription of a physician." The law left unclear who should determine which drugs should be sold by prescription only and on what grounds.[32]

In the first six months after the law's passage, the FDA set about issuing advisory statements about which drugs were so toxic or otherwise dangerous that they required the so-called caution legend. Pharmaceutical companies quickly realized that designating a product as for sale by prescription only saved them the trouble of meeting the act's more stringent standards for labeling and instructions for use. Withdrawing products from over-the-counter sale was so attractive a strategy that companies began to use it on drugs that had been in use for decades and posed none of the dangers associated with newer drugs such as sulfanilamide, which had sparked the law's passage. As one retail pharmacist noted, the 1938 law allowed a manufacturer "to confine a medicine he makes to a prescription though it be nothing more than charcoal or molasses."[33]

Other companies used the law's vagueness to go in the opposite direction, marketing powerful drugs for general use on the model of aspirin or vitamins. Despite widespread agreement that sulfa drugs, barbiturates, and amphetamines were exactly the sort of medications that the caution legend was meant to cover, over-the-counter sales of these drugs, both in drugstores and elsewhere, boomed in the 1940s, with disturbing consequences. In 1941, a new over-the-counter sulfa treatment for gonorrhea was accidently contaminated with phenobarbital, leading to some seventy deaths and many more injuries. By 1947, drug companies had introduced more than 1,500 different kinds of barbiturates, and hospitals reported a sharp upsurge in overdose cases. Amphetamines, known as pep pills and widely promoted among soldiers as a way to stay sharp during combat, raised similar concerns.[34]

While enabling manufacturers to maximize profits, the 1938 law's lack of clarity about what drugs should be sold with the caution legend created massive confusion for pharmacists and patients. The "uncontrolled and promiscuous use of the prescription legend label" meant that drugstore shelves now sold rafts of identical drugs, some labeled by one company as for use by prescription only, others packaged as safe for sale directly to the consumer. Old, familiar remedies were being sold by prescription, while powerful, potentially addictive drugs were being sold over the counter. Left "operating in a sea of doubt," as one observer put it, retail pharmacists had to sort out consumers' confusion, and the 1938 law made pharmacists, not manufacturers, liable for prosecution if consumers were harmed.[35]

FDA officials desperately wanted to impose a more consistent standard for what drugs required the legend designation, but the law was not written clearly enough to allow them easily to assert this power. In 1944, amid mounting concern about wartime use of both sulfa drugs and barbiturates, the agency had issued a rule restricting the legend designation to drugs known to be toxic or dangerous. Drug manufacturers immediately protested on the grounds that the FDA had no authority to impose this limitation. The rule remained in force, but companies continued to use the prescription legend for many products not considered in the least dangerous. Putting a stop to that practice required a case-by-case prosecution that that agency lacked the resources to undertake.[36]

Instead of pressuring the drug manufacturers or the medical profession to clear up the prescription drug muddle, the FDA went after the weakest link in the prescription drug chain of sale—pharmacists. In a landmark case that eventually went to the U.S. Supreme Court, the FDA filed suit against Sullivan's Pharmacy in Columbus, Georgia. Owner Jordan James Sullivan had built a substantial clientele by selling sulfa drugs over the counter to soldiers stationed at nearby Fort Benning so that they could treat themselves for gonorrhea. After two FDA agents posing as soldiers bought the drug, the agency charged Sullivan with violating the 1938 law because he repackaged the drugs, originally delivered in a bulk package with the appropriate caution and instruction labels, into a smaller container without the accompanying information. Overturning earlier court rulings in Sullivan's favor, the Supreme Court in 1948 upheld the government's position that the FDA had the power "to safeguard the consumer by applying its requirements to articles from the moment of their introduction into interstate commerce all the way to the moment of their delivery to the ultimate consumer."[37]

Invoking the *Sullivan* decision, Paul Dunbar, the head of the FDA's drug division, immediately announced the agency's intention to enforce a more stringent policy on the refilling of prescriptions in general. By long-standing tradition, a patient who had a prescription for a nonnarcotic drug could refill it whenever he or she wanted. Although medical and pharmaceutical societies had long objected to the practice, it remained widely accepted. As of the early 1950s, an estimated 40 percent of all prescription drugs were being dispensed as refills.[38] In an October 1948 speech to the National Association of Retail Druggists, the main trade association representing the nation's 50,000 independent drugstore operators, Dunbar announced the FDA's intention to put a stop to that practice. As Dunbar explained, the FDA wanted to enforce the prescription's importance "as a written expression of the physician's will and purpose that the individual patient for whom he is prescribing be furnished a specific quantity of a drug for use by that patient under the physician's direction and supervision." To continue to refill a prescription without consulting the physician made refilling the medication "in logic and in fact not distinguishable from an over-the-counter sale of the drug." To enforce that distinction, the proposed rules required a doctor's consent for each refill. Any pharmacist who violated the new rules could face hefty fines and imprisonment.[39]

Not surprisingly, pharmacists were outraged that the FDA seemed to be singling them out as responsible for the prescription drug mess. If pharmacists were going to be prosecuted for selling sulfa drugs over the counter or refilling prescriptions without a doctor's approval, surely they were entitled to clearer-cut guidance about which drugs should carry the legend warning. The refill controversy thus quickly broadened into a much bigger debate about how medicines were being dispensed. During the waning days of the Truman administration, two pharmacists who served as Democratic members of Congress, Representative Carl Durham of North Carolina and Senator Hubert Humphrey of Minnesota, began to hold hearings on the problems surrounding drug dispensing. Out of their deliberations emerged a set of changes to the 1938 law that came to be known as the Durham-Humphrey Amendments.[40]

In testimony reminiscent of Ruth deForest Lamb's "Chamber of Horrors" exhibit, members of the National Association of Retail Druggists sought to suggest that responsibility for the current chaotic state of the drugstore rested squarely on the drug manufacturers. They made their point with packages of sulfur ointment, paregoric, bromides, digitoxin, testosterone, belladonna, and strychnine, identical except that one bore the prescription legend and the other did not. Testified Los Angeles pharmacist Roy S. Warnack, "One of these packages and its content may not be sold lawfully without a prescription; while the other may be freely sold even to a child." Drugs bearing prescription labels, which were not supposed to carry instructions for use, did so in detail, while drugs designed to be sold over the counter carried only the vague statement for use "as directed by the physician." The most damning evidence came from the comparison between packages of barbiturates and sulfa drugs—medicines clearly meant for prescription use only—being sold for over-the-counter use, and boxes of completely harmless peppermint drops, calamine, and alum powder carrying the legend label.[41]

When their turn came, opponents of the bill, among them the American Pharmaceutical Association (the pharmacists' equivalent of the AMA), the American Drug Manufacturers Association, and the American Pharmaceutical Manufacturers Association, warned against the law as yet another bid on the part of a power-hungry FDA to restrain the exercise of free enterprise. All three groups argued that the problems surrounding prescription drugs could and should be resolved by voluntary collaboration among manufacturers, professional groups, and FDA officials. That such collaborations had so far failed, American Pharmaceutical Association representative Robert P. Fischelis argued, was the fault of retail pharmacists, who were not living up to their ethical responsibilities, and the FDA, which was intent chiefly on expanding its bureaucratic powers. The only problem that really needed fixing was the FDA's 1948 policy on refills, which went far beyond what the law intended.[42]

The members of the House committee, none of whom were pharmacists or physicians, had the difficult task of sorting through this contradictory testimony. Significantly, in doing so, they sought no input from individual consumers or consumer advocacy groups. This was hardly surprising, given that the second Red Scare was under way, and consumerists would soon be called before the House Committee on Un-American Activities to refute charges that they were communist sympathizers. In the absence of consumer testimony, the congressmen on the committee repeatedly tried to discern the proposed law's economic and social implications for the public, asking the various experts sent by professional and industry groups to speculate on its possible impact: Would it mean more or less costly medicines? Would it require patients to go to the doctor more often to get needed medicines? In asking those questions, explained New Jersey Republican Charles Wolverton, "I am looking at it from the standpoint of the patient or the consumer or whatever you wish to call him."[43]

In response, the expert witnesses offered dramatically different predictions about the amendments' impact on patient-consumers. Supporters suggested that the new law would likely have little or no impact on costs but would greatly benefit the public's health. Foes warned that the FDA would use its expanded powers to make all drugs available only by prescription, leading to higher costs. When the committee members asked to hear from doctors, they were told that the AMA's legislative committee was considering the bill. In fact, the AMA was so ambivalent about any government regulation of medical practice, even when intended to give doctors more control over prescription drug refills, that the organization never offered an opinion on the amendments.[44]

Congress ultimately passed the Durham-Humphrey Amendments, and President Truman signed the Prescription Drug Law on October 26, 1951. The measure represented a series of compromises among drug manufacturers, retail pharmacists, and agency officials. The law specified that the prescription legend was intended for a drug that "because of its toxicity or other potentiality for harmful effect, or the method of its use, or the collateral measures necessary to its use, is not safe for use except under the supervision of a practitioner licensed by law to administer such drug." Only such drugs would be labeled, "Caution: Federal law prohibits dispensing without prescription." But the all-important decision about which drugs should carry the legend remained firmly in the manufacturers' hands. The FDA's list of restricted drugs remained advisory only; companies retained the power to decide whether their products met the criteria set forth by the law, and if the FDA disagreed, the matter would have to be settled on a case-by-case basis in the courts.[45]

The law's supporters chose to emphasize the positives: the measure extended the special handling long accorded to poisons and narcotics to the new drugs of the 1930s and 1940s. The list of restricted drugs banned from over-the-counter sale included barbiturates, amphetamines, sulfa drugs, antibiotics, thyroid extracts, cortisone, and the sex hormones; with the exception of insulin, it also included drugs administered by injection. All prescription drugs now came under what the FDA referred to as the canceled check principle—that is, a prescription could be filled only once. To make refilling prescriptions easier, the new law allowed pharmacists to get physician consent via the telephone as long as written records of these calls were kept. Doctors also could specify on the initial prescription that it could be refilled multiple times. In a concession to the bill's opponents, the law allowed pharmacists to continue compounding prescriptions made up of unrestricted ingredients and refilling them at consumers' discretion. Thus if doctors wanted to write prescriptions for aspirin, the new law did not stop them.[46]

All the parties to the 1951 drug law believed themselves to be acting in patient-consumers' best interests. The law's more exacting definition of drugs to be sold by prescription only, the crackdown on selling popular new drugs over the counter, and the end to unlimited refills were justified as protective measures necessitated by the advent of more effective yet dangerous medicines. Explained an FDA staffer, the revamped regulatory system "protects the public health by keeping the physician in full control of the medication his patient receives." But from the patient's perspective, this control came at a cost.[47]

Ironically, the 1938 drug law's stricter labeling provisions, passed to facilitate informed consumer choice, made the prescription drug into the consumer equivalent of a black box: a product to be purchased and used on faith. Only physicians and pharmacists were deemed expert enough to be trusted with detailed information about the most powerful medicines. In other words, the 1951 amendments reinforced the idea of the trusting, compliant patient rather than the questioning, skeptical consumer when it came to the so-called legend drugs. This dearth of patient information about prescription medications stood in striking contrast to proprietary remedies, now increasingly referred to by the more respectable name of "over-the-counter" drugs. Clearly labeled with instructions for use, those products presented a sharp contrast to their prescription counterparts, which came with the minimum of information needed for their administration.[48]

Although it received little news coverage at the time of its passage, the Prescription Drug Law of 1951 would have major consequences for patient-consumers. In the name of protecting them from harm, the FDA simultaneously made the labor and expense of getting a prescription drug far more onerous and its contents more mysterious. The system established by the Durham-Humphrey Amendments, combined with the changes in patent law, led to a dramatic widening of the price differentials between the two kinds of drugs. Compared to its prewar counterpart, the 1950s prescription drug became a far more expensive product shrouded in a powerful mystique of secrecy. Free enterprise principles consequently worked not to allay the worries of the skeptical patient but rather to reinforce the absolute authority of the physician, an outcome that would become a central complaint of post–World War II medical consumerists.

The Healthiest Nation under God

With the "Good War" won and the Great Depression finally over, the free-market makeover of medicine proceeded rapidly in the early 1950s. Through investments in scientific research, hospital construction, private health insurance, and prescription drug regulation, the country's leaders hoped to resolve the problems that had plagued the interwar patient-consumer. For a brief time, American medicine ceased to be cause for national hand-wringing and became a source of Cold War pride; it served as a prime example of how the United States offered its people a higher quality of life than did its communist foes. As a Michigan physician testified in 1952 before the Commission on the Health Needs of the Nation, the free enterprise system had "enabled the United States to become not only the healthiest, but the best Nation, under God on this earth."[49]

Anyone inclined to question that statement did so at considerable risk. As the Cold War deepened, tolerance for what the interwar generation had termed "constructively critical" perspectives on capitalism in general and medicine in particular disappeared. Being too outspoken on consumers' behalf could be dangerous. Between 1944 and 1954, the House Committee on Un-American Activities listed Consumers Union in the *Guide to Subversive Organizations and Publications* and in 1953 forced the group's director, Arthur Kallet, to appear for questioning. That same year, the American Legion adopted a resolution declaring itself "unalterably opposed" to Consumers Union and its publication, *Consumer Reports*, without feeling any need to explain why. Similarly, critics of organized medicine faced charges that they were communist sympathizers. McCarthyism's "sledgehammer" fell hard on the medical left, including physician Harold Aaron, a longtime consultant to Consumers Union. Although Aaron remained associated with the group, Consumers Union removed his name from its masthead to protect the organization from red-baiting.[50]

The rising prices of both doctors' fees and prescription drugs would eventually bring consumer criticisms back into the realm of respectability. But as an unprecedented degree of prosperity took hold in the early 1950s, the spike in medical spending initially aroused little concern. Noted *Kiplinger's Washington Newsletter* in 1955, "People are still in a buying mood—with no letdown in sight." That this buying mood might and should extend to physicians' services and miracle drugs was hardly surprising. Wartime innovations in surgery and blood banking, significant advances in drug therapy, and hefty investments in hospitals and medical research seemed reason enough for Americans to want more medical care. And as economist Elizabeth Langford observed in 1957, compared to its prewar cost, medical care had shown "less increase than haircuts, shoe repairs, movie admissions, public transportation, laundry, and automobile repairs."[51]

Popular magazines and newspaper stories celebrated postwar medical progress, reinforcing the idea that rising expenditures on medicine made economic sense. At the peak of their readership, mass circulation weeklies such as the *Saturday Evening Post* and *Life* featured regular stories that combined medical miracles with the human-interest angle. In 1956, for example, the *Saturday Evening Post* published "Why Mac Isn't Dead," about a salesman saved after an automobile crash by the heroic efforts of the medical staff at a Norwalk, Connecticut, hospital. "After the accident his insides were so horribly mangled he seemed beyond hope," read the subtitle, "but fifty medical experts put him back together." Similarly, *Life*'s coverage of the development and distribution of the polio vaccine celebrated what became one of the great preventive successes of the 1950s. These stories reinforced the assumption that whatever their price, the medical advances of the Cold War period were worth every penny.[52]

The new medium of television also presented a generally positive view of medical progress. *Medic* (1954–56), the first TV medical drama, introduced viewers to the clinical and personal dramas occurring inside a big-city hospital. Its largely flattering-to-doctors content reflected the fact that the sponsoring network invited the Los Angeles County Medical Association to review all its scripts. In spite of that care, the show was canceled after it ran controversial episodes concerning childbirth and racial discrimination. But doctor dramas returned in the early 1960s to become a staple of television fare. Under the watchful eye of the AMA, shows such as *Dr. Kildare* (1961–66) and *Ben Casey* (1961–66) provided weekly displays of clinical acuity and interpersonal drama delivered by handsome young men in white.[53]

But along with media celebrations of medical progress emerged a sour undernote in postwar discussions of the medical profession. To the consternation of medical leaders, all the progress that free enterprise medicine had delivered did not dampen criticism. Returning veterans and their families had rising expectations about what American medical care should be like. Having promoted the superiority of free enterprise medicine over its socialized alternative, the medical profession faced new pressures to deliver on its promises of quality care for all.

In some respects, the resurgence of concerns about the cost and quality of medical care simply picked up where the interwar debates had left off. The complaint that old-fashioned family practitioners were being replaced by overly specialized and entrepreneurial physicians was by no means new. But in the mid- to late 1940s, this older tradition of lament about the demise of "good old doc" began to take on new significance as part of a broader Cold War debate. During the deeply isolationist era between the two world wars, comparisons of U.S. medical institutions to those of other nations had mattered little in American politics. But now that the nation had emerged as a postwar superpower—the leader of the "free" world—any failures to provide its citizens with affordable, efficacious, and safe care had potentially damaging political consequences. Not only was the Soviet Union eager to exploit American failings in any area, but Britain's new National Health Service suggested that capitalist democracies could pursue other pathways to universal health care. In short, medical problems that had represented only a domestic dilemma before World War II now became potential foreign policy issues as well.[54]

In this climate, barriers to care posed by income and race took on greater political significance. In the aftermath of a war supposedly fought to advance democracy, social divisions accepted as natural in earlier times now seemed far more troublesome. Even with generous taxpayer subsidies for hospital construction, medical research, and private insurance plans, free enterprise medicine remained out of reach for families of modest means. Already by 1952, when the Truman Commission took testimony across the nation, union leaders and social welfare experts were complaining that the rising cost of medical care was making it too expensive for many families. In a widely cited study of an upstate New York community, sociologist Earl Lomon Koos described a troubling class divide in public perceptions of medical progress: whereas the town's affluent residents spoke of "our" doctors and "our" hospital, their poorer neighbors referred to "their" doctors and "their" hospital.[55]

The enormous racial disparities in American medical care were even more problematic. At a time when Soviet leaders were exploiting civil rights issues to embarrass the United States, medicine provided a tempting target. Under New Deal spending programs, federal agencies had bowed to southern segregationists and allowed the creation of separate and unequal facilities for white and black residents. While funneling badly needed resources into black communities, this "deluxe Jim Crow" remained deeply disturbing to civil rights activists. The 1950 death of prominent black doctor Charles Drew, the architect of the highly successful wartime system of blood banking, after he was injured in a car accident raised troubling questions about the quality of care he had received in a "whites' only" emergency room. As court rulings began to challenge the idea of separate but equal facilities, the many forms of racial discrimination evident in medical care seemed all the more incongruent with American ideals.[56]

Had Cold War complaints about American medicine remained focused only on poor or black Americans, they might well have been ignored as problems that prosperity would eventually correct. Far more disruptive to medical confidence in the 1950s was a sense of dissatisfaction emerging from precisely the group assumed to be most advantaged by the free enterprise system, white middle-class Americans. As their expectations of medicine rose, so too did their dissatisfactions with the goods and services it had on offer.

That discontent reflected growing recognition of the paradox already apparent in the interwar period, that longer life expectancies and the luxuries associated with a mass-consumption economy increased the likelihood of dying from cancer and heart disease. On the one hand, the continued rise in the average American's life expectancy from sixty years in 1930 to seventy years in 1958 seemed a sign of progress. Even though demographers would later argue that better nutrition and public sanitation deserved the credit for this increase, the extension of life expectancy was often mentioned as proof that more money spent on individual medical care was a good investment. But on multiple fronts, postwar research also confirmed the "pathogenicity of progress" and highlighted larger cultural trends that the medical profession seemed ill equipped to address.[57]

During the 1950s, a rapidly expanding body of research linked cigarette smoking, one of the great success stories of twentieth-century consumer capitalism, with rising rates of lung cancer. The Framingham heart study, a large prospective analysis funded by the NIH, produced strong evidence for both smoking and a diet high in fats as factors increasing the risk of early death. Still other studies suggested that high levels of stress and anxiety were powerful sources of ill health, both physical and mental. As *Washington Post* reporter Nate Hazeltine wrote in 1951, modern science was showing that "many of man's present day ills" stemmed from "his relatively safe and soft living." The evolution from "the cave man to the office clerk" lay at the root of most modern illnesses.[58]

Unfortunately, reducing risk factors for chronic disease was not a goal that Cold War medicine was particularly well equipped to reach. Physicians were better-trained to diagnose and treat existing diseases than to prevent them in the first place. Now, as prosperity returned, bringing greater opportunities for smoking, drinking, overeating, and worrying, doctors faced an even greater challenge in "paving the roads that lead away from disease," as the 1937 American Foundation report phrased it. Moreover, the diagnosis of and treatments available for cardiovascular disease and cancer, two leading causes of death associated with long life and affluence, left much to be desired. While postwar physicians often blamed patients for being unwilling to make the lifestyle changes needed to avoid chronic illnesses, the profession's critics took a more cynical view: doctors did not emphasize keeping patients well because doing so would dry up the supply of "customers." Far more money could be made by promoting the expanding armamentarium of tests, procedures, and drugs than by preventing illness.[59]

Cold War medicine's alleged deficiencies in preventive care contributed to popular interest in alternative healing traditions. Despite the AMA's opposition, many state legislatures continued to allow the licensing of osteopaths and chiropractors on the grounds that citizens should be allowed to choose their own medical counsel. People disenchanted with mainstream medicine patronized Christian Science and naturopathy. While often at odds on other issues, alternative healing groups shared a common view that the mainstream medical profession depended too much on dangerous drugs and unnecessary surgery and neglected the mental and spiritual roots of disease.[60]

The interest in prevention contributed to the rising fortunes of the Rodale family's publishing empire. Established in the 1930s by J. J. Rodale, an organic farmer and health enthusiast, and carried on by his children, Rodale produced publications focused on the preventive and holistic aspects of health that the new biomedicine seemed to neglect. As J. J. Rodale wrote in his 1954 *Health Finder*, "Is there any good reason why we should not seek for a way to stay healthy—so healthy that we never need to visit a doctor or take pills?" Seeing a physician was not likely to be very useful, he continued, because "the ordinary doctor is so rushed and overworked today, especially because of the increasing of degenerative diseases such as cancer, heart trouble, [and] diabetes, that he has absolutely no time to give to healthy people and to showing them how to remain healthy." To fill that void, Rodale named his monthly magazine *Prevention* and used its pages to promote the virtues of careful diet and enlightened self-care as the means to stay out of the clutches of mainstream medicine.[61]

Other publishing success stories of the 1950s involved authors who emphasized the promise of "right living" as a corrective to the limitations of modern medicine. Nutritionist Adelle Davis delivered that message in her widely read 1954 book, *Let's Eat Right to Keep Fit*, which championed the idea of using specific nutritional approaches to treat common ailments. Although criticized both for her facts and for her breezy tone, Davis's book attracted a devoted readership, remaining in print until the late 1980s. The interest in "natural" health care also led to the extraordinary success of D. C. Jarvis's 1958 book, *Folk Medicine: A Vermont Doctor's Guide to Good Health*, which climbed to the top of *Publishers' Weekly*'s annual list of nonfiction best sellers in 1959 and 1960. In writing the book, Jarvis sought to share what he had learned from his patients, not his fellow doctors, about the natural processes of "resistance, repair, and recovery," or as he put it, the need for "working *with* nature, instead of against it." Among the simple remedies his informants touted was switchel, or honegar, a Vermont concoction of honey and apple cider vinegar.[62]

Most physicians dismissed Rodale and Davis as "health nuts" or "faddists" whose ideas were not worth the paper they were written on and regarded popular interest in switchel-drinking as yet more proof that the American people were too ignorant to be trusted with important medical decisions. But having embraced free enterprise as the foundation of the American way of medicine, postwar physicians had limited ability to check such enthusiasms. In the Cold War era no less than the late nineteenth century, medical liberty included not only the right to choose one's own doctor but also the right to doctor oneself with apple cider.

Even more destabilizing to the postwar doctor-patient relationship was a deeper current of cultural concern about medical authoritarianism. The question of how to reconcile scientific authority with individual autonomy, already being raised by interwar iconoclasts such as T. Swann Harding and James Rorty, became even more pressing in light of Cold War reflections on the dangers of both fascism and communism. In an influential 1949 study, *The Authoritarian Personality*, Theodor W. Adorno and his colleagues suggested that World War II had underlined the need to develop a more "mature" kind of democratic leadership watched over by a more critically informed citizenry. In the wake of both the trials of Nazi doctors and the advent of atomic weaponry, scientific authority was by no means exempt from this trend toward greater accountability. As Norman Cousins, the editor of the *Saturday Review of Literature*, argued in his 1945 book, *Modern Man Is Obsolete*, the atomic age required a "radical transformation" in education, the "primary aim" of which "should be the development of a critical intelligence." In light of wartime experience, the idea of passively following orders seemed inherently dangerous.[63]

The impassioned postwar debate over the differences between authoritarian and democratic cultures spilled over into discussions of medicine's leadership style. The insistence that true democracy required a more informed and critical citizenry cast the doctor-patient relationship in a new political light. On the one hand, it seemed evident that the growing scientific sophistication of Cold War medicine had increased the asymmetry between doctor and patient; even college-educated patients could not fully comprehend the rationale for tests, drugs, and procedures available for diagnosis and treatment. On the other hand, Americans, especially the new middle classes, were increasingly disinclined to accept an "ask no questions" kind of authoritarianism. While they respected the doctor's expertise, a growing number of patients wanted at least some explanation for what he was doing. As treatments became more powerful and prone to risks, such information sharing seemed all the more necessary.

This expectation may also have been fueled by the unsettled status politics of the 1950s. In his classic 1951 book, *White Collar*, sociologist C. Wright Mills argued that as middle-class men became salaried employees of big corporations—the "men in gray flannel suits," as Sloan Wilson's 1955 best seller dubbed them—they felt the pressures of workplace competition. This "status anxiety" bred envy of both physicians' autonomy and their rapid rise in income. Ironically, doctors, too, felt this status anxiety, with many complaining that their profession had become too focused on economic gain, that general practitioners were being pushed out by specialists, and that patients' need for comprehensive care was being overlooked.[64]

Distrust of the authoritarian physician fed into a broader disenchantment with modern consumer culture that emerged in the late 1950s. Cold War prosperity had promoted the quest for self-realization through the purposeful acquisition of the "just right" home, automobile, and refrigerator. But as social critics such as Vance Packard argued, this postwar fusion of expressive individualism and consumer culture easily degenerated into an empty, soulless materialism, to which the medical profession responded by prescribing a "pill for every ill."[65]

These currents of discontent help to explain why magazines and other forms of mass media simultaneously celebrated the march of modern medicine and perpetuated the theme of nostalgia for the "old-time" physician, a nostalgia beautifully illustrated in two famous depictions of doctors in the late 1940s. In 1947, the *Saturday Evening Post* reprinted Norman Rockwell's painting *The Family Doctor*, his painstaking, affectionate re-creation of the office of his personal physician, Dr. George A. Russell, whom Rockwell described as personifying "a whole band of hard-working men who deserve well of the republic—the family doctors." A year later, *Life* featured a photo essay by photographer W. Eugene Smith documenting three weeks in the life of Ernest Ceriani, a doctor in the small town of Kremmling, Colorado, whom Smith described as one of the "disappearing" breed of general practitioner. Smith concluded that doctors like Ceriani would soon be in short supply thanks to the tendency of medical schools to "present specialization as a glamorous occupation and general practice as the thankless chore of a drudge."[66]

In the decade after the war's end, therefore, American medicine found itself in a paradoxical position. Despite the extraordinary gains associated with both the new science and technology and the spread of consumer capitalism, the profession faced a restless patient population. Although medical leaders rejected many of the criticisms directed at American doctors, they realized that they needed to do a better job of meeting expectations. To that end, they embarked on an ambitious program of public relations.

But medicine's problems would prove difficult to resolve easily. As the dynamics of free enterprise medicine unfolded from the late 1940s to the early 1960s, they created their own distinctive set of shopping problems, some carried over from the interwar period, others quite new. In the eyes of postwar critics, the medical miracle became mirrored by the "therapeutic nightmare," a Cold War version of the old "doctor's dilemma" in which producing sick people appeared to be a better business model than keeping them well.[67] To the extent that physicians, hospitals, pharmaceutical firms, and other health-related businesses seemed wedded to that business model, their motivations became all the more suspect. Patients as well as doctors faced the danger of seeking surgical procedures and prescription drugs as a medical version of "keeping up with the Joneses." As a result, rather than nurturing a more passive generation of patients, the Cold War doctor's office and drugstore became breeding grounds for a new eruption of patient-consumer discontent.

{SIX}
The MDs Are Off Their Pedestal

In June 1957, Mr. and Mrs. Benjamin Hooper of Manorville, New York, paid a visit to the Suffolk County Medical Society. People of modest means—he drove a truck for the highway department, she was a telephone operator—they came to meet with the society's medical grievance committee to protest a large doctor's bill. But unlike the typical such case, the Hoopers' visit to the medical society became front-page news. A few weeks earlier, their son, Benny Jr., had fallen down an abandoned well in their Long Island backyard. Thanks to the new technology of television, people across the United States followed police and fire fighters' efforts to extract the boy from the deep shaft. Among the rescuers was Joseph Kris, a local physician who answered the police request for emergency medical assistance and remained at the site throughout the twenty-four hours of Benny's ordeal. At his suggestion, oxygen had been piped down to prevent Benny from suffocating, and after the rescue, he treated the child's minor lung infection at a local hospital. Described by the *New York Times* as a slightly stooped man dressed in "baggy trousers and battered hat," Kris was hailed as the "very picture of the country doctor," acting just as heroically as the policemen and the firemen involved in the "miracle rescue."[1]

But that kindly country doctor image shattered a month later when Kris sent the Hoopers an itemized bill for his services. One headline read, "Parents of Boy Rescued in Well Get Bill for $1,500 from Doctor," and described the Hoopers as "stunned" by the size of Kris's fee. As newspapers across the country reported the story in similar tones, "a storm broke over the doctor's head": he received threatening phone calls and telegrams, was denounced on the floor of the U.S. Senate, and got reprimanded by both the AMA and the Suffolk County Medical Society. Perplexed by the attacks, Kris explained that he had heard money was "pouring" into the Hoopers' household and felt he was entitled to some of it. At the grievance committee's urging, he agreed to cancel the bill.[2]

But in his book *The Doctor Business*, published a year later, journalist Richard Carter argued that Kris had been unfairly pilloried for doing what free enterprise medicine encouraged physicians to do—that is, to charge as much as the market would bear. For Carter, Benny's story illustrated a fundamental truth about contemporary American medicine: it operated according to the rules of "the bazaar," with predictable consequences: "abuses of the patient's person and pocketbook through unnecessary surgery, excessive fees, inadequate health insurance, professional neglect, and outmoded approaches to medical art and science." The time had come, Carter suggested, for "consumers" to work together and demand real change in "organized medicine's dollar policies."[3]

Carter's book was but one of many signs that the Red Scare's dampening of "constructively critical" medical consumerism was coming to an end and that "the M.D.'s are off their pedestal," as *Fortune* magazine declared in 1954. Paradoxically, this culture of complaint developed side by side with fulsome praise for medicine's spectacular postwar accomplishments, among them antibiotics, open-heart surgery, and the polio vaccine. As opinion polls and surveys revealed, Americans greatly valued modern science and respected individual physicians yet felt unsure whether to regard the doctor as "magician or mercenary."[4]

In theory, the Cold War doctor's office represented a masterful blend of business efficiency, scientific rigor, and personalized care. In practice, the proliferation of uncoordinated and expensive services generated conflict over both the size of the doctor's bill and the quality of services it included. Having been promised a medical order consistent with the highest ideals of both capitalism and democracy, a growing number of Americans felt dissatisfied with the results. So in spite of determined efforts to improve doctor-patient relationships, the medical profession found itself in an increasingly hostile environment of public and political opinion by the early 1960s.

The New and Improved Doctor's Office

This souring of the public mood would have been hard to predict in 1950. Thanks to a combination of research advances and professional reforms, medicine had all the markings of a scientific success story in the early Cold War years. Propelled by a dramatic reorientation of medical culture around research-oriented biomedicine, physicians could now draw on a continually expanding array of new treatments. As American medicine matured, physicians had good reason to think that they had entered a new "golden age" in which science and professionalism would be perfectly reconciled. Nowhere did those gains seem more evident than in the expansion and modernization of the doctor's office that took place in the 1940s and 1950s.

At the heart of Cold War medicine's transformation was the rapid growth of its research base. Thanks to investments in hospital building, research funding, and new drug development, American researchers began to be leaders rather than followers in the global pursuit of medical innovation. Whereas before 1940, groundbreaking discoveries had come along perhaps once a decade, they now seemed to appear continuously. Paralleling nuclear physics's understanding of the universe, medical science appeared to have made great strides forward in its mastery of the human body. In contrast to the physicists' accomplishments, which had ushered in a new age of nuclear fear, the medical arms race, as contemporaries termed it, offered more benign prospects for progress: "a chain reaction, in which discovery breeds discovery," as Alan Gregg, longtime director of the Rockefeller Foundation's medical sciences division, described it.[5]

This reorientation toward research transformed the culture of American medicine in general and medical education in particular. Elite medical schools now competed fiercely to hire faculty who could win research grants and produce innovations that would then secure more funding. Doctors who displayed such aptitude quickly came to dominate medicine's hierarchy of prestige. They not only trained up a younger generation of researchers dedicated to the same values but also changed expectations of how all physicians should practice. Whereas only a talented minority of "medical mandarins" might invent a new diagnostic technique, surgical procedure, or drug regimen, many more physicians could be trained to use them. The new medical regime established first in academic medical centers and their hospitals thus quickly moved outward to reshape the doctor's office.[6]

That reshaping began with a radical overhaul of medical education. To ensure that young physicians were better prepared to deliver a higher standard of care, the medical school curriculum expanded to include much more coursework in basic science. At the end of their four years of medical school, graduates now faced a battery of rigorous exams administered by the National Board of Medical Examiners, which verified that they had mastered the knowledge they needed. Students then moved on to a required year of internship, during which they learned to put that knowledge into practice. For those bent on becoming specialists, an additional one to three years of residency became standard.[7]

The postwar explosion of medical knowledge accelerated the trend toward specialization already under way before 1940. Specialty training became far more demanding, as a rapidly expanding network of specialty boards sought to clarify the difference between a real specialist and mere dabblers in a particular field. The number of specialty boards mushroomed from eighteen in 1950 to fifty-one (including subspecialties) a decade later. By 1960, 57 percent of all American physicians in active practice were full-time specialists, and the number seemed destined to grow as fewer medical students envisioned general practice as a desirable career goal.[8]

While a great boon in terms of treatment options, the accelerating pace of innovation and specialization steadily shortened the length of time that any particular medical advance might remain the standard. This speeding-up of knowledge production was reflected in the proliferation of medical journals; by the late 1950s, American physicians could choose among approximately 1,600 publications publishing around 110,000 articles a year. This "information explosion," as Vannevar Bush termed it in 1945, inspired a growing genre of medical writing aimed at helping physicians keep up, including the *Annual Review of Medicine* associated with Stanford's medical school; the serial *Medical Progress*, edited by the former editor of the *Journal of the American Medical Association*, Morris Fishbein; and frequent revisions of the *Merck Manual*, the busy physician's desktop guide to the latest and best forms of treatment. The information explosion also deepened physicians' reliance on representatives from drug companies to keep them abreast of the latest therapeutic trends.[9]

As the profession's scientific and educational standards increased, so, too, did its economic rewards. While specialists continued to earn significantly more than general practitioners, postwar prosperity lifted all physicians out of the economic insecurities that had plagued the profession during the Great Depression. Physicians' median income rose from $3,758 in 1929 to $22,100 in 1959. Although physicians still earned substantially less than high-level corporate executives, their incomes began to outpace those of other professional groups such as lawyers and dentists, making "the superior economic position of doctors" a source of envy. Because doctors had to work so hard, economists Herman Somers and Anne Somers observed, "most Americans do not begrudge doctors their high rewards." Yet these gains came with a significant price, both literally and figuratively.[10]

In many ways, then, the problems of the interwar medical order caused by uneven standards of medical education and specialization seemed to have been neatly solved by the 1950s. At the same time, postwar physicians still felt pressure to maintain their offices as "show windows" in order to compete for the most desirable groups of patients—that is, affluent families able and willing to pay more for medical services. Doing so required blending new technologies of diagnosis and treatment with a satisfying degree of personal care. While not as dramatic as the development of a new drug or vaccine, a well-run office contributed significantly to professional success.

Success started with the choice of a good location. As they had in the interwar period, physicians followed the broader population movements of the affluent middle class, overall their most reliable source of business. While the traditional "doctors' districts" in central cities continued to exist, many physicians, particularly those just setting up practices, joined the flow of postwar families to rapidly growing suburban areas. A 1954 *Medical Economics* survey discovered that the physicians involved in "shopping center practices"—medical offices located in or near newly built suburban shopping malls—tended to be five to ten years younger than their urban counterparts. At the same time, specialists began to depart from the old medical convention—"the specialist hangs out his shingle in the heart of town" while "the family doctor sets up a practice in a residential section"—and opened up second offices in the suburbs where they practiced several days a week. Among the first to relocate were obstetricians and pediatricians drawn to suburban neighborhoods filled with rapidly growing young families. According to one woman, she had gone to a city specialist to have her first child, thinking that guaranteed the best care; but when she was pregnant with her second child, traveling to the city became too difficult, and her child's pediatrician "was so good that he strengthened my confidence in shopping-center doctors generally."[11]

As they moved to the suburbs, some physicians built their own offices rather than renting space in strip malls. In their 1955 book, *Doctors' Offices and Clinics*, architects Paul Hayden Kirk and Eugene D. Sternberg noted the new collaboration between doctors and architects brought about by the postwar building boom, and journals such as *Progressive Architecture* frequently carried articles on the resulting designs. As befit the profession's strong commitment to individualism, medical office plans came in every combination from the single office designed for the solo practitioner to the medical clinic housing ten to twenty doctors. The suburban version of the "medical arts building" also proved popular. Easily built using a modular plan of uniform suites that provided the right mix of spaces for reception, examination, consultation, billing, and laboratory work, this became an attractive and comparatively inexpensive alternative to the purpose-built doctor's office.

Doctors' offices needed to be easily accessible by bus and provide "ample parking space" for cars, advised a 1954 *Medical Economics* article. Suburban doctors chose locations near bus stops for the benefit of stay-at-home wives whose husbands took their families' cars to work, while city doctors arranged patient discounts at nearby parking garages. Using a design created for Italian dictator Benito Mussolini, one enterprising San Francisco surgeon built a 1,200-car parking garage for patients and rented spaces out to other dentists and doctors in his neighborhood. "No parking problem here," he happily noted.[12]

The effort to make the office accessible and welcoming reflected doctors' ongoing efforts to cut down on house calls. Young physicians entering practice in the 1950s were frequently warned that making too many such visits would limit their success. Although family practitioners continued to make house calls, usually for very young or very old patients, the locus of medical care steadily shifted to their offices. Whereas in the 1930s, doctors saw four out of ten patients in the home, by the early 1960s, that number had fallen to one in ten. In a 1961 *Time* interview, a New Jersey pediatrician dismissed making house calls as "a bad habit" that was "as outdated as the horse and buggy," although she admitted that she made them occasionally "just as a favor to a good patient."[13]

Given the impetus to wean patients away from the house call habit, it became all the more important for physicians to make their offices easy to find. But unlike drugstores, which could use dramatic signage to attract patients, doctors' offices had to do so more subtly. The stylish doctor's building of the 1950s featured a modernist look characterized by strong lines with patterned brick and wood trim to give visual interest. While eschewing the automatic door openers found in modern drugstores, medical offices sought to limit steps or install elevators to provide ease of access for "cardiacs and other disabled patients" daunted by climbing stairs.[14]

Doctors also courted patients by showing concern for their privacy. Plans for doctors' offices often featured landscaping that functioned as a privacy screen as well as offering soothing views. Designers recommended natural light for waiting areas but suggested installing venetian blinds to shield patients from outside scrutiny. Soundproofing was advocated to prevent visitors from overhearing conversations. Some offices were set up so patients came in one door and went out another without having to go back through the waiting room. One architect's 1955 plan for a doctor's office in Tampa, Florida, included a separate reception area for "Negro patients" that "could, in another part of the country, be used perhaps for children."[15]

While seeking to make their office spaces more comfortable, doctors felt pressure to shorten patients' wait times. As a 1955 article on "how to have a well-run appointment system" noted, "the biggest single complaint of patients" is not the size of fees but rather "time wasted in the waiting room." Anecdotes abounded about the backlash against long waiting times. For example, a Detroit surgeon found his bill returned unpaid with a note from a male patient who had a 3:00 P.M. appointment but was not seen until 5:00 P.M.: "If I can wait, I guess you can wait too." Business and professional people understood the concept that time is money all too well and felt entitled to criticize physicians with excessive wait times as "un-businesslike." Thus, as a doctor explained, "a good appointment system frees [the doctor] from the strain and pressure of a reception room crowded with impatient and ill-tempered people" and was "certain to pay off in patient goodwill."[16]

Postwar doctors usually relied on female "medical assistants," who might also be registered nurses, to keep appointment schedules and manage offices. In her 1958 handbook for medical assistants, Miriam Bredow explained their role: "She builds up the doctor's reputation and, incidentally, his practice by creating an atmosphere of friendly good will in his office." Each morning, the assistant placed on the doctor's desk a list of that day's patients and their medical files. Throughout the day, she worked to keep him on schedule, and when she could not, she helped soothe patient discontent. She also transcribed the doctor's notes, entered test results, and tended to the billing.[17]

To make office visits more efficient, some physicians began to have patients complete health questionnaires while waiting in the reception area. The most widely used of these was the Cornell Medical Index, introduced in 1949 and used well into the 1970s. Patients answered four pages of questions such as "Have you coughed up blood?" and "Do you sometimes get out of breath just sitting still?" Such surveys did not replace a proper history taking, explained a 1955 *Medical Economics* article, but rather helped the doctor to "interview the patient with more dispatch and efficiency" and "reassured [patients] about the thoroughness of the exam."[18]

Once ushered into an examining room, Cold War patients were likely to encounter a far wider range of diagnostic and treatment equipment than had been available in the 1930s. The physical exam now included not only the trusty stethoscope, used to listen to heart and lung sounds, but other instruments designed to peer into the ears, nose, and throat. A sphygmomanometer would be employed to measure the patient's blood pressure. Depending on the patient's symptoms, a vaginal or rectal exam might also be performed. Based on the history and initial examination, the doctor would then order further tests, such as a urinalysis to detect excess albumin and sugar, blood work to count the different kinds of cells and measure iron levels, bacteriological cultures to confirm an infection, X-rays and fluoroscopes to scan bones and organs, and an electrocardiogram to evaluate cardiac function.[19]

While some doctors preferred to refer patients to commercial laboratories or hospitals for diagnostic tests, others chose to invest in the equipment needed to perform these assessments in-office. Successive editions of Bredow's handbook for medical assistants included more detailed instructions for doing X-rays, urinalysis, blood work, metabolic tests, and bacteriological cultures. Those instructions dealt with an expanding array of complex devices and instruments, such as the Sahli-Adams Plano-Parallel Hemometer (for checking hemoglobin levels), the Jones Waterless Motor-Basal (for measuring basal metabolism rates), and the Beck-Lee electrocardiograph (for assessing cardiac function). Medical device companies appealed to this do-it-yourself mentality, advertising an impressive array of new tools in medical journals. One, the Leitz Rouy-Photrometer, allowed the nurse to do forty "common clinical tests" right in the doctor's office, which meant "No waiting for results."[20]

Along with diagnostic tests, physicians could offer their patients a vastly expanded range of office-based treatments. Chief among them was the rapidly expanding armamentarium of powerful prescription drugs. Many patients went to their doctors hoping to obtain one of the many new "miracle" drugs, among them antibiotics for bacterial infections, cortisone to treat various types of inflammation, antihypertensive drugs to control high blood pressure, and psychoactive drugs to lessen anxiety. In addition to writing prescriptions, physicians performed procedures such as injections, irrigations, vaccinations, and minor surgeries. Depending on the specialty, they might also give inhalation therapy, electrotherapy, light therapy, and radiotherapy.[21]

In addition, new technologies changed the way that physicians kept the records so essential to building a successful practice. Starting in the 1940s, companies such as Histacount, Colwell Publishing, and Remington Rand offered doctors a widening array of preprinted forms, ranging in size from five-by-eight-inch cards to eight-by-eleven-inch sheets, along with the filing equipment to store them. Providing space for both clinical and billing information, the forms could be customized for the use of either general practitioners or specialists. Postwar physicians were also early adopters of the electric typewriters, adding machines, dictation devices, and copiers being developed by IBM and Xerox. Interspersed with ads for drugs and medical devices, journals such as *Medical Economics* and *Modern Medicine* carried promotions for the latest in business equipment that promised to enhance practice management.[22]

By the 1950s, then, affluent Americans had access to a new and improved style of office practice that promised to deliver superior care. Patients would find their doctors' offices conveniently located and provided with ample parking; wait (but not too long) in a comfortable waiting area; be examined and treated according to the latest and best in medical science; and depart with a carefully prepared bill. When done right, the postwar doctor's office would combine the efficiency of the factory with the logic of the department store to deliver a satisfactory experience and a desirable "package of services," as Michael Marks Davis termed it.[23]

But this new and improved doctor's office remained out of reach for many Americans. The outflow of physicians to the suburbs only worsened the class and race barriers to access already evident before World War II. Postwar improvements bypassed poor inner-city neighborhoods and the poorest of rural areas, which were lucky to have a doctor at all, much less one who provided magazines in the waiting room or kept to appointment times. So when optimists waxed enthusiastic about the improvements in care being offered in the Cold War doctor's office, they were speaking only for a privileged majority.[24]

Be Sure You Investigate Him

Ironically, all the improvements offered to affluent patients in the 1950s by no means obviated the necessity for careful doctor-shopping. In spite of the upgrades to medical education, specialty training, and treatment options, the quality of service delivered in doctors' offices remained highly variable. Cold War patient-consumers, no less than their interwar predecessors, had to learn to distinguish good care from bad. Advice given to patients about how to find a good doctor remained consistent: "find a doctor before you need him" and "be sure you investigate him," recommended the AMA's *Hygeia*.[25]

The necessity for doctor-shopping was impelled by the profession's deep commitment to individualism, which left individual doctors considerable latitude in how they practiced medicine. As medical educators were the first to admit, the standards taught in the best medical schools and praised in the pages of medical journals did not necessarily match the reality of what many doctors did. An extensive study of general practice conducted in North Carolina in 1953 and 1954 documented the wide variance in doctors' behaviors: when assessed on their skills at taking histories, performing physical exams, and keeping accurate records, only 8 percent of those observed performed well, while 44 percent showed significant deficits in technique. Delivering this sober message, the study's authors emphasized that they had no reason to assume that this variance was peculiar to North Carolina.[26]

By tolerating so much unevenness among its practitioners, the profession inadvertently promoted the necessity for doctor-shopping. Wrote Walter Alvarez in 1953, "We doctors, like all human beings, can be good, bad, or indifferent," so patients needed to learn to spot the difference. Since the profession could not provide uniformity in medical skills, it had to emphasize patients' choice of the "right" doctor as a prerequisite to getting good care. In essence, the 1950s culture of medicine encouraged its own brand of medical consumerism. In a 1953 talk, "Evolution of the Doctor-Patient Relationship," physician J. H. Means noted how by emphasizing the importance of personal choice of physician, the profession had helped to create a new kind of patient. When he had started in practice in the 1910s, "having chosen a doctor the patient was on the whole expected to stick by him," but "certainly patients have no such feeling today—they go shopping about from one doctor to another without a qualm, unless perhaps an economic one."[27]

This trend was reflected in the instructions that patient-consumers received about how to pick a good doctor. A 1942 *Hygeia* article outlined what remained the standard message for the next fifty years: every adult had a duty to find a good doctor before he was needed and to "investigate" his credentials carefully. Explained author Greer Williams, "The way to judge a doctor is the way doctors judge each other"—that is, using the highest standards of professional competence. Surprisingly, given *Hygeia*'s ties to the AMA, Williams warned that "one cannot rely solely on the American Medical Association or medical society membership to make a doctor competent or to keep him competent." Instead, patients needed to do their own research, verifying that a physician had attended a "recognized" medical school, interned at an "accredited" hospital, and now had admitting privileges at another such hospital. An appointment to a local medical school and membership in a specialty society were also signs of quality. Cautioning that some doctors might resent being asked about credentials on the first visit, Williams pointed out that patients could obtain this information in advance from publicly available sources.[28]

Other newspaper and magazine articles expanded on techniques for investigating doctors. Savvy patients were told to get lists of physicians from local hospitals, medical societies, and medical schools and then look up each name in the *American Medical Directory*, "the bible of the profession," which could be found at the local public library. According to a 1954 article in *Changing Times*, "By reading up on a man on your list, you can find out how old he is, what schools he attended, how long he has practiced, to what professional associations he belongs, and what honors have come to him." Well-informed patients searching for specialists needed to appreciate the importance of being board certified and learn to decipher the mysterious abbreviations that often followed a doctor's name, such as FACS (Fellow of the American College of Surgeons) or FACOG (Fellow of the American College of Obstetrics and Gynecology).[29]

The most frequently repeated advice to postwar patient-consumers was to seek out well-trained general practitioners to coordinate their medical care. Acknowledging that people most often wanted that sort of doctor, the *Changing Times* article suggested choosing members of the American Academy of General Practice, a newly formed group dedicated to raising standards for general practitioners. But that advice proved increasingly hard to follow as the number of generalists plummeted: by 1963, 65 percent of all practicing doctors were full-time specialists. In place of an old-fashioned general practitioner, postwar patients were told to find a general internist, arguably the most broadly trained of specialists, to be their primary care physician. Families with young children also began to rely heavily on pediatricians and obstetrician/gynecologists for more general medical advice. Whether general practitioner or specialist, the *Changing Times* article suggested, the real insider's method was to find "the doctor's doctor"—that is, the practitioners doctors used for their own families, for as everyone knew, "sick doctors are fiends for good medical care!"[30]

After a patient had chosen a doctor, the need for vigilance by no means ceased. Advice givers offered tips on what to look for on the first visit to assure themselves of a practitioner's trustworthiness. To that end, *Changing Times* posed a long list of questions about the doctor's office and how it was run as well as about the doctor himself: "How does he go about his job? How thorough is his examination? Does he answer your questions? Do you like him?" As in the interwar era, advice givers urged patients to look beneath the surface of appearances. While a shabby or unclean office was unacceptable, a lavishly furnished office filled with shiny equipment did not necessarily signify a good doctor. Likewise, the article advised, "He need not be as handsome or as impeccably dressed as the doctors in the cigaret [*sic*] ads, but you will naturally favor the doctor with the neat appearance." The physician should be friendly and take time to get to know the patient but not talk too much or waste time with gossip or jokes.[31]

Finally, patients were told to judge a doctor by his willingness to speak openly and freely about financial issues. "Always ask the doctor his fees for any medical care he proposes to give you and *always tell him your financial status*," Williams suggested in 1942. Some doctors were "shy" about the subject, so patients should be prepared to bring up the question. *Changing Times* noted, "You can be even more sure of your ground" when the doctor's waiting room displayed the AMA plaque that "invited" patients to speak frankly about fees.[32]

In many respects, the postwar advice about how to find a good doctor paralleled the strategies of savvy consumption advocated by groups such as Consumers' Research and Consumers Union. Just as no "intelligent" consumer would buy an automobile or home appliance without doing research on its quality, no "intelligent" patient should choose a physician without carefully evaluating his credentials and reputation. As the demands for deference to physician authority multiplied, so too did the necessity for placing that faith wisely. But it was worthwhile effort: "doing it the hard way will pay off in knowledge that you have done your best to obtain the most adequate medical care you can afford," concluded the *Changing Times* article.[33]

The efforts evidently paid off in that Americans started to visit the doctor more often: between the late 1920s and the late 1950s, the average number of visits per year doubled from 2.5 to 5. At the same time, their expectations of care were also on the rise, as service industries in general became more important to the overall economy. What a later generation of economists would characterize as the "postindustrial" service economy was already well developed by the 1950s. As Richard Rutter wrote in 1956, the phrase "at your service" had become an "apt way to describe the post-war economy." Between 1945 and 1955, spending on "the better intangibles of life" doubled from a little over $40 billion to $91 billion. By the mid-1950s, services accounted for a quarter of the gross national product. The biggest gains occurred in the category of "personal business," which included taxes, insurance, legal advice, and investment counseling, followed by medical spending.[34]

Despite medicine's high status, physicians still faced comparisons with other providers of hard-to-understand goods and services, particularly among their more affluent patients. During the prosperous 1950s, middle-class Americans, especially married couples, found themselves courted by banks, investment firms, and insurance companies that promised them fiscal security. They also interacted with a wide variety of specialized salespersons and repair personnel—real estate agents and car salesmen, appliance repairmen and auto mechanics. Service providers sought to win over and retain consumers with promises of reliability, expertise, and the "personal touch." While doctors' status as lifesavers and scientists gave them some insulation from the "customer is always right" ethos, they could not escape invidious comparisons with this competitive world of personal service. Thus, how doctors delivered their services—the cost, the financing, the experience of visiting the office or (worse) going to the hospital—became an area for concern. Moreover, those issues interested men as well as women, thus making medical costs a significant part of couples' budgeting decisions.[35]

The need to please a pickier generation of consumers was evident in the AMA's expanded program of public relations. The Whitaker and Baxter campaign to promote the "American way" of medicine was the start of a much broader AMA effort to get its members to take more care in patient management. Although lay critics often dismissed these measures as window dressing, they suggest just how much the need to enhance the physician's reputation as a service provider mattered to Cold War medical leaders. In a 1955 how-to guide for county medical societies, the AMA's Department of Public Relations explained, "In recent years doctors have been shaken from their saintly pedestals of yore." It continued, "Branded unjustifiably as modern-day 'sinners' by the press and the public," doctors have been accused of a "negative, do-nothing" response to calls for reform; "rebuked for a cold, impersonal attitude toward patients"; and "reproached for the actions of a few unethical medical men." Combating these public misconceptions required that the profession "first put its house in order, eliminating the causes for public criticism." To help in that endeavor, the Department of Public Relations not only provided these manuals but also published a weekly newsletter, *The PR Doctor*, to share ideas about how to improve patient satisfaction.[36]

In addition, the AMA promoted a wide range of patient-friendly programs to be run out of county medical societies. Those groups were urged to set up a call system to help patients locate physicians in emergencies, to create a grievance committee to hear and resolve patient complaints over fees and other issues, to arrange for free care of the very poor, and to cultivate good relations with local charitable groups, newspapers, and radio stations. The AMA also encouraged individual members to eliminate one of the most common sources of patient complaint by discussing their fees more openly. To help in that effort, the AMA provided members with plaques for office display that read, "To all my patients—I invite you to discuss frankly with me any questions regarding my services or my fees. The best medical service is based on a friendly mutual understanding between doctor and patient."[37]

By 1953, about a quarter of the country's almost 2,000 county medical societies had set up grievance committees. A 1955 survey of 1,125 societies found that most had put in place call services, grievance committees, "press codes of cooperation," and plans to provide medical care to the poor. Nearly a fifth of the societies ran speakers' bureaus as well as radio programs, more than 100 sponsored television programs, and 48 published public relations newsletters. More county societies had public relations committees than had ethics committees. Although many physicians initially resented the dues increases required to fund these public relations efforts, they soon came to see their benefits. A member of New York's Westchester County Medical Society recalled thinking, "It seemed to me that a $15 hike in annual dues was a pretty steep price just to mollycoddle chronic complainers and malcontents," but only six months into the new program, he changed his mind, not only because his patients seemed happier but also because they paid their fees more willingly, thus offsetting the dues increase.[38]

The Bitter Pill

The single biggest factor contributing to the sense that postwar medicine was confronting a public image problem was what public relations professional John Newton Baker described as the "bitter pill" of its "tremendously increased cost." Critical scrutiny of the doctor's bill was almost inevitable, given the profession's dramatic economic gains. Ironically, some of the same measures doctors adopted to make their billing seem more reasonable made it easier for patients to complain about the size of fees.[39]

The postwar debate about the "bitter pill" of cost reflected the growing attention to shifts in consumer spending more generally. As that spending grew more essential to the American economy, the Consumer Price Index became a closely watched measure of the nation's fiscal health. From the late 1940s onward, the index posted increases in spending on medical services, including doctors' services, hospital bills, and drug costs, at almost double the rate of other categories of consumption. Medical increases outpaced big durable items such as automobiles and home freezers as well as more frequent expenditures on food and clothing. As the economist Joseph Garbarino commented in 1959, "No other major category of items has increased in price so rapidly," increases that were bound to raise concerns given the "social significance" of the goods in question.[40]

In the public mind, the dramatic increase in medical costs was easily conflated with doctors' newfound prosperity. Despite their efforts to become more businesslike, interwar doctors had not been noticeably wealthier than their professional peers. Even into the 1940s, doctors retained a reputation for being indifferent businessmen for whom "the financial side of medical practice is extremely distasteful," as Miriam Bredow explained in her 1943 handbook for the medical secretary. But as medical fees and physician incomes rose in tandem during the 1950s, the profession's reputation as being above money began to fray. At a time of growing white-collar anxiety, the comparative freedom doctors enjoyed when deciding what to charge evoked resentment.[41]

To soften that resentment, postwar physicians used the same arguments made back in the 1920s to explain "the high cost of keeping alive." Becoming a doctor was an expensive undertaking, requiring many years of training and access to high-priced technologies, costs that had to be passed on to the patient. In addition, patients had to expect to pay more for drugs and procedures that worked far better than their predecessors; even at a much higher cost, "the product is a better buy than ever before," as economists Herman Somers and Anne Somers put it in 1961. Doctors pointed out that Americans were paying more for their homes and their cars, so why not their medical care as well?[42]

Still, rapidly rising medical bills fueled a growing debate over how doctors were determining their fees. Hospitals seemed to be the starting point for the spike in costs. Thanks to both expanded hospital construction and insurance coverage, rates of hospitalization for medical care rose dramatically between 1930 and 1960. As of 1958, 24 million Americans, one in eight of the total population, visited the hospital each year; in addition to surgery, a rising proportion came for nonsurgical treatments for conditions such as heart disease and cancer.[43] Even as hospital stays became shorter, the growing technological sophistication of care kept expenses rising. Hospitals modernized not only their clinical facilities but also their accounting systems, and they reshaped their billing practices to take advantage of expanding third-party insurance coverage.

In a panel discussion at the annual meeting of the American Hospital Association (AHA) in 1955, Dr. E. Dwight Barnett, a professor of medical administration at Columbia University, described what he saw happening. Imitating surgeons, all the physicians involved in patient care now wanted to submit separate bills for treatment, including radiologists, anesthesiologists, and pathologists. In effect, Barnett noted, the hospital was becoming "a hotel for horizontal persons, with a department store of independent but uncoordinated services offered," a system to which patients would surely object. Fellow panelist and science writer Donald Dunham agreed, saying that if he got separate bills from every doctor who treated him while in the hospital, "I would need another bill—from a psychiatrist."[44]

Despite warnings about its negative consequences, the new billing culture spread outward from hospitals to the billing practices of physicians in general, but not in a particularly orderly or understandable way. Although some doctors gave considerable thought to how they set their fees, many apparently did not. A 1954 AMA survey showed that most doctors simply charged what other practitioners in their community did—the "usual and customary rate." One doctor implied that asking why doctors charged a particular fee was silly: "A tonsillectomy is worth $75 because that's just what it's worth!" While general practitioners tended to charge relatively uniform fees, surgeons and other specialists used a sliding scale that pegged rates to patients' perceived ability to pay. During the 1950s, a generational difference began to emerge: older surgeons used the sliding scale primarily to discount care for low-income patients, while younger ones used it to set fees above the standard rate for patients who possessed hospitalization insurance.[45] Fees also varied across medical regions. Physicians in different parts of the country pegged the usual and customary rate at widely varying levels. Surgeons in the West, for example, charged more for procedures than their northeastern counterparts.[46]

This seemingly unscientific approach to fee setting seemed at odds with the profession's commitment to scientific and ethical rigor. In a 1950 editorial in *Medical Economics*, Sheridan Baketel warned of the potential damage to public trust. He began with three documented examples of unusually high surgical fees: $950 for a hysterectomy, $750 for an unspecified "emergency operation," and $1,600 for an appendectomy. While physicians might dismiss such inflated charges as very rare, "the public takes no such broad view of the matter," Baketel stated. Citing estimates that anywhere between 1 and 15 percent of doctors overcharged, he suggested that "the filthy few who ruin our public relations should be cut out or otherwise controlled." To that end, Baketel urged his physician readers to support the work of medical society grievance committees and to "avoid even the *appearance* of charging exorbitant fees." Cartoons, one of the most popular features of *Medical Economics*, made a similar point. A 1950 cartoon, "Our Name Is Mud," showed a "fee gouger" in a shiny new car, his head shaped like a money bag with dollar signs on his eyes, tossing mud on the "Medical Profession in General."[47]

Awareness of patient discontent fueled the AMA's efforts to get members to discuss their fees in advance. To sweeten the bitter pill of rising costs, some doctors borrowed tactics from other service industries. For example, a California obstetrician reported in a 1953 issue of *Medical Economics* that his auto mechanic had given him the idea of giving expectant parents an advance estimate of the costs of a normal delivery; complaints about his fees had consequently declined. "Patients appreciate having the question of medical costs put on a businesslike basis," and the forms "make for better cooperation and understanding all around." For similar reasons, many physicians began to itemize their bills to make clearer what specific services patients were receiving. Again using the auto mechanic analogy, *Medical Economics* ran a cartoon, "Be Wise: Itemize," that compared the doctor's indignation over an auto mechanic's bill devoid of itemization with a patient's reaction to the doctor's bill equally lacking in detail.[48]

In an article aptly titled "Show Them What They're Paying For," a Kansas physician recounted how his billing practices had been transformed by a conversation overheard at a ladies' canasta party. "I was in his office just two hours and I got a bill for $36," one woman complained, "and the only thing it said was 'For professional services.'" Another card player chimed in, "In *my* husband's business they break down a bill into separate items [b]ut I guess doctors are too high-hat for that." A third concluded, "Well the strategy's easy enough to see through. If everything was in black and white, they couldn't hide behind the 'professional services' line. We'd *know* we were being over-charged." To counter such opinions, the doctor and his medical assistant developed a service slip that made it easy to itemize the patient's bill. Whereas previously patients had been "apt to kick if a bill runs over $25," the doctor noted, now they paid without argument. The itemized bill had other benefits as well: one woman commented on the "thorough checkup" she had received, while a man noticed that the doctor offered a metabolism test and made an appointment to get it.[49]

In response to fee issues, some medical societies also began to think more systematically about how to standardize billing practices. Their interest reflected the growing burden that insurance paperwork imposed on a doctor's practice. For example, instead of using words to describe the presenting problem, physicians were encouraged to use the codes from the International Classification of Diseases, which had been substantially revised in the 1940s. Even more ambitious were state medical societies' efforts to develop fee scales based on the relative amount of time and skill a procedure required. The systems developed by the California Medical Association and the Kansas State Medical Society were especially influential in this regard.[50]

While improvements such as itemization, disease coding, and the use of relative value scales might be portrayed as sincere efforts to explain costs to patients, the new billing culture was primarily driven by the needs of hospitals, insurance companies, and medical providers to manage an ever-more-complex system of insurance payment. In 1960, insurance coverage for routine office visits remained relatively rare outside prepaid group plans, but almost half of all Americans had hospital insurance plans that would cover care by their personal physicians during a hospitalization; applying for this reimbursement became an increasingly important aspect of doctors' private practices. Whereas the 1943 edition of Bredow's handbook for medical secretaries devoted only a paragraph to medical insurance, the 1959 edition had a whole chapter on the topic, including both the Blues and their commercial competitors.[51]

For all the praise heaped on private insurance as the "American way" to finance care, its logistics caused increasing frustration for both doctor and patient. Until the mid-1960s, when insurance companies and the AMA agreed on a standard claim form that could be used for all types of insurance, doctors' offices had to contend with a bewildering variety of forms that had to be completed to the insurer's idiosyncratic specifications. Meanwhile, as Bredow noted in the 1959 edition of her handbook, "many patients are not at all aware of what their contracts cover," frequently confusing hospitalization and medical care provisions. Patients also failed to notice exclusions for preexisting conditions, so that "time and time again claims are disallowed because the patient consulted the doctor, before the waiting period had elapsed, for a condition that existed at the time he took out medical-care insurance." In 1959, she suggested that patients bring their contracts to their doctors' offices to be deciphered and, in the 1966 edition, that they present insurance cards that specified the covered services.[52]

The Debate over Unnecessary Surgery

Because they were both easy to count and expensive, surgical procedures figured prominently in the 1950s debate over the nation's rising medical costs. As the number and cost of operations rose, unnecessary surgery became the focal point for concerns about overtreatment and overbilling. In 1953, these worries erupted in a very public controversy that resulted in more bad publicity for the medical profession.

The controversy centered on an article in *U.S. News and World Report*, a weekly magazine aimed at giving businessmen "news you can use," as its motto promised. In that spirit, *U.S. News* featured a lengthy interview with Paul Hawley, the director of the American College of Surgeons and formerly the chief surgeon in the European Theater of Operations during World War II and the medical director of the Veterans' Administration. Known for speaking bluntly, Hawley detailed the downside of medicine's entrepreneurial culture, in particular four unethical practices motivated solely by the desire to make more money: fee splitting (getting a share of the surgeon's fee for referring a patient), ghost surgery (having another physician operate in one's place without the patient's knowledge), unnecessary surgery, and overcharging. Asked if he thought some doctors operated only for money, he replied, "I don't think it. I know it—and I can prove it!" Fee splitting was common, Hawley explained, because general practitioners felt they were underpaid in relation to the specialist, "who gets all the gravy." To discourage unnecessary procedures, the American College of Surgeons was urging hospitals to have physician committees review pathology reports to confirm the necessity for surgery. Hawley suggested that this process be expanded into a "medical audit" that included all the tests and procedures ordered in the hospital.[53]

Although Hawley held physicians accountable, he also blamed patients, especially women, for the increase in unnecessary surgery. He opined, "Some women, it seems, love to be operated on," and he suggested that fear of cancer lay behind the rash of hysterectomies. Echoing Katharine Kellock's 1935 advice, he warned people to spend more effort when initially choosing physicians, to switch doctors if they spotted the telltale signs of unethical behavior, and to report suspicious behavior to the local medical society.[54]

Somewhat paradoxically, Hawley also recommended that physicians give patients more of a partnership role in the healing process. Noting that "medicine hasn't outgrown its phase of druidical priesthood yet," he observed, "the attitude of 'never mind, the doctor knows best' still goes." Until recently, physicians had not known very much themselves, and secrecy was necessary to hide that fact from the patient. "Now, with better education of the people and the sounder scientific basis of medicine itself, there is no longer any reason why you shouldn't sit down and explain everything to a patient." When asked if "all this crusading against unethical practices in medicine [was] going to undermine public confidence," Hawley conceded that it might but argued that no "great evil" could be corrected "without bringing it out into the light." When the reporter asked, "Would you stress the point that no doctor should recommend an operation for a patient that he wouldn't recommend for himself?," Hawley agreed and concluded, "I have had as little surgery done on me as possible."[55]

Hawley's interview provoked a furious outcry from his fellow physicians that itself became a news story covered by the *New York Times, Reader's Digest, Harper's,* and the *New Republic.* Members of the American Academy of General Practice voted to censure Hawley and asked the AMA to pursue disciplinary action against him. At the AMA's June 1953 meeting, delegates introduced eleven resolutions denouncing him. A special committee appointed to review the controversy issued a report chastising Hawley on the grounds that "destructive critical comments serve no useful purpose" but recommended against censure on the grounds that the AMA should support the right of free speech. The committee also urged physicians to support the AMA's work to improve public confidence in the profession, a sentiment echoed by its incoming president, Edward J. McCormick, who called on county medical societies to "continue to expel from our ranks those who are unethical, dishonest and unfair."[56]

Lambasted for having presented only one side of the story, *U.S. News* allowed the American Academy of General Practice's president, Dr. R. B. Robins, to present a rebuttal. Robins contended that Hawley had grossly exaggerated the extent of physicians' unethical behavior but agreed with his advice that patients needed to be careful when picking doctors, insist on itemized bills, and make use of local grievance committees. Hawley remained unrepentant, pointing out that everything he said in the interview had also appeared in the pages of the *Journal of the American Medical Association* and other medical periodicals. While medical journals largely sided with the AMA, the national news media tended to present Hawley as the more believable authority.[57]

In the wake of the Hawley Affair, as it came to be known, the AMA set up a special committee on medical practice to investigate the ethical lapses he cited and hired a prominent survey research firm, Rollen Watterson Associates, to interview both physicians and patients about the issues of money and trust. In 1954, the committee submitted a lengthy report that did not mention Hawley by name but confirmed his statement that fee splitting was widespread and detailed the reasons for its ubiquity. Interviews with physicians showed that "many are deeply affected by economic insecurity, by public hostility, by conflicts within the profession, and by the feeling that they are not accurately represented by their leadership." Interviews with patients suggested that their faith in the medical profession was corroded by suspicions about its business ethics. Although praising the skill and generosity of individual physicians they knew, laypeople expressed deep skepticism about the economic motives of the larger medical profession. But presented with this evidence, the AMA committee could offer no solutions other than encouraging more internal surveillance by local medical societies and more use of grievance committees—measures that had already proved wanting.[58]

Playing out as it did in the national press, the unnecessary surgery debate reinforced the message that patients needed to maintain the "be sure to investigate" mentality not just when selecting doctors but also when evaluating their treatment recommendations. In a 1954 article, "Unjustified Surgery," Greer Williams warned readers that they needed to learn the difference between "commercial" and "conservative" surgeons: "The doctor who does unjustified surgery is usually a good salesman," able to convince patients and himself that there is "something they 'ought to have out.'" Commercial surgeons consulted by neurotic patients eager to be operated on "cheerfully adopt the motto, 'Give the lady what she wants.'" In contrast, conservative surgeons viewed surgery as a last resort and did not hesitate to refuse operating on neurotic patients who demanded care. As Williams made clear to readers, savvy patients needed to beware of the commercial sort and patronize only the more honorable conservative surgeons.[59]

Even though rates of surgery overall were equal for the two sexes, lay critics tended to portray women as the chief culprits in the rise of unnecessary surgery. Echoing Hawley's assertions, Williams wrote that "the chief victims of unjustified surgery in the United States are neurotic women." The increase in hysterectomies got more attention in the magazine articles than the simultaneous rise in appendectomies, tonsillectomies, and gall bladder removals. In 1953's "Hysterectomy: Medical Necessity or Surgical Racket?" Lois Mattox Miller wrote, "Where the hysterectomy is clearly needed, it is a lifesaving, health restoring operation," but it had become far too casually done. As evidence, she cited surgical audits in which physician reviewers found that in between one quarter and one third of the cases examined, no evidence existed to justify the operation. Like Williams, Miller presented the conservative surgeon as the educated patient's better choice. Women needed to realize, as the Johns Hopkins surgeon Lawrence Wharton explained to her, that physicians often required less skill to operate than "to carry out a painstaking diagnostic study and advocate a conservative course."[60]

While unnecessary surgery attracted the greatest attention, it was by no means the only area of concern about overtreatment. A 1954 story on the front page of the *Washington Post* summarized papers from the First Interstate Scientific Assembly of Physicians in the District of Columbia and Virginia under the headline, "Doctors Told They Abuse, Overuse Drugs and Blood." According to the piece, "Medical spokesmen yesterday shook 'the skinny finger'" of blame at "practicing physicians, for overuse and abuse of vitamins, hormones, antibiotics, surgery and even human blood," and characterized treatments as a function of medical "fashion" rather than hard science. Other articles pointed to another kind of "doctor's dilemma"—"how to keep up" with the "flood of new medical knowledge—on which the life of a patient may depend," as Leonard Engel put it in 1959. The fact that busy practitioners had so little time to follow the burgeoning reports of modern scientific medicine made them all the more susceptible to reports of new—and lucrative—tests and procedures.[61]

For all the progress in biomedicine, determining the scientific indications for and efficacy of specific treatments remained extremely hard even for physicians. Arguments about what did and did not work were typically based on a small group of cases, often presented by doctors in favor of the particular approach under study. The idea of the random controlled trial was in its infancy. In response to these problems, researchers both within and outside the medical profession began to call for better data collection and studies of the comparative worth of different therapeutic approaches, but to little immediate effect. Meanwhile, laypeople attempting to determine the value of a particular treatment might well find that experts disagreed over its worth.[62]

The Tarnished Image

The heated arguments occurring within the medical profession did little to reassure skeptical patient-consumers about either the cost or efficacy of medical care. In such a climate, the advice simply to "defer to your doctor" became all the more problematic. By the mid-1950s, physician and lay writers alike urged patient-consumers not to assume the latest, most expensive care was necessarily the best care. Meanwhile, a few commentators came forward with even more searing indictments of the profession's failings.

A particularly scathing account of the doctor's tarnished image appeared in the March 1952 issue of *Redbook*, a general-interest magazine trying to build readership by providing provocative articles on topics such as racial prejudice and nuclear fear. In that spirit, novelist and essayist Philip Wylie, well known for his acerbic 1942 best seller *Generation of Vipers*, delivered a hard-hitting assessment of the modern doctor in "The Doctors' Conspiracy of Silence." In the United States today, Wylie wrote, "the 'noble art' of Medicine is too much practiced as a *business* in which life and death are commodities," and the medical profession, "which is supposed to keep its own house clean, too often looks the other way when you and I and our loved ones suffer or even die because of medical greed, needless medical stupidity, or plain medical crime." Wylie insisted that the vast majority of doctors were indeed good and honorable but argued that even they failed their patients by refusing to discipline the few corrupt or incompetent practitioners, leaving patients to suffer at the hands of "men with medical degrees who are, actually, criminals, psychopaths, sadists, demented by senility, dope addicts, and so on." But "*the real wrong,*" he argued, "*lies in the fact that the body of physicians and surgeons, who are best fitted to judge one another, usually maintain an utter silence about all such wanton ravishment of the public.*" After giving his readers advice about how to choose an honest, qualified physician, Wylie concluded dramatically, "I stand steadfast against a racket which is beneath men who occasionally are privileged to reach out and touch the hand of God."[63]

Defenders of American medicine continued to dismiss such criticisms as overreactions to the misdeeds of a few bad apples, maliciously magnified by an unscrupulous press trying to sell magazines. But the medical effort to downplay the signs of discontent was countered by academics who began to investigate American attitudes toward doctors via opinion polls and social surveys. These studies added additional weight to the arguments about the troubled state of the doctor-patient relationship.

The crudest available tool for assessing public sentiment was opinion polling, an increasingly popular practice. As part of its public relations effort, the AMA commissioned several such polls, of which the most widely cited was a 1956 study conducted by the Chicago firm Ben Gaffin Associates. The study documented a striking division of opinion that would be repeated in subsequent polls: respondents trusted their personal physicians far more than the medical profession as a whole. For example, while 84 percent of those surveyed said that their own doctors did not overcharge, 43 percent believed that doctors in general charged too much. Equally striking was the response to the statement, "My doctor operates more than necessary": 95 percent said no regarding their personal physicians, but one-third believed it was true of other doctors. Fifty-five percent of lay respondents voiced specific criticisms of the medical profession, most commonly about "fees, hurrying patients, coldness, and lack of frankness"; 43 percent agreed with the statement that "doctors have the idea they are always right."[64]

The Gaffin Associates also interviewed physicians and members of other professional groups. On some points, physicians proved even more critical of their colleagues than was the public. Eighty percent of physicians agreed that doctors did not give their patients as much time as they would like, compared to 60 percent of laypeople. In response to "Most doctors try to hide other doctors' mistakes," 58 percent of the doctors agreed, compared to 54 percent of the public. Likewise, representatives of two groups with enormous influence over public opinion and public policy, newspaper editors and lawyers, tended to be very critical of organized medicine, with 64 percent of editors and 41 percent of lawyers agreeing that "the AMA is not doing a good enough job of getting along with the public." The Gaffin study suggested why the AMA found the perception of a discontented public so hard to counteract:

not only did more than half of all the respondents question the quality of personal service offered by doctors, but influential opinion makers believed the public was dissatisfied with the medical profession's leadership as well.[65]

Recognizing that opinion polls offered too limited—and, some observers argued, too easily manipulated—an assessment of a complex subject, medical societies and private foundations also funded more in-depth studies of the doctor-patient relationship. Unlike interwar social science, which had focused primarily on collecting data about household budgets or days spent sick, these new studies approached the patient-doctor encounter with more interest in its sociological and psychological complexity. Their findings reinforced the perception that there was trouble in the Cold War doctor's office.

One of the earliest and most widely cited such studies was Columbia sociologist Earl Lomon Koos's portrait of "Regionville" (a pseudonym for a small town in upstate New York), a study bankrolled by the Commonwealth Fund. Koos's interviews suggested that the postwar profession's refusal to make house calls and prescribing of expensive medicines had made doctors seem more uncaring. He also documented a marked class difference in attitude; when asked if they had been dissatisfied with a recent medical encounter, 11 percent of upper-income respondents and 20 percent of middle-income respondents replied yes, compared to 38 percent of the lower-income respondents. In a follow-up study of nearby Rochester, funded by the NIH, Koos found that patients were less upset about the cost of medical care, which they accepted as "not to be out of line with the general high cost of living," than they were about its quality: 64 percent expressed concern that "modern, technic-centered medical practice lacked the human warmth of the old-time general practitioner (who possibly knew less about medicine but more about his patients)." Younger households, those where the father was under age forty, expressed this criticism even more strongly than older households. Said a young middle-class matron, "If we could feel that we *mean* something to Doctor ———, I'd be happy with him." Instead, she noted, he had to look at her chart or ask the nurse to remember her name. "It's like running through an assembly line to go to his office. . . . I'm sure, though, that he knows his medicine—from that point I'm satisfied."[66]

From his research, Koos concluded that "the 'halo' of the physician" had been "subject to considerable battering" for both economic and emotional reasons. Avoiding blame directed at doctor or patient, Koos presented their problems as the unintended consequence of their "differing subcultures" and "different languages"; "dissatisfaction resulted from a lack of communication between the physician and his patient." The growing focus on prescriptions and procedures threatened to reduce the quality of the doctor-patient relationship. "Most patients and families see the physician as a purveyor of services related to a given symptom. Their view is not much different from the one they hold of the garage mechanic, who is asked to repair the lights, the horn, or the carburetor of the car when these cease to function properly." But healing was a much more complicated matter. If doctors were to have better relationships with their patients, they had to become better teachers and explain "the why and how of illness," Koos concluded.[67]

While Koos emphasized the class dimensions of the problem, other postwar social scientists focused more on the interpersonal dynamics of the doctor-patient relationship and the growing imbalance between the knowledge and power of both parties. Some social scientists suggested that this asymmetry necessarily reinforced doctors' authority and the patients' passivity; in his influential 1951 formulation of the "sick role," sociologist Talcott Parsons argued that illness required patients to step outside their "mature" selves and trust in their physicians as children did parents. Yet as Parsons noted, grown people did not so easily give up that adult identity. Other social scientists and clinicians, among them psychologist Carl Rogers and psychiatrist Thomas Szasz, began to make a different argument: the growing asymmetry of knowledge and power between doctor and patient heightened rather than diminished the need for shared decision making, particularly in the case of so-called educated or intelligent patients—that is, patients similar in educational and class background to doctors.[68]

That argument was front and center in a 1950 research study Ernest Dichter prepared for the California Medical Association and the Alameda County Medical Association. Born in Austria, Dichter received a doctorate in psychology from the University of Vienna in 1934, training in an anti-Freudian form of motivation-based personality theory. Like many Jewish academics, he fled Europe for the United States, arriving in 1937. Following the lead of his mentor, Paul Lazarsfeld, Dichter set up his own market research firm in 1946, specializing in qualitative research using what today would be called focus groups.[69]

In his 1950 study, Dichter described his adopted country as in the midst of an upward evolution from "immaturity and emotionality to maturity and rationality" and consequently in need of leaders who were "more mature, more far sighted, better cooperators than the others." Unfortunately, Dichter observed, doctors were not meeting that leadership challenge very effectively. Rather than portraying patients as the chief source of the problem, Dichter suggested that many doctors were "in general insecure, and behaved in many instances emotionally and immaturely," especially when they encountered better-educated, more assertive patients. While Dichter certainly leveled criticisms at patients, his study implied that they were evolving toward maturity more quickly than their physicians.[70]

A number of the laypeople Dichter interviewed voiced their wish to be treated like grown-ups. Explained one interviewee, "He definitely wasn't the right doctor for me. Like a New York bus conductor he rarely answered any questions and never explained anything to the patient—why he did what he was doing." Instead of helping the patient "understand what's wrong with me" and how to address the problem, the doctor "wrapped himself in a mystical, weird silence which removed him to a god-like distance and height." Dichter attributed these kinds of complaints to both rising levels of schooling and an increase in consumer savvy: "Patients, being part of the world we live in, have changed with this world. They no longer simply accept the authority of the doctor. They have become more sophisticated in every respect." He also noted, "In our commercial studies we have found that people ask many more questions about advertising and products' services than they used to" and that they had become "more conscious of the powers having influence over them." This questioning attitude inevitably carried over into the doctor's office. In Dichter's view, today's patients "are better informed; they have read more popular medical articles [and] have read about new discoveries." In sum, "the patients of 1950 are no longer the patients of 1914 or 1920."[71]

The same themes emerged in the 1954 study that the AMA commissioned from Rollen Watterson Associates for which Dichter acted as a consultant. Based on hundreds of interviews with both doctors and patients, Watterson's final report described how rising expectations for medical science were contributing to patient confusion and discontent: "Today the word 'science' has some of the connotations of magic in the non-scientific man's vocabulary." Wherever he looks, modern man hears that "science reveals a new substance to make his teeth whiter, a way to estimate his fitness for a job, a chance to cruise around the solar system." Given the extravagance of such claims, "It is not easy for him to understand where science leaves off and science fiction begins." Physicians tended to suffer because the patient's "science fiction expectations may become attached to his doctor who is the only real live scientist he knows,—a dispenser of 'wonder drugs' and a performer of 'life-saving operations.'"[72]

For most people, the Watterson study observed, the doctor was akin to a priest, who "works with forbidden things, things beyond most people's knowledge." Likewise, the doctor "thinks that in order to keep his patients' confidence he must live up to a superman role, and build the illusion that medicine is an exact science and doctors infallible." To retain patient confidence, the doctor could be tempted to subscribe to the "god-complex," the sense that he is "God's right hand man." One doctor stated, "If you tell [patients] you don't know, they lose faith in you." But a doctor should never forget, the report pointed out, that "if you don't tell them and they find out, they not only lose faith; they are disillusioned and even vindictive." The same doctor also mentioned the mass media's role in this process of disillusionment: "Magazine editors whose business it is to gauge public response and thereby build circulation will not hesitate to exploit this bitterness." Nowadays, when a doctor approached the treatment room door, he did not know "whether the patient on the other side thinks he is a god or a crook."[73]

Similar results came from a study conducted by Richard H. Blum, a psychologist affiliated with the Stanford Research Institute, in the late 1950s, again on behalf of the California Medical Association. Based on five years of interviews with patients and physicians, Blum described a pervasive lay "disenchantment" with the new physician. While portraying patients as motivated by complex combinations of envy, anger, and fear, he suggested that physicians' unskillful handling of those emotions helped contribute to "the bitter fruits" produced by a broken doctor-patient relationship, among them "treatment failures, patients quitting their doctor, the majority of citizens critical of doctors and medical care, patients not paying doctors' fees, patients turning to nonmedical healers, and fast-rising rates of malpractice suits."[74]

Based on such studies, social scientists concluded that American medicine was suffering from what they termed a "cultural lag." Physicians' attitudes and behaviors were badly out of step with the postwar public's mood. From these social scientific "diagnoses" emerged calls for the medical profession to rethink its approach to the patient-citizen. On the one hand, the new work presented patients as a bundle of complex and sometimes unrealistic desires, often in dire need of guidance from their physicians. On the other hand, it suggested that physicians needed to improve their own maturity levels, and as the expert party to the transaction, they had all the more obligation to do so. To this end, Dichter told a group of physicians in 1958, the doctor needs to "regard himself as more a business man and less a saint" and to "accept the fact that today's patient has grown up and can read current medical articles."[75]

This message found a receptive audience among some medical educators. The social scientific critique of the doctor-patient relationship helped encourage educational reforms aimed at improving physicians' skills of appreciating the "whole patient." To that end, a number of medical schools, including Harvard and Case Western, adopted a more "comprehensive" approach aimed at teaching students to communicate more effectively with patients. As H. Jack Geiger, a medical student at Case Western, wrote in a 1956 *New York Times* article, "The Patient as a Human Being," the new curriculum reflected the insights of Dichter and Koos. "A good deal is now known about patients' preconceptions, desires and feelings," he wrote, and what they wanted was a cross between the "good old fashioned family doctor, radiating interest, warmth, sincerity and understanding" and "the cool, precise clinician, the specialist fortified by electrocardiograms and X-rays and laboratory tests, the man who 'knows his medicine.'"[76]

Other physicians suggested the even more radical idea of enlisting educated patients as partners in the healing process. In a 1956 article, "The Basic Models of the Doctor-Patient Relationship," published in the prestigious *Archives of Internal Medicine*, psychiatrists Thomas Szasz and Marc Hollender suggested that possibility. They argued against the existence of a single model for the doctor-patient relationship and in favor of three distinct variants: the "passive" mode, which pertained in emergencies; the "guided" relationship, in which the physician simply told the patient what to do; and the "mutual" relationship, in which the two had "approximately equal" power and acted as a team. Szasz and Hollender suggested that all three models had their place but clearly regarded the "mutuality model" as the highest form, since it "requires a more complex psychological and social organization on the part of both participants." While it was "rarely appropriate" for children, the "mentally defective," the "very poorly educated," or the "profoundly immature," the more similar the background of doctor and patient, the "more appropriate and necessary this model of therapy becomes."[77]

Blum's study highlighted the impact on medicine of the "at your service" mentality of the 1950s. While physicians felt no kinship with the banker or the auto mechanic, that comparison came more naturally to patients. Some laypeople, Blum observed, viewed the doctor as "a professional employee of the patient." Having paid for the doctor's services, the patient felt entitled to ask for "full explanations of the reasons for the doctor's recommendations or actions." In contrast, "the average physician," according to Blum, "often assumes the patient should be subservient" and "may forget that the doctor is an intelligent employee who is offering service in exchange for money." As the size of patients' bills grew, so, too, did their expectations of what they were getting.[78]

Still, many physicians found the concept of patient as partner or doctor as employee far-fetched, to put it mildly. As a 1960 article in *Medical Economics* about Blum's work noted, physicians "got their backs up" when confronted by social scientists looking for the "hidden motives in what you and your patients do" and "explaining you to yourself in the complex and sometimes pretentious jargon of biosocial science." From this perspective, the strategy of according patients' demands more attention seemed a dangerous form of mollycoddling bound to make the practice of medicine even more difficult. An occasional patient might be sensible, but the patient public as a whole was not to be trusted to make rational therapeutic or economic decisions about medical care.[79]

In equating patient discontent with neurotic behavior, medicine's defenders returned to a strategy used in the interwar period to dismiss the "guinea piggers" as unstable individuals with authority problems. But by the late 1950s and early 1960s, that argument was becoming increasingly tenuous. The image of physicians as all-powerful, fully knowledgeable experts conflicted with another concern: that the profession was becoming too easily swayed both by therapeutic fashion and by an inability to resist patient demands. Blaming patients for unnecessary treatments meant conceding that scientific men of medicine were too weak to avoid being pushed around by neurotic, immature patients. If, in fact, doctors knew what was best, why did they agree to treatments that were wasteful or ill-advised? Why did the "cool, precise clinician" give in to the inflated demands of *Reader's Digest*–toting patients? This argument also evaded the question of the medical profession's complicity in raising patients' expectations of medical miracles. Too often physicians seemed more than willing to promote any and all new treatments so long as they profited from them. Nor did doctors appear to be as resistant to commercial influence as they needed to be, given the powerful influence that the pharmaceutical industry now seemed to wield over their prescribing patterns.

In discussing these issues, both doctor and lay writers turned to retail metaphors to try to grapple with medicine's problems. Defenders of physicians' fees often used comparisons with other aspects of consumer culture to explain why their economic methods differed from those of the department store. "The physician doesn't have a high-test treatment or a bargain-basement special," explained a 1960 article in *Medical Economics*. "Every patient gets the best brand of care, regardless of what he pays." As C. Marshall Lee Jr., a Boston physician, explained, "This is one of the biggest reasons why doctors often have a hard time explaining their fees to patients." The consumer had been conditioned to buy goods "as his means and judgment dictate"—for example, to choose the $5 hat over the $200 hat. "But no doctor may offer a patient his second-best skill, judgment, or effort. It is his best, whether the patient is affluent or needy." As a result, "Everybody gets a $200 hat, regardless of what he pays."[80]

Physicians frequently contrasted patients' griping about medical bills with their cheerful willingness to pay for leisure and entertainment goods. "We all know the family that apparently can't pay a $150 surgical fee, yet manages to own a $250 television set," Charles Miller wrote in 1950, but "there's no use preaching that a repaired hernia is more important than Hopalong Cassidy." Likewise, a 1955 *Medical Economics* editorial, "Most Fees Are Modest," suggested that patients could hardly call charging $350 for a hysterectomy (the median rate at that time) "exorbitant" when nowadays "they'll spend $300 on accessories for a new car, and sometimes twice that on a high-fidelity phonograph." Using data from the Department of Commerce, the journal published a chart in 1955 comparing the amounts Americans spent "for being well" (drugs, hospitals, physicians' services, and other health care) and "for well-being" (personal care, tobacco, alcohol, and recreation). Readers liked the graphic so much that *Medical Economics* made available reproductions suitable for framing and hanging in their offices. Wrote one physician, "The chart would be worth a thousand words in dealing with the occasional patient who complains unreasonably about the fees charged him."[81]

In responding to the growing volume of complaints about rising fees, physicians articulated an unflattering view of the American public. The problem with the medical system, they argued, lay not in the way providers set fees, which were eminently fair and reasonable. Rather, it lay in patients' entrenched unwillingness to accept personal responsibility either for maintaining their health or for managing their personal finances. Expecting quick fixes for complex medical problems, American patients demanded the latest in new and improved medicine but then did not want to pay its fair price. From the doctor's standpoint, patients' constant "kicking" about doctors' bills reflected their immaturity.

But evidence of many physicians' own prosperity complicated their ability to adopt the halo-and-wings defense to justify their higher fees. As doctors' incomes rose dramatically in the 1950s, allowing them and their families to enjoy a better lifestyle than their Great Depression predecessors, they inevitably attracted envy. As Herrymon Maurer noted in a 1954 *Fortune* article, doctors were becoming wealthier and displaying that wealth. "In some circles physicians are labeled 'the new rich,' and Cadillacs are supposed to have displaced Buicks as 'the doctor's car.'" As doctors' incomes continued to rise over the 1950s, the profession faced a new dilemma, aptly captured in a 1960 *Medical Economics* article, "How Prosperous Should You Look?," contrasting the behavior of two successful surgeons, one who lived a lavish lifestyle and "was always bragging" about his wealth, and one who was "so sensitive to what people might think that he drives an old Chevy and lives in a boxlike house." As the article suggested, it was hard to navigate "between the extremes of ostentation and self-denial."[82]

While women frequently figured as the archetype of the "neurotic" patient demanding unnecessary treatment, the examples of patients who suffered the pangs of both therapeutic disappointment and economic resentment were often men. Selig Greenberg's 1960 article, "The Decline of the Healing Art," for one, began with a story about a male friend. Under considerable personal pressure at work and home, the friend felt run-down and had trouble sleeping. He made an appointment with his doctor, who performed a complete and expensive checkup and then informed the man that there was nothing wrong with him. When he still felt poorly, the friend went back, only to have his doctor dismiss them as "neurotic symptoms." Asked by the "hurried and harried" doctor if anything was bothering him, the friend was reluctant to unburden himself, feeling that he had already taken up too much time, and left unsatisfied. "On the way out, the sight of the doctor's Cadillac parked at the curb stirred an added resentment toward a profession that—as he sees it—gets rich at the expense of other people's misery."[83]

According to Greenberg, "Money became the focal point for his grievances although in fact—like many others—his disenchantment was largely due to the feeling that he had been treated with condescension and denied his rightful share of sympathy and affection." At a time when psychosomatic ailments were on the rise, the pressures converging on the doctor's office made that sense of being cared for harder and harder to find. With fewer physicians now working longer hours, the result was "a kind of hit-or-miss medicine" in which "the busy physician has little time to look beyond the organic symptoms of troubled patients." As Greenberg suggested, "Poor medicine is inevitable when crowded schedules force a doctor to get through with a patient in five or ten minutes." Under those constraints, the healer had no time to probe for insight. "Instead his watchword becomes, 'When in doubt prescribe.' An antibiotic or tranquilizer serves as a substitute for painstaking diagnosis and clinical judgment—and a source of relatively effortless income for the doctor." The consequences appeared in the form of "our huge consumption of sedatives and tranquilizers, in the dismal trek from specialist to specialist, in the resort to exorcism by surgery, in the crowded schedules of our all-too-few psychiatrists, and in the packed warrens of our mental hospitals."[84]

So despite their protestations, doctors found it increasingly difficult to escape the idea that they bore a new and onerous responsibility for patient satisfaction. The postwar profession presented its ability to deliver more and better goods and services—prescription drugs, diagnostic blood tests, X-ray technology, cancer treatments, and the like—as the mark of what made the American version of free-market medicine superior to its "socialized" counterparts. Providing those new and improved products was a demonstrable way of showing that one was a "man who knew his medicine." Much as physicians might want to do otherwise, they could not deliver goods such as prescription drugs or surgical procedures without becoming implicated in their cost and effectiveness. Moreover, along with this product- and procedure-heavy style of practice came expectations about how it was delivered: Did the sum total of the tests and procedures add up to a coherent whole that satisfied patients' expectations?

Presented with a model of medicine cast in a free-market mold, postwar patients assumed the role of disgruntled customer. Having cast its lot with free enterprise, the medical profession found it hard to ignore the buyers' remorse about the new medicine. In evading the hated yoke of government, doctors had made themselves responsible for the disappointments as well as the successes of the new medical department store. Having embraced the market, they now had to live with its consequences.

A Crisis in American Medicine

In October 1960, just weeks before the presidential election, a special issue of *Harper's* hit the newsstands and soon sold out. Drawing together themes that had been developed over the past decade, the editors declared the existence of a "crisis in American medicine." The special issue suggested a grim picture: the rush toward specialization and technologically based care had produced a very expensive, uncoordinated system of health care in which the "whole patient" was being lost. At a time when Americans desperately needed family doctors to guide medical decision making, their numbers were shrinking. The mainstream medical profession continued to resist efforts to redress growing problems of cost, quality, and access. In the words of distinguished microbiologist René Dubos, "Medicine today is like a mighty and glamorous ocean liner with powerful engines and luxurious appointments but with a defective compass and an absurdly small rudder." After finishing the special issue, *Harper's* readers might well have conjured up images of the *Titanic*. Whereas in the 1930s, the nation's problems had been characterized as a "medical muddle," the *Harper's* forum marked the first but certainly not the last time that they would be declared to represent a state of crisis.[85]

In a radio forum held soon after its release, AMA representative James Appel denounced the *Harper's* issue as "a mixture of truths, half-truths and distortions" and insisted that "there is no crisis in American medicine today," although he noted that one might well be "on the way" if Congress passed the new Medicare bill then under consideration. But the special issue was quickly republished in book form, and its arguments inspired more commentary in local newspapers, on television shows, and at medical society meetings. It also prompted many letters to the editor; the editors noted that not only did 75 percent of the laypeople agree with the issue's negative views, but "half the physicians we heard from concede that a medical crisis exists and disagree strongly with the way their societies are coping with it."[86]

Harper's declaration that medicine was "in crisis" reflected growing media attention to the rate of medical inflation. A 1959 article in the *Washington Post* carried the startling headline, "Per Capita Health Cost Up 359% since 1929," while a 1960 *New York Times* piece noted a "42% Rise Reported in Medical Costs" since 1953. The AMA protested that the numbers behind these headlines were incorrect, hiring an economist to show that when properly controlled for inflation, the costs of medical care were actually down, but the U.S. Labor Department remained unpersuaded. Medical leaders also tried to put the rising rates of medical spending in context by comparing them with other statistics about consumption—for example, that Americans spent more on chewing gum than on medical research and more on tobacco and alcohol than on medical care.[87]

But the issue of rising medical costs continued to attract extensive press coverage. Realizing it had a hot topic to promote, *Reader's Digest* ran ads in national papers for its July 1960 issue featuring an article titled "7 Ways to Cut Your Medical Costs," providing vital information at a time when "the price of medical care is at an all-time high, and rising." Insurance companies also emphasized the "high cost of being sick," citing a recent *U.S. News and World Report* article that found only one in ten Americans had sufficient hospitalization insurance. For example, Bankers Life and Casualty Company used the one-in-ten statistic to promote its White Cross insurance plan, which "pays you $100 a Week extra!" Likewise, Blue Cross/Blue Shield ran ads touting its "service benefits" as "the best bet against rising hospital and medical costs."[88]

As part of the larger discussion of medicine's "tarnished image," the late-1950s commentary included a growing sense of dissatisfaction with the new product that was supposed to "solve" the problems of the patient-consumer, the private insurance plan. The first and most glaring problem remained the large number of uninsured people. With only about a quarter of the work-force in unions as of 1960, many workers labored in industries that offered no fringe benefits of any sort; for those lucky enough to have insurance, it usually ended with retirement. The growing concern for the elderly was captured in a 1960 *Washington Post* article. Reporter Eve Edstrom visited the Golden Age Club of Washington, D.C., and found people angry about doctors who billed for phone calls, charged $50 for looking at an X-ray, and offered only minor discounts on their large fees. As one reported to Edstrom, "I told my doctor I was a poor widow lady living on Social Security and he said he would reduce the bill by $10—if I paid within 30 days." After the difficulties of caring for her elderly mother, another woman, described as a housewife with a "comfortable Chevy Chase home," stated, "I am shopping for another doctor for my family because we can't afford the one we have had for 18 years."[89]

Nor were those Americans covered by private insurance necessarily happy with its workings, as medical reporter Robert Plumb documented in a 1957 series of articles for the *New York Times*. Since the great majority of insurance plans only covered hospital care, physicians frequently admitted patients to the hospital to treat them and charged more for services delivered there because the insurance plan would provide reimbursement. Insurers then passed those costs on to subscribers in the form of higher premiums and de-ductibles. Patients with insurance still ended up with substantial bills, while those without it had to cover the whole cost, often at the same prices charged to the insured. Insurance companies repeatedly asked for raises in subscrib-ers' premium rates, prompting questions about the economic controls, or absence of them, in medical practice. As physicians repeatedly pointed out, they had no control over what hospitals charged for care. But as a report com-missioned by the New Jersey Banking Commission noted in 1960, physicians "are the ones who admit the patients to the hospital, who determine how long he must stay, who set the standards for the services they must have available [and] the extent of the usage of those services." So try as they might to deflect responsibility for the rising costs, doctors had difficulty avoiding the blame.[90]

Given that many experts connected the cycle of rising costs to the fee-for-service system, some lay reformers urged "smart" patients to consider the alternative of a prepaid plan, in which patients paid a fixed amount each month entitling them to preventive care from a coordinated team of medical specialists. By the late 1950s, such plans were available in the largest American cities, including Los Angeles, Washington, D.C., and New York; roughly 4 percent of the 110 million Americans with medical insurance had this type of coverage.[91] In *The Doctor Business*, Richard Carter promoted prepaid plans as the best solution to the nation's medical problems.

But patient-consumers' enrollment in such plans remained limited. In part, their availability was constrained by location and occupation. Many large corporate employers only offered insurance plans on the fee-for-service model. The expansion of prepaid plans faced daunting opposition from local medical societies, as evident in the long-running battle between the Health Insurance Plan of Greater New York and the Richmond County Medical Society over hospital privileges for the plan's physicians. In addition, patients did not necessarily see the group plans as appealing. As sociologists discovered, some patients felt that they could be just as impersonal as their fee-for-service counterparts. Moreover, having been told that doctor-switching was the best safeguard against medical abuse, patient-consumers tended to distrust plans that made it hard for them to quit doctors they did not like.[92]

So extensive were public worries about medical care that they became an important factor in the presidential election of 1960. Aware of the public concern, candidate John F. Kennedy made it a campaign issue, and his advocacy for what later became Medicare may well have helped him win a very close election. Meanwhile, worries about unnecessary surgery and the Cold War "doctor's dilemmas" converged with intensifying debates over medical professionals' use of the prescription pad. Concerns about the new doctors' drugs fused with those about the "doctor business" to create enormous pressures for change in the 1960s.

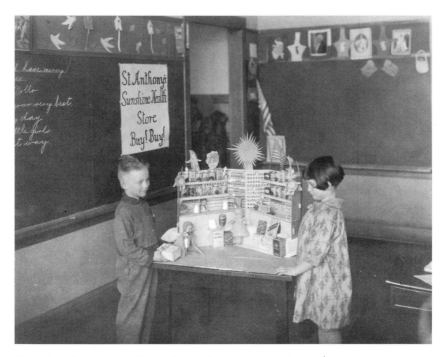

St. Anthony's Elementary School, Fargo, North Dakota, mid-1920s (Institute for Regional Studies, Fargo). This photograph shows a health education exhibit created by a third grade class at a Fargo elementary school. The accompanying sign, which reads, "St. Anthony's Sunshine Health Store, Buy! Buy!" suggests the association of good health with wise shopping, symbolized here by a tempting array of packaged foods and canned goods. Although often associated with big cities, the equation of careful consumption with health promotion had clearly spread to small towns such as Fargo, which in 1920 had a population of 22,000.

	100%	100%	100%	100%	100%	100%	100%
	$6.45 PER CAPITA	$7.54 PER CAPITA	$21.32 PER CAPITA	$21.20 PER CAPITA	$11.14 PER CAPITA	$36.09 PER CAPITA	$53.89 PER CAPITA
ALL OTHER SERV.	4.9%	7.7%	10.2%	13.6%	5.3%	14.4%	9.5%
PUBLIC HEALTH	2.6%				3.7%		
DENTISTS	10.2%	12.2%	10.3%	2.4%	8.5%	3.4%	2.6%
				7.4%			12.6%
HOSPITALS	16.8%	7.4%	14.7%	18.2%	10.3%	16.0%	
							28.7%
DRUGS AND MEDICINES	28.0%	44.2%	29.8%	27.2%	41.4%	23.5%	
						18.7%	20.4%
PHYSICIANS	37.5%	27.7%	33.7%	31.2%	30.8%	24.0%	26.2%
	CHESTER CO. TENN. 1930	TOOMBS CO. GA. 1930	SHELBY CO. IND. 1928	FRANKLIN CO. VT. 1929	LEE CO. MISS. 1930	SAN JOAQUIN CO. CALIF. 1929	PHILADELPHIA PENNA. 1928

THE PERCENTAGE COMPOSITION OF THE MEDICAL BILL IN SEVEN
SURVEYED COMMUNITIES

"The Percentage Composition of the Medical Bill in Seven Surveyed Communities"
(I. S. Falk, C. Rufus Rorem, and Marta D. Ring, *The Costs of Medical Care* [Chicago:
University of Chicago Press, 1933], 164). As part of the first full-scale study of medical
economics in the United States, the Committee on the Costs of Medical Care collected
household budget information in seven different communities between 1928 and 1930.
This chart shows the relative amounts that those households spent on dentists, hospitals,
physicians, and medicines. The high proportion of spending on medicinal drugs, most of
which were bought without a prescription in this era, suggests why many physicians viewed
the drugstore as an unwelcome competitor for the patient-consumer's dollar.

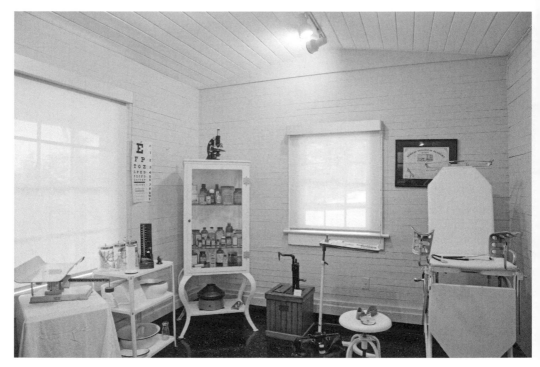

Re-creation of 1930s doctor's office, Mobile Medical Museum (George F. Landegger Collection of Alabama Photographs in Carol M. Highsmith's America, LC-DIG-highsm-05217, Library of Congress, Prints and Photographs Division). As office-based practice became more central to their success, physicians began to devote more attention to the arranging and furnishing of their workspaces. Since medical ethics forbade any form of advertising, the office's function as the "doctor's showroom" was all the more important. In order to attract and keep patients, doctors were advised to provide both a cheerful, comfortable waiting area and a clean, functional examining room. This re-creation of a 1930s doctor's office in Mobile, Alabama, features the kind of medical tools and furnishings that an interwar patient would likely have seen on a visit to a general practitioner.

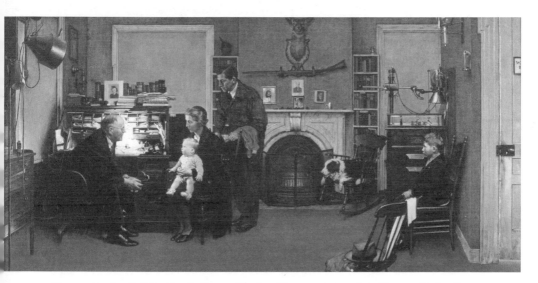

Norman Rockwell, "The Family Doctor" (printed by permission of the Norman Rockwell Family Agency, © 1947 the Norman Rockwell Family Entities). The artist Norman Rockwell frequently included the family doctor in his nostalgic evocations of everyday American life. Like many of his works, this painting was based on a painstaking re-creation of the subject, in this case the office of Dr. George Russell, Rockwell's own personal physician in Arlington, Vermont. A local couple posed with their baby as patients; the dog belonged to Dr. Russell. When asked if it was proper to have a dog in a doctor's office, Rockwell replied, "Nobody ever seemed the worse for it." Like Eugene Smith's photo essay "The Country Doctor," which appeared in *Life* a year later, Rockwell's affectionate portrait of the family doctor eulogized a style of medical practice that seemed to be fast disappearing in the post–World War II period.

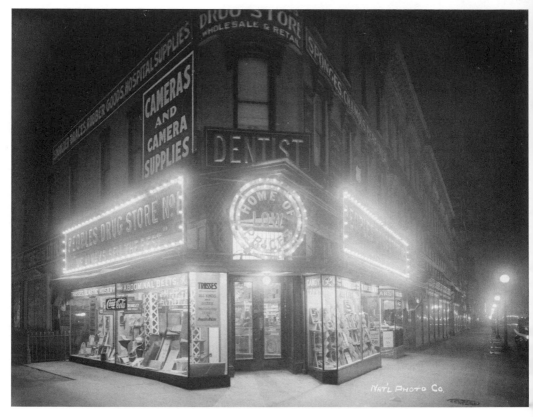

Peoples Drug Store, 7th & K Streets NW, Washington, D.C., ca. 1919 (National Photo Company Collection, LC-DIG-npcc-28982, Library of Congress, Prints and Photographs Division). Founded in 1905 by Malcolm G. Gibbs, the Peoples Drug Store chain originated in Washington, D.C., and expanded to more than 500 stores in the eastern United States. At its opening in 1909, the flagship store at the corner of 7th and K Streets gave away leather cigar cases and mirrored compacts to its first customers. Describing it as "a department drug store," a 1922 *Washington Post* article titled "The Once-Ubiquitous Peoples Drug Stores" observed, "You can't miss the display from the sidewalk and can even see it from an automobile or passing street car. It is just like a page in a paper." This photograph taken at night shows the brightly lit marquee that helped make the drugstore an inviting destination after dark.

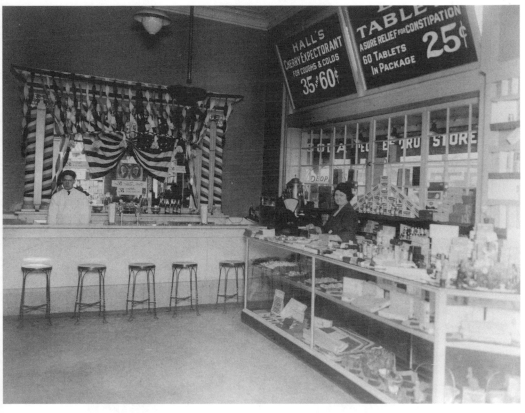

Interior of Peoples Drug Store, 14th and Park Streets, Washington, D.C., ca. 1922
(National Photo Company Collection, LC-USZ62-129897, Library of Congress, Prints
and Photographs Division). This photograph of the new Peoples store in the Mt. Pleasant
area of Washington prominently featured the soda fountain and perfume counter. Like
many chain stores, Peoples expanded its food offerings to include not only ice cream
and carbonated drinks but also sandwiches and baked goods. While featuring food and
perfumes, the prominent display of ads for Hall's Cherry Expectorant and constipation-
relieving tablets reminded customers that for all its frills, selling medicines still remained
the store's central purpose.

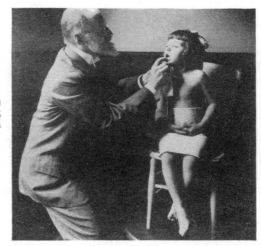

Dr. Bertram Burp, Noted Horse Doctor, and ex-cigarette endorser, is head of the Advertising Clinic in Vienna.

"The effect of yeast on my *pocketbook* is remarkable"

ARE you troubled with sheriffs in front of the eyes?

Hot flashes? Hoof and Mouth disease? Rubber checks?

Falling of the bank account? Goldman Sachs under the eyes?

All these conditions come from a sluggish Republican party.

Go to the polls, young man, and vote a straight anti-prohibition party . . . and

in the meantime, rise in the world by eating Yeast.

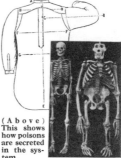

(Left) "I was badly run down," writes Lizzie Lapoopkawa, "by a Mack Truck. After taking 37 yeast cakes, I licked hell out of the truck driver, and haven't been run down since."

(A b o v e) This shows how poisons are secreted in the system.

Before and After Using Vallee's Yeast

"The effect of yeast on my *pocketbook* is remarkable" (*Ballyhoo*, November 1932, 26). Like *Mad Magazine* would do a generation later, the 1930s humor magazine *Ballyhoo* featured many satires about advertising. A popular theme was the use of modern medicine to turn insignificant symptoms into urgent problems requiring the frequent purchase of a manufacturer's product. In that spirit, this cartoon lampooned the Fleischmann's Yeast Company's use of medical testimonials as a health boon. The doctor is humorously styled as "Dr. Bertram Burp, Noted Horse Doctor, and ex-cigarette endorser" affiliated with "the Advertising Clinic in Vienna." Dr. Burp's Viennese connection reflected Fleischmann's heavy reliance on prominent European physicians because the AMA had convinced American doctors not to cooperate in such campaigns.

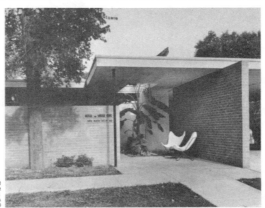

exterior view of
entrance and carport
at extreme right (right);
large waiting room
looking north (below)

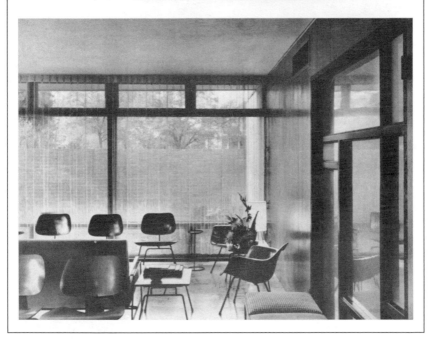

Doctors' office, Gonzales, Texas, mid-1950s (Paul Hayden Kirk and Eugene D. Sternberg, *Doctors' Offices and Clinics, Medical and Dental* [New York: Reinhold, 1955], 60, 61). Designed by architect R. Gommel Roessner, this office built for two general practitioners illustrates the postwar preference for streamlined design and the heightened concern for patient privacy. In the notes accompanying the plan, the architect wrote, "Waiting room with large glass windows is protected from the street by a high wall."

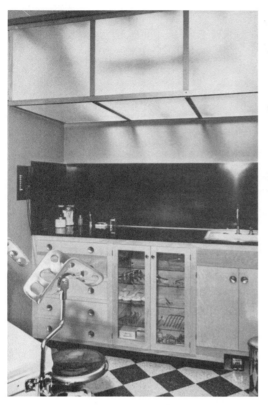
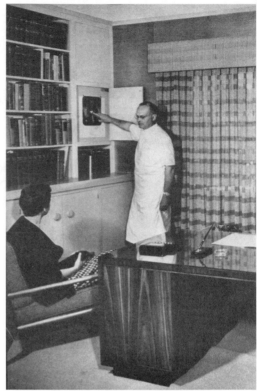

A doctor's office, San Jose, California, 1955 (Lois Hoffman, "Planning Paid Off in This One-Man Office," *Medical Economics* 32 [August 1955]: 129, 131, 134). When he moved from downtown San Francisco to the outskirts of San Jose, Dr. M. James Whitelaw, an endocrinologist specializing in treating infertility, worked with an architect to plan his "one-man office." Featured in a 1955 *Medical Economics* article, these photographs show how different spaces functioned to help the physician do his work more effectively. In the examining room, the doctor first saw the patient in a clean, well-lighted room equipped with the latest diagnostic tools. In his office, he had a comfortable yet dignified setting in which to discuss the examination results, including a lightbox where he could display an X-ray for the patient. Finally, in her office, the doctor's nurse had access to the latest office technology for the keeping of patient records and preparing of bills and insurance forms.

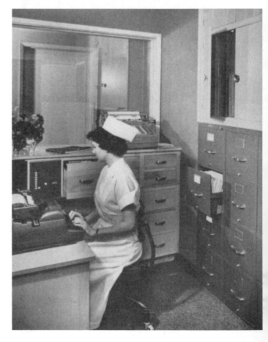

ORVILLE S. WALTERS, M. D.
218 GRAND BUILDING • MCPHERSON, KANSAS

Name_____

Date_____

Office Visit_____		
Physical Examination_____		
Medication_____		
Urinalysis_____		
Blood Count, White Cells_____		
Blood Count, Red Cells_____		
Blood Count, Differential_____		
Hemoglobin_____		
Sedimentation Rate_____		
Electrocardiogram_____		
Electrocardiograph Exercise Test_____		
Basal Metabolism_____		
Gastric Analysis_____		
Blood Sugar_____		
Kidney Function Test_____		
Blood Test_____		
Skin Test_____		
Office Surgery_____		
X-Ray_____		
Total_____		

Itemized doctor's bill, 1951 ("Show Them What They're Paying For," *Medical Economics* 28 [January 1951]: 203). As medical fees rose after World War II, *Medical Economics* urged its physician readers to provide patients with itemized bills detailing all the services delivered during an office visit. In a 1951 article, a Kansas doctor shared the form that he and his office assistant had devised after a businessman patient complained about being handed a big bill with no explanation for what it covered. Although intended to help reconcile patients to the cost of care, the itemized bill also created an opportunity for patients to question both the necessity for and price of specific procedures.

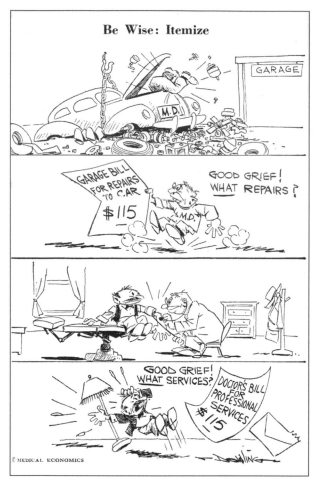

Be Wise: Itemize

Medical Economics was famous for the number and quality of its medically themed cartoons. While some were meant purely for amusement, others aimed to reinforce the journal's editorial advice to its physician readers.

"Be Wise: Itemize" (*Medical Economics* 29 [April 1952]: 69). "Be Wise: Itemize" reflected the journal's efforts to persuade doctors to build better relationships with their patients by explaining fees in advance of treatment and itemizing their bills. By making the comparison with the auto mechanic's bill, this cartoon drew on physicians' own experiences as consumers to help them see the patients' point of view.

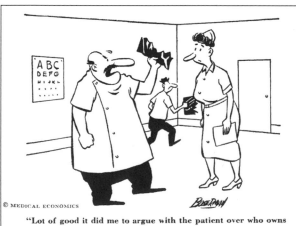

"Lot of good it did me to argue with the patient over who owns the X-ray film. He got the biggest half."

"Lot of Good It Did Me to Argue . . ." (*Medical Economics* 29 [October 1952]: 131). Having paid that itemized bill, some patients then felt entitled to have access to the results, such as laboratory findings and copies of X-rays. The growing advice to seek a second opinion before embarking on possibly unnecessary and expensive treatments reinforced that trend. A 1952 cartoon offered a comical view of the conflict between doctor and patient that resulted from the latter's sense of entitlement to a copy of his X-ray.

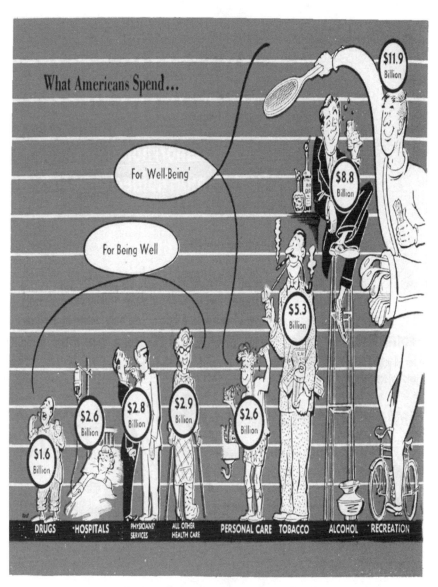

"What Americans Spend" (*Medical Economics* 32 [October 1955]: 48). At the same time its editors urged physicians to do a better job justifying their fees, *Medical Economics* also criticized patients for their unwillingness to pay medical bills as promptly and cheerfully as they did other expenses. This chart, copies of which readers could purchase to give their patients, contrasted how little Americans spent on "being well" with how much they lavished on "well-being," including tobacco, alcohol, and recreation.

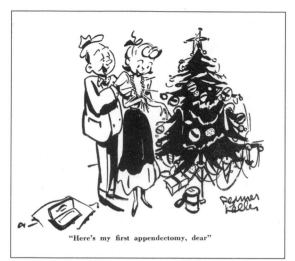

"Here's my first appendectomy, dear"

Reamer Keller, "Here's My First Appendectomy, Dear" (*Medical Economics* 26 [December 1949]: 121). While warning physicians against being perceived as "fee gougers," cartoons in *Medical Economics* sometimes reinforced popular fears about the medical profession's increasingly entrepreneurial orientation. In this 1949 cartoon, Reamer Keller jokingly represented the connection between the doctor's first appendectomy and his ability to buy his wife a nice Christmas gift. Appendectomies were one of several operations that figured prominently in the 1950s debate over unnecessary surgery.

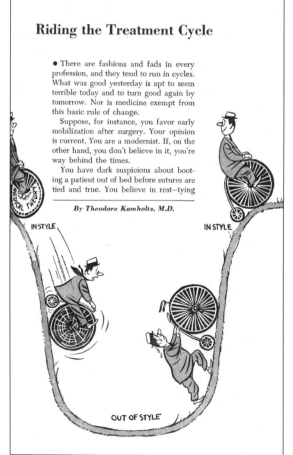

Riding the Treatment Cycle

● There are fashions and fads in every profession, and they tend to run in cycles. What was good yesterday is apt to seem terrible today and to turn good again by tomorrow. Nor is medicine exempt from this basic rule of change.

Suppose, for instance, you favor early mobilization after surgery. Your opinion is current. You are a modernist. If, on the other hand, you don't believe in it, you're way behind the times.

You have dark suspicions about booting a patient out of bed before sutures are tied and true. You believe in rest—tying

By Theodore Kamholtz, M.D.

IN STYLE

IN STYLE

OUT OF STYLE

Theodore Kamholtz, "Riding the Treatment Cycle" (*Medical Economics* 29 [February 1952]: 89). Physicians concerned about the escalating speed of therapeutic change often used the language of "fashion" and "fad" to call for caution. In the post–World War II period, as the pace of new drug and procedural innovation quickened, so too did references to what this physician referred to as the "treatment cycle," in which "what was good yesterday is apt to seem terrible today and to turn good again by tomorrow." As the article noted, some physicians "rode" the treatment cycle as a way to attract patients and justify higher fees. Awareness that physicians followed fads and fashions in treatment contributed to patient-consumers' sense that they needed to do their own due diligence before following their doctors' recommendations.

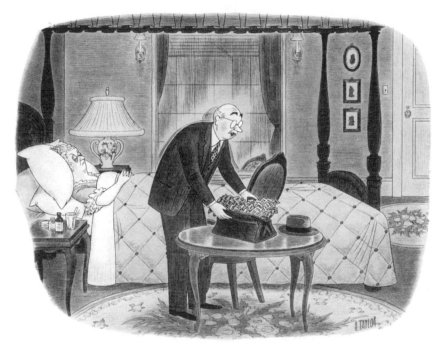

"Pshaw! I grabbed the wrong bag."

Richard Taylor, "The Wrong Bag" (*New Yorker*, September 19, 1959, 35; used by permission of Richard Taylor/The New Yorker Collection/The Cartoon Bank). In the 1950s, cartoons commenting on the growing prosperity of physicians appeared in mainstream publications such as the *New Yorker*. Richard Taylor's "The Wrong Bag" portrayed a doctor arriving on a house call only to discover that he had grabbed the "wrong" black bag: instead of the one carrying his medical instruments and medicines, he had mistakenly picked up the one stuffed with cash. One of Taylor's best-known cartoons, it served as the cover for a book of his collected work, *The Wrong Bag*, published by Simon and Schuster in 1961, and was also reprinted in Walter Goodman's 1966 article "The Doctor's Image Is Sickly," discussed in Chapter 8.

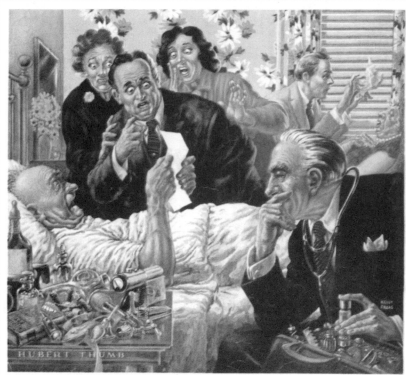

PRESENTING THE BILL—reproduced here, is one of a series of original oil paintings "Practising Medicine For Fun and Profit", commissioned by Park-David

Great
Moments
in
Medicine

Once the crisis has passed . . . once the patient has regained his strength . . . once the family is relieved and grateful . . . that's the time when the physician experiences one of the great moments in medicine. In fact, the *greatest moment* in medicine! Mainly, the moment when he presents his bill! That's the time when all of the years of training and study and work seem worthwhile. And there's always the chance that the shock might mean more business for him!

Park-David scientists are proud of their place in the history of practicing medicine for fun and profit, helping to provide doctors with the materials that mean higher fees and bigger incomes. For example, our latest development . . . tranquilizer-impregnated bill paper . . . designed to eliminate the shock and hysteria that comes when the patient gets a look at your bill. Not only will he remain calm when he sees what you've charged . . . now he won't even *care!*

COPYRIGHT 1959—PARK-DAVID & COMPANY, WITH THE BLESSINGS OF THE AMA

PARK-DAVID

Kelly Freas, "Great Moments in Medicine: Presenting the Bill," 1959 (MAD #48 © E.C. Publications, Inc.). Like the depression-era humor magazine *Ballyhoo, Mad,* which began publication in 1952, traded heavily on satires of contemporary advertising. In this 1959 spoof, artist Kelly Freas lampooned Parke, Davis & Company's well-known advertising series titled "Great Moments in Medicine." But instead of Parke, Davis's inspiring scenes of medical achievement, Freas portrayed the patient's shock on seeing his bill. The bottles and gadgets surrounding him suggested the many itemized services that contributed to the size of the doctor's fee.

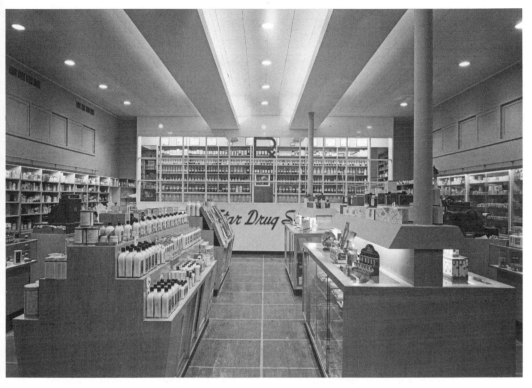

Interior of Star Drug, Kingsbridge Rd., Bronx, New York, 1946 (Gottscho-Schleisner Collection, LC-G612-T-48415, Library of Congress, Prints and Photographs Division). In the postwar period, drugstores continued to invest heavily in improved store design and product selection to hold their own in a competitive retail landscape. Following the lead of their supermarket rivals, many drugstores gradually began to introduce the concept of self-service. Unlike the old-style store, in which consumers had to ask the clerk for an item, self-service let them make their own choices from the drugstore's shelves. This Bronx, New York, store shows the beginnings of that shift, with its sleek, well-lighted aisles offering many tempting products for shoppers to consider. The shift to self-service placed an even greater premium on effective advertising campaigns and eye-catching packages to serve as "silent salesmen" in the clerk's place.

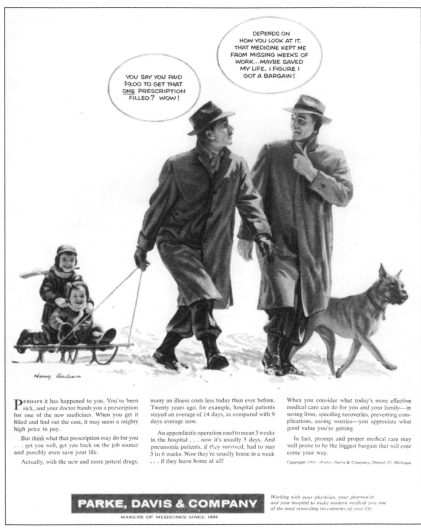

"I Figure I Got a Bargain" (*Life,* January 14, 1957, 105; Parke, Davis & Company, 1957).
As prescription drug prices rose precipitously in the 1950s, so too did the volume of patient complaints about the cost. To help counter that discontent, the Parke, Davis pharmaceutical company developed a series of advertisements aimed at explaining why the new drugs were worth their higher price. In this 1957 advertisement, the message is presented as a conversation between two middle-class fathers spending time with their kids and pets. As one dad tells the other, even at a higher price, he figures that the prescription drug was a good investment compared with the potential cost of lost workdays or a hospital bill: "I figure I got a bargain."

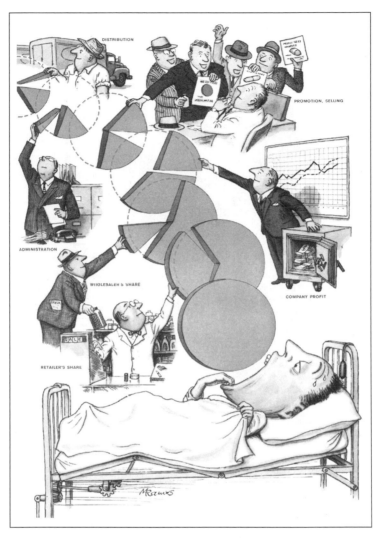

Michael Ramus, illustration for "A Big Pill to Swallow" (*Life*, February 15, 1960, 99). The "it's a bargain" argument did not put an end to complaints about the rising price of prescription drugs. In an article about the Kefauver hearings, which began in 1959, *Life* included this drawing showing the many parties who claimed a share of the drugs' rising costs. The article's subtitle reminded readers that "the wonder-drug makers get handsome profits from their captive customers." As was often the case in cartoons about rising medical costs, the patient shown "swallowing" the cost is a male.

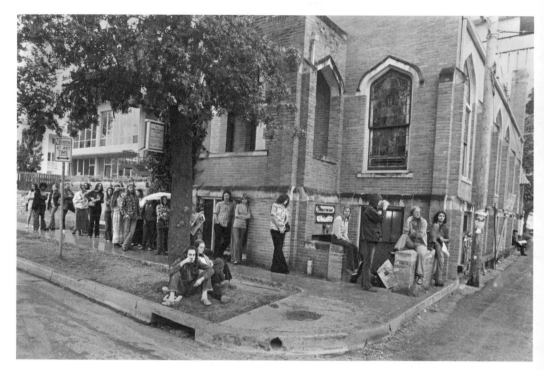

Alan Pogue, "The Line outside the People's Free Clinic," 1972 (© 2015 Alan Pogue).
The People's Free Clinic of Austin was founded in 1970 by volunteer doctors and nurses
working out of a Congregational church's basement. The clinic served college students
attending the nearby University of Texas at Austin as well as immigrant workers. The clinic
was open only two nights a week, and this photograph shows the long line of prospective
patients waiting to be seen. Like many such clinics, the People's Free Clinic shifted its focus
after 1980 to concentrate primarily on the needs of uninsured and underinsured Austin
residents.

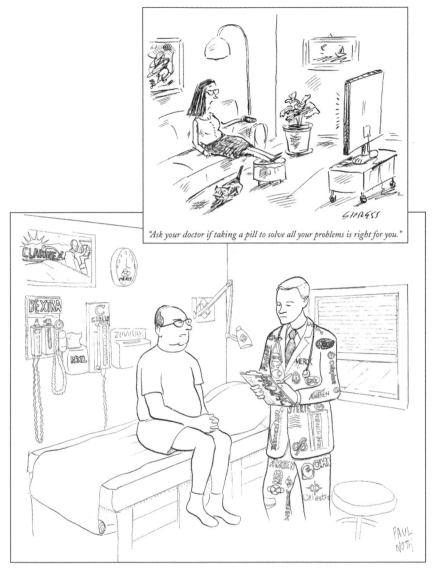

"Ask your doctor if taking a pill to solve all your problems is right for you."

(*top*) David Sipress, "Ask Your Doctor if Taking a Pill to Solve All Your Problems Is Right for you" (David Sipress/The New Yorker Collection/The Cartoon Bank); (*bottom*) Paul Noth, untitled (Paul Noth/The New Yorker Collection/The Cartoon Bank). Of the many ways that medicine has changed over the last two decades, the erosion of traditional restraints on prescription drug advertising has prompted perhaps the most satiric commentary. Although drug companies have portrayed this advertising as a beneficial service to consumers, comedic opinion has reflected a more skeptical view of its intentions. David Sipress's 2007 *New Yorker* cartoon evokes the long-standing concern that drug advertising promotes an unrealistic faith in the existence of "a pill for every ill." Paul Noth's 2008 comparison of doctors to race car drivers suggests another persistent worry: that physicians have come to function too well as sales representatives for pharmaceutical companies.

{SEVEN}

A Big Pill to Swallow

In the winter of 1951, Washington, D.C., lawyer Walton Hamilton came down with a nasty strep throat. To treat it, his physician prescribed a powerful new antibiotic, Chloromycetin. When he went to fill the prescription, Hamilton was shocked to discover that a four-day supply of the drug cost eight dollars, a steep price at that time. He asked his doctor to see if there was a cheaper brand, but the same drug made by other companies cost exactly the same amount. Hamilton grudgingly bought the Chloromycetin but complained about the price to his wife, Irene Till, an economist who worked at the FTC. While little came of their conversation at the time, their concerns would eventually find an outlet during the investigations into the pharmaceutical industry overseen by Senator Estes Kefauver from 1959 to 1961. Hamilton's bad day at the drugstore presaged a growing sense among American consumers that the expense of prescription drugs had become a "big pill to swallow," as a 1960 *Life* article contended. Like doctors' bills, the cost and quality of prescription drugs became a central issue as medical consumerism began to recover from the chilling effects of the Red Scare.[1]

The late 1950s debates over the rising cost and escalating use of the new "doctors' drugs" contributed to the larger unrest in the doctor-patient relationship. Along with unnecessary surgery, the overuse of prescription drugs emerged as a common complaint about the changing culture of the doctor's office. Having solidified their exclusive right to prescribe the most powerful kinds of drugs, physicians now found themselves held responsible for concerns about both the prices and the safety of these medications. Perhaps more than any other single issue, the economic ties between doctors and the pharmaceutical industry became the focal point for worries that commercialism was corrupting medical professionalism.

Those controversies played out not only in the doctor's office but also in the drugstore. Hamilton's eight-dollar antibiotic was part of a prescription drug boom that was turning what was once a loss leader into an economic powerhouse. As the new patent rules and drug regulations took hold, drugstores enjoyed exclusive sales on the "legend drugs" that cost more and came with very little information for patients. Meanwhile, trends in other parts of the drugstore were headed in the opposite direction. Following the lead of their supermarket competitors, drugstores gradually adopted a system of self-service for packaged medicines that reflected greater confidence in consumers' shopping skills. Formerly suspect proprietary products were recast as "over-the-counter" drugs safe enough to be sold directly to consumers without clerks' guidance.

Shopping in the postwar drugstore thus came to reflect the same tension between the exercise of self-expression and the deference to scientific expertise that was unsettling the doctor-patient relationship more generally. The principles governing the front end of the store—the calculated mix of sundries and common remedies of everyday life, advertised with enthusiasm—differed markedly from the order of business prevailing behind the prescription counter. The greater transparency of the over-the-counter drug, clearly labeled and openly advertised in a competitive retail environment, contrasted sharply with the state of the prescription drug, shrouded in the mystery of the trade secret and shielded from price competition. The faith in the educated consumer, able to read labels and make good choices, stopped short of the pharmacy department.

The widening distinction between over-the-counter and prescription goods reflected in the Cold War drugstore brought about an ironic reversal of fortunes. Whereas before 1940, the proprietary industry had been the focal point for criticism, its ethical counterparts became the chief object of critical consumerism's concerns after World War II. Miracle drugs, patient-consumers soon learned, came with significant costs, in terms of both expense and side effects. Both pharmaceutical executives and medical leaders insisted that these problems were minor blemishes on the otherwise outstanding performance of the free enterprise system. But the widening disparity between how the two different kinds of medicines came into patients' hands would become the focal point for a revival of medical consumerism.

From Counter Service to Self-Service

The drugstore's transformation occurred at a time of unprecedented prosperity in the United States. During the quarter century starting in 1949, the quantity of goods and services produced increased fourfold, while the average family income doubled. Whereas during World War II, doing more with less had been a virtue, now shopping with no other end in mind than enjoyment became a quasi-patriotic act. Retailers competed for customers, making consumer convenience and choice their watchwords, while manufacturers tailored products to suit individual tastes, symbolized by the rainbow of colors that Americans could now choose for their automobiles, their kitchen appliances, and even their toilet paper.[2]

Drugstores played a prominent role in the postwar retail revival. Having survived the Great Depression with a reputation for being recession-proof, they were well positioned to take advantage of the new buying mood. Sales surged as the economy grew, and the success of the new prescription drugs soon brought additional profits. Many owners invested part of those profits in adding and updating stores. Although old-style pharmacies continued to exist into the 1950s, the new growth came primarily in the form of more promotional drugstores, both independents and chains. Meanwhile, all drugstores faced increasingly stiff competition from other retailers, chief among them the supermarkets, eager to cut into the "retail cream."[3]

In a competitive retail environment, store design took on even more importance. Drugstores aimed for a strong presence at street level to draw in customers. Following the broader architectural trends of the era, the Cold War drugstore favored strong, streamlined designs with imposing facades. Architect Robert Fash's design for a New York City Whelan's store, featured in the 1944 *Architectural Forum*, exemplified the "slick, shiny" look of the postwar drugstore, complete with an impressive marquee to lure customers from the street. Another architect's 1948 plan for a suburban drugstore signaled a retreat from the "garish facades" of the old "toothpaste temples" in favor of an impressive storefront, "well glassed for light and display" to attract customers.[4]

Postwar stores were modernized in other ways to promote convenience and comfort. New floor plans included multiple entrances to allow access from multiple directions. In the late 1940s, the trendsetting Walgreens chain made entry even easier by introducing the first automatic door opener, the "In-a-matic," which competitors soon copied. Inside the store, other new technologies such as air-conditioning and fluorescent lights enhanced shoppers' comfort. Overall, 1950s stores appeared far brighter and more spacious than their predecessors.[5]

By far the most radical change in the postwar drugstore occurred not in its physical plant but in its style of selling. Starting in the 1940s, first in the western United States, then in other parts of the country, stores began to transition from traditional counter service, in which clerks helped customers with purchases, to self-service, in which customers selected their own goods and took them to cash registers to pay. After years of economic uncertainty and wartime privations, Americans seemed eager to shop without the guidance of store employees. As retailers' studies showed, when left to make their own choices, shoppers spent more than when they were served by clerks. Initially reluctant to give up counter service, chain drugstores eventually did so because their retail competitors gave them no choice.

The pressure to adopt self-service came from the drugstore's leading postwar rival, the supermarket. First introduced in the southeastern United States by the Piggly Wiggly chain in the 1910s, self-service groceries such as Grand Union, A&P, and Kroger began to proliferate in the 1940s. The shift to self-service coincided with supermarkets' aggressive expansion of the health and beauty products they carried. Goods such as shampoo, body soaps, and toothpaste were easy to sell and had much higher profit margins than food (18 percent compared to 3 percent). "What made the grocer climb the fence into the drugstore's field," observed *Business Week* in 1952, was "profits." Between the early 1940s and the early 1950s, the number of grocery stores stocking personal-care products rose from 37 percent to 85 percent. The grocery store that sold only food, like the drugstore that only sold drugs, was "beginning to go the way of the dodo," as a *New York Times* business reporter wrote in 1952. By 1955, drugstores' share of toiletry items had fallen from 45 percent to 30 percent, primarily as a consequence of rising sales in self-service grocery stores.[6]

Self-service grocery chains were also eager to cut into drugstore sales of health-related products such as vitamins and aspirin. In 1939, the new Kroger grocery chain headquartered in Ohio had announced plans to sell its own brand of vitamins. In neighboring Indiana, where Kroger had many outlets, the Board of Pharmacy declared that Kroger stores could not sell vitamins because they were not licensed as pharmacies. After a lengthy court battle, the state supreme court ruled in 1943 that vitamin products were to be classified for sale by the claims carried on their labels: if a vitamin was labeled for "the prevention, treatment or cure of disease," it was a drug to be sold in a drugstore; if it was labeled "not for medicinal use," it could be sold in a grocery store. Other states either adopted the Indiana compromise or ruled that vitamins were food products.[7]

In the 1950s, similar battle lines developed over the sale of aspirin and other commonly used medicines. By upgrading standards for drug regulation, the 1938 Food, Drug, and Cosmetic Act inadvertently made it easier for retailers to argue that there should be no restrictions on where consumers could buy over-the-counter remedies. Given that the FDA had greater powers to ensure that such products were safe and accurately labeled for self-medication, there was no reason their sales should be limited to drugstores. Taking advantage of the "proprietary exemption," general retailers began to expand their sales of over-the-counter medications. As drugstore profits began to suffer, state pharmacy boards tried to intervene by forbidding supermarkets to sell products such as aspirin; their efforts set off a chain reaction of lawsuits and legislative battles involving state pharmacy boards, supermarkets, and trade groups such as the Proprietary Association, the chief representative of the over-the-counter industry. At the heart of these legal disputes was the question Should the "proprietary exemption" be narrowed or widened, and in making that determination, how should the law balance the competing goals of encouraging free enterprise and protecting the public's health?[8]

While not the only product involved in these controversies, aspirin figured prominently in many of these lawsuits. First made by a German chemist in 1853, then rendered therapeutically usable by Bayer's Felix Hoffman in 1899, acetyl salicylic acid, better known as aspirin, was powerful and versatile in its uses. Once aspirin lost its patent protection in 1917—it was one of the few proprietary remedies to have such a patent—many companies began to manufacture and sell it. As the promotion and use of aspirin expanded, so too did the range of cultural baggage that it carried. On the one hand, aspirin became an icon of safe self-medication as a "harmless" but powerful drug that belonged in everyone's medicine cabinet. The popular press hailed aspirin as the "king of drugs" and "the original miracle drug." On the other hand, aspirin acquired some negative associations as well. Even when used as directed, it could cause gastric bleeding and allergic reactions. When used carelessly, "aspirin can be deadly," as a 1944 article warned. In 1955, incidents of accidental aspirin poisoning prompted the FDA to require the label warning, "Keep this and all medications out of the reach of children." Finally, its widely variant pricing led to warnings against overpaying, as did a 1957 *Reader's Digest* article that warned, "Don't be an ass about aspirin."[9]

For all these reasons, aspirin figured prominently in post–World War II battles over where over-the-counter drugs should be sold. The restrictionists pressed for a narrow definition of the proprietary exemption: it should apply only to drugs under patent or otherwise "secret" in their formulation. They argued that all medicines, including aspirin, posed significant risks to the unwary patient-consumer and thus should only be sold in drugstores where a pharmacist could supervise their use. In support of that position, restrictionists noted the problems associated with taking aspirin: allergic reactions, potential for deliberate or accidental overdose, and side effects such as stomach bleeding. Their opponents advocated for what became known as the "common usage interpretation," which defined the proprietary exemption to cover "all harmless, pre-packaged medicines properly labelled for use." In their view, the FDA now did a sufficiently good job ensuring drug safety and accurate labeling that such restrictions did not benefit the patient-consumer; rather they were designed solely to protect the economic interests of retail pharmacies. Anti-restrictionists pointed to surveys that showed people buying aspirin in drugstores rarely got any counseling from the pharmacist, a trend hastened by the growing trend toward self-service. Many of the problems with aspirin—child poisonings, suicide attempts, and bleeding stomachs—occurred with bottles purchased at the drugstore and not the supermarket.[10]

In the end, while the restrictionists won a few battles in a few states, they ultimately lost the war. At a time of Cold War celebration of free enterprise, state courts and legislators agreed that sufficient regulation of over-the-counter drugs now existed to guarantee that packaged goods were safe and adequately labeled for use. Legal opinion largely concurred with the view that restricting aspirin sales was not justified by concern for consumers. As a 1954 article in the *Yale Law Journal* explained, striking down those restrictions worked to "serve consumers' convenience" and "may expand manufacturers' markets." The only possible harm was to the drugstore owner, who had little right to complain. "While holding his drug patronage captive, he has been free to expand his merchandising in all directions." The author concluded that "his plight does not seem tragic enough to justify sheltering him from competition through use of the technical definition—a legislated monopoly masquerading as a health regulation."[11]

With the courts ruling in favor of more competition, supermarkets made significant inroads into drugstore profits from products such as toothpaste, vitamins, and aspirin. Drugstores initially responded by trying to improve their clerks' selling techniques. A 1952 Bristol-Myers training film sought to help druggists capitalize on the "one major asset . . . that the supermarket hasn't got—[a] personal relationship with the customer." Using the "Candid Camera" technique—a hidden camera that recorded the uncensored conversations of everyday life—television personality Allen Funt spent seven months filming his efforts to sell Bristol-Myers's products at forty-three different drugstores, documenting exactly how hard it was to do so. In a typical sequence, he made a "strenuous effort" to sell Ipana toothpaste, only to have the consumer stubbornly insist on buying Squibb's brand instead. Thus, even as the film tried to extol the power of personal selling, it demonstrated how time-consuming and unsuccessful such efforts could be.[12]

As the power of sales clerks ebbed, the argument for self-service grew more compelling: left to their own devices, shoppers bought more products. But even with the supermarket threat, the shift to self-service did not come easily to drugstores. Customers might be deemed to have sufficient knowledge to select their own socks or cereal, but medicines were a different matter. Drugstores had long derived their selling advantage from the premise that patient-consumers needed expert supervision in choosing medications. Like their medical colleagues, most pharmacists took a dim view of consumer rationality, swapping stories about dim-witted customers, such as the woman who returned a package of foil-wrapped rectal suppositories because they were "too hard to swallow."[13]

Yet chain drugstores eventually accepted the new selling philosophy due to consumers' growing distaste for personalized selling. Counter service came to be seen as an old-fashioned style of shopping unsuited to the postwar generation. Having the freedom to roam throughout the store, examining and comparing products without interference from clerks, made shopping a more pleasurable activity. As a 1953 advertisement sponsored by the Brand Names Foundation promised, "Today you can often serve yourself faster and better than someone else can help you—and brand names are the reason!" Rising levels of education also contributed to the embrace of self-service. In 1940, half of all Americans had high school diplomas; by 1960, that number had topped 60 percent. Many American high schools included courses on consumer education as a standard part of their curricula. Postwar consumers consequently seemed intelligent enough to be able to read labels and compare packages of medicine without the assistance of clerks.[14]

By the early 1940s, the United States had several hundred self-service drugstores, almost all of them in the western part of the country, where perennial labor shortages made them especially appealing. On a 1949 trip to California, Charles Walgreen Jr. visited a self-service Sav-On store and came away so impressed with what the trade journal *Advertising and Selling* christened the "drugstore of the future" that he returned to Chicago determined to introduce the idea in some Walgreens stores. In a 1952 company newsletter, Walgreen summed up the advantages of the new system: customers spent more at self-service stores, they were willing to travel farther to shop at one, and the reduction in labor costs increased the bottom line.[15]

Still, the conversion to self-service posed difficulties that slowed its pace. In old stores, installing the open-shelf system required expensive remodeling. Owners also had to worry more about shoplifting. They tried installing turnstiles to deter potential thieves only to find they deterred customers from entering the store. Chains faced the added complication that their self-service stores generally charged lower prices than their older stores that still practiced counter service, thus undercutting business in the latter. Resolving these problems proved costly, in both economic and personal terms.[16]

But the trend toward self-service continued, due to the higher profits shown by stores adopting the new system, which saw their sales volumes boosted by at least 20 percent and in some cases as much as 50 percent. Moreover, the gains occurred throughout the store: sales in the prescription department grew along with sales in the self-service sections. Combined with the lower labor costs, these advantages led more and more drugstore owners to make the change. By 1953, the number of fully self-service stores had exceeded 600, while another 7,000 stores had introduced self-service into some of their departments. Regional differences remained strong: 40 percent of self-service stores were in the West, with only 3 percent in New England. The idea of "every customer a clerk" steadily gained ground in the 1950s, seemingly a fitting tribute to American independence and intelligence.[17]

Creating a self-service drugstore necessitated rethinking not only store design but also advertising strategies. In the counter-service era, manufacturers had worked to imprint brand-name preferences in customers' heads so that they could ask for products by name—"I'll have a bottle of Bayer aspirin" or "Give me some Phillips' Milk of Magnesia." Now customers needed to be primed to pick the product off the shelf without the guidance of clerks, making familiarity with and discrimination among brand names and company reputation all the more critical. As the Brand Names Foundation pointed out in 1953, those familiar names were becoming "probably the world's most efficient salesclerks."[18]

The effort to grab patient-consumers' attention started with the appearance of the product itself. Instead of sales clerks, companies increasingly relied on eye-catching packages to serve as "silent salesmen." Starting in the 1940s, package designs became critical to drawing consumers' attention. In 1948, the McKesson Company created a whole new "American look" for all its product lines and ran advertising in magazines and newspapers to familiarize consumers with the change. Similarly, Rexall's redesigned its "family of products" and publicized the new look in a national advertising campaign featuring comedian Jimmy Durante. To entice shoppers once they were in the store, manufacturers and retailers invested heavily in point-of-sale displays that sought to make products look irresistible. For similar reasons, manufacturers competed fiercely to get their products positioned on shelves at eye level to provide a greater selling advantage.[19]

The power of these silent salesmen depended heavily on influencing consumers' preferences. Always a robust feature of the industry, spending on over-the-counter drug advertising skyrocketed after World War II, penetrating the national mind-set to an unprecedented degree via television. Initially, TV ads were conceived simply as radio scripts with visuals added. Like radio, early TV shows had single sponsors, so audiences saw *The Adventures of Ozzie and Harriet* courtesy of Listerine and *The Colgate Comedy Hour* courtesy of Colgate toothpaste. By the late 1950s, that tradition had given way to the selling of advertising time in units, or "spots," so that companies could place their commercial messages on multiple shows.[20]

In the spot format, television drug ads repeated many of the same themes used in pre-1940 print advertising, such as claims that a product was "doctor-approved," contained a unique "scientific ingredient" that made it effective, or eliminated specific symptoms such as headache, indigestion, or fatigue. But important changes occurred as well, as the "fear sell" so popular during the Great Depression fell out of advertising fashion. Instead of bombarding consumers with references to disease and death, TV ads experimented with more lighthearted elements such as animation and graphics to catch viewers' attention.[21]

With the new doctors' drugs now presenting a far stiffer kind of competition, over-the-counter medicines often chose to emphasize the convenience of their use and the speed with which they worked. Alka-Seltzer, a combination antacid and pain reliever, did well with this new approach in its 1951 ad campaign featuring an animated character, Speedy. With a squeaky voice provided by veteran radio actor Dick Beals, Speedy's singsong "Plop, plop, fizz, fizz, oh, what a relief it is" became one of the best-known jingles of the decade and remained iconic into the 1970s. Alka-Seltzer commercials devoted little time to arguing that the product was safe, perhaps confident that viewers' faith in federal regulation ensured little worry about the issue. In fact, Alka-Seltzer made no mention of physicians or science; consuming the product was likened to drinking a cola or other refreshing beverage rather than taking medicine.[22]

While it boosted sales dramatically and earned a spot in the advertising industry's canon of "ads that worked," Alka-Seltzer's use of cartoon characters and likening of medicine to a soft drink did little to lessen critics' worries about the misleading character of over-the-counter drug advertising. The 1938 Wheeler-Lea Act had given the FTC authority to regulate over-the-counter drug advertising on consumers' behalf. But due to its limited staff and competing priorities, the agency's disciplinary process remained slow and cumbersome. Those problems were evident in the FTC's prosecution of the J. B. Williams Company for its promotion of Geritol, a tonic introduced in 1950. In both print and television ads aimed at women and the elderly, the company claimed that the product's iron-rich formula relieved symptoms of fatigue. In 1959, the FTC challenged Williams's advertising on the grounds that such claims were misleading, since iron deficiency constituted only one small factor in causing fatigue. As the case dragged on for years without resolution, Geritol's makers made no changes to their marketing strategy.[23]

Meanwhile, critics railed against the misleading quality of over-the-counter drug advertising and called for stricter regulation of product claims. In 1958, a Rutgers pharmacy professor appeared on television and declared deceptive ads were "as potentially dangerous as a loaded gun." The cause received further attention from Warren G. Magnuson, a Washington State Democrat who chaired the Senate Commerce Committee, who threatened to push the FTC to regulate the advertising industry if it did not police itself more adequately. In response, the National Association of Broadcasters passed a new code of advertising in 1959 aimed at eliminating the worst abuses. For example, the new code banned "white coat" ads in which actors pretending to be physicians or nurses promoted products, a move welcomed by both the AMA and the American Pharmaceutical Association, which had long objected to faux invocations of medical authority. Although strictly voluntary, the National Association of Broadcasters code, which covered all three major networks and 303 television stations, appeared to be a major step in the right direction. As a 1958 *New York Times* editorial reported approvingly, "After January next it will no longer be possible for any actor or announcer to put on a white coat and pose as 'science.'"[24]

Nevertheless, experts and politicians continued to regard over-the-counter drug ads with grave suspicions. Despite the addition of cartoon characters and the subtraction of white-coated pitchmen, they also remained very unpopular with viewers. An early 1960s survey by Columbia University's Bureau of Applied Social Research found that drug commercials were far and away the most disliked category of television advertising, regarded as "exaggerated, in bad taste, and repetitive." Moreover, as concerns about drug addiction began to grow, critics suggested that the heavy exposure to slogans about "fast, fast, fast relief" and the magical quality of medicines helped to promote the use of illicit drugs.[25]

Yet over-the-counter products retained one characteristic that enhanced their consumer appeal: affordability. In a supercharged economic environment in which supermarkets competed with drugstores and national companies fought for brand-name recognition, prices remained low. While retailers avoided the scorched-earth tactics of the Great Depression, in which companies used price cutting to run each other out of business, they practiced other forms of price competition, such as coupons and two-for-one sales, to attract customers. As a result, prices for over-the-counter medicines rose but still remained far lower than those for prescription drugs. Those low prices, along with ease of access, ensured that packaged medicines remained a critically important product line for the postwar drugstore.

The Doctors' Drugs

The transformation of the drugstore's front end, including the shift to self-service, the cultivation of the silent salesman, and the advent of televised drug advertising, contrasted dramatically with the other revolution occurring behind the prescription counter. At the same time that the shelves of over-the-counter medicines were opening up to self-service, patient-consumers' access to prescription drugs became even more constrained. Instead of encouraging choice and convenience, the dispensing of the doctors' drugs reinforced the ideal of the all-powerful doctor and meekly passive patient, illustrating the growing tension between personal autonomy and deference to expert authority.

Prescription drugs became increasingly important to the postwar drugstore's profitability as scientific advances, business reorganization, and patent protection fostered a dramatic increase in their prices. Prescription pharmaceuticals became one of the boom industries of the postwar era. Companies posted record profits between the late 1940s and the early 1960s, by far the greatest profit rise in the ethical firms' century of existence. Dominated by a handful of powerful companies, the American industry increased tenfold in size and assumed a commanding role in not only the national but also the international drug trade.[26]

As a consequence, prescription drug sales became far more important to the drugstore's balance sheet. In the interwar years, prescription drugs had functioned primarily as what retailers refer to as loss leaders—they brought customers into the store to buy other, more profitable goods, among them proprietary remedies. After World War II, the prescription department became an economic asset in its own right. As the president of Sterling Drug, J. Mark Hiebert, observed at a 1956 meeting of the wholesale druggists' association, "The market in this country for prescription drugs is 'growing like Jack's beanstalk.'" The per capita average (the number of prescriptions divided by the total population) had increased from 1.4 in 1938 to 2.54 in 1948 and 3.2 in 1955. "Dollar-wise," he noted, these changes represented an eightfold increase, or a 225 percent increase from 1948 to 1955, and prescription drugs and over-the-counter ethical preparations brought in a record $1.2 billion that year.[27]

Moreover, the expanding sales of doctors' drugs did not necessitate the kind of expensive remodeling that self-service required. The prescription department remained in its traditional location at the back of the store and still used the semi-open plan to allow consumers to admire the bounty of drug products while providing pharmacists some privacy for preparation and packaging. As the pharmacists' labor shifted from compounding drugs to relabeling medicines already made up by pharmaceutical companies, this privacy became all the more valuable.

Although the look of the prescription counter changed relatively little, the conduct of business behind it certainly did. The regulatory system created by the Durham-Humphrey Amendments posed new barriers to the easy acquisition of prescription drugs. While its measures had been adopted in the name of the public good, little coordinated effort was made to explain them either to physicians or to patient-consumers. The result was a wave of complaints directed at both the FDA and the drugstore pharmacist.[28]

The tighter restrictions on refills were a case in point. The Durham-Humphrey Amendments put an end to the long-standing practice of letting patients refill nonnarcotic medicines at will. The law's requirement that pharmacists obtain physician confirmation before refilling any prescription annoyed not only patients but also physicians. As interim FDA medical director Irvin Kerlan wrote to the AMA's Council on Pharmacy and Chemistry in November 1952, "We have noted a number of articles about annoyances resulting from telephone calls by pharmacists to physicians regarding the refilling of prescriptions." Kerlan suggested that to reduce the friction, the AMA urge its members to adopt a revised prescription form that let physicians indicate whether the remedy could be refilled. As this system caught on, it reduced aggravation, but significant new restraints remained on patient-consumers' ability to get refills.[29]

Likewise, pharmacists had heightened responsibilities for explaining how patients should take their prescriptions. By law, a prescription drug was defined as a medicine whose labeling and instructional information were intended only for the doctor and the pharmacist. Any company that violated that principle and provided too much information to the patient could face legal action. Yet to correctly take the medicine, patients had to have some instruction on its use. In theory, physicians were supposed to explain all these details during the office visit; in practice, many relied on pharmacists to provide that guidance.

Thus the post-1952 system of drug delivery presented pharmacists with many challenges. On the one hand, they needed to give patients information without appearing to threaten physicians' authority. The medical profession remained very alert to any sign of "counter servicing"—that is, pharmacists trying to infringe on prescribing prerogatives. On the other hand, pharmacists faced much more direct pressure to keep patient-customers happy by answering their questions than did physicians. At the point when patients were paying for their new, often expensive prescriptions, their requests for information were hard to dodge. Pharmacists thus had to exercise considerable ingenuity to make prescription drug service more consumer-friendly without running afoul of either the FDA or the medical profession.

One simple way pharmacists tried to increase satisfaction with prescription service was by enhancing the packaging of drug products with the use of accessory or special labels. Although detailed instructions for use were forbidden, reminders such as "For external use only" or "Shake well before using" were not. First introduced in the late 1800s, accessory labels became even more popular with the invention of self-adhesive brands in 1935. As pharmacists strove to improve their service to patient-consumers, they put increasing time and effort into this aspect of packaging. This effort was evident in the extensive array of labels that the New Jersey Board of Pharmacy introduced in 1947, inspiring other state boards to follow that lead. Patients increasingly came home with prescriptions that carried simple, brightly colored stickers designed to provide reminders about important information.[30]

Pharmacists also honored patient-consumers' requests for written copies of prescriptions. As the 1951 edition of Remington's textbook stated, many states required pharmacists to keep a record of prescriptions and gave patients a "qualified ownership" of them, meaning that they could request copies. According to the authors, "In those cases where the patient makes a bona fide request for a copy, it should be furnished": "Not only would this seem to be the patient's right, but it is also conductive to the maintenance of good will relations between the patient and the pharmacist." After passage of the Durham-Humphrey Amendments, the Indiana Pharmaceutical Association asked the FDA for clarification on this issue, and the agency telegraphed in reply, "There is no provision in federal law prohibiting pharmacist from giving customer a copy of prescription, provided it is clearly marked as a copy" and might include "any refill instructions appearing on original prescription." Pharmacists stamped customers' copies with the phrase "Not to be refilled without a physician's consent" and took care to give them only to patients or "known members" of their immediate families.[31]

Finally, pharmacists and physicians facilitated the switch from Latin to English for writing prescriptions. In part this change reflected the medical profession's abandonment of Latin as fewer students possessed command of that language. But it also reflected consumer preferences as well. The 1948 edition of Remington's textbook acknowledged the impact of medical consumerism: "At one time it was believed advisable to withhold from a patient the names and properties of the medicinal agents administered, but in this day of more specific medicines and greater intelligence among people generally, there is less of the mysterious and more of assured confidence in the relation between patient and physician, based upon the evident efficiency of the treatment rendered."[32] At the same time, growing industry reliance on complex chemical and brand names made prescriptions sufficiently hard for laypeople to decipher that the resort to Latin was unnecessary.

For all the innovations pharmacists adopted to try to ease its introduction, many patients did not like the new prescription drug system. As the Durham-Humphrey Amendments' stricter requirements came into force, the FDA received angry letters in which consumers protested that they now had to get prescriptions for drugs that formerly had been available over the counter. In May 1953, Mrs. Joseph Dabes of Groton, New York, wrote asking why she "was unable to buy antihistamines, whereas arsenic and alcohol are available without prescription," and demanding to know who "elects or appoints" the people who made such decisions. Members of Congress also relayed complaints from the public about the new law. Ohio Republican representative William H. Ayres contacted the FDA in August 1952 on behalf of a constituent who wanted to know why he could no longer get his drugs "refilled as formerly."[33]

FDA officials politely replied that it was manufacturers who decided whether to label a drug for use by prescription only and that Congress had required the change in the refill policy. In this fashion, the agency reminded grumblers that it was free enterprise and democracy at work here, even though the results were not necessarily to consumers' liking. As the volume of complaints rose, the agency's commissioner, Charles Crawford, decided in 1952 to create a "consumer consultant program" to help publicize the logic behind the Durham-Humphrey Amendments. Staffed by women, the program focused on women's clubs and home economists. In 1955, the FDA set up a Citizens' Advisory Committee, allowing prominent business leaders and home economists to provide the agency with advice on consumer issues more generally; prescription drug issues figured prominently in the committee's work.[34]

Side Effects

But try as they might to placate unhappy consumers, the pharmacy profession and the FDA faced a difficult task. Perhaps inevitably, as the volume of prescription drugs consumed rose, so too did a sense of their imperfections. On a number of grounds, including safety, price, and potential for abuse, the so-called wonder drugs came in for a rising volume of negative scrutiny. Ironically, whereas prewar medical consumerism had primarily focused on the dangers of the proprietary branch of the drug business, now its focus shifted increasingly to the prescription side.

That shift in attention reflected the new drugs' potency. The "legend drugs," which could be administered only under a doctor's supervision, were far more effective than their prewar counterparts; indeed, many of these drugs remain in use to this day. But their efficacy came with problems that became more apparent as doctors prescribed them to more people. Three areas emerged as particular points of consumer concern about the doctors' drugs: what side effects they might produce, how much they cost, and how they were being advertised to physicians. The lack of satisfying answers to those questions combined to make the prescription drug business a fertile breeding ground for postwar consumer consciousness.

Long before the 1950s, doctors and patients had understood that powerful drugs could have unpleasant and even dangerous side effects. The first modern "magic bullet," Paul Ehrlich's salvarsan, an arsenical preparation introduced in 1910 to treat syphilis, had such horrific side effects that sufferers often preferred the disease to the cure. Likewise the sulfonamides, wide-spectrum antimicrobials that became the "miracle drugs" of the 1930s, turned out to be hard on the kidneys and triggered allergic reactions in some people, especially when taken in large doses.[35]

By the late 1930s, the term "side effect" had entered the medical dictionaries as a recognized problem of modern therapeutics. Harold N. Wright and Mildred L. Montag's 1939 *Textbook of Materia Medica, Pharmacology, and Therapeutics* explained, "The effects which are not desired in any particular case are referred to as 'side effects' or 'side actions' and, in some instances, these may be so powerful as to limit seriously the therapeutic usefulness of the drug." Even aspirin, a nonprescription drug widely perceived as safe, had demonstrated its possible hazards. As stronger "doctors' drugs" came on the market in the 1940s and 1950s, popular awareness of their unintended and unwanted effects grew as well. Indeed, all the wonder drugs introduced during the Cold War, including antibiotics, corticosteroids, and psychoactive drugs, came with the risk of formidable side effects.[36]

Penicillin's introduction during World War II became the stuff of medical mythology thanks to its ability to bring wounded soldiers back from the brink of death. But as the drug's use expanded, so too did awareness that for about one in ten people, penicillin triggered an immune system overreaction that in rare cases could cause anaphylactic shock and ultimately death. In 1953, the *Journal of the American Medical Association* carried an article reporting on the "increasing frequency" of fatal reactions to penicillin, and newspapers and magazines began to warn the public about the problem. Those warnings increased after the FDA released a 1957 report attributing at least seventy-two deaths and more than a thousand "life-threatening" reactions to penicillin's use. As the tag line for Nate Haseltine's *Washington Post* story on the 1957 report warned, this wonder drug was "not always a life saver."[37]

Other new antibiotics turned out to pose dangerous risks to a small percentage of users. Perhaps the most frightening example was chloramphenicol, widely known by the brand name Chloromycetin, the drug Walton Hamilton was given for his strep throat in 1951. A powerful antibiotic introduced in 1947 by Parke, Davis, it worked well against a broad spectrum of microorganisms. However, it also put patients at risk for potentially fatal forms of anemia. Despite physicians' reports of the problem, the company denied the drug's dangers and continued aggressively to promote its use. In 1952, California physician Albe Watkins, whose ten-year-old son had died after taking chloramphenicol, presented the FDA with more than forty such cases he had collected from fellow doctors. The FDA confirmed that the risk was real and warned physicians to be very careful in using the drug. But chloramphenicol remained on the market until the 1970s, when a safer drug with similar broad-spectrum efficacy became available.[38]

Dangerous side effects also accompanied the use of cortisone and other steroids. Along with penicillin, the isolation of the adrenal gland's essence was considered one of the great achievements of postwar pharmaceutical research. Corticosteroids had many uses, including the treatment of rheumatoid arthritis and skin diseases. But patients on steroids had to endure discomfiting side effects, including peptic ulcers, weight gain, and the facial swelling dubbed "moon face." Economist John Blair, who played an important role in the Kefauver drug investigations, got interested in drug issues in large part due to his family's experience with steroids. When close relatives began taking cortisone to reduce the pain of rheumatoid arthritis, it had "fearful side effects that nobody had warned them about—peptic ulcers and moon face, where your head swells up like a basketball," Blair recalled; in addition, it was so expensive that it became a major financial drain. Even worse, some cortisone products could cause psychotic symptoms, as Berton Roueché recounted in a compelling 1955 *New Yorker* article about the drug's "ugly side." The central character in his story was a high school teacher who took powerful doses of adrenocorticotropic hormone to treat a dangerous inflammation of the arteries, only to become manic-depressive as a side effect. As a professor of medicine explained to Roueché, "We are dabbling in the unknown with dangerously potent tools." The story was turned into a 1956 movie, *Bigger Than Life*, starring James Mason.[39]

New psychoactive drugs presented equally worrying potential for addiction. Reassured that the new drug laws bestowed safety, doctors and patients alike embraced the use of a wide variety of new medications capable of relieving mental distress. In 1955, Meprobamate, the first of the so-called minor tranquilizers, was sold under the trade names Miltown and Equanil and enjoyed spectacular success. Cleverly marketed to a weary postwar generation as a safe "feel good" drug, Miltown became a staple of 1950s popular culture, including its enthusiastic promotion by talk show host Milton Berle. In years to come, new products such as Librium and Valium would enjoy similar bursts of popularity. As more and more Americans made use of prescription tranquilizers, commentators anxiously wondered about their addictive quality; while manufacturers insisted that this risk did not exist, some patients' experiences suggested otherwise.[40]

The side effects associated with the new drugs to treat schizophrenia and other major mental disorders were even more frightening. When first introduced in American mental hospitals in the early 1950s, chlorpromazine, marketed under the brand name Thorazine, seemed to be the very definition of a medical miracle: patients who had been violent and delusional became calmer and more rational. But the drug's benefits came along with many serious side effects, including extreme sedation, blurred vision, seizures, muscle spasms, and involuntary movements of the body known as tardive dyskinesia. While facilitating the discharge of patients from public mental hospitals, the drug regimens came under intense criticism in the 1960s as the chemical equivalent of a straitjacket.[41]

As more patient-consumers began taking the powerful new drugs, they learned firsthand what had long been common knowledge among pharmacists and physicians: strong drugs could have equally strong side effects.

Popular magazines took up the theme that patients needed to be more fully educated regarding these dangers. In 1952, the popular magazine *Science Digest* explained to its readers that "any medicine can hurt some people," mentioning the "dual role of good and bad effects" to be found in cortisone, penicillin, and streptomycin. A year later, *Good Housekeeping* warned, "Many patients develop a sensitivity to the miracle drugs" and noted that taking Chloromycetin over a long period of time had produced fatal cases of anemia.[42]

Yet in spite of these risks, physicians had no clearly defined responsibility for informing patients about the possible side effects of their medications. On the contrary, many doctors felt that sharing such information was a bad idea. As they saw it, telling patients about possible side effects did more harm than good: it might either dissuade the patient from taking the medicine or, in a reverse placebo effect, make them imagine side effects where none really existed. Given this medical opinion, pharmacists had to be careful about supplying such information to consumers lest they be accused of undercutting doctors' authority. Thus the dramatic postwar rise in per capita consumption of prescription drugs occurred without a corresponding increase in information for patients about what drugs they were taking, much less about the risks involved. This lack would become a focal point for medical consumerists' advocacy efforts from the late 1950s onward.

Patient-consumers' sense of outrage was only deepened by the significant jump in the product's price. Consumers were being asked not only to take their pills on blind faith but also to pay much more for the privilege. While prescription drugs had traditionally cost more than over-the-counter preparations, the difference in price had not been huge: as of 1929, the average cost for a prescription was 85 cents. As the new regulatory system and patent protections took hold, the price of the doctors' drugs rose steeply: from an average of $1.11 in 1939 to $3.08 in 1959. That rise was reflected in the Consumer Price Index, where the percentage of the consumer's shopping basket of goods represented by prescription drugs jumped nearly twenty points between 1948 and 1958. While a 1958 survey found that the majority of prescriptions remained under $3, about 15 percent cost far more—from $5 to $10 for a single course of treatment.[43]

Patient-consumers who read the newspaper's business pages were also likely to know that pharmaceutical companies were posting record profits. The industry's spectacular gains perhaps inevitably led to increased scrutiny of its business practices. Although discovering new drugs required large investments in research development, most medications could ultimately be produced cheaply and in large quantities. In essence, drugmakers' profit margins reflected a huge markup that could be preserved as long as the product remained under patent. And as Walton Hamilton's experience with Chloromycetin reflected, companies competed by offering different brands of the same drug but charged the same—often substantial—price.

Pharmaceutical companies also faced criticism for their growing sway over physicians' prescribing choices. Both proprietary and ethical drug companies had long sought to win doctors' patronage, but after World War II, company efforts to build medical loyalty to particular brands of antibiotics, steroids, or tranquilizers took on unprecedented scale and scope. To this end, physicians were deluged by direct-mail advertisements, and medical journals contained page after page of print ads. Companies also greatly expanded the number of detail men sent to visit hospitals and doctors' offices to promote their product lines.[44]

Moreover, the techniques used to influence postwar physicians became much more like those used on consumers in general. Harry Dowling, the chair of the AMA's Section on Experimental Medicine and Therapeutics, noted the change in a 1957 speech to his fellow doctors. "Within recent years," he observed, "the drug industry has discovered that the techniques that had been used so successfully in the advertising of soaps and tooth pastes and of cigarettes, automobiles and whiskey could be used successfully to advertise drugs to doctors." Marketing to physicians had become "flamboyant," "incessant," and "without question confusing." He concluded, "The battle front of today has shifted, and false advertising to the public is no longer the major issue" but instead "false advertising to the doctor."[45]

In their defense, ethical houses such as Pfizer, Merck, and Eli Lilly insisted that their marketing was both needed and appropriate. As they emphasized, their detail men were highly professional, "well trained to provide skilled advice to the busy physician." But other aspects of the new pharmaceutical marketing seemed more akin to the promotional drugstore's methods than some doctors found palatable. Having been imbued with the tradition that advertising and professionalism did not mix, they looked askance not only at print advertising but also at sponsored social events at medical meetings and the free samples and giveaways brought by detail men, whom one commentator dubbed "Santa Clauses." This uneasiness reflected the fear that the ethical pharmaceutical companies, long an ally in the doctors' war against misleading advertising and commercial excess, had begun to adopt the tactics and mind-set of their proprietary counterparts. Observers both within and outside the medical profession began to worry about the negative impact of the new-style drug promotions on physician prescribing habits and the doctor-patient relationship.[46]

The controversies surrounding price and advertising contributed to what the trade journal *Printers' Ink* summed up in 1959 as the "special vulnerability of the drug field." Unlike other types of goods, "the consumer, or patient, has no real choice": he had to buy exactly what the doctor ordered. As a result, "there is a tendency to resent the whole situation because [the patient] feels forced to buy and forced to pay, whatever price is charged." Even if the prices charged for most drugs were "not exorbitant," the types and quantities needed by certain groups, such as the chronically ill and the elderly, made for a hefty price tag. Finally, what *Printers' Ink* described as the "coming of the profits" had triggered critical attention to the industry: between 1946 and 1959, sales had increased from half a billion dollars to more than $2 billion, and the industry was reporting profits as almost 20 percent of sales, compared to an average of 7.4 percent for all manufacturing industries. While industry representatives justified those profit levels as "legitimate rewards for a job well done," others, including politicians and advocates for the elderly, not surprisingly disagreed. "Tremendous political forces are coming to bear, and all marketing may be affected," the article concluded.[47]

Pharmaceutical companies responded to these criticisms with a strong defense of their industry's conduct and motives. In a 1959 speech, Austin Smith, president of the Pharmaceutical Manufacturers Association, marshaled arguments that would be repeated frequently in years to come. Prescription drugs, he pointed out, represented a comparatively small part of the rising cost of medical care, far less than doctors' fees and hospital charges. By treating ailments that formerly required surgery and hospitalization, their use saved money overall. The prices charged for these valuable commodities reflected the high cost of discovering and testing new drugs. All in all, Smith insisted, drug prices were fair and reasonable given the value of the product itself, and he hinted that the attention being given to consumers' complaints about the high costs of their medicine might be the work of advocates for socialized medicine. The American pharmaceutical industry would continue to produce lifesaving drugs only "if freedom to compete, to succeed and to serve remains with us," Smith concluded.[48]

To get this message across to both practicing physicians and patients, pharmaceutical companies greatly increased their lobbying and public relations efforts. Much as the AMA had started to do in the late 1940s, the industry realized that it needed to be more active in shaping public opinion.

The companies most involved in prescription drug manufacture reorganized to create a stronger trade association, the Pharmaceutical Manufacturers of America. They also invested more heavily, both as individual companies and through the association, in institutional advertising. Even though the drug laws passed in 1938 and in 1952 had not forbidden the advertising of prescription drugs directly to consumers, ethical firms still felt the need to proceed carefully with such measures out of deference to doctors' aversion to the idea. To advertise without appearing to do so, they concentrated on institutional advertising that promoted the value of the new drugs and the companies producing them.[49]

For example, in a 1950s version of an infomercial, Pfizer paid to have a special advertising section on antibiotics run in the Sunday, March 31, 1957, edition of the *New York Times*. Similarly Parke, Davis celebrated "great moments" in medicine and pharmacy in an elaborate series of advertisements that were suitable for display by physicians and pharmacists. Parke, Davis also developed a series of ads that spoke more pointedly to patient-consumers about the fairness of prices for new drugs: one pictured a man returning to the office after being cured of tuberculosis; another showed a mother watching a formerly sick child take a ballet lesson. A 1957 ad that ran in the *Saturday Evening Post* showed a man saying that even at nine dollars, the prescription drug that had cured him was really "a bargain" because it kept him from missing work.[50]

Less Than Wonderful

But many commentators remained unpersuaded that drug prices were a bargain. The rising cost of the new prescription drugs, along with escalating concerns about their safety, contributed to a growing volume of negative news coverage about the pharmaceutical industry. In 1954, the same year that *Fortune* magazine observed that doctors were "off their pedestals," *Business Week* described the prospects for the doctors' drugs as "less than wonderful." With Joseph McCarthy's investigations into "un-American" activities finally at an end, critics could comment on their business practices without fear of congressional scrutiny.[51]

As in the 1930s, a coalition of journalists and politicians found common cause in pointing out the dangers that an insufficiently regulated pharmaceutical industry posed to the American public. For Democrats eager to contest the Republican domination of national politics, the issue had particular appeal. Citing constituents' concerns, especially among the elderly, Democratic members of both the House and Senate began to raise questions about drug costs. Among those interested were some very powerful figures who headed up important committees that in the wake of a major reorganization of Congress had considerable power over agency budgets. In this climate, the New Deal concerns about cartelization as a threat to competition reemerged as a political issue that Democrats were ready to exploit.[52]

The FTC's investigation into drug price-fixing illustrated the shifting political climate. The agency's staff first got interested in antibiotic pricing in the early 1950s, in response to Walton Hamilton's experience with Chloromycetin. As a Ph.D. economist with many years of regulatory experience—he had served on the CCMC and later helped develop the Justice Department's 1937 antitrust suit against the AMA—Hamilton's complaints about his eight-dollar prescription were founded in substantial knowledge of how medical markets worked. He was quick to suspect that the antibiotic's high price was not an accident but, rather, represented an informal kind of price-fixing that allowed all the companies making the drug to make a tidy profit. When he shared that opinion with his wife, Irene Till, who held a doctorate in economics and worked at the FTC, she agreed with his hunch and passed the story along to her supervisor, John Blair. Blair concurred that the matter was worth investigating, but before the inquiry could get under way, the newly installed Eisenhower administration restructured the FTC, leading to Till's firing and Blair's demotion in 1953.[53]

As prescription drug prices continued to rise, congressional Democrats began to press the FTC to restart the investigation into drug pricing. Senator Magnuson took a particular interest in the issue after a trip to Sweden during which he discovered that American-made drugs cost patients there only 20 percent as much as in the United States. Finally, in August 1958, the FTC issued the results of its investigation and formally charged six drug companies with price-fixing of the newer broad-spectrum antibiotics, among them chlortetracycline, oxytetracycline, and tetracycline. In 1963, after years of hearings and arguments, the FTC commissioners eventually ruled against the drug companies.[54]

The publicity generated by the "wonder-drug price probe," as the *Washington Post* dubbed it, overlapped with an even more broad-ranging inquiry into the drug industry initiated by another powerful senator, Estes Kefauver. First elected in 1948, the Tennessee Democrat achieved national attention in 1950 as chair of a Senate committee investigating organized crime, including the rise of the Mafia; the first televised congressional hearings, they were watched by an estimated 20 million Americans. Largely as a consequence of that performance, Kefauver was chosen as Adlai Stevenson's vice presidential running mate on the 1956 presidential ticket. After the Democrats lost, Kefauver took over as chair of the Senate Subcommittee on Antitrust and Monopoly.[55]

Under Kefauver's direction, the committee reviewed price policies in a wide range of industries, including automobiles, steel, professional sports, bread, and milk. To run his committee, Kefauver hired former FTC staff members familiar with the problem, among them Irene Till and John Blair. After the committee finished its work on the steel and automobile industries, Till suggested that it turn its attention to prescription drugs. Starting in 1959, Kefauver's subcommittee spent two years collecting testimony from more than 300 witnesses, including pharmaceutical company executives, physician researchers, and practicing physicians. In addition, the staff did its own investigatory fact-finding.[56]

The result was a mass of published testimony and a lengthy 1961 report highlighting the negative consequences of the postwar expansion of the pharmaceutical industry, in particular its new patent, pricing, and promotional methods. The Kefauver hearings reinforced the concurrent FTC price-fixing probe, and with the 1960 national election looming, media coverage of prescription drug issues, much of it offering an unflattering portrayal of the industry, mushroomed. Kefauver became such a focal point of industry concern that the *F-D-C Reports*, a trade newsletter aimed at the drug and cosmetic industry, offered its subscribers daily reports on Kefauver's activities.[57]

Based on the committee findings, Kefauver and his Democratic allies called for sweeping reforms of the patenting, pricing, and advertising of prescription drugs. His proposals met with fierce resistance both from the pharmaceutical industry, which defended its practices as essential to the supply of more and better drugs, and from the AMA, which objected to further government encroachment on physician autonomy. These drug battles spurred a revival of critical consumerism, as the need for personal vigilance, once cast primarily as necessary when purchasing proprietary medicine, was expanded to cover prescription drugs as well.

For those already inclined to be "constructively critical" of the medical profession's approach to prescription drug use, the media coverage of the Kefauver hearings provided considerable fodder. Between 1958 and 1963, the *New York Times*, the *Washington Post*, and the Associated Press and United Press International wire services carried almost 400 articles about the Tennessee senator and his drug investigations. Weekly newsmagazines and more highbrow monthlies such as the *Saturday Review* and the *Atlantic* provided extensive coverage as well. The press reported at length not only on Kefauver's charges but on pharmaceutical executives' and the AMA's rebuttals as well.[58]

Some of this coverage portrayed Kefauver's arguments in negative terms. For example, *Washington Post* columnist George Sokolsky, a longtime supporter of the National Association of Manufacturers, dismissed the Senate committee's 375-page report as "babystuff, uninformative and not very helpful." He concluded, "Of course drugs are expensive; so are tombstones."[59] On balance, however, the press coverage reinforced the impression that the pharmaceutical industry's business practices deserved such intense scrutiny. Moreover, in a few cases, journalists directly contributed to the committee's investigations. The investigative reporting of *Saturday Review* science editor John Lear provided the committee with some leads, among them the revelations that the FDA's Henry Welch had financial investments in the companies he was regulating. In 1962, using material supplied by Kefauver's staff, the *Washington Post*'s Morton Mintz broke the story on the thalidomide tragedy that spurred the passage of drug reform legislation. Media coverage of the drug controversies in the late 1950s and early 1960s thus reinforced the idea that serious problems existed in the prescription drug business and that the "intelligent buyer" needed to beware.[60]

These critiques of the pharmaceutical industry gained attention in part because they coincided with a much broader questioning of American consumption patterns that arose in the late 1950s. The most influential of these came from journalist Vance Packard, the author of three best sellers that explored deceptive advertising, status seeking, and wastefulness as features of the American way of life. Companies were not delivering new and better products, Packard suggested, but instead promoting a deliberate kind of planned obsolescence. To sell more products at ever-higher prices, firms misrepresented minor variations in design as major improvements while simultaneously blocking useful innovations that might bring real progress in cheaper forms.[61]

While discovering new drugs seemed a more serious business than changing the tail fins on automobiles or offering appliances in new color combinations, industry critics saw parallels to Packard's argument. As far back as the turn of the twentieth century, some physicians had warned that therapeutic practice was becoming too responsive to fads and fashions; the sophisticated marketing campaigns aimed at doctors in the 1950s only increased those concerns. Following Packard's lead, physician experts voiced the fear that new and more expensive drugs were not always demonstrably better than the older, cheaper ones and that advertising budgets, not clinical efficacy, seemed to be driving changes in physicians' prescribing habits. In 1954, *Business Week* quoted a pharmaceutical researcher using antibiotics to describe what came to be known as the "drug life cycle." "Sales of a new antibiotic start slowly, then pick up as doctors begin to adopt it." Then "pretty soon a national magazine runs a whoopdedoo article, and the sales shoot skyward." Sales peak but "begin to dip when a few doctors express doubts," and "then the news gets out that the antibiotic has made a patient ill." In short order, the price and volume of sales drop, and the drug company is left with a "steady profit but no bonanza."[62] Testifying before Congress in 1961, Dale Console, former director of research at Squibb, claimed that drug products were starting to "change like women's hemlines" and warned that "rapid obsolescence is simply a sign of motion, not progress." During the same hearings, Johns Hopkins University pharmacologist Louis Lasagna expressed doubts about the constant parade of supposedly new and improved drugs: The "problem of 'built in obsolescence' of drugs" reflects the "miserable quality of drugs that are issued each year," he lamented. "The advertising agencies are being asked to sell to the medical profession a whole bushel basketful of sows' ears for silk purses each year." It was no wonder, he concluded, that "advertising excesses" were followed by "so-called product failures and that obsolescence sets in."[63]

Although common to all drug classes, the dangers of the therapeutic cycle and systematic overselling drew more censure in relation to some medications than others. The minor tranquilizers offered a case in point. Starting with the 1950s debate over Miltown, the idea that drugs were being used to medicate "ordinary problems of living" brought what psychiatrist Gerald Klerman in 1970 dubbed "pharmaceutical Calvinists" out in force. So, too, did the use of hormone extracts to offset the effects of aging. In the 1930s, controversy had centered on John Brinkley's goat gland extract for men; in the late 1950s and 1960s, it focused on women as doctors began to prescribe synthetic estrogen products for menopausal patients. The "vain" female consumer attempting to reverse the normal aging process became a convenient symbol of the forces driving overmedication.[64]

In explicating the therapeutic cycle, many commentators in the late 1950s and early 1960s assigned patients a large share of the blame. Paralleling the commentaries on unnecessary surgery, critics emphasized the public's foolish pursuit of perpetual youth and happiness and its eagerness to find "a pill for every ill" as the root cause of prescription drug overuse and misuse. In antidrug jeremiads, the Miltown-popping American of the 1950s strongly resembled the yeast-eating, elixir-guzzling mark of the pre-1938 era. But at a time when physicians were insisting that patients should trust their doctors' choice of prescription drugs, the evidence of the medical profession's failure to be constructively critical of drug company promotions seemed particularly troubling.

While the majority of doctors still felt confident that their scientific training made them impervious to therapeutic fashions or false advertising of any sort, many professional leaders were less sure. In a widely cited 1961 article, Charles May chided his fellow physicians because "the traditional independence of physicians and the welfare of the public are being threatened by the new vogue among drug manufacturers to promote their products by assuming an aggressive role in the 'education' of doctors." According to Haskell J. Weinstein, the former medical director of a Pfizer division, the doctor "has been taught, one might almost say brainwashed, to think of the trademark name of the drug at all times." In place of objective information about the drug's efficacy or cost, "he is seduced with gimmicks of all sorts in an attempt to make him loyal to a particular company or a particular drug, with relatively little attention being paid to the specific merits of the drug in question."[65]

The potential dangers of misleading prescription drug advertising were compounded by the growing fragmentation of American medical practice, which meant that general practitioners were as likely to be prescribing potentially addictive psychoactive drugs or risk-laden antidiabetic remedies as their specialist colleagues. As a consequence, pharmacological experts within the profession worried that the goal of rational prescribing—the right drug in the right amount at the right time—was retreating even further from the medical profession's grasp. Once viewed as impervious to misleading advertising, the American doctor now seemed in danger of becoming as confused as his patients.

Having become exclusive guardians of the doctors' drugs, the medical profession faced increasing responsibility for patients' use and misuse of these medications. Before 1938, patients had only themselves to blame when they fell for a misleading advertising campaign and purchased an ineffective or unsafe proprietary remedy. But with the creation of the new prescription drug system, patients had to depend on physicians to select drugs; the medical profession acted as "learned intermediaries," to use the legal term introduced in the 1960s, guarding patients against unwise and dangerous choices. Doctors became increasingly responsible, at least in some patients' eyes, for the price, efficacy, and side effects associated with prescription drugs.[66]

The rapid pace of drug development increased the evaluative burden on the physician. As Leonard Robinson noted in a 1960 article in *Coronet*, twenty-five years earlier, an average of only six new drugs arrived on the market each year; now, that number was one drug every day. "The range of possible secondary effects in modern drugs is now so great that even doctors sometimes have trouble keeping track of which *good* drug can cause which *bad* reaction." Robinson concluded that given doctors' difficulties in evaluating drugs, patients should not even try. But if as witnesses before the Kefauver committee testified, physicians were struggling to perform their due diligence as informed consumers, their patients' faith in them would seem to be misplaced. The influential journal *Science* noted in 1960 that doctors had no "convenient index of information that would allow them to sort out the misleading from the meaningful messages among the barrage of promotion to which they are subject (about a pound of mail a day plus regular visits from the companies' 'detail men')."[67]

One response to these concerns was the creation of a Consumers Union publication for physicians, the *Medical Letter on Drugs and Therapeutics*, which began biweekly publication in January 1959. The *Medical Letter* was started by Arthur Kallet, coauthor of *100,000,000 Guinea Pigs* and a founder of Consumers Union, and Consumers Union's longtime physician consultant, Harold Aaron. As an alternative to drug advertising and detailing, their journal aimed to provide "concise, authoritative, and unbiased appraisals of both new and old drugs." Like *Consumer Reports*, it accepted no advertising, depending entirely on subscriptions for its operating income. As a favorable notice of the new publication in *Science* reported, one could now pay $12.50 for an annual subscription and learn "what is a valuable addition to the therapeutic armamentarium and what is not."[68] The publication initially met with resistance within the medical profession. Some doctors were suspicious of Kallet and Aaron, labeling them communists and "therapeutic nihilists." Representatives of the drug and advertising industries derided the publication, asking, "Who gave these guys the right to tell everyone how good or bad drugs are?" But within a year of its first issue, the journal had 14,000 subscribers, and the number continued to grow in the 1960s. While intended as a service to physicians, the *Medical Letter* also became a resource for lay consumerists as well, who used the publication to stay up-to-date on the latest drug information.[69]

Criticism of the prescription drug industry also helped Consumers Union emerge from the shadow of the second Red Scare. From its earliest issues, its monthly *Consumer Reports* had contained articles on over-the-counter drugs; during the 1950s, the publication slowly widened its coverage to include prescription drugs. In 1961, the organization published *The Medicine*

Show, a compilation of those articles.[70] While acknowledging the value of the new drug discoveries, the book warned that they were being promoted overzealously. As Consumers Union head Dexter Masters wrote in the preface, a long, hard look at drug advertisements suggested that "we are here in the presence of something irrational." To protect themselves, consumers needed to become more aware "of the differences between genuine advances in medical research and the 'miracles' of drug advertising." The chapters on prescription drugs sought to provide "a guide for laymen to the half-revealed world that lies beyond the prescription pad." After describing the growth in direct-mail advertising to physicians, pharmaceutical-company-sponsored activities at medical conventions, and the use of detail men, the book warned that "the spirit, the values, and the tactics of the patent medicine promoter now hold sway over the 'ethical' drug."[71]

This critical message was by no means confined to Consumers Union's publications; it also found its way into mainstream mass-circulation magazines such as *Life*. In February 1960, the magazine featured "A Big Pill to Swallow," which repeated the essence of the *Medicine Show* argument for a much wider audience. Lavishly illustrated with photos, charts, and diagrams, the article summarized the recent business history of the pharmaceutical industry as an explanation for the high costs of prescription drugs. "Unlike other major industries, this one has the advantage of selling to captive consumers—sick people who cannot shop around but must buy what the doctor orders." The article concluded that the Kefauver hearings might eventually bring a lowering of prices, particularly by encouraging the substitution of generic for brand-name medications. "But in the long run it is up to better informed consumers to insist on being less captive and to pressure the doctors into using a finer discrimination." Otherwise, Americans would just go on "digging deep" into their pocketbooks every time they needed a prescription drug.[72]

By the early 1960s, the tenets of critical consumerism in the drugstore had returned to public prominence. But in contrast to the pre-1940 era, the politics and practice of skeptical consumerism now focused on the doctors' drugs as opposed to over-the-counter medication. Rather than critiquing proprietary companies and consumer choice of over-the-counter medicines, the new crusade focused on the role of doctors as patient advocates and educators. Politicians and journalists devoted more attention to doctors' shortcomings than to those of laypeople. At the same time, the controversy revisited older debates about how to regulate the special goods sold from behind the prescription drug counter. As *Science* commented in 1960, "The basic issue, rarely stated clearly by either side, seems to be whether the industry should be allowed to run itself as a normal business, or whether its special position justifies the federal government's taking steps to see that it is run as a public service." The industry was in many ways a victim of its own success: its business methods attracted attention precisely because they generated such high profits—the "fourth highest among American industries, more than double the 11 percent average of all industries."[73]

These developments resulted in a new generation of shopping problems: high prices, undisclosed side effects, and doubts about the trustworthiness of physicians' therapeutic judgment. These tensions were all the more evident given the trends toward convenience and transparency that prevailed on the other side of the prescription counter, where over-the-counter drugs were more clearly labeled and accessible. Questions arising about the pricing and promotion of the new doctors' drugs deepened concerns about how much patients could trust their physicians' advice. The Cold War drugstore thus laid the foundations for a new wave of drug activism. With rising concerns about the cost of medicine more generally, the discontents of the 1950s evolved into a new and more radical era of protest in which the patient-as-watchdog concept would move from the margins to the mainstream of American culture.

PART THREE

A Consumers' Revolution?

The 1960s to the 1990s

{EIGHT}

The Patient Must Prescribe for the Doctor

In 1966, Walter Goodman, a senior editor at the *New York Times*, began a lengthy article on the current troubled state of American medicine with the lament, "What ever became of good old doc?" Underneath a photograph of a top-hatted nineteenth-century physician, Goodman mused, "Whereas the relations between patient and family doctor in the days when the latter treated every ailment that came up might well have been rich in human resonances, the relationship between patient and specialist today is about as resonant as that between a car owner and a transmission mechanic." The cartoons accompanying the article were equally provocative, showing a doctor whose familiar black bag was now stuffed with cash, another who was thinking about his upcoming golf game while examining his patient, and another who "flaunted" his economic success by driving a very expensive automobile.[1]

To explain why the "doctor's image is sickly," Goodman ran through a litany of problems with the "new" medicine. As more and more doctors specialized, Americans found it hard to find the kind of personal family physician they trusted. They wondered if they should trust medical advice, given that "doctors have proved themselves to be approximately as gullible as laymen when it comes to wonder drugs" and "continue to inflict a great many questionable operations" on patients, at least those with health insurance. Precisely because American patients had such high regard for science and medicine, perceptions of "prestige and scorn" were appearing "hand in hand." The stalwart opposition by the AMA to reforms intended to improve drug safety, discourage cigarette smoking, and extend medical insurance to the elderly and the poor "has helped spread abroad the idea that the interests of America's doctors and of America's patients are not identical."[2]

Goodman's article prompted a deluge of furious letters from doctors protesting his argument and his imagery. A young doctor driving a Volkswagen while paying off his medical school loans wrote that he was "damned angry at being included in Mr. Goodman's stereotype of the 'rich, Cadillac-driving doctor.'" Another physician wrote, "Everyone keeps checking the M.D. plates outside the golf club; does anyone report the lineup of M.D. plates outside the hospital at 3 A.M.?" He also regretted that "too many nonprofessionals have taken it upon themselves to elaborate on 'the truth about your doctor.'" While medical professionals lambasted Goodman, laypeople applauded him: wrote Doris Gordon of Atlantic City, New Jersey, "Hooray for the Goodman article. Everyone already knows what you have said so well. I only hope that the sick doctors will read it."[3]

Goodman's provocative article appeared amid a sense that not only medicine but all of American society was starting to unravel. Dragged down by entrenched racism and a misguided war in Vietnam, "the Great Society has become a sick society," as Arkansas senator William Fulbright put it in a widely cited 1967 speech.[4] Despite the reforms adopted during the liberal Kennedy and Johnson administrations, social conditions, including medical care, seemed to be worsening instead of improving. Characterizations of the American medical system as in crisis persisted even after landmark legislation aimed at correcting its worst flaws: the 1962 Kefauver-Harris Amendment to increase drug safety and the 1965 creation of Medicare and Medicaid to fill in the gaps left by private insurance. As disaffected young radicals began to argue, those liberal solutions only reinforced the defects inherent in the "medical-industrial complex"; real change for patients required a rejection of free enterprise medicine altogether.

Starting in the mid-1960s, health care became the centerpiece of intense political arguments about the causes and symptoms of the "sick society" and its "sick care" system. All parties to that debate—radical, liberal, and conservative—came to the conclusion that in order to improve, health care providers and institutions had to become more responsive to patient-consumer voices. During the turbulent years between 1965 and 1975, the ideal of "doctor knows best" came under withering attack from multiple directions. The time had come, as one doctor said in 1969, that "the patient must prescribe for the physician."[5]

As medical authority came under attack, many new interested parties entered the national discussion about the doctor-patient relationship, including welfare mothers, radical feminists, and Black Panthers. Radical critiques of scientific knowledge intermingled with grassroots activism to inspire more egalitarian models for the doctor-patient relationship. Amplified by larger political and intellectual trends, activists spearheaded a "revolt of the patients" that brought the concept of the patient as watchdog into the mainstream of American medical politics. But despite gaining some notable public victories, the post-1968 version of medical consumerism failed to dismantle the medical-industrial complex. As the fire of the 1960s faded, much of what would be done in the name of the empowered patient-consumer bore little resemblance to what patient activists originally had in mind.

From Great Society to Sick Society

Perhaps no set of reforms better embodied the limits of 1960s liberalism than the health care legislation associated with the Kennedy and Johnson administrations. The election of Democrats to the presidency in 1960 and 1964 resulted in significant new efforts to address the problems that had developed in the doctor's office and drugstore: the 1962 Kefauver-Harris Amendment, which raised standards for the safety and truthful advertising of prescription drugs, and the 1965 Medicare and Medicaid bills, which created government insurance programs for the elderly and the poor. Far from dampening discontent, these solutions left untouched some of the most troublesome features of free enterprise medicine at the same time they heightened patient-consumers' expectations of change.

Those expectations had been fueled by John F. Kennedy's 1960 victory on promises to attend to the medical needs of the elderly and to advance consumer protections. In March 1962, Kennedy outlined before Congress an ambitious agenda for consumer reform. Consumers, he noted, accounted for two-thirds of the nation's spending but "are the only important group in the economy who are not effectively organized, whose views are often not heard." Kennedy argued that the federal government had to do more to advance consumers' rights, which he enumerated as the right to safety, the right to be informed, the right to choose, and the right to be heard, a formulation that became known as the Consumer's Bill of Rights.[6]

At the head of Kennedy's list for immediate action was drug safety. Citing Kefauver's investigations, the president asked Congress to strengthen the power of the FDA on the grounds that "the physician and consumer should have the assurance, from an impartial scientific source, that any drug or therapeutic device on the market today is safe and effective for its intended use" and that its "accompanying promotional material tells the full story—its bad effects as well as its good." But Kennedy's public rhetoric did not match his political willingness to push forward with drug reforms. At the time of the consumer's rights speech, Kefauver had drafted a tough bill providing for changes in the patent system, more oversight of drug pricing, tighter regulation of drug advertising, expanded warnings about side effects, and more rigorous testing of new drugs. Both the pharmaceutical industry and the

AMA strongly opposed Kefauver's proposals, and the Kennedy administration backed away and signaled its support for the much weaker bill crafted by Senate Republicans.[7]

Furious at this defection, Kefauver staged an effective countermove. For months, his staff had been collecting information about the international tragedy unfolding around thalidomide, a drug prescribed to reduce nausea and anxiety in pregnant women that turned out to cause severe fetal deformation. Despite intense industry pressure to approve the drug, the FDA's Frances Kelsey had refused to do so, citing its potential dangers, so very few Americans were among the almost 10,000 women harmed by the drug. In July 1962, Kefauver's staff handed over their thalidomide files to Morton Mintz of the *Washington Post*, who shared Kefauver's skepticism about the drug industry. After Mintz broke the thalidomide story, newspapers and magazines across the country took it up.

In the face of headlines about the controversy, President Kennedy had little choice but to back a stronger bill, and what became known as the Kefauver-Harris Amendment passed Congress in October 1962. But even with the thalidomide case to use as political capital, Kefauver and his supporters won only a partial victory. To be sure, what they did get was extremely important. The FDA was now empowered to require experimental proof that new drugs were both safe and effective before they went on the market as well as to reassess all drugs currently in use, both prescription and over-the-counter. The 1962 law also transferred oversight of prescription drug advertising from the FTC to the FDA, a reform long desired by drug reformers. In 1938, when reformers had made that request, Congress had declined on the grounds that "men of science" needed no special protection from misleading advertising; after the testimony presented during the Kefauver hearings, legislators were easier to convince that the FDA needed more authority to ensure accuracy of prescription drug labels, packaging, and advertising.

Yet other key parts of Kefauver's bill, including the provisions for patent reform and price control, were stripped from the legislation to enable it to pass. The 1962 law thus left in place the existing system of pricing and patent protections that underwrote the high cost of prescription medications. Other administrative efforts, such as the FTC's efforts to prosecute price-fixing of drugs, had comparatively little effect. The industry's argument—"of course drugs are expensive; so are tombstones," as George Sokolsky put it—seemed to prevail. Moving oversight of prescription drug promotion from the FTC to the FDA did not solve the problem of pharmaceutical company influence over doctors' prescribing habits, while the new informational guidelines the agency developed for doctors and pharmacists highlighted the absence of similar information for patient-consumers. The problems left unresolved by the 1962 amendments, including the absence of price controls, pharmaceutical companies' influence over physician prescribing patterns, and patients' lack of warning about side effects, would spur more congressional investigations, journalistic exposés, and consumerist complaints in the decades to come.[8]

The same sense of forward progress hampered by concessions to the medical status quo marked the other landmark health care legislation of the Great Society, the passage of the bills creating Medicare and Medicaid in 1965. It took Kennedy's assassination in 1963 followed by inspired political maneuvering by his successor to bring those programs into existence. In 1960, Kennedy had campaigned on a promise to create a public program that would cover hospital insurance for the elderly. With strong backing from organized labor, his administration launched an unprecedented grassroots effort to build public support for the plan, culminating in an elaborate rally held at New York City's Madison Square Garden in May 1962. The AMA responded with a public relations effort reminding Americans of the dangers of socialized medicine; its campaign featured an up-and-coming actor-politician named Ronald Reagan, who warned that if Kennedy's plan succeeded, "you and I are going to spend our sunset years telling our children and our children's children, what it was like in America when men were free." In July 1962, the administration's bill met defeat in the Senate by four votes at the hands of a coalition of conservative Democrats and Republicans who agreed that the reform was too costly and too threatening to America's free enterprise principles.[9]

Even more committed to health care reform than Kennedy, his successor, Lyndon Baines Johnson, was determined to achieve it after his landslide election in November 1964. In his first State of the Union address, Johnson promised to pursue change that would better "match the achievements of medicine ... to the afflictions of our people." A skillful politician with his own party now firmly in control of both houses of Congress, Johnson and his ally, Wilbur Mills, an Arkansas Democrat who headed the powerful House Ways and Means Committee, combined opponents' plans with the White House's own to create two ambitious programs, Medicare for the elderly and Medicaid for low-income Americans. To get the support of the conservative Ways and Means Committee, Johnson's negotiator, Wilbur Cohen, promised that "there would be no real controls over hospitals or physicians." Johnson waved off his staff's warnings that this new "three-layer cake" was likely to be very expensive, and Congress passed the legislation in July 1965. Johnson traveled to Independence, Missouri, to sign it into law so that former president Harry Truman could be enrolled as the first recipient of Medicare.[10]

Johnson's victory represented a painful defeat for the AMA. At its next annual meeting, a journalist commented that "the atmosphere of gloom resembled nothing so much as descriptions of the French at Dienbienphu," the epic battle at which France lost control of Vietnam. While some AMA members initially threatened a boycott, the profession soon made its peace with Medicare, after realizing the economic benefits it would bring. To placate medical opposition, both programs honored the principle of fee-for-service billing at the "usual and customary rate"; in essence, taxpayers now funded a system in which the hospitals and physicians decided what to charge. As doctors who had initially opposed Medicare now raised their fees by as much as 300 percent to benefit from it, the profession's image as too money-oriented got strong reinforcement.[11]

While spending on Medicaid patients remained grudging, Medicare brought a much appreciated flow of funds into a health care system starting to feel the pinch of an economic slowdown. Operated on the "costs plus" system, Medicare represented an open-ended commitment to covering services rendered, incentivizing hospitals and physicians to upgrade facilities and provide more expensive treatments. Prior experience with private insurance could and did predict the results: billings and fees under public programs rose dramatically, becoming a worrisome drag on the federal budget and taxpayer generosity. Moreover, rising rates for Medicare reimbursement encouraged comparable trends for employer-based insurance plans. Thus, between 1965 and 1975, spending on medical care increased about 12 percent per year, while private spending grew at 10 percent each year. The amount of the gross domestic product spent on health care rose from 5.2 percent in 1960 to 8.3 percent in 1975. As the economy weakened in the early 1970s, these increases became a grave cause for political concern.[12]

Far from solving problems, the Great Society modifications of free enterprise medicine created new ones. Medicare and Medicaid helped to underwrite a massive expansion of product- and procedure-oriented medical care with no cost or quality controls over its delivery. Combined with the 1962 drug reforms, which did little to lower drug costs, the Great Society medical programs put the government stamp of approval on the ethos of "new and improved" medicine but made no effort to rein in its faults: the lack of coordination among care providers, the absence of quality standards, and the temptations of the Shavian "doctor's dilemma." As a new generation of critics started to point out, Great Society programs made huge concessions to business and professional interest groups while asking for little assurance of quality or cost-effectiveness in return.

Meanwhile, the AMA's positions on drug reform and Medicare and Medicaid did little to improve its public standing. In his 1966 *New York Times* article, Goodman specifically mentioned the AMA's political stances, including its opposition to the Kefauver-Harris Amendment, controls on cigarette advertising, and Medicare, "the most popular bill of the decade," as reasons why the doctor's image was "in a decided state of disarray."[13] As the economy stagnated and health care costs rose precipitously, not only liberal Democrats but moderate Republicans became more willing to challenge the AMA's political power. Simultaneously, a powerful push to do the same came from another direction, as far more radical groups of activists emerged whose criticisms of medicine would make those of earlier medical consumerists seem mild in comparison.

Medical Power to the People

In 1968, this rebellious mood emerged in the wake of the assassinations of Martin Luther King Jr. and Robert F. Kennedy, the urban riots following King's death, and the violent encounters between protestors and police at the Democratic National Convention in Chicago. As the social order seemed to be unraveling, a far more radical critique of American society in general and American medicine in particular began to emerge from what was informally termed "the movement." Activists with a shared commitment to social change organized in cities and towns across the United States, often in close proximity to colleges and universities. Loosely organized and famously fractious, the movement included student radicals associated with the New Left, militant factions of the civil rights movement, radical feminists, and environmentalists. For a variety of reasons, all of these groups sought to return "medical power to the people."[14]

Health and medicine became increasingly prominent issues as activist groups sought to broaden their base of support within the larger community. As a feminist activist explained in 1971, "Health is an issue that everyone can relate to . . . black, white, men, women, old, young, gay, straight. . . . All are messed over by the health care system in different ways and in different degrees."[15] Health issues served well to illustrate the ways that the American system had failed key groups of its citizens. The National Welfare Rights Organization and the Black Panthers thus began to call attention to the health harms associated with entrenched racism and poverty; feminist activists focused on medical paternalism and its threats to women's reproductive health; labor organizers trying to rebuild the union movement focused on unionizing hospital workers, many of whom were black and/or Hispanic; and environmental activists emphasized the toxic side effects of pollution as a threat to human health.

In their censure of medicine, the late-1960s generation echoed older consumerist complaints about the "marriage of medicine and business," as James Rorty had dubbed it back in 1939. But in their critiques they adopted a far more hostile attitude toward both modern science and modern capitalism than had their New Deal predecessors. Movement thinking reflected the influence of several different strands of radicalism, including the Third World liberation struggles inspired by Frantz Fanon and Che Guevara and the post-Holocaust critiques of Western culture produced by European philosophers such as Jean-Paul Sartre and Theodor Adorno. In their focus on the body, health activists also built on the counterculture's call for personal as well as political transformations; as philosopher Herbert Marcuse wrote in his widely read 1969 "Essay on Liberation," the development of a "free society" required not just an end to political repression but a deeper sense of personal "liberation" from the constraints of an "exploitative order."[16]

In this quest for liberation, activists viewed medical science as an enemy rather than an ally. Far from constituting neutral sources of useful truths, modern medicine and technology had become tools that the white male elite used to preserve the capitalist system. Like science in general, mainstream medicine had become a willing handmaiden to the "medical-industrial complex," a phrase that first appeared in the 1970 book *The American Health Empire*, written by the Health Policy Advisory Center collective. Medicine's capture by capitalist principles meant that "profit, power, [and] personal aggrandizement take precedence over the prevention of illness." As a consequence, the book argued, "health is no more the top priority of the American health industry than safe, cheap, efficient, pollution-free transportation is a priority of the automobile industry." Radical critics also decried the trend toward medicalizing human experience in order to treat it, expensively but often ineffectively, with prescription drugs and surgical procedures. As historian-philosopher Ivan Illich suggested in his widely read 1975 book *Medical Nemesis*, modern medicine itself had become a prolific source of iatrogenic or doctor-inflicted injuries. The radical feminist magazine *off our backs* made a similar point far less elegantly by dubbing the AMA the American Murderers' Association.[17]

While deeply critical of scientific expertise, the new health activism nonetheless derived much of its effectiveness from the leadership of radicalized doctors, nurses, and dentists. Particularly important was the Medical Committee for Human Rights, founded in 1964 by physicians involved in the civil rights movement. In the late 1960s, this organization began to take a leading role in movement health politics as a coalition builder, bringing together white New Left groups with black and Hispanic groups such as the National Welfare Rights Organization, the Black Panthers, and the Young Lords. By 1971, about forty chapters of the Medical Committee existed. Another very important organization was the Health Policy Advisory Center, better known as Health-PAC, a group of physicians and academics created in 1968 to provide politically useful research and analysis. Health-PAC's *Bulletin* provided trenchant New Left critiques of American health problems and promoted alliances among newly unionized health workers and the patients they served.[18]

While guided by what Health-PAC members Barbara Ehrenreich and John Ehrenreich labeled "professional radicals," the new health activism rested on a core belief that all patients should and could speak for themselves. The antidote to medical ills lay in helping the layman to "reclaim his own control over medical perception, classification, and decision-making," as Illich put it in 1975. And unlike earlier generations of consumerists, who assumed such control ought to be limited to "educated" patients, movement activists thought that every patient's views should be taken seriously. Whether a Medicaid recipient, mental patient, or middle-class housewife, patients had knowledge of their bodies and preferences for care that physicians should respect.[19]

To advance their principles, health activists drew on organizing tactics developed in the labor, civil rights, and student movements; their "politics of confrontation" deployed strikes, protest marches, and lawsuits to challenge the medical "establishment." As sociologists Marie R. Haug and Marvin B. Sussman noted in 1969, "Nowadays individual clients do not drop out; they get together, sit in, and confront the functionaries of service organizations."[20] In that spirit, protesters began to show up at the annual meetings of the AMA, the American Psychiatric Association, and the AHA. The protest tradition started in 1963, when the Medical Committee for Human Rights organized a demonstration against racial discrimination in medicine, and grew livelier over the rest of the decade. At the 1968 AMA meeting, a reporter described the "crocodile of pickets undulating across the street," among them "hippies, yippies, kooks, religious maniacs, health food nuts," and a sprinkling of physicians. Protesters carried signs that said "Give better medical care to the poor" and "Prescribe love as the best therapy" and chanted "Hip, hip Hippocrates / Up with service, down with fees." These protests could become quite elaborate. At the AMA's 1974 annual meeting, the Gray Panthers, an advocacy group for older Americans, staged a minidrama imploring the organization to "have a heart." With TV cameras and photographers in attendance, four Panthers dressed as medics arrived in a white ambulance-like van to administer resuscitation to another member impersonating the "sick AMA"; after removing wads of dollar bills from the AMA's chest, the "doctors" finally found the organization's "heart" and saved it.[21]

Along with such street theater, health activists conducted sit-ins at medical schools and hospitals, organized strikes of hospital workers, and held teach-ins about institutional racism in the health care system. Among the most publicized such events was the 1969 takeover of Lincoln Hospital's Mental Health Services, in which a group of more than 150 workers, many of them black and/or Puerto Rican, seized control of the Bronx facility. During the two weeks they occupied the hospital's administrative offices, the protesters drew attention to the institution's failures to treat both staff members and patients with respect and demanded more worker and community control over its policy.[22]

In addition to directly challenging the medical establishment, activist groups sought to build alternatives to it. One favored solution was the expansion and democratization of the community health clinics created under the aegis of various Great Society programs, including the Community Mental Health Centers Act (1963) and the Economic Opportunity Act (1964). By 1973, that funding had created approximately 325 community mental health clinics and 150 general clinics offering medical services in underserved neighborhoods. In addition, movement groups set up their own clinics, frequently with the word "free" in their titles, starting with the Haight Ashbury Free Clinic, founded in 1967 to care for the young people who came to San Francisco to celebrate the Summer of Love. Far less securely funded than their Great Society counterparts, the free clinics numbered an estimated 400 by the early 1970s, including "people's clinics" founded by the Black Panther Party and feminist health clinics that provided birth control and abortion services. Along with coffeehouses, food cooperatives, and alternative newspapers, free clinics became one of the most visible signs of the counterculture's existence.[23]

Although they differed in how much they challenged medical professionalism, both types of community health clinics shared a commitment to developing a more democratic alternative to the traditional doctor's office. Some clinics charged nothing, relying on charitable donations and government grants to cover their expenses. Others used a sliding scale determined by the patient's circumstances but still charged far less than regular physicians.

As *The Seed*, an alternative newspaper, explained to its readers, Chicago's free clinics "are run to provide decent medical care for people who might not otherwise even SEE a doctor." Warning that patients who could afford to pay should not try to take advantage of the clinic's generosity, the paper concluded, "Don't fuck them up, nobody needs freeloaders."[24]

Community clinics also departed from business as usual by concentrating on neighborhoods and groups traditionally underserved by free enterprise medicine: the poor, people of color, addicts and alcoholics, young runaways, gays and lesbians, and women. Theirs was an alternative medicine aimed at correcting the racial and moral blind spots of mainstream medicine. Thus community clinics sought to address problems such as lead poisoning and sickle-cell anemia that afflicted inner-city black neighborhoods; to provide nonjudgmental treatment of people suffering from drug overdoses, sexually transmitted diseases, and septic abortions; to dispense contraceptive devices and abortion referrals to single and married women alike; and to acknowledge the special emotional and physical needs of gay men and women.[25]

In the same spirit, the new-style clinics fostered a more comfortable and inclusive atmosphere that minimized the social distance between doctor and patient; their goal, as one clinic physician explained, was "medicine without the hassle." Although many clinics were located in dilapidated buildings and run on shoestring budgets, staffers delivered care in settings "designed to be warm and inviting, and most important, non-threatening." To avoid the "little tin god" syndrome, clinic workers departed from traditional medical etiquette, either by having both doctor and patient use their first names or by having the physician refer to the patient as Mr., Mrs., or Ms. The result, as one visitor noted, was an "atmosphere strikingly different from that found in the usual clinic, doctor's office, or hospital"; "it is often impossible to tell the difference between the patients, the doctors and nurses, and the community volunteers," and "the waiting rooms resemble more of a social gathering place than a clinical setting."[26]

In the same spirit, clinic workers sought to demystify medicine by explaining procedures in terms patients could understand, whether they were poor inner-city residents or college students. As Ava Wolfe, a pediatrician working at a free clinic in the Georgetown neighborhood of Washington, D.C., explained to a journalist, "The idea is to get the parent to take an active part in the examination and the diagnosis." Not only do "patients have a right to know what is being done to them or to their children," but through the process they would "learn more and more to keep themselves healthy." Feminist health clinics took special pride in making women feel more knowledgeable about their bodies by teaching them to examine their own vaginas and cervixes. An *off our backs* article summed up their motto: "Anatomy: Dig Yourself."[27]

In addition to offering individual services, many clinics sought to encourage collective efforts at prevention. For example, the Black Panther Party's "people's clinics" not only provided medical care but also helped clients with housing problems, offered free breakfasts for children, and provided screenings for sickle-cell anemia. Other clinics offered classes in nutrition, child rearing, stress relief, self-defense, consciousness-raising, yoga, and meditation. Waiting rooms featured information about local community groups and health-related political issues that clients might want to support.[28]

Last but not least, community clinics sought to replace medical hierarchy with a more democratic, participatory kind of governance. For clinics funded by the U.S. Office of Economic Opportunity, that objective was federally mandated; the program's guidelines specified "maximum feasible participation" by the recipients of assistance. In practice, this rule came to mean that in order to receive federal funds, an agency's governance board had to have at least 51 percent of its members be either eligible for or receiving the services offered. Free clinics had no such bureaucratic mandate, yet they aspired to even more egalitarian principles of organization. Many of them operated as collectives in which patients, community volunteers, and medical staff all had an equal voice. For both types of clinics, community participation and control proved difficult to sustain; those goals were undercut by conflicts among community members and clinic staff as well as between lay and professional workers. In order to survive, many clinics eventually abandoned some of their egalitarianism. But overall, community clinics maintained a much more open and responsive style of governance than did a hospital or a traditional doctor's office.[29]

In the early 1970s, many activists pointed to community health clinics as a viable alternative to the American "sick care system." According to *Health Rights News*, the newsletter published by the Medical Committee for Human Rights, "The free clinics are a model for community control, absence of fees, and innovations in preventative medicine"; "whatever health care looks like in the future will bear the strong stamp of the free clinic movement." Not everyone agreed; physician H. Jack Geiger wrote in 1971 that the people running these clinics were "playing house, not responding to real needs." Many hospitals and physicians remained hostile to the clinics, making it difficult for them to refer patients who needed more specialized care, while the police and public health departments prosecuted clinics for violations of city and state health codes. In one celebrated example, Los Angeles police officers staged a raid on the Feminist Women's Health Center and arrested its founders, Carol Downer and Colleen Wilson, for practicing medicine without a license, though they were eventually acquitted of the charges.[30]

As funds dried up and the political climate turned more conservative, the predictions that community health centers would transform American medical care proved unfounded. They did not, as health activists had hoped, put an end to fragmented, fee-for-service medicine. But many centers founded in this era survived, remaining an important source of care for low-income and uninsured Americans to the present day. Moreover, their commitment to medical democracy encouraged a broader trend within medicine to rethink its authoritarian customs and to treat patients with respect. Finally, the community health movement's efforts to advance the medical rights of poor and underserved groups helped lend a new seriousness to medical consumerism.[31]

Given that activists sought to liberate health and medicine from the corruption of the capitalist marketplace, their adoption of the term "consumer" to describe empowered patients might seem paradoxical. But in the context of the early 1970s, referring to patients as consumers made strategic sense. For activists committed to changing power relationships in the clinic and hospital, the word "patient" was deeply suffused with the values of medical paternalism. As alternatives to "patient," groups tried out different terms, among them "client" and "survivor." In the end, "consumer" emerged as the preferred term even among radical groups. Thus when representatives of the Black Panthers, radical feminists, the Young Lords, and the Medical Committee for Human Rights were denied entrance to the 1970 AMA meeting, they agreed to form the Consumer Health Coalition to continue working together. With benefit of hindsight, the pitfalls of conflating patient rights with consumer rights would become all too evident. But in the still optimistic days of the early 1970s, "consumer" appealed because of its capaciousness: not only did it suggest a big tent under which very different groups might come together, but it also formed a bridge to a larger public that activists hoped to mobilize for change.[32]

We Can All Be Naders

Referring to empowered patients as consumers seemed all the more strategically sound as consumerism underwent its own political transformation in the late 1960s. Like health activism, the resurgence of consumer activism built on while it critiqued Great Society reforms. With Democrats in control, Congress in the 1960s passed a series of laws aimed at reducing air, water, and soil pollution; improving consumer product labeling; ensuring the safety of children's toys and sleepwear; and reforming consumer credit laws. It had also expanded the regulatory power of existing federal agencies, such as the FDA and the FTC, as well as creating new bodies, including the National Transportation Safety Board (1967), the Environmental Protection Agency (1970), the Occupational Safety and Health Administration (1970), and the Consumer Product Safety Commission (1972).[33]

Still, like health activists, the new generation of consumerists felt that these liberal programs remained too weak to offer real protection. According to a 1973 book, *The Consumer and Corporate Accountability*, liberal consumerism conceived of the problem as created by a few "bad apples in the barrel"—that is, a minority of irresponsible entrepreneurs who "polluted the honest business atmosphere and spoiled it for the legitimate businessmen." In contrast, the new consumerism believed that corporate capitalism itself had become a prolific source of harm, evident in industrial pollution, hazardous products, and the illnesses they caused. By documenting the impact of this "corporate power" on "life, death, and the pocketbook," the new consumerists aimed to raise standards of corporate accountability as well as to promote more sustainable consumption patterns.[34]

The new consumerism's appeal was reflected both in the growth of existing organizations, such as the National Consumers League and Consumers Union, and in the creation of new ones, such as Public Citizen and the Center for Science in the Public Interest. So many groups existed by 1968 that they decided to create an umbrella organization, the Consumer Federation of America, to coordinate their efforts; from 60 founding members it had expanded to include 160 organizations by the mid-1970s. Targeting a wide variety of topics, including product safety, consumer credit, and advertising to children, the federation coordinated national lobbying efforts and began to rate members of Congress on their commitment to consumers.[35]

Within the broader consumerist movement, groups emerged that had a particular interest in health issues. The Center for Science in the Public Interest, founded in 1971, concentrated on food and nutrition policies. The Center for Medical Consumers and Health Care Information, founded in 1976, concentrated on the safety and effectiveness of new drugs and medical procedures. Women's health concerns inspired so many different groups that in 1975 they formed their own advocacy network, the Women's Health Lobby (later renamed the National Women's Health Network) to coordinate their efforts. But perhaps the single most important advocacy group was Public Citizen's Health Research Group, founded by Ralph Nader and Sidney Wolfe in 1971. Like Health-PAC, the Health Research Group engaged in fact-finding and critical analysis, using that information as the basis for intensive lobbying. By working its ties to sympathetic legislators and journalists, the Health Research Group came to have a political clout out of proportion to its small size and funding. Its approach to protecting what Nader termed "body rights" helped to bring medical consumerism into the mainstream of American politics.[36]

The Health Research Group's success resulted in no small part from Nader's outsized personality and intellect. The son of Lebanese Christian immigrants, the Harvard-educated lawyer achieved national celebrity in 1965 when he published *Unsafe at Any Speed*, a searing exposé of safety issues in the American automobile industry. General Motors's attempts to discredit Nader (he was followed by detectives and tempted with prostitutes) not only increased his popular standing but resulted in a court settlement for the company's "overzealous surveillance" that provided him the funds to start his first organization, the Center for Study of Responsive Law, in 1968. He attracted a like-minded cohort of young lawyers, Nader's Raiders, whose actions seemed proof that a small group of committed activists could bring about significant change. As an admirer wrote in 1971, their work inspired confidence that "we can all be Naders."[37]

From the outset, medicine and health figured prominently on the Naderite agenda as a natural extension of the concept of "body rights" he had articulated in *Unsafe at Any Speed*. As Nader wrote in the preface, "A great problem of contemporary life is how to control the power of economic interests which ignore the harmful effects of their applied science and technology." To counter their influence, society needed "to protect the 'body rights' of its citizens with vigorous resolve and ample resources." Like the automotive industry, medicine was a prolific source of "designed-in dangers"; in addition, in Nader's view, it was failing in its professional responsibilities to protect the public. One of the first reports completed by the Center for Study of Responsive Law, *One Life—One Physician: An Inquiry into the Medical Profession's Performance in Self-Regulation*, concluded that the profession's self-discipline was not so much "inadequate" as "non-existent."[38]

Even more important to the evolving Naderite critique of medicine was the influence of Wolfe, a 1965 graduate of Case Western Medical School. When Nader met him in 1970, Wolfe was working as a NIH researcher and serving as cochair of the Washington, D.C., chapter of the Medical Committee for Human Rights. Fearing that the Medical Committee for Human Rights was losing momentum, Wolfe decided that partnering with Nader might offer a better platform for advocacy. In 1971, the two men founded the Health Research Group as the medical division of Public Citizen, and Wolfe became the organization's director. The Health Research Group quickly became one of the most visible consumer health advocacy groups, a position it continues to occupy.[39]

While more inclined to challenge scientific authority than the pre-1965 generation, the Health Research Group's approach had some striking similarities to the 1930s version of medical conservatism. Like the New Deal generation, Nader and Wolfe believed that patient-consumers needed independent groups to pressure government and business to protect the public interest. At the same time, individuals also needed to assume the role of "a searching and inquiring patient." The key to both efforts rested on gaining access to better information, a theme that would become a hallmark of 1970s medical consumerism. By becoming better educated and forceful in demanding their rights as patient-consumers, Americans could not only protect themselves from abuse but also improve the whole health care system. "There needs to be some kind of force that will give the patient a greater choice," Nader explained in 1974, and "that force, in part, is information."[40]

The Health Research Group illustrated the power of aligning New Left critiques of the medical establishment with a more Washington-insider style of pressure-group politics. According to a story about Nader that appeared in the *Washington Post* in 1970, "The public is discovering that by bottling its anger and then squirting it out under controlled pressure at carefully selected targets it can erode the walls of special privilege behind which vested interests have operated so long with impunity."[41] The "bottled anger" also had more impact because the new consumerists expressed greater concern for the health needs of the poor and of minority groups.

A 1970 editorial written by Theodore Cron, a colleague of Nader's and founder of another advocacy group, the American Patient, articulated the sense of common cause between poor and minority patients and their more affluent counterparts: the patients' rights movement had started with the goal of "bringing better health service to our minority poor" but in the process had discovered that "the deprived consumer[s] of health service" included not only "indigent, black, and angry ghetto-dwellers" but all Americans. Doctors were shocked to learn "that many well-heeled, white consumers have also 'had it up to here' with the health establishment and want some changes made." "Health deprivation is now recognized among all our people, of every color and station," Cron concluded, and "if only we can one day provide *excellent* care with the same egalitarian spirit, we will have accomplished a great deal for the American model consumer."[42]

In the early 1970s, the new consumerists recycled old arguments about medicine's failings with growing success. Their argument that the medical profession's inability to maintain internal standards lay at the root of both high prices and poor service found an increasingly receptive audience of judges and politicians. While rejecting the radical aspects of health activism, policymakers became more willing to reconsider their traditional deference to the medical profession and the health care industries that supported it. As a result, consumer activist groups seemed to achieve a new level of political clout: to become "giant killers," as Michael Pertschuk, the former head of the FTC, styled them.[43]

Let the Seller Beware!

The giant killers' odds of defeating the corporate Goliaths seemed promising in the early 1970s. As *Newsweek*'s correspondents covering national politics and business affairs announced in their 1969 book, *Let the Seller Beware!*, the United States was in the midst of a "consumer revolution." Powerful congressional Democrats, including Senators Edward Kennedy from Massachusetts, Warren G. Magnuson from Washington, and Gaylord Nelson from Wisconsin and Representative John E. Moss from California, sponsored hearings and drafted legislation regarding issues of concern to patient-consumers, including national health insurance, heightened regulation of prescription drugs, and oversight of medical practices. Even more ominously from the medical profession's point of view, Republican leaders also began to adopt the language of consumerism to advance their policy ends—in particular, halting the steep rise in public spending on medical care.[44] Likewise, federal regulatory agencies such as the FDA and the FTC felt increased pressure from both members of Congress and patient advocacy groups to act on patient-consumers' behalf. Even federal organizations that had never faced grassroots pressure before, such as the NIH, suddenly found themselves embroiled in public controversy. In this hypercharged political climate, one well-written letter, one threatened lawsuit, or one provocative news story could disturb the steady state of political business as usual.[45]

That sense of institutional instability was heightened by changes occurring in the judicial branch of government. The Naderite disposition to use legal authority to check medical autonomy was by no means an isolated phenomenon. A more liberal generation of jurists came to the bench, where they proved more sympathetic to the need to rethink the power relations between doctor and patient. After a century of deferring to the expansion of medical judgment, courts shifted from assuming that the "doctor is right" to insisting that the "patient has rights," as a legal historian observed. Simultaneously, changing views of product liability heightened a legal focus on manufacturers' responsibilities to the end user of their products, a trend with clear implications for potentially hazardous prescription drugs and medical devices.[46]

This legal revolution occurred gradually and unevenly. Although nothing in the Constitution seemed to guarantee a legal right to health care, many of the document's provisions could be and were reinterpreted to suggest that patients had rights regarding how they were cared for. Legal activists pushed not only to widen the scope of medical malpractice laws but also to expand patients' rights to privacy and due process under the law. While the courts protected prescription drugs and medical devices from the trend toward strict liability by recognizing the physician's role as a "learned intermediary" overseeing their use, that ruling directed new attention to the means by which risks were communicated from manufacturer to doctor and doctor to patient. As jurists' and juries' views on all these topics shifted, trial lawyers started to win cases that in the past might not even have been brought to trial. The fear of the lawsuit, in turn, gave pharmaceutical companies, hospitals, and doctors new cause to take seriously patients' assertions of their rights.[47]

All of these political and legal developments received coverage from journalists eager to get a reputation-enhancing story. As in earlier periods of patient unrest, the press recognized that stories about medical controversy attracted popular interest. While often dismissive of its more radical elements, mainstream journalists presented many aspects of patient-consumer unrest in the early 1970s with respect and sympathy. One particularly dramatic example of media attention came in the spring of 1970 when for the first time in television's history a major network devoted two hours of prime-time coverage to the health care crisis.

Promoted as a look at the "health industry as perceived by the consumer," the documentary *Health in America* was prepared by the CBS News staff, who spent months investigating why "the problem of health care has even perfectly healthy people worried sick." Reporters visited trouble spots all over the country, including a rural Indiana town that had no practicing doctors and Chicago's Cook County Hospital, where an overwhelmed staff sought to help very poor, very sick inner-city residents. Journalists also visited the bedside of a "Mr. Average American," a Los Angeles salesman with no health insurance who had just received a $1,017.85 bill for a routine hernia operation. The commentary suggested that all these problems—the absence of care for rural folk, the neglect of ghetto residents, and the financial burdens on middle-class families—stemmed from the same source: the misguided American faith in the superiority of "the single, free-enterprise virtuoso physician." That faith had encouraged a dysfunctional medical culture dominated by "the 'corner grocery' hospital" needlessly duplicating expensive services and the "push-cart peddler doctor" promoting "treatment piece by piece." The time had come, the documentary concluded, for Americans to reconsider that faith.[48]

As lead reporter Daniel Schorr recalled, the documentary provoked "a massive spasm of telephone calls, telegrams and letters that made it clear we had touched a raw nerve." The AMA lodged a formal protest and asked (unsuccessfully) for equal time to rebut the documentary. Physicians wrote to protest their portrayal as "arrogant, money-grabbing entrepreneurs" and to warn that "socialized medicine" would rob Americans of their cherished freedom of choice. "Believe me," wrote one doctor's wife of government control of health care, "this is *not* our dream!" But just as passionately, many viewers wrote to praise *Health in America* for taking a critical look at American medicine "long past due." One woman declared, "I am a very conservative Republican, but would vote for socialized medicine today if given the opportunity." Another viewer labeled it "the most important series ever aired on television" and commented on the AMA's negative response, "Does anybody want to cut down the money tree?"[49]

In light of all the tough talk about medical responsibility and accountability, deference to medicine's authority no longer seemed axiomatic. For a brief period, changes in the political climate, new currents in legal thinking, and the attentiveness of sympathetic journalists seemed to give the new-style health activism an impact out of proportion to its numbers and resources, producing a kind of "intellectual euphoria," as activist Barbara Ehrenreich recalled, in which fundamental change appeared to be on the horizon. While the moment soon passed, activists scored some significant victories in legitimating the concept of the empowered patient-consumer, among them the creation of the Patients' Bill of Rights, the provision of a patient leaflet for oral contraceptives, a broadened definition and practice of informed consent, and the expansion of patients' rights to health information.[50]

The Patients' Bill of Rights

Of all the new ideas generated by health activists in the late 1960s and early 1970s, perhaps the most ambitious was the concept of the Patients' Bill of Rights: a statement of the new, egalitarian principles on which patients would interact with physicians and hospitals. While its ideals proved hard to implement, the promulgation of the Patients' Bill of Rights represented a significant milestone in the legitimation of medical consumerism.

Although its exact origins are unclear, the idea for a Patients' Bill of Rights arose out of concerns about how inner-city hospitals treated poor people of color. Such a document was meant to have a twofold purpose: to help individual patients be more assertive about their care and to put hospitals on notice that outsiders were watching for abuse and neglect. In this manner, the Northwestern Health Collective in Chicago presented patients entering Cook County Hospital with a leaflet that began, "The doctor and the hospital are *not* doing you a favor to see you," and then explained that patients had rights to "informed consent, confidentiality, and privacy." The brochure also included questions that patients might want to ask their doctors, such as, "Is this treatment for my benefit or for research?"[51]

In 1970, the National Welfare Rights Organization, a group formed in 1966 to address the concerns of poor Americans, adopted the idea of a Patients' Bill of Rights as an organizing tool. Charged with devising new forms of health advocacy, the organization's Health Committee came up with the idea of preparing such a document and pressing its acceptance on national professional groups. Working with the Medical Committee for Human Rights, the Health Committee drafted a list of demands based on the Health Left's critique of mainstream medicine. They included not only the recognition of individual rights to privacy and personal autonomy but also structural changes, including universal access to medical care regardless of race or income, protection from use as experimental subjects, and governance boards on which consumers occupied 51 percent of the seats.[52]

The National Welfare Rights Organization first presented its demands to the AMA, requesting that the organization consider amending its code of professional ethics to include recognition of patients' rights. When the AMA failed to respond, the next stop was the Joint Council for the Accreditation of Hospitals, which was in the process of revising its accreditation guidelines. Since only institutions it accredited could receive Medicare and Medicaid funding, getting that group to acknowledge the demands would constitute a major step forward. In April 1970, after meeting with representatives from the National Welfare Rights Organization, the Joint Council's board agreed to create a "consumer advisory board" and to include a Hospital Patients' Bill of Rights in the preamble to the new accreditation standards.[53]

The Joint Council's consumer advisory board disintegrated within a year, and the Bill of Rights remained a voluntary statement of principle rather than a requirement for accreditation. But simply getting this particular medical Goliath to acknowledge David's existence encouraged the National Welfare Rights Organization to pressure the AHA to adopt the Patients' Bill of Rights. In September 1970, activists set up picket lines at the AHA's annual meeting and, with media attention squarely focused on them, threatened to disrupt the conference if they were not allowed to meet with the delegates. Organizers invited National Welfare Rights Organization representative Geraldine Smith to address the assembly, where she received a polite if chilly hearing. After the meeting, the matter was turned over to the AHA's Committee on Health Care for the Disadvantaged for review. In 1972, that committee presented its own draft of the Bill of Rights and recommended its adoption by the full association. After further revision, the document was approved by AHA delegates in February 1973.[54]

The AHA version had none of the more radical measures included in the National Welfare Rights Organization's original draft; gone, for example, were the demands for community control and the acknowledgment of the right to health care. Yet while softened in important respects, the Bill of Rights nonetheless represented the first of what today are called performance standards written from a patient's point of view. The text specified that all patients were entitled to receive "considerate and respectful care"; to be advised of their diagnosis, treatment, and prognosis "in terms [they] can be reasonably expected to understand"; to receive sufficient information to enable them to grant informed consent prior to any procedure; to refuse treatment; to get a "reasonable" and timely response to requests for care; to be apprised of any research or experimentation that the hospital proposed to undertake and to refuse to participate in such studies; to be assured of the privacy and confidentiality of all treatments and medical records; and finally to examine their bills and have all charges explained.[55]

While described as a Patients' Bill of Rights as opposed to a Consumers' Bill of Rights, the 1973 document clearly paralleled the language and intent of Kennedy's 1962 speech on consumers' rights. In essence, the document's provisions defined in a medical setting what it meant to possess "the right to safety, the right to be informed, the right to choose, and the right to be heard." In a broader sense, it evoked standards of what constituted "good" professional service—respect, information, privacy, even itemized bills—that had been articulated by earlier generations of discontented patients. In urging hospitals to adopt these principles, the AHA acknowledged an idea that would become central to 1970s medical consumerism: "an informed patient is a more receptive patient" as well as "less likely to be dissatisfied with the outcome of the treatment," as the AHA guide to the Bill of Rights summed it up.[56]

But while the Patients' Bill of Rights undoubtedly represented a significant milestone in medical consumerism, its limitations were immediately apparent. First, the document constituted a voluntary guide to behavior rather than a legally binding contract. Hospital attorneys immediately registered their dislike of the bill's vague language; according to one, it "is likely to mean one thing to the patient, another to the hospital and still another to the practicing physician," an imprecision all too likely to result in lawsuits. In cruder language, a hospital administrator argued, "Spelling out the patient's rights gives every shyster lawyer in town an invitation to sue you."[57]

For their part, patient advocates lamented the deletion of key items— most notably, universal health insurance and community control of medical institutions—from the original list of demands. Noted Walter Lear, a physician member of the Medical Committee for Human Rights, commitments to provide access and continuity of care were meaningless in a highly fragmented health care system where many patients lacked insurance coverage. Without more patient control of hospitals, the Patients' Bill of Rights would serve merely as "a public relations strategy for diverting attention from the hospital's failure to deliver services humanely and to accord due respect to the legal and economic rights of its patients."[58]

The bill also received bad reviews from the ethicists who were starting to weigh in on the troubled state of the doctor-patient relationship. Psychiatrist Willard Gaylin, a cofounder in 1969 of the new Hastings Center for Bioethics, published a harsh commentary describing the Patients' Bill of Rights as a "well-intended, though timid, document" that "perpetuates the very paternalism that precipitated the abuses." He complained, "In effect, all that the document does is return to the patient, with an air of largesse, some of the rights hospitals have previously stolen from him." Gaylin warned patients not to rely on hospitals or doctors to watch out for their rights: "It is not for the hospital community to outline the rights it will offer, but rather for the patient consumer to delineate and then demand those rights to which he feels entitled" and to use the courts and the legislatures to get those rights.[59]

Hospital officials' commentaries on the Patients' Bill of Rights also reflected a sense of its futility. A Pennsylvania hospital administrator responded, "We have more important things to do than promise we'll be nice to people," while a Memphis hospital staff member asked, "Why not just post the Golden Rule?" Many hospitals refused to accept the document even as a voluntary guideline, and as of 1975, only a third had adopted any version. In "Whatever Happened to the Patients' Bill of Rights?," *Medical Economics* referred to it as "one of the world's most unpublicized documents." When asked whether his hospital had adopted the bill, one physician board member replied, "Lord, I don't know. What is it—some kind of consumer-reports thing?" On January 9, 1973, the text inspired comedian Johnny Carson to deliver a *Tonight Show* monologue in which he chided the AHA for not including "the right of a comatose patient not to be used as a doorstop" and "the right of a patient, no matter what the extenuating circumstances, to refuse to be given a sponge bath with 'Janitor in a Drum.'"[60]

As critics rightly pointed out, the Patients' Bill of Rights constituted a weak weapon. Although it had value as an educational tool, making patients aware that they might make demands on and ask questions of caregivers, the Bill of Rights imposed no real obligation to answer those questions. In other words, patient-consumer activists and bioethicists might argue strongly for the existence of basic body rights as human rights, but if the courts did not recognize such rights, health care practitioners and institutions had little incentive to make changes that might require real effort or expense. As activists warned, posting the Bill of Rights served more as a public relations gesture than as an agenda for change.

Despite all the criticism and scorn, the concept of spelling out on paper the standards of service and information-sharing that patients deserved had considerable appeal. Among the most enthusiastic adopters of the Patients' Bill of Rights were state legislatures, which had become frustrated by hospitals' and physicians' unwillingness to undertake needed reforms. Pennsylvania, Colorado, Minnesota, and New York were among the states that adopted formal bills of rights and required that hospitals present them to patients on admission. In addition, the Department of Health, Education, and Welfare began to require adoption of the Patients' Bill of Rights before hospitals could receive certain kinds of reimbursements.[61]

Moreover, elements of the Patients' Bill of Rights began to take on more force as advocates worked to give them greater legal substantiation. Even more than the protest marches, threats of lawsuits made health care institutions start to take patients' rights more seriously. Using what became known as "judo politics"—turning opponents' power against them—activist groups and lawyers started to look for settings in which to pose legal challenges to medical authority.[62] In mental hospitals, birth control clinics, and surgical suites, new definitions of informed consent began to be put into practice. Simultaneously, federal agencies found themselves under pressure not only from activists but also from researchers concerned about the ethical status of their own work. As critics would later lament, signing consent forms and undergoing commitment hearings too easily ended up being perfunctory gestures that served more to rationalize the exercise of medical authority than to temper or challenge it. But in the optimistic days of the early 1970s, activists' ability to raise awareness of patients' rights in general and the principle of informed choice in particular was a heartening development.

The Patient Information Leaflet

Not surprisingly, information about prescription drugs and their risks emerged as a leading issue in the campaign for expanding patients' rights to make informed choices about treatment. As standardized products, drugs offered an easier target for consumer activism than the far more individualized forms of medical services. Already by the 1950s, the patient's right to be apprised of prescription drug side effects had emerged as a consumerist complaint. Ironically, the reforms put in place by the 1962 Kefauver-Harris Amendment only made the absence of this information for patients more noticeable. This lapse became all the more consequential with changes in product liability law, which exempted drug manufacturers from the duty to warn patients about potential hazards because of the physician's role as their learned intermediary.

The 1962 law stipulated that prescription drug packaging material "shall present a true statement of information in brief summary relating to side effects, contraindications . . . and effectiveness." In the wake of the bill's passage, industry representatives battled the FDA over exactly what needed to appear in this "brief summary." Representatives of the Pharmaceutical Manufacturers Association and the Pharmaceutical Marketers' Council threatened to call for public hearings on the agency's proposed guidelines, effectively delaying their implementation for years. In response, the FDA created a Reconciliation Committee of agency staff members and pharmaceutical company representatives, and in 1968 they finally agreed on regulations defining the "brief summary" and "fair balance" that were "very tough, very explicit, and not well-liked by the industry," according to an FDA official. Many physicians objected to the guidelines as an encroachment on their right "to make a choice and to practice medicine as [they] see fit," wrote John Adriani, the chair of the AMA's Council on Drugs.[63]

In the meantime, this "brief summary" was intended only for the use of the physician and pharmacist, not the patient. In theory, the former were supposed to pass the risk information on to the latter. In reality, studies suggested that neither pharmacists nor doctors were doing an adequate job of educating patients about their medications. The inattention to patients became all the more consequential as courts began to adopt the doctrine of "strict liability," which imposed new burdens on manufacturers to warn consumers of product hazards. Prescription drugs were exempted from that more demanding standard on the grounds that they were essential but "unavoidably unsafe" products that consumers needed to use but could not fully understand; thus the manufacturer's duty to warn was to the physician, not the patient directly. The "learned intermediary" doctrine reinforced the idea that patients had to rely on doctors to guide safe drug use. Physicians' failure adequately to explain medication risks to their patients thus became a key issue for patient advocates.[64]

The public debate about these issues came to center on concerns about the side effects associated with oral contraceptives. In part, the pill emerged as the test case for patient information about prescription drugs because of the strength of the women's health movement, which had made reproductive health one of its leading concerns. Also, the pill attracted attention because it was a contraceptive rather than a treatment for disease and because safer forms of contraception existed, meaning that the pill's popularity seemed a matter more of personal choice than of medical necessity. Finally, as "unavoidably unsafe" drugs went, it appeared to be particularly risky. Within five years of the FDA's approval of the pill in 1960, more than 6.5 million American women were taking it. By 1966, the FDA had received enough reports of serious side effects such as blood clots and strokes associated with its use that they appointed a panel to review its safety. The panel found the evidence inconclusive but nonetheless argued for the need to test the effectiveness of lower doses of the pill's key ingredients. For the burgeoning women's movement, this cautious response seemed evidence of the FDA's lack of concern about women's health issues.[65]

In 1969, feminist activist Barbara Seaman published *The Doctors' Case against the Pill*, which helped make the safety of the oral contraceptive a cause célèbre among second-wave feminists. In Seaman's view, "the deceptively easy act of swallowing the innocent-looking pill is, in fact, an act of *uninformed* consent." The absence of vital information about dangerous side effects such as stroke constituted "the silence that could kill you." She noted that while few physicians shared information about risks with their female patients, many were telling their wives to stop using the pill. This situation was all the more reprehensible because safer, highly reliable forms of contraception were available. Seaman argued that women needed to receive better information about the safety and effectiveness of all their contraceptive options before they could make truly informed choices.[66]

In 1970, after Gaylord Nelson held Senate hearings on the pill's safety and under intense pressure from feminists and some physicians, the FDA decided to issue a special patient package insert aimed at ensuring that women knew about the pill's potential side effects and their warning signs. This was not the first time the FDA had required a patient insert: in 1968, it had ordered makers of an asthma inhaler to include a written warning that excessive use could cause breathing difficulties. But requiring a warning about the birth control pill received significantly more attention. Bowing to industry pressure, the FDA kept its first leaflet very short: it was seven sentences long and mentioned only the risk of blood clotting disorders. Women wanting more information were advised to write to the AMA for a more detailed brochure. Despite its limitations, activists still hailed the insert as a significant victory for the women's health movement and for medical consumerism in general.[67]

The controversy over oral contraceptives marked a significant turning point in the long-running consumerist campaign to challenge the black box exemption for prescription drugs. At a time when informative labels were being added to clothing, food, and other consumer products, it seemed that the same would soon be true of prescription drugs as well. The dangers of contraceptive pills underlined the status of prescription drugs as "unavoidably unsafe" products that came with serious risks. The fight for the contraceptive leaflet was the opening salvo in what would turn out to be a long struggle to ensure that patients were informed about the potentially hazardous side effects of their prescription drugs.[68]

Informed Consent

The argument made during the pill debate—that patient-consumers could grant informed consent only if the risks of the treatment had been fully and formally disclosed to them—gained power as a legal principle in other aspects of medical care as well. Of all the protections included in the 1970 Patients' Bill of Rights, the demand for informed consent had perhaps the most far-reaching implications. Of course, consent to treatment was not a new principle. Since the nineteenth century, courts had approached the doctor-patient relationship as a quasi-contractual agreement based on fiduciary obligations that required patient consent. Growing concerns about malpractice lawsuits had already led physicians and hospitals to document consent from patients undergoing diagnostic and therapeutic procedures. But as of the late 1960s, the procedures for obtaining consent and sharing information with patients remained highly variable across institutions and specialties. Physicians exercised great discretion in deciding what information to share and what to withhold, confident that they knew best what patients needed to know.[69]

That sense of complacency began to disintegrate in the mid-1960s as a consequence of highly publicized revelations about ethical lapses in medical experimentation. In 1966, physician Henry K. Beecher published a landmark article in the *New England Journal of Medicine* documenting the extent of nontherapeutic experimentation in American prisons, orphanages, mental hospitals, and institutions for the mentally handicapped. Concerned about the kinds of problems Beecher had documented, the U.S. surgeon general issued new guidelines governing research with human subjects, and the NIH began to implement stricter controls on investigators receiving federal research dollars. In doing so, they were also responding to pressure from congressional leaders, among them Democratic senator Walter Mondale of Minnesota, to increase federal oversight of medical research.[70]

Then, in 1972, journalist Jean Heller brought further attention to one of the cases Beecher had described: the U.S. Public Health Service's Tuskegee Syphilis Study. Black men with syphilis enrolled in the study during the 1930s had later been discouraged from receiving new treatments—in particular, penicillin—so that the study could be completed. In the wake of the Tuskegee scandal, the federal government moved belatedly to create a new system of institutional review boards so that future research involving human subjects would be conducted only with the patients' knowledge and consent.[71]

The concerns over research ethics quickly spilled over into clinical practice as well. For a younger generation of lawyers and jurists, the revelations of abuse seemed all the more reason to enhance the legal protection of patients' rights. As Alan Stone, a psychiatrist and legal expert observed, lawyers perceived "the traditional doctor-patient relationship" as one "in which the doctor and the patient are unequal bargaining partners in a contract for services." Lawyers sought to use the law "to force the doctor to give the patient knowledge that will make him or her an equal bargaining partner."[72]

The result was a tidal wave of legal decisions that defined and expanded the doctrine of informed consent, in which the courts laid down higher standards for what physicians needed to tell patients. They had a duty to disclose to patients, in the words of AMA's legal expert Leslie J. Miller, the "nature and the risks involved in treatment" as well as "alternative treatments that might be used." Subsequent cases would add the duty to disclose the risks of refusing treatment. Much as medical insurers bowed to "reasonable and customary practice" when setting fees, the courts initially used the profession's own standards for what patients should be told as the measure of informed consent. Patients could not win a malpractice suit as long as their doctors did what a "reasonable medical practitioner" would have done under similar circumstances. But starting in the early 1970s, some courts began to use a different measure, that of the "reasonable patient." Also known as the "material risk" approach, this theory held that informed consent required disclosure of any risk "that a reasonable person" would be likely "to attach significance to" in deciding to undergo treatment. Here, the standard was not what the medical profession thought sufficient but rather what patients deserved to know, a position far more compatible with the patients' rights movement.[73]

Through the 1970s, the courts remained divided over which rule prevailed. The majority of states and some federal courts stuck with the reasonable doctor, but a significant minority, including New York and Massachusetts, often trendsetters in health law reform, adopted the "material risk" standard. Huge variations from state to state resulted, requiring doctors and hospitals to pay careful attention to which standards applied, and the situation provided new opportunities for patients and lawyers to exploit the informed consent doctrine to win malpractice suits. As a result, the doctrine of informed consent became "an area to be feared by every practicing physician and every medical research investigator," in the words of legal expert William Curran.[74]

The legal reframing of standards for informed consent helped legitimate health activists' demands for more information about treatment alternatives. For example, Rose Kushner and other breast cancer advocates began to challenge the radical mastectomy as the sole option for treatment, citing surgeons such as George Crile and Thomas Dao who believed it to be unnecessary. Women, they argued, should be afforded a two-step process of giving consent rather than being forced to permit the doctor to biopsy the tumor and remove the breast during a single operation. Many surgeons as well as the American Cancer Society initially dismissed that request, but by the late 1970s, both the National Cancer Institute and the American Cancer Society had come to accept the argument that women had the right to know more about treatments and their rates of effectiveness. The advocates' victory illustrated how informed patient-consumers could bring about significant changes in medical thinking.[75]

The growing institutional importance attached to informed consent was evident in the increasingly complicated forms that patients were asked to sign before receiving treatment. Although many states accepted verbal consent as adequate, hospitals and physicians were aware that in case of a malpractice suit, written documentation could be very useful to the defense, so signed consent forms came into widespread use. As some critics pointed out, real informed consent meant more than simply a signature on a piece of paper filled with incomprehensible legal jargon. But other commentators suggested that the written forms represented a step in the right direction; if nothing else, they opened up new opportunities for patients to ask questions.[76]

In this legal climate, the rights of patients to refuse treatment also received greater validation. Traditionally, such cases had centered on patients whose religious beliefs precluded medical treatment, as in the refusal of Jehovah's Witnesses to receive blood transfusions. But as the use of new technologies such as respirators and feeding tubes became more common in the 1950s and early 1960s, some people began to object to having their lives prolonged if they became terminally ill. Support grew for documenting one's wishes in what we now call an advanced medical directive or living will. Luis Kutner, a prominent human rights lawyer who helped found Amnesty International in 1961, drafted the first living will in 1967 and published it in the *Indiana Law Journal* two years later. The idea gained wider public exposure in 1973, when advice columnist Dear Abby (Pauline Phillips) lauded its value. Further legal validation of the concept came during the 1976 Karen Ann Quinlan case, in which the courts ruled that a woman's parents had the right to disconnect life support for their brain-dead daughter.[77]

Many of the landmarks in the legal rebalancing of power between doctor and patient rested on reinterpretations of older traditions related to malpractice, negligence, and consent. But some also involved more sweeping efforts to reinterpret the place of constitutional rights in medical settings. For example, legal advocates for the mentally ill argued that involuntary commitment as it was currently practiced in the United States represented a violation of the constitutional rights to due process and habeas corpus. Arguing that mental patients were essentially "prisoners of psychiatry," their advocates won important legal modifications to commitment procedures and standards for treatment. Even more innovative—and controversial—was the Supreme Court's 1973 acceptance in *Roe v. Wade* of the right to privacy as the fundamental grounds for granting women the right to an abortion until the third trimester of pregnancy.[78]

The legal profession's oversight of medical practice on patients' behalf thus widened dramatically in the 1970s. In the words of lawyer Andrew Dolan, that decade saw "the explosion of all those areas we now lump together under the heading of patient rights." In 1978, the Center for the Study of Civil Liberties and Civil Rights began to publish the *Patients' Rights Digest* to keep advocates up-to-date on the latest legal opinions and regulatory developments. Along with the legal changes concerning malpractice, the expanding definition of patients' rights helped make health law a growing specialty, as reflected in the proliferation of textbooks devoted to the subject as well as the addition of courses on health law in both law schools and hospital administration programs. In time, those developments would also produce significant backlash, as rates of malpractice and malpractice insurance rose precipitously. But in the short run, the ease with which patients could secure legal hearings for their concerns seemed to underline the optimistic view that a new era of protecting patients' rights had arrived.[79]

Shoppers' Guides to Health Care

Along with patient information leaflets, informed consent forms, and living wills, consumer advocates pursued other, more mundane goals in their quest to be better informed about their medical care. Thus one hallmark of the early 1970s health consumer movement was the attempt to create new kinds of "buyer's guides" that would help patient-consumers find the kind of medical services they wanted. The idea of a "people's guide" to medical care originated with the Health Left. Building on the long tradition of relying on family and friends to find good doctors, movement members thought to do the same. Thus activists in Berkeley, California, created a guide to local hospitals, and the Boston Women's Health Collective originally came together to create a list of "reasonable" doctors in their community. In the same spirit, many alternative newspapers listed local clinics likely to be hospitable to their readers. In this collation of information, activists included information about fees and hours as well as other aspects of care, such as the doctor's attitude toward contraception and drug use.[80]

Moreover, in a political climate increasingly concerned with transparency, consumer activists felt more emboldened to demand that both government and business interests disclose their financial stakes in particular transactions. This approach became a favored form of "judo politics" among Naderite activists, who looked for ways to turn the existing machinery of bureaucratic oversight to consumers' advantage.[81] A natural place to insist on greater transparency was the setting of insurance fees. Steadily rising insurance premiums and the lack of accountability for their increase had emerged as a sore political point in the late 1950s. With the fusion of patients' rights and third-wave consumerism, the demand for explanations became harder to ignore, in part because it fit with a growing strain of conservative thinking.

These converging interests were evident in the 1971 "shoppers' guide" to hospitals conceived by Herb Denenberg, Pennsylvania's insurance commissioner. A law professor at the University of Pennsylvania and Nader protégé, Denenberg had been appointed to the post by newly elected governor Milton Shapp. Like many Democratic governors, Shapp wanted to make the state's department of insurance more protective of policyholders as opposed to insurance companies. During his tenure as commissioner, Denenberg used his regulatory power to force insurance companies to disclose more information to consumers. Known in business circles as "Horrible Herb" as a consequence of his combative style, his motto was "the public has been screwed long enough."[82]

Denenberg's 1971 *Shoppers' Guide to Hospitals in the Philadelphia Area* grew out of his battles with Blue Cross/Blue Shield of Pennsylvania. During a hearing about how hospital rates were set, Denenberg learned that Blue Cross had an agreement with Philadelphia hospitals not to disclose their rate agreements to the public. Denenberg suggested that such information be made public, an idea highlighted by a reporter from the *Philadelphia Inquirer* in his coverage of the hearings. The article used the phrase "shopper's guide," and the positive reaction it received led Denenberg to order hospital and insurance officials to provide him the information needed for a cost comparison. His office printed up a one-page foldout listing daily rates, bed capacities, and average length of stay, plus data on "unsafe beds" gleaned from annual reports by Pennsylvania's Department of Health, Education, and Welfare.[83]

Denenberg's foreword stressed the philosophy behind the guide: "Much of this information is supposed to be public information, but nonetheless it has often not been available or has not been publicized despite its usefulness." Patients clearly deserved to know which hospitals failed to meet safety standards. "Although 'shopping' for a hospital may not be in vogue, greater dissemination of information and wide public awareness might contribute to more hospital economy, especially if the public begins to question costs that appear to be out of line with what others are charging." He concluded, "The public may not be in a position to shop for a hospital, especially in view of a doctor's requirements and his hospital connections, but it is entitled to information that will permit comparisons."[84]

Encouraged by the public response, Denenberg went on to produce a series of "shoppers' guides" to life insurance, medical insurance, and other financial services. He also developed a "shoppers' guide to surgery" that laid out fourteen rules for avoiding unnecessary operations. While his efforts gained positive notice in newspapers and magazines, Denenberg aroused increasingly fierce enemies who portrayed him as "antibusiness." He resigned as commissioner in 1974 to run unsuccessfully for the U.S. Senate. Denenberg went on to become a journalist, a field for which his muckraking style proved a much better fit. He pioneered the "shame on you" style of reportage that has since become a staple of the American news industry. Meanwhile, the concept underlying the guide—the public reporting of information collected by the government and its regulatory agencies—eventually proved to be a potent policy tool, appealing not only to Democrats but also to Republicans.[85]

Around the same time that Denenberg was developing his consumer guides, in 1973, members of Public Citizen joined with a neighborhood group funded by the National Center for Urban Ethnic Affairs to develop a directory of physicians practicing in Prince George's County, Maryland. Addressing complaints patients had been making since the 1930s, they noted how uninformative the doctor listings in telephone books were and set out to provide a more informative alternative.[86] To compile it, the group developed a list of questions that they wanted answered. They started with the standard facts that patients had been advised to get about their doctors for decades, such as information on board certifications, as well as mundane details such as their office hours. But the survey also included questions regarding matters patients might be afraid to ask about: how long on average the doctor spent with each patient, what lab tests and immunizations he or she offered, and whether he or she prescribed birth control pills (since many doctors still refused to prescribe them for unmarried women). The survey also asked about fees: what the doctor charged for an office visit and when payment was expected. Finally, the survey asked how the doctor handled patient complaints about treatment or billing issues: Did he or she meet with the patient, have office staff or a nurse deal with the matter, or refer the complaint to the medical society?[87]

After developing the questionnaire, the group then asked local doctors to complete it. They began, logically enough, with the referral bureau operated by the Prince George's County Medical Society, which had been created in response to the AMA's outreach program. But the society refused to provide such a list, explaining that "their 'practice' was not to release lists of their doctors to the public" because such lists "had been 'badly misused' in the past." Fifteen other local medical organizations proved no more helpful. Even the local health advisory planning committee, set up under the 1966 law—"a federally funded, supposedly consumer-controlled organization charged with planning health facilities development in Prince George's County," as the directory group pointed out—refused to share its list, "describing instead its own extraordinary difficulties securing its list of practicing doctors." The Public Citizen group ultimately compiled its list using the AMA directory, a national directory of specialists, and a local medical directory available only to physicians provided them by a sympathetic "health department doctor."[88]

Over four days in July 1973, a group of volunteers tried to contact the 560 doctors whose names appeared on the list. Some responded courteously, while others were hostile and uncooperative, "even shocked at our treating them as equals, e.g. merely asking them to either respond to our questionnaire or be listed as uncooperative." According to the volunteers, "Many doctors told us we had no right to ask them about their practice"; they considered the group's action an "invasion of privacy" and felt no obligation to provide such information. Some cursed the callers ("Get the hell off the phone you damn S.O.B."), while others threatened lawsuits, "claiming that we were defaming them if we printed the fact that they would not cooperate with our project."[89]

Meanwhile, the Prince George's Medical Society told its members that it had no knowledge of the survey (although it had been contacted about providing a list of members) and advised them that publishing any information about fees constituted a form of "indirect advertising" and thus was prohibited in the state. When the doctors who had cooperated with the survey were asked to review their entries, many changed their minds about participating, in large part, the Public Citizen volunteers believed, because the medical society pressured them to do so. Of the 461 actively practicing doctors reached by the group, only 25 percent cooperated, compared to 57 percent who refused; another 18 percent simply did not respond to the survey. The names of all the nonresponders were listed in the back of the directory.[90]

The introduction, written by project director Rob McGarrah, explained that the directory had been created because useful information about physicians was too hard to find: "Most people can find out more about a car they plan to buy than they can about a doctor who may hold their life in his hands." Hoping to alert its readers to what was coming, *Medical Economics* published a condensed version of McGarrah's introduction in March 1974, explaining that its readers needed to become acquainted with "the thinking behind it—

the rationale that could sweep the country and put *you* in the next directory, ready or not." The Prince George's directory, the *Medical Economics* article explained, was only the beginning: consumer groups in thirty-two states were gearing up to do their own directories.[91]

In a follow-up article on the Prince George's directory that appeared in *Medical Economics*, James Reynolds faulted the interviewers for not making clear that they were affiliated with Nader's group: some doctors answered the survey because they thought it came from either the health department or the regional health planning board. A spot-check of the entries revealed some inaccuracies, testimony "either to the slipshod way the directory makers went about their business or to the inherent difficulty of keeping a directory up-to-date or both." At the same time, Reynolds suggested that physicians had badly overreacted to the request. Doctors who agreed to be listed did not find themselves deluged with demanding, difficult patients; in fact, three-quarters of them said that their patients said nothing at all about the directory. A few doctors even went on record as supporting the idea behind the directory. One did so because he thought that "too many physicians put themselves on a pedestal," while another said, "I'm enough of a consumerist to think it serves a useful function."[92]

Consumer Reports, not surprisingly, took a very positive view of the directory movement. "The medical profession itself," it wrote in 1974, "has done little to inform prospective patients of physicians' qualifications or pertinent facts about their practices. The burden of gathering the information and distributing it to the consumer has fallen, at least for now, on the consumer." To encourage other consumer groups to develop such directories, *Consumer Reports* included a list of potential questions: in addition to queries about the doctor's credentials, the list included questions about billing, waiting times, technologies offered, answering services, office staffing, and willingness to prescribe generic drugs and contraceptives: "Do you usually advise patients about possible side effects of drugs you prescribe? Do you allow patients to view their medical records if requested?"[93]

In the wake of the Prince George's experiment, similar directory projects were begun around the country. But for all their appeal as a form of consumer empowerment, patient-oriented directories faced daunting logistical problems. They were difficult to compile and keep up-to-date, and local consumer groups lacked the resources to keep them going. To forestall the creation of consumer directories, some medical societies, including the one in Prince George's County, issued their own directories, leaving out the questions they found objectionable.[94] But in the end, the most significant impact of the

Prince George's directory controversy came from an unexpected direction, in the form of a new FTC lawsuit. The case came to the attention of the FTC due to the media attention showered on the Prince George's controversy as another example of consumerist Davids taking on an establishment. At the time, the agency was in the midst of a broad-based study of how professional standards were being used to deny consumers information not only in medicine but in other fields as well. In 1975, the FTC filed a suit against the AMA, challenging the ban on physician advertising that the medical society had cited as its grounds for refusing to cooperate with the directory. As the next chapter will discuss, the AMA lost that suit in 1982, ending its long-standing prohibition on the advertising of medical services. The results of that landmark legal decision would bear little resemblance to what patient-consumer advocates had initially wanted in the way of information.

In the late 1960s and early 1970s, some high-profile activist successes seemed to suggest that a new day of consumer power in the drugstore and the doctor's office had at long last arrived. While imperfect in scope and execution, the Patients' Bill of Rights, the patient leaflet for the contraceptive pill, the new attention to informed consent, and the new-style health shopper's directories, represented an important turning point in what it meant to be an educated patient. Through these new tools, key precepts long associated with critical medical consumerism—the idea that patients needed to be informed and consulted about their care—received powerful external validation from politicians, regulators, and judges.

The threat of regulatory rulings and lawsuits encouraged change where prior appeals to political conscience and professional ethics had failed. With the courts in ferment, the specter of an army of angry patients, ready not just to protest but to hire lawyers, became a concrete fear for physicians, hospitals, and insurance companies. Average Americans came to believe that "we can all be Ralph Naders"—or Barbara Seamans, Jane Roes, Sidney Wolfes, and Herb Denenbergs. Grassroots activism, legal trends, and political pragmatism converged in the early 1970s to give the concept of patients' rights greater visibility and legitimacy.

But even at the movement's peak, empowering patient-consumers both as a group and as individuals ran into powerful resistance. By the mid-1970s, the limits of grassroots activism and its ability to form big-tent alliances among different interest groups had become apparent. Already weakened both by internal dissent and by external harassment by local and federal law enforcement agencies, the New Left began to face a New Right determined to counter alleged immorality and political subversion. For their part, business and professional leaders learned the art of co-optation, adopting what they deemed the more "reasonable" of protesters' demands in order to lessen the pressure for truly radical change.

In short order, sweeping critiques of medicine and capitalism gave way to a more domesticated version of medical consumerism. The energies unleashed during the previous decade were redirected back into the existing culture of "new and improved" medicine. Providing patients with more information and choice about the products and procedures available to them became a means of ensuring greater patient compliance as well as of avoiding lawsuits. Both patients and doctors were encouraged to assume more responsibility for being educated consumers. But this "new and improved" version of medical consumerism proved to have no magic cure for the problems that patients faced in the rapidly changing medical marketplace of the late twentieth century.

NINE

Get Ready for a New Breed of Patients

In 1974, *Medical Economics*, the journal dedicated to keeping practicing physicians up-to-date, carried an article advising readers to "get ready for a new breed of patients!" Author Donald L. Cooper, the medical director of Oklahoma State University's Health Center, warned his fellow doctors that new college graduates were going to be far more assertive patients than their parents had been. Physicians should expect these young people to "insist that you explain what you're doing," practice "doctor-switching" to get the care they wanted, and contemplate suing for malpractice when they did not. Appreciative of modern technology, especially computers, they would expect "all the latest treatments" at the same time they had a great interest in alternative medicine. "If you want to get along with the new breed," Cooper advised, "I urge you not to pooh-pooh offbeat techniques like acupuncture, hypnosis, and meditation." Last but not least, he predicted that they would be casual about paying their bills.[1]

Cooper's was but one of many such observations during the 1970s. Popular as well as medical periodicals marked the progress of what was variously termed the patients' rights movement, medical consumerism, or simply the "big change." While few Americans seemed ready entirely to reject mainstream medicine, many appeared to share the anger toward the medical establishment expressed by the Health Left. As Robert J. Bazell explained in 1971, health radicals had "plucked a responsive chord, for, as few politicians have failed to notice, Americans of almost every social and political persuasion are fed up with the health care they receive." The protests lodged on behalf of the poor, people of color, and women provided an opening for a much broader spectrum of complaints about medicine's failings. The radicalism of the few promoted a greater sense of entitlement among the many to complain about their care. In the midst of what one doctor described as the profession's Cuban Missile Crisis, physicians found it increasingly hard to ignore patients' complaints.[2]

Although frequently treated as if they were brand-new, the demands made by this new breed of patients had plenty of precedent. Previous generations of patient critics had also asked for more information about the cost, value, and risks of proposed treatments as well as for more respect as the doctor's partner. But the members of the 1970s cohort enjoyed greater success than their predecessors in getting those demands met. What was different this time around was not only the ferocity of the patient revolt but also the political climate in which it occurred. After almost a decade of political assassinations, urban riots, student unrest, and building bombings, concepts formerly viewed as extreme started to seem more reasonable. Compared to protest marches and hospital sit-ins, patients' requests for information or consultation did not appear so impolite.

Among those converted to the reasonableness of these requests were political leaders, who began to see endorsing some facets of medical consumerism as beneficial to their goals. The patients' cause provided politicians a powerful weapon to override long-standing traditions of physician autonomy that they now viewed as economic liabilities. Some of the stakeholders adopting consumerist rhetoric sought to slow health care spending, while others wanted to make sure it continued to increase. For mixed and often contradictory reasons, the new breed of patients became a justification for dismantling protections that had long shielded the doctor's office and the drugstore from certain kinds of market competition.

Over the course of the 1970s, old debates about how much information American patients needed to make good medical choices took on new policy significance. As hippies gave way to yuppies and Watergate increased distrust of government, embracing patient-consumer empowerment became an appealing solution for groups on the political left, right, and center. Politicians who could agree on little else endorsed the philosophy of giving patient-consumers more information and choice so that they could help push medicine toward greater efficiency, higher quality, and lower prices. By replacing uncritical deference to medical authority with the educated oversight of patient watchdogs, medical consumerism seemed to offer a promising cure for medicine's failings. But enlisting patient-consumers in the cause of transforming a dysfunctional health care system would be far harder than anticipated.

A Riled-Up Generation

Behind the gradual transformation of medical consumerism from an outsider to an insider tradition lay a perception that many Americans were fed up with the cost and quality of health care. The grassroots efforts of health radicals and Naderites appeared to constitute the tip of a much broader iceberg of discontent. Medical leaders continued to characterize that discontent as unfair and unwarranted but had difficulty denying that it existed. As Austin Smith, chairman of the board of the Parke, Davis pharmaceutical company, lamented in 1972, "Consumers are misinformed and riled up; and sensationalism and criticism are everywhere in evidence."[3]

This perception arose not simply from media coverage of patient protests and sit-ins but also from contemporary opinion polls and social science surveys. As in the 1950s, these assays of public sentiment helped shape the sense that the doctor-patient relationship was in transition. Starting in the mid-1960s, polls and surveys provided evidence that patients were coming to the doctor's office in a less deferential mood than before. Polls conducted by Louis Harris and Associates and the National Opinion Research Center showed a precipitous drop in the percentage of Americans who expressed "a great deal of confidence" in medicine's leadership—from 66 percent in the mid-1960s to 49 percent a decade later.[4] This decline reflected a broader "confidence gap" affecting all sectors of American society in the 1970s. Physicians could take some comfort from the fact that their loss of trust paled in comparison to that of other institutions, especially the military, business, and Congress, which started out with lower numbers and fell even more sharply. But given the importance of trust to the doctor-patient relationship, the confidence gap posed a very personal challenge to the medical profession.[5]

Polling results suggested that Americans continued to feel a complicated mix of admiration for and resentment of the medical profession. As in the 1950s, members of the public respected and trusted individual physicians yet remained skeptical of organized medicine. In late 1971, one poll found that 84 percent of Americans had "a fair amount of confidence" that they could get good medical care for themselves or their families; however, a 1972 survey reported that 40 percent of those interviewed had experienced a "negative medical care experience," and more than two-thirds felt that the physician had been at fault. A 1975 Harris poll found that 15 percent of respondents believed that someone close to them had been a victim of malpractice. Echoing the complaints of the 1950s, 38 percent of those interviewed in a 1976 study were unhappy about their out-of-pocket expenses for medical care, 28 percent felt that they had to wait too long to see the doctor, and 18 percent were dissatisfied with the information they received about "what was wrong with you or what was being done for you."[6]

Social scientific studies based on more in-depth interviews with patients seemed to confirm Cooper's observation that patients were starting to judge their medical care with a more critical eye. In part, these findings reflected the fact that the researchers conducting these studies started with a less deferential attitude toward medicine than did their counterparts in the 1930s or the 1950s. This "new breed" of researchers was far more willing to assume that laypeople could and should play a significant role in medical decision making. Their work helped to perpetuate the belief that a noteworthy shift in medical culture was under way. As sociologist Marie Haug noted in 1976, "The 'revolt of the client' and the demand for accountability signify a growing public suspicion that neither the expertise nor the goodwill of the professional are to be taken on trust, at face value."[7]

The researchers coming of age in the late 1960s were also more attentive to class and race differences. Their work documented the long-term consequences of the postwar free enterprise ethos that had left poor neighborhoods bereft of physicians' offices and dependent on underfunded inner-city hospitals. Social scientists also showed a greater willingness to believe that all patients, including those who lacked much in the way of formal education, had the capacity to make informed judgments about their care. In a 1969 study of people covered by Medicaid, Arnold Kisch and Leo Reeder found that patient judgments of what constituted good medical care matched those of more expert observers, concluding, "A sample of supposedly 'ignorant' clients" was able to differentiate between good and bad care. Similarly, researchers were more likely to interpret patient doctor-shopping as a strategic effort to get better care rather than as a symptom of irrationality.[8]

For all this new social scientific attention to class and race, popular understandings of the new breed of patients tended to assume, as Cooper did, that their revolt originated with the baby boomers—the wave of young people born after the end of World War II. Admirers cast the boomers as bold, independent freethinkers with a genuine passion for social justice and distaste for crass materialism, while critics portrayed them as the spoiled, narcissistic products of Dr. Spock and the boob tube. In either case, it seemed natural that a generation that had originated the motto "Don't trust anyone over thirty" would approach their doctors with a more combative spirit. Friend and foe alike tended to attribute the boomers' assertiveness with their physicians as the consequence of three long-term trends: educational advantages, unprecedented enjoyment of prosperity, and exposure to mass culture.

In explaining why baby boomers were so rebellious, observers frequently pointed to their rising level of educational attainment. By 1970, more than 70 percent of Americans between the ages of eighteen and thirty had at least a high school degree. Not only were younger Americans better educated than their parents, but they had been brought up to have particularly high expectations of science and professionalism. As economist Robert Herrmann wrote in 1970, "The new generation will have little use for so-called consumer advisers who are either poorly informed or seek to promote some special interest." To win trust, Herrmann concluded, "consumer educators must perform with the expertise and concern for their client's best interests characteristic of true professionals."[9] Younger people were likely to expect physicians to do the same.

Likewise baby boomers had come of age in an affluent "mass society" dominated by new forms of popular culture. As the first generation to grow up with television, observers suggested, the boomers' "heavy exposure" to mass media and its advertising inclined them to be cynical and skeptical about everything. Herrmann singled out the popularity of *Mad* as both a source of and a reflection of this youthful skepticism. Inspired by the depression-era satire magazine *Ballyhoo*, *Mad* exposed its devoted readers to irreverent parodies of over-the-counter medicine advertisements and satires of medical professionalism such as Kelly Freas's "Presenting the Bill," which spoofed Parke, Davis's "Great Moments in Medicine" series.[10]

While baby boomers got the most media attention as the face of the new breed of patients, more discerning commentators noted the importance of another age group, the elderly. Now living longer and wanting to stay healthier, their interest in consumerist issues was evident in the growth of a wide variety of groups, including the National Council on Aging, the American Association for Retired Persons (AARP), and the Gray Panthers. Like Betty Friedan, who was forty-two when she wrote *The Feminine Mystique* in 1963, older women constituted a powerful source of support for women's health activism. So while commentators tended to fixate on the baby boomers as the driving force behind the new patient, medical consumerism had a far broader generational base of support.[11]

Consumer Protection in the Watergate Era

The nation's political leaders were among the older Americans impressed by the need to placate a riled-up generation of unhappy patient-consumers. Even as the tumults of the 1960s began to subside, the political momentum they set in motion continued to unfold. The need for institutional transparency and accountability received powerful reinforcement in the wake of the Watergate scandal that led to Richard Nixon's resignation in 1974. Against this backdrop, the political struggles over health care issues intensified, and competing groups sought to enlist empowered consumers in their pursuit of change.[12]

Buoyed by grassroots developments, in January 1971, Senator Ted Kennedy, a Massachusetts Democrat, and Representative Martha Griffiths, a Michigan Democrat, introduced the Health Security Act, proposing a single-payer system of national health insurance. Even more ominously from the medical profession's point of view, Republican leaders also began to advance alternatives to fee-for-service medicine. Both to counter Kennedy's bill and to contain costs, President Nixon in 1972 announced his own "national health strategy" built around prepaid group medical plans now renamed "health maintenance organizations" (HMOs). Over the strong objections of the AMA, Republicans and Democrats united to pass the 1973 HMO Act, which provided federal subsidies to start more such plans. Republican governors, including Nelson Rockefeller in New York and Ronald Reagan in California, set up incentive plans to start more HMOs.[13]

Growing bipartisan support for cost containment and physician accountability spurred other significant legislative initiatives in the 1970s. Congressional Republicans and Democrats agreed to require more oversight of the care provided by Medicare and Medicaid, voting in 1972 to strengthen the power of "professional service review organizations" (PSROs) to monitor and discourage unnecessary care; based on the idea of having doctors watch over other doctors, these groups were appointed to conduct "utilization reviews" very similar to the medical audits Paul Hawley had proposed back in the 1950s. According to Joseph A. Califano, secretary of health, education, and welfare during the Carter administration, the PSROs would ensure that care was "medically necessary, provided according to professional standards, and rendered at the appropriate level and length of stay of institutional care." In 1974, Congress passed the Health Care Planning Act, establishing regional health policy agencies charged with cutting down on the duplication of expensive medical technology such as CAT scanners and strengthening the PSROs' influence; to protect patients' interests, these agencies had to include consumer representatives in their decision making. In response to consumer complaints, state and federal legislators increased critical scrutiny of the health insurance industry, questioning both its rate hikes and its refusal to cover specific forms of care, such as mental health treatments and childbirth. Finally, in 1974 Congress passed the Employee Retirement Income Security Act, which set minimum standards for employee health insurance plan coverage. Although all these 1970s reforms would ultimately prove disappointing, their passage signaled a new political resolve to make physicians, hospitals, and insurance companies more accountable for the cost and quality of their services.[14]

The implementation of the 1962 Kefauver-Harris Amendment also contributed to a heightened sense of federal protection for patient-consumers. As the law mandated, the FDA conducted a systematic review of all drugs on the marketplace. The agency started with prescription medications, appointing a series of panels to review their safety and efficacy in what became known as the Drug Efficacy Study Implementation. In response to repeated legal challenges by pharmaceutical manufacturers, including several that reached the U.S. Supreme Court, the courts upheld the FDA's authority to remove ineffective medicines from the market. In 1984, with only a handful of cases remaining unfinished, the FDA declared its review complete. A total of approximately 3,500 prescription drugs were examined, and 1,100 of them (30 percent) were deemed ineffective and removed from the market.[15]

In 1971, the FDA began the parallel process of evaluating over-the-counter drugs for safety and efficacy, setting up panels to study seventeen categories of drugs that included somewhere between 100,000 and 500,000 products (depending on how combination drugs were counted). In April 1973, the first panel report on antacids appeared, soon followed by reviews of laxatives and diarrhea remedies, pain relievers, and medicines for motion sickness. The over-the-counter review was largely completed by the late 1970s, having met with far less industry resistance than its prescription drug counterpart because drug company officials saw it as helping rather than hindering sales. As the president of the Proprietary Association said in 1974, "When the review is completed, the consumer will have even greater assurance that any [over-the-counter] medicine he buys will be safe, properly labeled, and capable of affording relief for minor illness and discomfort."[16]

As the FDA executed the new powers granted it under the 1962 Kefauver-Harris Amendment, the U.S. Congress moved to extend its regulatory reach to include medical devices. Originally proposed as part of the 1962 reforms, that provision had been deleted due to industry opposition. As concern grew about the many new medical devices coming onto the market, Congress in 1970 set up a special committee to investigate the problem and make recommendations. The Dalkon Shield controversy helped spur legislative action. An implantable contraceptive device introduced in 1971 as a safe alternative to the pill, it soon proved not only ineffective but dangerous, due to its association with severe pelvic infections and septic miscarriages. Fifteen women died as a result, and some 200,000 more filed lawsuits against its maker because of injuries received from its use. To forestall future such tragedies, Congress in 1976 passed the Medical Device Amendments, which extended the FDA's regulatory oversight to include medical devices. As President Gerald Ford said at its signing, the new law eliminated "the deficiencies that accorded FDA 'horse and buggy' authority to deal with 'laser age' problems." Although patient advocates saw the new law as far too industry-friendly, its passage marked a significant widening of the agency's oversight.[17]

During the same years that the FDA's powers were expanding, the FTC was in the midst of its own institutional transformation. While not as dramatic as the FDA's accomplishments, the FTC's reforms nonetheless brought about significant changes in the advertising of over-the-counter drugs. As part of a larger revitalization process, the FTC launched a new effort to restrain advertising excess as a danger to free-market principles. Its staff began to argue that claims made without some reasonable basis violated section 5 of the Federal Trade Commission Act, which stated that "unfair or deceptive acts or practices in [or affecting] commerce" were illegal. If a company could not produce some proof for its advertising claims, it was breaking the law and might be required to undo its "deception" through corrective advertising and affirmative disclosure.[18]

In 1973, the FTC won two significant legal battles based on the new approach. After litigation dating back to 1959, the agency got a fine of $800,000— one of the largest ever in FTC history—levied against the makers of Geritol for its misleading claims about relieving fatigue. The FTC also won a critical battle over Pfizer's television advertising for Un-burn, a sunburn remedy, by convincing the commissioners to adopt a new standard for substantiation: companies needed to present either a literature review of scientific studies or their own product testing to back up their claims or risk being accused of misleading advertising. What became known as the "Pfizer doctrine" underscored the importance of accurate advertising in a healthy market economy: "Given the imbalance of knowledge and resources between a business enterprise and each of its customers, economically it is more rational, and imposes far less cost on society, to require a manufacturer to confirm his affirmative product claims rather than impose a burden upon each individual consumer to test, investigate, or experiment for himself."[19]

With similar goals in mind, the agency used the expanded powers granted it by the 1975 FTC Modernization Act to write trade regulation rules for the entire over-the-counter drug industry. The guidelines allowed some leeway for making claims so extravagant that consumers knew not to take them seriously, but if a manufacturer implied that scientific evidence backed up its product claims, it had to provide that proof. For example, Bufferin ads claimed that the headache product was "a faster pain reliever or gentler to the stomach than aspirin." But as the FTC argued, "showing glass models of people with Bufferin and aspirin tablets crumbling in their stomachs and reforming in their heads" did not constitute credible proof that the product worked faster than others. Moreover, the guidelines held that if Bufferin was going to compare its product favorably to those containing aspirin, it had to disclose the fact that it, too, contained aspirin.[20]

By the late 1970s, the business backlash against what some described as the "consumerist" takeover of the FTC halted the expansion of its advertising oversight. The agency became a particular target of conservatives who opposed the expanding role of big government; to them, the FTC had become a "national nanny," wasting time and tax dollars on seemingly inconsequential complaints about laundry detergents and Cheez Whiz. In the face of that resistance, the FTC eventually shifted its focus from misleading advertising to consumer fraud. But the substantiation guidelines remained, as did the perception that over-the-counter drug advertising had become more informative and less deceptive.[21]

Even more radical was the FTC's challenge to the AMA's ban on physician advertising. The refusal to advertise was a hallmark of the physicians' professionalism, the mark of what made them different from "mere" trades. Over the years, critics, including medical consumerists, had complained about how unevenly the AMA and its constituent societies enforced the ban; it was often used to harass physicians who criticized fee-for-service practice while members in good standing were allowed to skirt the rules. But consumerist critics, who shared with physicians an intense dislike of advertising, wanted a stricter, fairer application of the no-advertising principle rather than its revocation. Thus the FTC's crusade against the AMA illustrated a great irony: in the name of giving patient-consumers more information, the FTC sought to give them more advertising.

The frustrations consumer activists encountered in preparing their guide to physicians in Prince George's County, Maryland, helped to inspire the FTC suit. As part of its general review of advertising, agency staffers had begun to focus on professional bans on advertising as a barrier to healthy market competition. In 1975 the FTC filed its first suit against the American Bar Association, quickly followed by one against the AMA.[22] The FTC's action reflected the neoliberal view that advertising served as a valuable form of information that allowed prospective buyers to make better choices. From their perspective, "advertising" meant the kind of straightforward disclosure of fees, office hours, and services that medical consumerists had had so much trouble prying out of the Prince George's County Medical Society.

The FTC regulators essentially sided with the consumerists' position that like buyers of any good or service, prospective patients deserved the right to know more about medical care. Agency officials also shared the 1970s enthusiasm for the role of the patient watchdog in making medicine more efficient. "One possible way to control the seemingly uncontrollable health sector," the FTC's Michael Pertschuk wrote, "would be to treat it as a business and make it respond to the same marketplace influences as other American businesses and industries." In its landmark 1977 decision, *Bates v. State Bar of Arizona*, the U.S. Supreme Court agreed with the FTC's logic. As the majority opinion held, "Advertising [is] the traditional mechanism in a free-market economy for a supplier to inform a potential purchaser of the availability and terms of exchange"; thus, advertising might benefit the administration of justice. The justices also ruled that "commercial speech serves individual and societal interests in assuring informed and reliable decision-making."[23]

In the same spirit, Congress endorsed the concept of information as solution with passage of the 1976 National Consumer Health Information and Health Promotion Act. That law gave the secretary of the Department of Health, Education, and Welfare new powers and responsibilities to keep Americans informed about their health and health care. Anne Somers, the chair of the task force whose report prompted the legislation, noted that it marked the first time that the federal government formally recognized "the responsibility of government to provide the individual with the necessary information to enable him to advance and protect his own health and to promote social attitudes conducive to motivating people to translate such information into personal practice and life style." As a result, "one of the major missing links in United States health policy is beginning to be forged."[24]

Thus by the late 1970s, the right of patients to be informed, a central tenet of critical medical consumerism, had received powerful reinforcement in national health care policy. After years of scorn and doubt, the idea of the patient as watchdog, entitled to information as a means to "protect his own health," as Somers put it, had come to be accepted as a policy tool. With even physicians starting to be more supportive of patient education, optimists might well have concluded that at long last the playing field of decision making had been leveled. The celebratory tone surrounding what some were starting to refer to as the consumer health information "revolution" certainly encouraged this conclusion. But as would soon become evident, the information solution would not prove a magic cure-all for the health care crisis.

The Passive Role of the Patient Is Passé

The government embrace of consumer health education came in the midst of a grassroots information revolution already well under way. Building on a long tradition of self-health and do-it-yourself enthusiasms, 1970s patient-consumers sought out new sources of medical advice, which authors and publishers were happy to provide them. As the author of a 1978 guidebook for patients noted, "Consumers (sometimes known as patients) fed up with the patronizing attitude of many physicians, are insisting, with considerable success, that they deserve not just a piece of the action, but a piece of the knowledge," so much so that "the passive role of the patient is passé."[25]

In that spirit, the new breed of patients defied long-standing medical sensibilities by openly staking the right to consult physicians' reference materials. Whereas libraries had previously treated such items as intended solely for doctors, patients now begged to differ. A particular favorite of the 1970s health consumer was the *Physicians' Desk Reference* (PDR), an annual compilation of prescriber information for prescription drugs. In a 1974 interview, Gloria Steinem, the founding editor of *Ms.*, described the PDR's appeal: "I could never get doctors to explain to me very fully what the side effects of drugs might be," but after receiving a copy of the volume from a woman doctor, Steinem felt better prepared to look after herself. Her enthusiasm was widely shared. Public libraries noted an upsurge in requests for the book, and by the late 1970s, annual sales topped 150,000 copies. As a pharmacology professor noted in the 1983 *American Journal of Public Health*, the PDR's status as "a brisk seller in lay book shops" suggested that "the patient is attempting to and actually succeeding in looking over the shoulder of prescribers."[26]

Another standard tool for the aspiring patient watchdog was the *Merck Manual of Diagnosis and Therapy*. First published in 1899 by the Merck pharmaceutical company, the book presented a convenient compendium of the chief symptoms and recommended treatments for many common disorders. Although its publishers intended it for professional readers, laypeople soon discovered that booksellers would order copies for $7.50. The *Merck Manual's* indispensability to the well-informed citizen was indicated by its inclusion in Stewart Brand's 1968 *Whole Earth Catalog* (along with *Consumer Reports*, the *I Ching*, and the complete works of Buckminster Fuller), as one of the tools essential for self- and community improvement.[27]

In addition to raiding the doctor's reference shelf, the new breed of patients also sought out popular advice literature written with their interests in mind, an inclination that publishers rushed to satisfy. The number of health-related titles published increased to about 1,000 per year by the end of the 1970s. New print and paper technologies allowed the production of better-quality paperbacks, which in turn fostered publishing on more specialized topics. At the same time, mass-market magazines and newspapers carried a similarly diverse array of coverage; the number of pages devoted to health and medicine in the *Readers' Guide to Periodical Literature* increased nearly tenfold over the decade. Much as popular culture in general was becoming more segmented by audience, so, too, were the health-related offerings on bookstore shelves and magazine racks. There was something for everyone, from people interested in herbalism and natural food to those wanting to evaluate the latest pharmaceutical innovation or surgical procedure or to learn about how to manage a particular illness.[28]

In the early 1970s, a still-vibrant counterculture contributed to the growing diversity of health information. One such source was the many alternative newspapers started by activists dissatisfied with the mainstream press. By 1970, more than 600 such papers and three different alternative news services reached an estimated subscriber base of 5 million. These publications carried articles critical of mainstream medicine and supportive of alternative medicine and self-help. Some even developed medical advice columns, such as the *Berkeley Barb*'s Dr. Hip Pocrates and the *Great Speckled Bird*'s Aquarius, M.D.[29]

Dr. Hip Pocrates, whose real name was Eugene Schoenfeld, was so popular that his column was syndicated and carried in eight different papers. Grove Press's 1968 compilation of his columns, subtitled "advice your family doctor never gave you," was one of the first movement-oriented entries in the health publishing field, intended to attract readers who liked their medical advice "irreverent, direct, instructive, tuned in, and 'where it's at.'" Random House sought to reach a similar audience in 1972 with the *People's Handbook of Medical Care*, written by the physician brothers Arthur and Stuart Frank, veterans of the Medical Committee for Human Rights. In addition to offering uncensored information about recreational drug use and sexually transmitted diseases, the Franks discussed "what to do if you are hit with a billy club" and what first aid measures to use for tear gas exposure.[30]

The women's health movement proved an even more prolific source of advice literature. Determined to give women alternatives to the stereotypes and misinformation common in mainstream medicine, many groups developed educational materials, some of which made the transition from mimeographed handouts to print text. Feminists published newsletters such as *Health Right* and the *Monthly Extract* and covered health issues in magazines such as *off our backs* and *Ms.* In a few cases, feminist guidebooks found commercial publishers and became widely available in bookstores and libraries.[31]

The most successful of these guidebooks was *Our Bodies, Our Selves*. In 1969, frustrated at the poor quality of the available information on women's health, especially its reproductive aspects, twelve feminists who called themselves the Boston Women's Health Collective decided to do something. Recalled Nancy Hawley, one of the original authors, "We didn't have the information we needed, so we decided to find it on our own." First published in a newsprint edition by the New England Press in 1970 as *Women and Their Bodies*, the volume sold 250,000 copies without any advertising. In 1973, Simon and Schuster published a revised, expanded edition under the new title *Our Bodies, Ourselves*, and it became a best seller. Combining a critique of medical paternalism with detailed advice about contraception, childbirth, and menopause, the book quickly became a classic of second-wave feminism and has remained in print ever since.[32]

The health publishing boom also helped bring alternative medicine into wider circulation. As the "confidence gap" between patient and regular physicians increased, the latter's ability to dismiss other healers as quacks and charlatans weakened. Whereas prior to 1960, groups such as Consumers' Research and Consumers Union had maintained their distance from nontraditional approaches, the rise of the counterculture made it increasingly acceptable, even fashionable, to experiment with acupuncture, homeopathy, and herbal medicine. Similarly, many people viewed better nutrition as a key to disease prevention and wanted to avoid pesticide residues on their food.[33]

These trends were reflected in the rapid expansion of the Rodale publishing empire. Founded in 1930 by Jerome Rodale and carried on by his son, Robert, Rodale published books and pamphlets promoting organic farming and natural health, including the monthly magazine *Prevention*, started in 1950 to serve readers interested in a healthy diet and exercise. In the late 1960s and 1970s, the market for Rodale publications expanded rapidly. Adopting what in the magazine trade was known as "slick" format, *Prevention* raised its circulation numbers dramatically and earned a spot on public library magazine shelves.[34]

In addition to consumer guides aimed at readers with countercultural sympathies, the 1970s saw an increase in more consumer-friendly guidebooks written by doctors. Intended to replace the old-style family medicine handbooks made popular by Morris Fishbein and Walter Alvarez, the new-style volumes openly acknowledged that contemporary medicine had flaws that made getting good care a challenge and endorsed medical consumerism as essential for navigating a complex and confusing health care system. Unlike traditional medical advisers, who either ignored or ridiculed the idea that consumerist values had any place in medicine, 1970s physician authors accepted the premise that the generic consumer rights articulated in the 1960s—the rights to safety, information, choice, and voice—applied to medical products and services as well. As physicians Francis Chisari and Robert Nakamura and nurse Lorena Thorup wrote in their 1976 book, *Consumers' Guide to Health Care*, the "consumer's right to know as much as possible about the product or service he pays for" applied to "health care as much as breakfast cereals." Further, "the consumer has the right to expect the provider of medical services to demonstrate his credentials of training and experience, his availability when needed, his awareness of current developments and his fee on an hourly or some other reasonable basis."[35]

While accepting that consumers had the right to know more, new-style guidebooks also recognized that many patients lacked the knowledge needed to properly evaluate the quality of their medical services. Consumer health education could fill that gap, providing patients with the tools to make better decisions. In other words, patients needed what Chisari, Nakamura, and Thorup called "enlightened consumerism." To this end, the new-style consumer literature provided readers with guidelines and checklists designed to help assess how well their doctors were doing their job. The *Consumers' Guide to Health Care* included a list of questions that a doctor should ask when taking a medical history and suggested that patients ask questions designed to assess whether a doctor was keeping up-to-date, such as "What medical journals do you read?" and "How often do you attend medical lectures and seminars?"[36]

The same spirit was evident in one of the most popular guides, 1976's *Take Care of Yourself: A Consumer's Guide to Medical Care*, by physicians Donald M. Vickery and James F. Fries. Linking the do-it-yourself spirit to the more dignified-sounding goal of "health promotion," Vickery and Fries sought to level the informational playing field between patients and doctors so that the former could do a better job of managing their health. Vickery and Fries encouraged patients to seek out information about the drugs and treatments that their doctors suggested, singling out Consumers Union as a particularly reliable source of information, an endorsement hard to imagine happening a decade earlier. These authors also introduced a decision-making tool that would later become common in many medical advice books: flow charts that laid out the criteria for when self-help was acceptable and when a doctor's care was required.[37]

Vickery and Fries also validated the legitimacy of doctor-shopping, stressing that the savvy patient-consumer needed to take great care in the initial selection of a physician. In that regard, much of their advice echoed that of pre-1960 writers: patients should not base their choices on "the social status of the office address, the depth of the carpet, the clothing of the staff, or the hair style of the physician." But Vickery and Fries departed from traditional wisdom by encouraging laypeople to "rely upon your friends' experiences with their doctors." In essence, they were early proponents of what today is known as peer-to-peer reviews, now a standard means of evaluating doctors and hospitals.[38]

Finally, Vickery and Fries acknowledged that patients often had good reason to switch doctors. As they argued, "For the 'free market' to work effectively, you must be willing to 'vote with your feet.'" On the one hand, they cautioned patients against changing doctors out of annoyance over waiting room delays, since physicians who were more responsive to their patients were more likely to fall behind schedule: "You may need this special attention later," they pointed out, so "take something useful to do" and do not get upset if the doctor runs late. On the other hand, Vickery and Fries encouraged patients to refuse to tolerate poor medical service, providing a list of tip-offs that should give rise to concern: visits that did not involve physical exams, doctors who wanted to give patients injections at every visit, and doctors who prescribed "three or more medicines of different types daily," advice that reflected how uncommon polypharmacy—taking multiple prescription drugs at the same time—was in the 1970s. "Be wary when any service costing a significant amount of money is promoted enthusiastically even though you were not aware of the need." Last but not least, "if you cannot communicate effectively with your physician" and "your questions are not adequately answered, go somewhere else."[39]

In their willingness to advise patients on how to avoid being "hustled," Vickery and Fries offered a *Consumer Reports*–style combination of insider information and practical advice. The approach worked, judging by sales of the book, which went through four editions and sold more than 5 million copies, earning a place on the *Publishers' Weekly* list of "hidden supersellers"—that is, older books that continued to sell better than many newer ones. It was only one of a host of similar books and articles offering variations on the same message: this was a new era of "patient power" in which information went hand in hand with personal decision making. As Shirley Linde, author of the *Whole Health Catalog: How to Stay Well Cheaper*, wrote in 1978, "It is a time for the patient to stop feeling ignorant of his body and of his health; to stop blindly accepting whatever he is told," a time "to ask questions, to read, to understand," and "to make the final decision concerning his own body."[40]

This message carried over into more specialized health writings aimed at people coping with specific diseases. If well people needed to be better informed about their medical choices, sick people presumably had an even greater interest in doing so. For decades, voluntary health associations such as the American Lung Association and the American Cancer Society had been producing educational materials to fulfill that need. Now, with the popularity of medical consumerism, the mainstream publishing industry sought to do so as well. The listings in the *Readers' Guide to Periodical Literature* for cancer, diabetes, heart disease, and other medical conditions expanded dramatically in the 1970s and 1980s. By 1981, when Alan M. Rees and Blanche A. Young published a sourcebook on consumer health information, it ran to 354 pages, including separate chapters on women's and elders' health issues and on individual diseases such as cancer, diabetes, and cardiovascular disease.[41]

Along with market segmentation by disease, the consumer health literature also focused on specific products and procedures. As might have been predicted given prescription drugs' long-standing status as a focal point for consumer worries, the literature on these medications exploded. Consumers Union continued to revise and update its popular guide, *The Medicine Show*, which faced growing competition from other books and consumer newsletters aimed at keeping patients abreast of the latest information. One especially popular new authority was the 1976 book *The People's Pharmacy*, written by Joe Graedon, who earned a master's degree in pharmacology and then decided to provide more accessible drug information to consumers because, as he wrote, "people are fed up with being treated as objects by doctors who often do not care about, or can't even discuss in easy-to-understand language, the medicines which they prescribe." He urged consumers to become more knowledgeable about the drugs they were taking because "there is no such thing as a safe drug." In 1978, Graedon and his wife, anthropologist Teresa Graedon, began to write a syndicated column, also titled "The People's Pharmacy," and in the early 1980s, they got their own show on National Public Radio.[42]

In addition, persistent concerns about unnecessary surgery led to a raft of articles and books that sought to educate patients on the need to obtain a second opinion before undergoing any operation. Repeating the cautions issued by earlier doctors such as Bertram Bernheim and Paul Hawley, surgeon Lawrence P. Williams published *How to Avoid Unnecessary Surgery* in 1971 to help Americans avoid the one-sixth of all operations that experts felt were entirely unnecessary. According to the volume's preface, "Mr. Ralph Nader recently stated that medicine is an industry and the patient is the consumer," but unlike other services, the consumer "is faced with a lack of available information by which to judge who is the best doctor and which is the best hospital." Moreover, Williams agreed with Nader's assessment that medicine had virtually no "quality control."[43]

Other books concurred with Williams's caution and sought to educate patients to be more critical consumers of medical procedures, among them Lawrence Galton's *The Patient's Guide to Successful Surgery* (1976), George Crile's *Surgery: Your Choices, Your Alternatives* (1978), and Myron K. Denney's *Second Opinion* (1979). Feminist guidebooks took special pains to warn women against "hip-pocket operations" such as hysterectomies. The value of the second opinion quickly expanded to include treatment plans in general; patients were encouraged to conduct the equivalent of their own medical audits. To facilitate doing so, consumer advocates urged patients to obtain copies of their medical records. A 1978 booklet published by Public Citizen's Health Research Group, *Getting Yours: A Consumer's Guide to Obtaining Your Medical Record*, explained both how to obtain one's records and the benefits of "a more open physician-patient relationship, and avoidance of repetitive costly tests and procedures."[44]

Thus by the mid- to late 1970s, what the medical profession had deemed heretical in the 1930s—doctor-shopping, doctor-switching, reliance on other consumers' evaluations, asking for second opinions, and requesting copies of one's medical records—had been recast as the reasonable actions of mature adults. Whereas Katharine Kellock's 1935 suggestion that patients look up articles about their ailments in the *Index Medicus* had been dismissed as too radical, by the 1970s this kind of patient initiative was viewed as not only appropriate but even essential to getting good care. Moreover, the idea of patient choice had widened to include not only physicians but also the packages of services that they recommended. In this context, behaviors formerly considered inappropriate or neurotic were now accepted as right and fitting. As Donald Vickery wrote in the foreword to the 1981 *Consumer Health Information Source Book*, "The individual is the key decision-maker in health practice and medicine."[45]

Yet as librarians and other information specialists were already beginning to note, opening the floodgates of information did not alone guarantee its wise or efficient use. According to Rees and Young, the massive quantity of health-related materials now available "does not reach the public in any effective or systematic manner." Many groups provided consumer health information with little or no coordination of their efforts, and no widely accepted guidelines existed to evaluate its quality. Professional disagreements over many issues, from the role of fiber in the diet to the best surgical treatments for breast cancer, carried over into the literature read by laypeople. In other words, the consumer health revolution mirrored the fragmentation and confusion of the health care system as a whole.[46]

Moreover, health educators realized that they still competed with another very powerful but not very reliable source of information: television. As Anne Somers noted, a 1971 Harris poll showed that 29 percent of Americans got most of their health information from television advertising, while another 25 percent cited television news stories as their primary source. Content analysis suggested that only about 30 percent of that screen time offered "useful" information, while the remainder was "inaccurate or misleading." Even with the FTC's efforts to upgrade the standards of television advertising, commercials remained a source of pervasive but low-quality messages about health.[47]

The antidote to this fragmentation and unevenness of quality was better collection and curation of good information. Thus 1970s medical consumerism gave rise to repeated calls for improved information databases, an idea that dovetailed with the growing use of computer-assisted technologies. While some groups called for the creation of separate consumer health databases, others suggested simply opening up those originally created solely for expert use. This cycle of information disclosure, dissatisfaction, and pressure for more disclosure became one of the most important consequences of the 1970s patient revolt.

Physicians and the New Patient

While the news that the "passive patient is passé" aroused enthusiasm in many quarters, it did not receive a uniformly warm welcome from the medical profession. Along with Republican presidents and governors backing HMOs, members of Congress mandating PSROs, and the FTC suing the AMA over its advertising ban, the arrival of 1970s-style medical consumerism deepened the sense that physicians' autonomy had come under siege. After two decades of increasingly strident attacks and political setbacks, doctors now had to contend with patients arriving for appointments with *Merck Manual* in hand. As Pieter Joubert and Louis Lasagna wrote in 1975, "It is obvious to the physician who is in contact with reality that the era of drug therapy surrounded by a cloud of mystery and patient ignorance is fast disappearing." In the current climate, "more and more, patients want to know what is wrong with them, what is being done about it, and why; and what the relative risks and benefits of treatment are."[48] Many physicians felt bewildered by this more assertive kind of patient as well as angered by the new forms of government interference being justified on consumers' behalf.

At medical meetings and in the pages of professional journals, doctors struggled to make sense of the new medical consumerism. Not surprisingly, given the profession's size and complexity, the approximately 135,000 doctors treating patients as of 1975 held a variety of opinions on the subject that reflected their ages, personalities, specialties, and geographic locales.[49] Some doctors remained deeply hostile to medical consumerism, which they saw as the work of a tiny minority of malcontents abetted by a liberal-dominated media. Some admitted that patients had legitimate complaints but viewed the consumerist watchdog approach as entirely the wrong way to address them. Finally, a significant minority welcomed the rise of patient engagement, agreeing with lay critics that the patient-as-partner approach was essential to making a complex medical system work better. In their discussions of the new breed, doctors revisited many of the same issues that Alvarez and other physicians had raised in their responses to critics such as T. Swann Harding and Ernest Dichter. But for the most part, those earlier arguments occurred in private correspondence or the occasional editorial.

In contrast, the 1970s debates over the competing imperatives of individual autonomy and deference to scientific expertise burst into far more public view. Particularly revealing was the coverage of medical consumerism that appeared in *Medical Economics*, the journal most widely read by physicians in private practice. Throughout the 1970s, it carried frequent articles and editorials that attested to physicians' contradictory reactions to the new breed of patients. On the one hand, the articles often portrayed medical consumerists as irrational, ill informed, and vaguely ludicrous; on the other hand, the pieces also warned that physicians needed to improve their standards of personal service and communication skills in order to dampen patient discontent.[50]

The journal's treatment of the women's health movement exhibited the uneasy mix of ridicule and curiosity that marked its coverage of medical consumerism. In 1973, Washington, D.C., cardiologist Michael J. Halberstam, a frequent contributor to *Medical Economics*, wrote a half-comic, half-serious article, "When Women's Lib Marches into Your Examining Room." Starting with the warning to "be prepared for hairy legs and unshaven axillae," he went on to detail the very different kind of patient that the women's health movement was bringing to the doctor's office. These women would ask "hard questions about the pill and the I.U.D." and would want to know if the doctor had done a test for venereal disease and consider him negligent if he had not. Feminist patients, he concluded, were good at reminding their doctor "that he isn't God and that lots of his patients aren't going to think of him that way anymore."[51]

In a 1974 interview with Gloria Steinem, Herbert Klein, the senior editor of *Medical Economics*, allowed her to make the case for patient empowerment with less pushback. In essence, Steinem offered up a medical version of the Golden Rule: "It would be helpful if a doctor asked himself in each instance if he would want to be treated the same way he treats his patients." Using the familiar car analogy, she pointed out the absurdity that "most people do, in fact, know more about what makes their cars run than how their bodies work." Doctors had to learn to think of educated patients not as enemies but as allies; patients who question "can help doctors to be better doctors."[52]

In comparison, Ralph Nader received much harsher treatment from the journal, first in a lengthy interview conducted by executive editor A. J. Vogl and Washington correspondent James Reynolds and subsequently in a follow-up commentary by Halberstam. Halberstam's article, written in the form of an open letter to Nader, succinctly summarized why his ventures into medicine left doctors convinced that "you don't know what you're talking about." To begin with, consumerist methods encouraged a distrust of medical authority that would only hurt patients. Halberstam criticized Nader's demand that hospitals disclose their mortality rates on the grounds that "scientific studies in medicine have consistently correlated positive outcome with the patient's faith in his physician or his therapy." Hence "to publicize one's own failures—as opposed to enumerating them, as physicians already must do in consent forms—is to help ensure failure." Likewise, Halberstam criticized Nader's call for ratings for doctors, which the cardiologist likened to "trying to rate wives": "one man's ideal may be another's nightmare."[53]

More fundamentally, Halberstam argued that applying *Consumer Reports*-style evaluations to medicine was misguided because "placing oneself into the hands of a hospital or a physician isn't the same as buying a seat on an airplane." Unlike medical care, which was highly variable and personalized, "objective data" for automobiles "are more reliable." Consumer buying guides to physicians and hospitals were pointless. Finally, Halberstam questioned the legitimacy of consumer groups such as Public Citizen setting themselves up as judges of the medical profession, asking, "Who are the watchbirds watching you?" In short, Halberstam concluded that while doctors might not be perfect, they were still better judges of what was good care than the lawyers flocking to join Nader's Raiders.[54]

While many physicians shared Halberstam's skepticism about the patient's role as watchbird, they found other aspects of the medical consumerist message much harder to dismiss. For decades, the profession had insisted that the personal relationship between individual doctor and patient constituted the greatest strength of American medicine. Having made personal service their touchstone, doctors could ill afford to ignore the many signs that the public was unhappy with the profession, or to imply that patients did not deserve information or respect. As had happened in earlier periods of popular unrest, medical leaders suggested that doctors needed to respond to patient concerns by getting their own medical house in order.

One line of physician response conceded that health activists had a point: physicians' overreliance on technology and search for cures had caused them to lose sight of the "whole patient." Proponents of this view echoed the concerns lodged by medical educators such as Francis Peabody in the 1930s and John Whitehead in the 1950s but did so with a much keener sense of the profession's vulnerability: in light of the growing confidence gap, doctoring needed to change in order to survive. That transformation should begin with training doctors to communicate more skillfully with their patients.

Two widely read books, Mack Lipkin's *Care of Patients* (1974) and Eric Cassell's *The Healer's Art* (1976), made the case for listening to patients with greater patience and dexterity. Internists Lipkin and Cassell presented mea culpas for the overly technical bent of modern medicine and urged their fellow doctors to learn how to work better with patients. As Lipkin argued, the goal was to balance the technology with the human side of medicine, a process that would require engaging the patient in the healing process. In similar terms, Cassell noted "the extraordinary ability that people have to make themselves well" and suggested that physicians should actively work to mobilize it.[55]

The belief that working with the new breed of patients required a different kind of doctor helped propel major changes in medical school admissions policies and curricular offerings. Reflecting the assumption that a diverse patient population might communicate better with doctors more like them, medical schools increased admissions of nonwhite and female applicants. Once enrolled, prospective doctors took coursework that tried better to balance the imperatives of technology-driven medicine with the need to tend to the whole patient. Medical students began to work with patients as early as the first year; they were taught how to conduct a thorough patient inter-view as part of a "problem-oriented medical record." Medical schools also started to require courses in the medical humanities, the social sciences, and the rapidly expanding field of bioethics that exposed students to critiques of modern medicine.[56]

This "rehumanization effort," as the *New England Journal of Medicine* termed it, paralleled a growing debate within the profession about how to accommodate the "new breed" of patient. That argument came into full view in late 1976 with what became known in medical circles as "the Cousins affair." In November of that year, the prestigious *New England Journal of Medicine* published "Anatomy of an Illness (as Perceived by the Patient)," written by Norman Cousins, longtime editor of the *Saturday Review*. The article and the medical response to it represented a turning point in the profession's acceptance of the "educated" patient.[57]

According to Franz J. Ingelfinger, editor of the *New England Journal*, Cous-ins's was only the second article written by a layman to appear in the journal since its founding in 1812. In the piece, Cousins described an illness he had suffered over a decade earlier. In 1964, less than a week after returning from a taxing trip to the Soviet Union, he had succumbed to a mysterious ailment that left him in great pain and increasingly unable to move. The various spe-cialists consulted ultimately agreed that he suffered from an autoimmune disorder in which his body's collagen or connective tissue had begun to break down. Told he had perhaps a 1 in 500 chance of surviving, Cousins was admit-ted to a New York hospital for a last-ditch round of treatment. At that point, he recalled, "It seemed clear to me that if I was to be that 'one case in 500' I had better be something more than a passive observer."[58]

Cousins turned his skills as an author and editor to the scientific litera-ture on autoimmune disorders and devised a simple treatment regimen for himself: he moved from the hospital to a hotel (one-third as expensive, he noted, and a place where he could sleep unmolested), watched funny mov-ies and reruns of *Candid Camera*, and took an IV drip of vitamin C. Within a week, he had significantly improved; within a month, he was back at work. Throughout his self-treatment, Cousins had the full support of his internist, a longtime friend. Cousins wrote, "If I had to guess, I would say that the principal contribution made by my doctor to the taming, and possibly the conquest, of my illness was that he encouraged me to believe I was a respected partner with him in the total undertaking."[59]

Cousins explained that he had waited more than a decade to share his story because he did not want to raise false hopes about his unusual treatment regimen. He likely also realized that his narrative would not have gotten a sympathetic medical hearing in the mid-1960s; it is hard to imagine that an elite medical journal would have published a story about a patient partnering with his doctor to design his own treatment at that time. But in the late 1970s, after a decade of patient revolts, that idea that a man of Cousins's standing—an educated writer, editor, and public intellectual—felt entitled to read medical journals and to try alternative treatments such as vitamin drips and funny movies no longer seemed so outrageous.[60]

The fact that physicians saw Cousins as more of their social equal than a hirsute feminist or a welfare mother undoubtedly contributed to the positive response his article got from physicians. He received more than 3,000 letters, the vast majority of them positive, from doctors around the world. Their reactions, Cousins later wrote, suggested "an important new mood in American medicine" that was marked by "genuine signs of a desire to inform and educate and not superimpose." More concretely, five medical schools invited him to join their faculties. Cousins eventually became a lecturer at the University of California at Los Angeles School of Medicine and a much-sought-after speaker at medical society meetings.[61]

To be sure, not all physicians approved of Cousins's argument, testifying to the difficulty the new breed of patients had in gaining acceptance. In a letter to *Commentary*, Yale surgeon and author Richard Selzer described himself as "outraged by the shabbiness and lack of control that Norman Cousins exhibits in his presentation." Selzer continued, "I am sadder, even, at the sheep-like acquiescence" of the journal in publishing the piece and of the medical schools who invited him to teach. Other physicians chided Cousins for believing that he had "to attack and embarrass medicine and physicians" to make his point and warned that the *New England Journal of Medicine* and the UCLA Medical School "will forever have the albatross of Cousins about their egregious necks."[62]

But the Cousins affair became less an albatross than a turning point in that it marked a new awareness of and acceptance by physicians that the patients' revolt had permanently altered the landscape of American medicine. While it might be safe to ignore the demands of radical feminists or Black Panthers, the kind of medical consumerism embraced by educated, white, middle-class men could not be so easily dismissed. Many doctors might be resentful of the changes under way, but the profession's leaders, particularly those involved in medical education, sought to accommodate the new reality. In that spirit, the AMA's House of Delegates passed a resolution in 1978 supporting programs that "inform consumers and patients about the costs and benefits associated with potential and alternative courses of treatment and emphasizing self-help programs directed at well and worried-well individuals."[63]

Hospitals were especially enthusiastic converts to the patient education cause. Once chiefly the domain of public schools and colleges, the field of health education rapidly expanded to include hospital-based programs. As treatments for various ailments became increasingly complex and technologically sophisticated, enlisting patient assistance in carrying out those treatments became ever more vital. It seemed only logical that patients would do better recovering from complex surgeries, managing blood sugar levels, and enduring chemo- and radiation therapy if they had more information about and involvement with the treatment plan and its likely course. Fostering a generation of "activated patients" made sense in the highly technological world of modern medicine.[64]

Hospital administrators also saw patient education and advocacy programs as a good way to improve patient satisfaction and enhance the institution's public standing. Studies of medical malpractice suits, which were on the rise, suggested that many originated with poor communication between doctor and patient. By improving hospital efforts at gaining and keeping patient trust, education programs could reduce the number of such lawsuits. For similar reasons, many hospitals set up patient advocacy programs, hiring people (usually women) trained in communication skills to resolve situations in which patients were unhappy with their care.[65]

Although patient education was most visible in hospital-based settings, the idea carried over into medical practice more generally. Keith Sehnert, a Virginia internist, began a "course for activated patients" in 1970 and five years later published *How to Be Your Own Doctor (Sometimes)*. Participants attended two-hour classes once a week for between twelve and sixteen weeks, learning, according to Sehnert, to "accept more individual responsibility for their own care and that of their families"; to master "skills of observation, description, and handling common illnesses, injuries, and emergencies"; and "how to use health care resources, services, insurance, [and] medication more economically and appropriately." By transforming patients from passive to active partners in care, such programs promised not only to save money but also to make better use of the physician's time and training.[66]

This concept of patient education was compatible with the emphasis on self-help and personal initiative that had long characterized medical consumerism. Yet it did not prove the quick fix to patient discontent that proponents so optimistically predicted in the 1970s. The promotion of patient education glossed over the continued divisions between patient and physician perspectives on what constituted rational or appropriate "self-help" or "self-care." As critics noted, such programs too easily became a tool to secure the individual patient's compliance rather than to improve the overall quality of care. Patient education goals tended to be "medicocentric"—that is, to define problems and analyze data only from a physician's point of view. As one health educator noted in 1977, "The patient's perspective has received less emphasis in practice than it has lip service among the planners of patient education programs, clinicians, and researchers." In short, patient education programs did not necessarily produce more satisfied or compliant patients.[67]

In Search of the Medical Yardstick

While the challenge of medical consumerism stimulated efforts to educate doctors and patients to better work together, medicine's Cuban Missile Crisis produced another line of response: the quest for more reliable measures of what medical treatments worked. As Halberstam had noted in his 1974 critique of consumerism, the absence of such measures made medical care inherently difficult to evaluate and thus to improve. But even as he made that observation, researchers were attempting to develop a science of "outcomes research" that would provide more objective assessments of medical care.

Like the quest to train physicians to appreciate the whole patient, the search for medical yardsticks capable of distinguishing good from bad treatment had a long and distinguished medical pedigree. Starting with Ernest Amory Codman in the 1910s and continuing on with Paul Hawley in the 1950s, medical reformers had advocated that doctors perform more rigorous audits of their work to determine which treatments worked best. In the 1960s, the concept of the medical audit intersected with the enthusiasm for "systems thinking" that emerged in business and government circles. A key figure in this synthesis was Avedis Donabedian, a physician and public health professor at the University of Michigan, who published an influential 1966 article, "Evaluating the Quality of Medical Care," in which he proposed a formal process of evaluating outcomes to measure quality. If not as powerful as the gold standard of the randomized clinical trial for medicinal drugs, Donabedian-style outcomes research still promised a more scientific approach to evaluating procedure-based treatments than currently existed.[68]

In the late 1960s, researchers took up the challenge of studying surgical practice in more systematic ways. Surgery was a natural starting point for such research, given the long history of worry about the extent of unnecessary procedures. Earlier studies had already pointed to significant differences in the extent and type of procedures performed. By applying more sophisticated methods of collecting and analyzing statistics, researchers hoped to get a better idea of the extent and cause of variations in surgical practice.[69]

The work of John Bunker, a Stanford anesthesiologist, was particularly important in terms of both method and findings. In the early 1960s, Bunker began to use a computer so that he could analyze outcomes from massive samples of surgical cases from the United States and Great Britain. In 1970, he published the results of his analysis in the *New England Journal of Medicine*. Bunker's research documented American physicians' greater willingness to operate compared to their British counterparts, who achieved equally good outcomes with less surgery. He suggested that the difference was a function of the fee-for-service payment system dominant in the U.S. Thus Bunker's study confirmed what lay and medical critics had been saying since the late 1930s: the economic structure of American medicine encouraged physicians to operate when doing so might not be necessary.[70]

Other studies supported and extended Bunker's findings. Reviewing surgical practice patterns, Eugene G. McCarthy, a public health professor at Cornell, estimated that at least 17 percent of all nonemergency operations were unnecessary. By comparing survey data collected from American and English physicians, medical sociologist David Mechanic documented that the former ordered far more diagnostic tests than the latter when presented with the same symptom patterns. Looking at medical practice more generally, Jack Wennberg, a physician on the faculty of Dartmouth Medical School, documented striking regional variations in treatment standards. The Dartmouth Atlas, as his study came to be called, confirmed that despite their standardized training, physicians in different communities treated the same types of ailments very differently.[71]

Supporters of this kind of systematic review pointed to its potential to help improve decision making and thus to bolster physician autonomy and authority. Better documentation of treatment outcomes—what today is referred to as "evidence-based medicine"—would help stiffen individual physicians' spines and give them the confidence to refuse patients' requests for unnecessary surgery. It would also allow the profession to deal more confidently with third-party payers wanting justification for medical recommendations. Both Bunker and McCarthy testified to that potential at 1975 Senate hearings on unnecessary surgery overseen by Utah Democrat Frank Moss. The Moss committee ultimately praised the potential of physician-directed systems of quality control to solve the twinned problems of overtreatment and rising medical costs.[72]

But this more rigorous study of outcomes by no means worked as quickly or cleanly as its promoters hoped, either to bolster physician autonomy or to bring restive patients under control. Both the potential and the limits of evidence-based medicine were evident in *Medical Economics*'s coverage of Bunker's study. In a 1973 article, "What Makes Americans So Operation-Happy?," John H. Lavin and Linda C. Busek gave an extensive, largely positive report on Bunker's work yet also emphasized the difficulties of applying such insights to the individual doctor-patient relationship.

On the one hand, the article presented a wide spectrum of physician opinion suggesting that the medical profession bore a great deal of responsibility for the problem of overtreatment. The "elements creating America's high incidence of surgery" included "the profit motive, fee-for-service, outmoded ideas and training, ritual and patient pressure, inadequate surgical training, and low hospital standards." At the same time, physicians believed that far from being a cure for what ailed American medicine, patients were in fact a big part of the problem. The "do-something syndrome" was a national characteristic of Americans. As Kerr White, a Johns Hopkins internist, put it, "Americans take a fix-it approach, the same attitude they show when they take their cars to the service station. 'Take something out or put something in, but fix it.' They want whatever will make them better—fast." Even Bunker noted, "We've oversold the product and patients themselves are calling the tune, even though they don't really know enough to do so. We knuckle under, because if we don't they'll go to another doctor who will."[73]

This diagnosis of the fundamental causes of overtreatment was by no means new to the 1970s; for decades, both medical and lay critics had pointed to excessive patient demand as the root problem. As journalist Greer Williams had observed in 1954, the entrepreneurial surgeon lived by the motto "Give the lady what she wants." The trend toward more educated and empowered patients was simply making an old problem far worse: the new consumerism of the 1970s increased the likelihood that more patients would demand treatment that was expensive and ill-advised. Nor could the profession escape culpability for patients' unrealistic ideas about their physicians. As Ingelfinger wrote in 1976, "The public's expectations of what medicine can do, expectations generated by offices of public relations, the media and biomedical researchers themselves, are in part responsible for the distrust of medicine and the public's propensity to sue members of the health-care establishment when anticipated cure or relief fails to materialize." The overselling of medical science, in effect, had helped create the mind-set of the modern health consumer.[74]

The Limits of Information Sharing

While physician reformers revisited the unnecessary treatment debates in light of the new consumerism, another contentious set of arguments was emerging over prescription drugs. Among the many thorny issues raised by a more equal partnership between doctor and patient was the difficult-to-resolve question of how to exchange information about drugs and their risks. At a time when the idea of patients' right to more information had been endorsed from the White House to the AMA House of Delegates, the argument that an exception had to be made for consumer guidance about prescription drugs remained surprisingly strong. The continued resistance to the idea of the patient information leaflet revealed that for all the apparent acceptance of medical consumerism, many physicians remained opposed to some of its most fundamental principles.

In 1975, the Center for Law and Social Policy, acting on behalf of a coalition of consumers' and women's groups, petitioned the FDA to expand the leaflet program it had begun in 1969 to allay concerns about oral contraceptives. The petitioners asked that all prescription medications be dispensed with information for patients about recommended uses, dosage, contraindications, side effects, and the like and further suggested that the FDA start with those drugs most likely to harm pregnant or nursing women or be liable to abuse, such as hypnotics, tranquilizers, and amphetamines. The petition contended that such a program was needed for many reasons: "Patients do not receive sufficient information about prescribed medication," physicians were "too rushed and overburdened" to discuss such matters with their patients, and medication was too freely "passed from one consumer to another" without sufficient awareness of the potential dangers involved.[75]

This petition arrived at a time when the Republican administration was positively embracing the idea of the patient as a "market actor." FDA commissioner Alexander M. Schmidt, a cardiologist, could see both the medical and the market logic for the argument "that there were certain drugs that the patient did need to know more about than he was getting." Thus Schmidt set up the Patient Prescription Drug Labeling Project to consider the idea. Echoing the commonly heard sentiment that a better-educated patient would be a more compliant patient, Schmidt justified the project as a means to "strengthen communication" by telling a patient "why it's important to take a drug, why he or she is getting it, why it should be taken as directed, why it shouldn't be discontinued without the physician's advice, what to avoid, [and] what side effects to report to the physician."[76]

Interest in the idea continued during the Carter administration, when the FDA began to hold hearings to solicit opinions from consumer groups, physicians, pharmacists, and industry groups. A wide range of consumer organizations testified on behalf of the patient information leaflet, including Public Citizen's Health Research Group, the National Women's Health Network, the AARP, and Consumers Union. In addition, many patient-consumers wrote to detail their experiences with prescriptions: for example, patients taking tetracycline who had not been warned that it might make them unusually susceptible to severe sunburn or patients narrowly avoiding serious accidents because they had not been told that a drug they were taking might make them drowsy. But the FDA also heard some strong consumer opposition to expanding the leaflet program, at least in relation to estrogen. In 1977, the agency decided that it needed to widen its mandatory warnings beyond oral contraceptives to include other estrogen products since strong evidence indicated their association with endometrial cancer. When the agency announced the plan, many women protested, largely because they feared that it represented the first step toward taking the drugs off the market.[77]

Concerned that consumer advocacy groups might not be representing what the majority of consumers wanted, the FDA conducted surveys of public support for the idea of patient leaflets. When the first survey was conducted in 1973, only half of respondents wanted additional information, but five years later, that number had risen to two-thirds. In addition, patients now expressed a preference for receiving the information both orally and in print—that is, they wanted to discuss drugs with their physicians and have leaflets for future reference. Convinced that the new breed of patients did indeed want more guidance about prescription medications, the FDA continued the leaflet project.[78]

The most determined resistance to the leaflet idea came not from consumers but from physicians, the pharmaceutical industry, and pharmacists. While all three groups affirmed their belief that patients had a right to more information about their treatment than they were currently getting, they objected to the idea that the FDA should give them that information. As a doctor opposing the FDA program wrote in the *Medical Times*, "No one will deny the right of a patient to learn all he *needs* to know about his treatment." Yet the rhetorical agreement that patients had a right to know masked deep divisions over exactly what patients had the right to know and who should tell them.[79]

Physicians were ambivalent about the idea of patient leaflets. On the one hand, they agreed that simply giving patients the same package insert that doctors and pharmacists got was a very bad idea; not only was that information hard to understand, but its long list of side effects might make them too frightened to take their medications. On the other hand, many doctors saw merit in the idea of a patient leaflet written by doctors to minimize the scare factor and to be distributed at their discretion. In a 1977 survey, Lawrence Fleckenstein found that 72 percent of doctors thought information leaflets were a good idea if done properly—that is, if patients did not receive the equivalent of the existing package insert. The AMA put such a plan into action by developing its own series of leaflets for members' use.[80]

Where doctors remained united was in their belief that the FDA should have nothing to do with the provision of patient leaflets. In their view, the agency's plan was a very bad one, first because it was mandatory and second because it came from the federal government. As editor William Barclay of the *Journal of the American Medical Association* wrote in 1977, "There is not a shred of evidence that [patient package inserts] will serve any useful purpose, and they may be just one more burden to a society already staggering under an insupportable mass of bureaucratic red tape." Likewise, in another editorial published in the journal the same year, Richard Dorsey wrote, "The only consequences of this program predictable with assurance are increased legal concerns for manufacturers, erosion of professional freedom for the pharmacist and physician, and higher drug costs for the patient." Given opinion polls suggesting that patients trusted physicians far more than they did the federal government, he noted the "irony of the government's intervening on behalf of the patient's 'right to know' in dealing with physicians."[81]

Pharmaceutical companies also emphasized the damage that leaflets might do to the doctor-physician relationship. In a critical 1976 commentary, the Pharmaceutical Manufacturers Association insisted, "It is not possible to convey sufficient information in lay language to untrained patients to enable them to intelligently enter into this decision-making process." The leaflet might "contain information which the physician may not want the patient to have access to"—for example, that Thorazine was being prescribed to treat schizophrenia. Moreover, the "full disclosure" precept ran the risk of frightening patients by disclosing unlikely side effects. "The necessary numerous cautionary statements certainly invite unnecessary patient fear, worry, anxiety, and drug defaulting." In short, the patient leaflet furnished the patient with a "how-to-kit," encouraging him to "bypass the physician and treat himself," to "become a self-styled 'authority' and [to] conclude the services of a physician are unwarranted."[82]

Last but not least, retail pharmacy organizations opposed the new program because it imposed the burden of providing the leaflets on pharmacists, not physicians. For practical reasons, the FDA had decided that pharmacists would be "best able to collate, store, and provide labeling to patients." But as pharmacists pointed out, this system encouraged physicians to do even less drug counseling with their patients. Moreover, critics suggested that providing the leaflet after the prescription was written undercut the idea that it improved consumers' choice of medications: noted one commentary, "Once a woman has left the doctor's office . . . her opportunity to participate in the decision is gone."[83]

Despite this opposition, the FDA decided in 1979 to proceed with the leaflet program, in large part because of strong backing from the agency's incoming commissioner, Jere Goyan, the former dean of the School of Pharmacy at the University of California, San Francisco. Justifying the decision to proceed despite industry opposition, Carol Scheman, the FDA's deputy commissioner for external affairs, stated, "We at the FDA find it incomprehensible that the public's right to know should include the amount of saturated and unsaturated fat in a coffee cake—but no explanation of the risks and benefits of prescription drugs." Citing the strong consumer support for additional drug information, the FDA asserted that the leaflets would not endanger but strengthen the doctor-patient collaboration, serving primarily as an "informational adjunct" to rather than a replacement for the doctor's advice.[84]

But the patient leaflet program never went into effect, instead falling victim to growing resistance to the prevailing consumerist trends. Conservatives saw the leaflet program as a perfect example of the kind of government red tape supposedly hobbling American business. In the late 1970s, the idea made the Commerce Department's list of the "twenty most burdensome regulations" imposed by the federal government. After Ronald Reagan's 1980 election as president, the leaflet program was immediately canceled. In its place, there arose a voluntary system of drug education that many critics found wanting. For all the lip service paid to consumer information, the means of its provision remained hotly contested.[85]

The Return of Caveat Emptor?

As the fate of the leaflet program portended, the more activist features of medical consumerism gradually faded in the second half of the 1970s. Although the principles of "watchbirding" and second-guessing physician opinion remained salient, the overall message shifted from "We can all be Ralph Naders" to "We can all be Norman Cousinses." As the hard edges of medical consumerism softened, few voices dared dispute the principle that patient-consumers had a right to more information and choice when shopping for medicine. At the same time, some commentators began to call attention to how the defanged version of medical consumerism helped to perpetuate some of the same features of the health care system that had led to the movement's genesis.

In her 1978 study of medical malpractice, lawyer Louise Lander articulated some of the "dilemmas of reform" that medical consumerism was producing. Echoing Halberstam's criticisms of the Naderite approach, she noted that while buying a medical treatment and a dishwasher might be the same in the sense that "either can turn out to be a mistake," they remained fundamentally different commodities. By adapting the methods of choosing a refrigerator to selecting a physician, "the consumerists' individualistic, every-man-for-himself economic model" was reinforcing what was wrong with American medicine. "To the extent that it is elevated to a long-range strategy buttressed by a theory of the medical marketplace," she wrote, "consumerism ratifies, even encourages, some of the most invidious trends in modern medical practice," including the tendency "to increasingly commodify the process of giving and receiving medical care." In essence, Lander argued, medical consumerism was reintroducing the idea of caveat emptor to medicine, thereby "encouraging doctors to act just like entrepreneurs, unencumbered by any social obligation to exercise ethical restraints over what they do to patients."[86]

While Lander's critique underlined the dangers of further commodifying an already overcommercialized transaction, other commentators stressed a different tension within medical consumerism—that between patients' rights and their responsibilities. By the 1970s, patients' rights had acquired greater moral and legal standing, as evident in the Patients' Bill of Rights and the rising standards for informed consent. But as the preface to *The Rights of Hospital Patients*, a 1975 publication by the American Civil Liberties Union, warned, patients needed to exercise those rights: "If they are only rarely used, they may be forgotten and violations may become routine." Having been declared more empowered and educated, patient-consumers now became more responsible for their medical fates. The growing acceptance of medical consumerism made it even easier to blame them both for the illnesses that necessitated treatment, and for medical encounters that turned out badly.[87]

The potential that medical consumerism had to turn into patient blaming was evident in John H. Knowles's "The Responsibility of the Individual," published in 1977 and frequently reprinted thereafter. The former director of Massachusetts General Hospital, Knowles had earned the enmity of his

fellow doctors for speaking out too frankly about the problems of misdi-
agnosis and overtreatment, opinions that cost him a position in the Nixon
administration. In the wake of that controversy, he was invited to join the
National Commission on Critical Choices for Americans, a bipartisan group
set up in 1973 to ponder solutions to the country's many problems, including
those of medical care. In his essay, which grew out of the commission's work,
Knowles showed the conservative side of the patient-has-rights viewpoint.[88]

In the United States, Knowles argued, "the idea of individual responsibility has been submerged to individual rights—rights, or demands, to be
guaranteed by government and delivered by public and private institutions."
But health could not be so guaranteed, because many of its determinants lay
solely in the individual's control. "Prevention of disease means forsaking the
bad habits which many people enjoy—overeating, too much drinking, taking
pills, staying up at night, engaging in promiscuous sex, driving too fast, and
smoking cigarettes." Americans felt they had a right to these activities, "but
one man's freedom in health is another man's shackle in taxes and insurance
premiums." Thus, Knowles argued, the "idea of a 'right' to health should be
replaced by the idea of an individual moral obligation to preserve one's own
health—a public duty if you will." To this end, "the individual then has the
'right' to expect help with information, accessible services of good quality,
and minimal financial barriers." This formulation was far more rational than
telling Americans that "national health insurance, more doctors, and greater
use of high-cost, hospital-based technologies will improve health" when in
fact "none of them will."[89]

In Knowles's conservative version of medical consumerism, Americans
had not a right to health but "a right to expect help with information," as a
Texas librarians' group wrote enthusiastically about his essay. The "inform
and educate" approach shifted attention away from structural problems over
which patients had no control and toward individual behaviors that patients
could presumably change more easily. The key to mastery began with more
and better information and more choice, solutions upon which liberals and
conservatives, politicians and policymakers, publishers and librarians could
all agree.[90]

This reformulation meshed well with the strategies advocated by medicine's professional leadership. First, physicians would be better trained in
the "healer's art"—listening to and communicating with their patients. By
cultivating a greater conception of the whole patient, they would avoid the
problem of being perceived as a "little tin god." Second, doctors would re-
gain their professional authority and in the process patients' trust by relying

more on outcomes-based research to decide what treatments would most benefit their patients. Books such as John Bunker, Benjamin Barnes, and Frederick Mosteller's *Costs, Risks, and Benefits of Surgery* (known colloquially as Bunker's Bible) would become the lodestar for proponents of this view. By putting their faith in outcomes research, physicians could prevent irrational and wasteful treatment.[91] By these means, it was hoped, physicians could turn empowered patient-consumers into allies instead of enemies. In a national medical culture that still believed that the best course was to "do something," doctors needed new kinds of authority and evidence to say no to patients who wanted the wrong kind of care, to resist the pressure to "give the lady what she wants."

Yet medical professionals remained deeply divided over many aspects of medical consumerism, from what types of information and choices patients should have to who was to blame when treatment went bad. As more radical changes roiled the economics of medicine, those divisions would become all the more apparent. By the late 1970s, the limits of the consumer health revolution were already becoming apparent. On one side, consumer advocates continued to warn that regulatory agencies remained too susceptible to industry lobbying groups. In their view, health consumers' menu of choices fine-tuned rather than restrained the medical-industrial complex. On the other side, conservative critics objected to the expansion of government regulation that consumer protection required. Consumers should have the freedom to make their own choices about their health and should not expect the "nanny state" to protect them or to pay for their mistakes. As conservative views gained traction, they paved the way for new kinds of entrepreneurship and cost control that disempowered both patients and their physicians in profoundly unsettling ways.

{TEN}

Shopping Mall Medicine

In late 1982, a new building bearing a large blue and white sign, "MedFirst—Physician Care—Open 7 Days a Week," opened on a busy street in St. Petersburg, Florida, between a shopping center and a McDonald's. On a Sunday morning that December, the sixteen patients waiting to see the young board-certified family physician on duty were interviewed by *New York Times* reporter Milt Freudenheim about why they had come there. Sylvia Peollmann, who had recently moved to the area, had gotten a brochure about the center a few weeks before and came for a checkup "because it was convenient." College student Arlene Krause, who had been bothered by an irritated eye, reported, "I was driving by and saw the sign." Alma Dixon came to get her blood pressure medicine because she knew that the office was open long hours on Sunday. From these patients' perspective, a visit to MedFirst clinic seemed a natural part of a consumer culture dedicated to providing quick and convenient service even on a Sunday, now that the old blue laws that kept businesses closed on the Christian Sabbath had been repealed.[1]

But as Freudenheim was well aware, extending that culture of convenience to patients represented a significant change in medicine. Behind that "revolution," as Freudenheim termed it, loomed a new kind of for-profit medical enterprise exemplified by Humana, MedFirst's parent company. After developing a profitable group of nursing homes and hospitals, Humana had decided to add clinics to the mix after its research division reported that between 25 and 35 percent of suburban American families had no family physician. To serve those families, Humana created the MedFirst division to provide conveniently located walk-in clinics that featured eye-catching signs, were open long hours every day of the week, and accepted credit cards for payment.[2]

While patients liked what Freudenheim called "shopping mall medicine," many physicians he interviewed did not. What the former viewed as a helpful accommodation to their busy lifestyles the latter saw as a dangerous arrangement. "It is fast-food medicine," said Donald D. Trunkey, the chief of surgery at San Francisco General Hospital. "It's convenience for the physician, convenience for the patient," but "it destroys the long-standing personal, human relationship a physician should have with a patient." That sentiment was repeated by both the AMA and the American Academy of Family Physicians, which warned that the new "docs in a box," as they came to be derisively known, could not offer the continuity of care that good medicine required. Yet the medical profession's ability to prevent such developments was diminishing. As a securities analyst specializing in health care explained to Freudenheim, recent Supreme Court decisions had eliminated traditional barriers to competition such as restrictions on physician advertising, and the peer pressure that had long blocked doctors from exploring alternatives to fee-for-service practice had greatly weakened. At the same time, the analyst noted, patients were becoming more educated and wanted to make their own decisions. "The doctor has been knocked off the pedestal," he concluded; "he ain't a god any more."[3]

Once again, the image of doctors falling off pedestals seemed an apt metaphor for the profession's plight. But in contrast to the Cold War era, when the pedestal phrase referred to ethical issues such as fee splitting, the late-twentieth-century version reflected unprecedented reductions in physician autonomy. With Ronald Reagan in the White House, the 1950s version of free enterprise medicine underwent another wrenching transformation as a consequence of two simultaneous and overlapping developments: a greater political determination to reduce medical costs in the public sector, and the advent of new corporate players in the private sector. Both sectors adopted managerial strategies that pressured doctors and hospitals to reduce costs and improve the quality of care in the name of patient-consumers.

The ethos of managerial medicine that emerged in the 1980s rested on a series of contradictions. Although frequently depicted as a return to a more competitive kind of medicine, the 1980s makeover reflected a huge increase in the power of both government and private industry to dictate terms of treatment to providers and institutions. While both public and private reformers insisted otherwise, the goal of cutting costs often seemed to trump that of improving quality or access to care, a suspicion fueled by the growing prominence of for-profit corporations and venture capitalists in health care delivery.

Change for patient-consumers came in piecemeal fashion. On the one hand, economic pressures on medicine resulted in attention to some long-standing areas of popular dissatisfaction. For example, in relatively affluent, densely populated neighborhoods, people could find more walk-in clinics open for longer hours. On the other hand, patients experienced significant losses as well. Faced with growing pressure to reduce costs, institutions and providers tried to adjust in ways that did not necessarily improve patient outcomes—by increasing the volume of care delivered, introducing new technologies, and shifting costs. While demonstrating a greater interest in patients as "customers," for-profit medical corporations encouraged an entrepreneurial medical culture associated with high costs, uneven quality, and financial barriers to access. Meanwhile, the logic of managerial medicine posed more and more bureaucratic limits on the choice of doctor and treatment.

The result was a growing sense of disconnect between the ideology of informed choice and the realities of 1980s medicine. At the exact moment that patients were being told to become more responsible for their medical choices, they encountered formidable obstacles to doing so. The contradictions between the imperatives of patient empowerment and managerial medicine were not long in revealing themselves and made the need for critical medical consumerism even more urgent.

Brave New Medical World

This drastic reordering of American medicine came as part of a much larger economic transformation. After decades of unprecedented expansion, the limits of the Second Industrial Revolution were finally reached by the 1970s. American manufacturing and the high-paying jobs associated with it declined precipitously in the face of foreign competition. In its place arose a new kind of postindustrial economy that relied on the personal service and entertainment sectors as engines for national growth. As economist Victor Fuchs wrote in 1979, it was an economy in which "the hospital, the classroom, and the shopping center have replaced the coal mine, the steel mill, and the assembly line as the major work sites of modern society." What financial writers christened the "health care industry" or "industries," a category that included hospitals as well as pharmaceuticals, played a leading role in this shift.[4]

Health care exemplified the kind of "sunshine" enterprises—businesses based on cutting-edge research that generated high-paying jobs, excellent profit margins, and seemingly unlimited growth—that were expected to lead the way to postindustrial prosperity. Reflecting the optimism of the era, John Bedrosian, the president-elect of the AHA, told a 1981 seminar on emerging medical technologies, "as you all know, health care in the United States today is big business." It was now "the country's second largest industry, surpassed only by food and agriculture." As he noted, "Americans are now spending more to get well and stay well than on national defense." Attesting to that shift, medicine's share of the gross domestic product rose from 6 to 9.5 percent between 1960 and 1980, or $254 billion.[5]

That promise of profitability brought a flood of new investment capital into the health care field. In addition to pharmaceuticals, which Wall Street had long rated a good buy, investors began to explore the potential of hospitals, nursing homes, commercial laboratories, and kidney dialysis. Perhaps the most dramatic—and unsettling—development was the emergence of for-profit health care companies such as Humana and the Hospital Corporation of America (HCA). Stories about new medical products and services and the investment opportunities they presented figured prominently on the financial pages of major newspapers and newsmagazines. This "monetarization," as economist Eli Ginzberg termed it in 1984, transformed the economic dynamics of medical care, particularly as they affected physicians.[6]

Prior to the 1960s, medicine's financial prowess had been acknowledged, but only as an anomaly in an economy dominated by manufacturing. The doctor's status as an independent professional seemed out of step with the kind of modern corporate capitalism responsible for bringing Americans more automobiles, appliances, and foodstuffs. By the 1970s, medicine seemed much less of a fiscal oddity. Not only was the economy far more service-driven in general, but physicians had become more dependent on pharmaceutical companies, medical device makers, and private insurance companies. As a result, the traditional view that medicine existed apart from corporate America became increasingly hard to sustain. At a symbolic level, that view was further undermined by a 1969 change in Internal Revenue Service policy that led many doctors to form professional corporations in order to take advantage of tax breaks. Now, along with their medical certifications, practitioners' listings included the abbreviation "PC." As the *New York Times* quipped, "my doctor the corporation" had become a fact of everyday life.[7]

Underlying these economic trends was the deepening of collaborations among universities, hospitals, pharmaceutical companies, and medical device makers that quickened the output of new medical goods to be sold. Building on breakthroughs in basic sciences such as genetics and immunology as well as applied sciences such as engineering, researchers working in both universities and industrial settings produced dazzling medical advances, many of which remain in use to this day. Covered not only on the front page but the business section as well, medical progress seemed ample proof that health care was destined to become the cornerstone of a vibrant postindustrial economy.[8]

The advances of this era combined sophisticated science with a generation of smarter machines. Many specialties came to rely on new computer-assisted imaging devices, starting with computed tomography (CT) scanners and followed by magnetic resonance imaging (MRI) devices. Other assistive devices expanded treatment possibilities in the surgical suite and the doctor's office. For example, in cardiology, pacemakers regulated unreliable heartbeats, better heart-lung machines facilitated longer operations, and new procedures such as coronary artery bypass surgery and balloon angioplasty repaired damaged heart vessels. In orthopedic medicine, better manufacture and installation of artificial joints opened up new possibilities for knee and hip replacements. In oncology, cancer treatments were revolutionized by more precise combinations of chemotherapy and radiation. Perhaps most dramatic of all, transplant specialists learned to suppress the natural immune response so that donated organs could replace failing kidneys, livers, and hearts. Meanwhile, pharmaceutical research continued to produce new and versatile compounds, including drugs that could prevent future disease by controlling risk factors such as high blood pressure, the wrong kinds of cholesterol, and insufficient insulin production.[9]

Moreover, medicine seemed in good position to continue this cycle of innovation. Academic medical centers had become vital hubs of basic science and clinical research. Their teaching faculty served to train the next generation of doctors, some to be researchers, continually improving methods of diagnosis and treatment, others to deliver those advances to patients, thanks to the expansion of public and private insurance plans. So in many ways, the shift toward a postindustrial service-based economy appeared to have put doctors in an enviable position of strength.

But in reality, medicine's situation was far more complex. Compared to its Cold War expansion, the post-1970 cycle of innovation unfolded under very different political and economic circumstances. The escalating cost of health care caused powerful interest groups to conclude that the business of medicine had become too important for physicians to manage on their own. Whereas these third-party payers had previously accepted a relatively limited role in dictating physician practice, they now began to assert much more power over the "doctor business." Major initiatives to that end emerged in the public sector, particularly in the reform of Medicare payment, as well as in the private sector, where corporations faced growing bills for employees' medical care.[10]

Perhaps the most important locus of change was the federal government, where political leaders faced the challenge of managing Medicare, the most expensive of public medical investments as well as a driver of rising medical costs in general. Washington's get-tough mood reflected the disappointing results of the previous decade's efforts at cost containment and quality improvement. The largely top-down approaches of the 1970s, such as federal efforts to expand HMOs, encourage centralized planning for new technologies, and mandate more medical quality control, had foundered on institutional resistance and lack of coordination. As health care costs continued to increase, more drastic measures seemed necessary. Politicians across the political spectrum declared the need for more fiscal responsibility from medical providers. Faced with taxpayer revolts and Rust Belt decline, political leaders could not afford to continue allowing doctors and hospitals to raise fees at will while avoiding accountability for their performance.[11]

The demand for increased accountability came not only from liberal Democrats, so long the profession's chief critics, but also from Republicans, who had traditionally supported the AMA's version of free enterprise medicine. That shift reflected the rising influence of neoconservative thinkers such as Milton Friedman, whose influential 1962 book, *Capitalism and Freedom*, included a long, critical discussion of medicine's professional powers. While few Republicans endorsed Friedman's suggestion that medical licensing be abandoned, they agreed that more exposure to market competition would make for better medicine. Moreover, as the party of fiscal conservatism, the GOP was deeply concerned about the drag that public spending on Medicare and Medicaid placed on a struggling economy. Republican leaders consequently embraced a position long associated with the Health Left: allowing doctors too much freedom to regulate their own affairs had created an expensive, wasteful health care system.[12]

Reflecting these concerns, in 1977 President Jimmy Carter shifted oversight of Medicare and Medicaid from the Social Security Administration to the newly created Health Care Finance Administration (HCFA, now called the Centers for Medicare and Medicaid Services), with the express intent of facilitating coordination and cost controls. In 1980, Ronald Reagan won election on a promise to bring government spending under control and, amid growing fears that the Medicare trust fund was headed for bankruptcy, directed his appointees to HCFA to make cost control a top priority.[13]

To that end, HCFA officials instituted a new system of Medicare funding based on the use of diagnostic related groups (DRGs). The brainchild of Yale researchers, the DRG system created fiscal incentives for hospitals to provide more cost-effective care. Analyzing the now extensive data available on payout patterns, the Yale team calculated the average cost of treatment for specific categories of illness. In essence, they conceptualized those treatments as standardized services and then estimated the projected cost of supplying those services to the average "case mix" that Medicare patients represented.

But instead of delivering that sum for treatment already provided, the DRG system worked prospectively, by giving hospitals a lump sum in advance. If an institution could treat patients more cost-effectively, it could keep the difference; if the care cost more, the hospital had to absorb the loss.[14]

New Jersey pioneered the DRG system in 1980, and it appeared to work reasonably well. Recalled its local manager, "Hospitals got paid, grandma was not thrown out onto the street prematurely by hospitals, and so it was generally viewed as a positive change despite all the predictions to the contrary." Based on that success, the Reagan administration decided in 1983 to adopt the DRG system for all hospital payments under Medicare; henceforth, reimbursement was based on a scheme of 467 categories of illness, with the final one covering whatever did not fit in the first 466. As the Reagan administration later justified it, the change represented "the response of a prudent purchaser concerned with creating incentives for efficiency and reducing the federal budget deficit."[15]

The results were dramatic: the annual growth in Medicare's hospital payments dropped from 16 percent to 6.5 percent by the late 1980s. The prospective payment system had such success in controlling hospital costs that Medicare administrators in 1992 adopted a similar approach to physician services, the Resource-Based Relative-Value Scale. That program aimed not only to slow down the amount Medicare spent on doctors' reimbursements but also to rethink the setting of "customary and reasonable charges," which greatly favored specialists over generalists. Like the DRG, the Resource-Based Relative-Value Scale concept helped to slow the rise in Medicare payments, and it, too, was adopted by private insurers. In general, Medicare's funding reforms accelerated a broader trend toward using payment mechanisms as a way to slow rising health care costs.[16]

At the same time these changes were unfolding in the public sector, growing pressures for cost control emerged in the private sector as well. In part, that pressure came from corporations worried about the escalating costs of employee health care plans. For example, as the American auto industry struggled to survive in the face of overseas competition, its union-negotiated medical plans became a source of concern. When Lee Iacocca took over the near-bankrupt Chrysler Corporation in 1978, he discovered that Blue Cross/ Blue Shield was the company's single biggest supplier of services. To stave off bankruptcy, he bargained with both the United Auto Workers and the insurance companies to reduce health care spending. During the late 1970s and early 1980s, other large employers, among them American Express and General Electric, looked to retool employee health insurance plans as a way to stay competitive. As an industry analyst observed in 1985, "The days of providing employees with unlimited access to health care facilities with minimal utilization review and virtually no pricing control are over."[17]

The rise of a new kind of corporate player in the medical field hastened the business community's conviction that traditional forms of financing and delivering medical care had become obsolete. For-profit health care corporations suggested that with the proper management, hospitals and clinics could be run in such a way that their quality could be improved and their costs controlled while returning healthy profits to their investors. The pathbreakers in this respect were Louisville-based Humana and Nashville-based HCA, which followed similar pathways to success: first they acquired a chain of regional hospitals, then they developed outpatient facilities to guide patients into those hospitals. Both companies sought to cut costs by streamlining care from the first patient visit through the hospital discharge and by using their size to obtain discounts on products and services. Humana eventually branched out into primary care and developed a line of insurance plans, while HCA stayed focused on hospitals and outpatient surgery.[18]

The success of Humana and HCA signaled a growing interest in health care as an investment opportunity. Starting in the 1980s, external investment in medical enterprises increased dramatically as health care stocks became a popular addition to investment portfolios. Many for-profit medical corporations looked to the stock market to find funding for start-ups and expansions. Between 1987 and 1997, health service companies initiated 233 public offerings, and their capitalization jumped from around $16 billion to $113 billion. As yet another sign of investor interest, the number of financial analysts tracking health care stocks grew from 152 to 559 over the same span. The new partnership between medical enterprises and Wall Street signaled what *New England Journal of Medicine* editor Arnold Relman dubbed the "new medical-industrial complex."[19]

Among the most visible elements of this new medical-industrial complex was a new kind of HMO. The template envisioned in the 1973 HMO Act had been a nonprofit company on the model of Kaiser Permanente, which ran clinics and hospitals where physicians worked as teams to offer high-quality preventive care. In contrast, the 1980s saw the development of for-profit HMOs that integrated existing providers into more cost-effective arrangements. Within these networks, local physicians and hospitals contracted to provide service following the HMO's guidelines for treatment and payment. The new-style HMOs used a variety of reimbursement methods to hold down physician costs: putting doctors on salary and paying them bonuses for cost-conscious treatment, paying doctors so much per patient (capitation) as an incentive to hold down costs, and enhancing oversight of clinical decision making to minimize expensive specialist visits and diagnostic tests. From only 12 percent of HMO enrollees in 1981, for-profit companies using these strategies had expanded to cover 62 percent of them by 1997.[20]

The initial successes of for-profit hospitals and HMOs raised fears that they would eventually come to dominate the whole industry. In fact, those fears were not realized. The for-profit companies recouped some dramatic initial savings but ultimately ran into the same problems of cost containment that plagued their nonprofit counterparts. By the end of the 1990s, venture capital enthusiasm for such companies had cooled. But the advent of for-profit health care corporations permanently altered medicine's economic landscape, adding a new competitive intensity to managerial strategies designed to attract patients and control costs.

In essence, the 1980s represented the end of the generous postwar funding for both hospitals and physicians that had helped finance the dramatic expansion of the medical-industrial complex. With remarkable equanimity, all the third parties responsible for financing medical insurance plans—state and federal governments, private employers, and insurance companies—declared that the old days of simply reimbursing hospitals and doctors for their "usual and customary charges" were over. As economist Uwe Reinhardt put it, "Physicians have lived like kids in a candy store," and now "we, the payers, want the key back." Both public and private insurers felt emboldened to set limits on what providers charged through a whole range of bureaucratic mechanisms. In the process, third-party insurance systems no longer simply funded medical care but also monitored and sometimes sought to deter it.[21]

All of these changes occurred despite the active resistance of the medical profession, which found its ability to protect physician autonomy greatly weakened. The new managerial medicine appeared at a time when medicine was struggling to come to terms with another legacy of the late 1960s patients' revolt: under pressure from the federal government, American medical schools had increased their admissions and recruited more women and minority students. Between 1965 and 1990, the ratio of physicians to patients jumped from 148 to 247 per 100,000 people. In the 1980s alone, the number of young physicians entering the profession increased by 30 percent. These new doctors had grown up in the turbulent 1970s and did not necessarily share the older generation's attachment to fee-for-service principles.[22]

As the profession became larger and more diverse, its ability to act as a unified force in policy debates declined precipitously. By the early 1980s, the

AMA had suffered a dramatic loss in membership and political clout. In the early 1950s, 75 percent of all American doctors belonged to the AMA; by 1987, that number had fallen to 43 percent and was continuing to decline. The AMA's losses reflected the splintering of physicians into competing special-ties. Already a problem before 1965, that fragmentation accelerated rapidly thereafter, a consequence both of medicine's growing technological sophis-tication and of the reimbursement schemes used to fund its delivery. Both public and private insurers favored specialists over generalists and rewarded different specialties at very different rates. As a result, the professional inter-ests of radiologists and cardiac surgeons increasingly diverged from those of pediatricians and psychiatrists. Although specialty societies worked hard to advocate on their members' behalf, there was no single "voice of American medicine" speaking for the profession as a whole.[23]

The arrival of DRGs and HMOs in the 1980s brought a profound sense of uneasiness to the medical profession, which had yet to recover from the upheavals of the 1970s. At medical meetings and in professional journals, doc-tors expressed shock and dismay over the new reimbursement schemes and managerial methods. At one 1986 symposium, speakers likened the doctor to "a grief stricken person who still is in the denial stage" and a "boxer reeling from his opponent's initial blow." Particularly hard to accept was the more corporate style of management, with its emphasis on third-party oversight and accountability. A profession long proud of its independence seemed to be losing its battle to remain so, hemmed in on one side by the federal government and on the other by Wall Street. The dismay inspired by this new economic order was captured in a satire of the Hippocratic Oath that appeared in the *New England Journal of Medicine*. In place of the traditional oath, which began, "I swear by Apollo the physician, and Asclepius, and Hy-gieia and Panacea and all the gods and goddesses as my witnesses," the "cor-porate version" said, "I swear by Humana and the American Hospital Supply Corporation and health maintenance organizations and preferred-provider organizations and all the prepayment systems and joint ventures, making them my witnesses, that I will fulfill according to my ability and judgment this oath and this covenant."[24]

Among the worst indignities associated with the new corporate-speak was the recasting of the doctor-patient relationship in the language of providers and consumers. Even before the coming of the corporation, physicians had taken a dim view of patients' roles as "intelligent buyers" of medical services. That skepticism turned into outrage as the ethos of managerial medicine spread. Writing to the *New York Times* in 1986, Connecticut physician Lee Sataline bitterly decried the new era of "corporate health care with cost containment and profit margins," in which "the white coat and black bag have been replaced by a pin-striped suit and attaché case." In a world ruled by these "new masters," Sataline observed, "physicians are referred to as 'Providers' and the patients as 'Consumers,'" a transformation that in his estimation added "a supermarket touch to the whole affair."[25]

Madison Avenue Medicine

Yet another blow to the medical profession's sense of autonomy came in 1982 when the U.S. Supreme Court finally ruled for the FTC in its lawsuit against the AMA over the issue of physician advertising. The FTC had filed that suit on the grounds that the AMA's advertising ban impeded consumers from getting the information they needed to make good medical decisions. For seven years, the AMA disputed the FTC's argument, only to have the courts agree that the ban constituted "a formidable impediment to competition in the delivery of health care services by physicians in this country."[26]

Having for decades defended traditional fee-for-service medicine as the free enterprise system at its best, the AMA was now hoisted by its own petard: regulators and jurists deemed advertising to be a healthy part of a free-market economy even for doctors. Thus in 1982, the AMA rewrote its code of ethics to profess, "There are no restrictions on advertising by physicians except those that can be specifically justified to protect the public from deceptive practices. A physician may publicize him or herself as a physician through any commercial publicity or other form of public communication." The doctor's office seemed poised to take on even more of a supermarket aura as a result.[27]

In fact, relatively few doctors rushed to adopt aggressive advertising campaigns after the ban was lifted. Older physicians retained their distaste for shilling, while younger physicians seeking to establish practices were a little more inclined to advertise but stuck to what came to be known as "yellow pages professionalism"—that is, providing more information in the yellow pages section of the telephone directory of the sort consumers had long requested: office hours, board certifications, range of procedures performed, forms of payment accepted. Some also began to add mild embellishments: pediatricians, for example, would tout their kid-friendliness. The exceptions were medical specialties that depended on performing a high volume of specific procedures, such as face lifts and hernia repairs, which did begin to advertise more robustly. One Houston cosmetic surgeon used billboards, magazines, and radio to build his practice, while two New Jersey surgeons changed their office telephone number to 1-800-HERNIAS to draw in patients.[28]

By 1995, almost 35 percent of physicians under the age of forty-five reported having done some form of print advertising, but many doctors continued to view such practices with distaste. As one told a *New York Times* reporter in 1990, "As a general statement, I think the more a doctor advertises, the less good he is." Meanwhile, advertising by price—what 1970s regulators had been most interested in encouraging—remained quite rare in the 1980s. Except in the cases of a few standardized surgeries, doctors did not try to attract patients by claiming to charge the lowest prices. Instead, they stuck to far less concrete promises to provide high-quality care in patient-friendly settings. So far as fees went, the new kind of physician advertising did little to advance the kind of price competition that the FTC and the courts had hoped to stimulate.[29]

More competitive kinds of medical advertising developed less among individual physicians than around hospitals and the expanding array of clinics and diagnostic facilities affiliated with them. Unlike the AMA, the AHA had never had a formal ban on advertising. As early as the 1910s, big-city hospitals promoted services and amenities to attract paying patients. As both medical consumerism and economic competition increased in the 1970s, hospital promotional campaigns expanded, prompting the AHA to issue its first formal guidelines for advertising practice in 1977. As more for-profit companies entered medicine, they spent heavily on advertising as part of their business strategy. With Humana investing around $20 billion a year in advertising, its nonprofit rivals felt pressured to respond in kind. As *Adweek* observed in 1985, "With the health care industry waging an all-out competitive brawl," institutions that had formerly spent little on advertising now began to do so. Thus the nonprofit Kaiser Foundation Health Plan, "historically a rather quiet $3.5 billion-a-year conglomerate," was now "getting ready to throw a few marketing punches of its own."[30]

As part of their competition with one another, health care groups tried to address some long-standing complaints from patient-consumers. Humana and many other hospitals picked up on people's problems in finding doctors and began offering physician-referral services by telephone. Unlike the emergency call systems that local medical societies had operated back in the 1950s, however, the new referral systems did not pretend to be equal-opportunity listings of their members but instead funneled patients to practitioners aligned with the referring hospital or clinic. Hospitals could contract with one company, Ask-A-Nurse, and pay between $35,000 and $180,000 per year for a "health information and referral service" staffed by registered nurses who steered callers to the contracting facility. Since only one hospital group could be licensed in each particular geographic area, this exclusivity was "intended to position the provider as a community leader in health care information and generate referrals for its physicians." By 1990, 190 hospitals in thirty-seven states used Ask-A-Nurse, and the company received 4.5 million calls from consumers. Overall, an estimated 75 percent of hospitals offered some kind of referral service by 1991; as the Internet expanded, many began to use web-based referral services as well.[31]

Hospital and clinic groups sought to attract patients by adopting other tactics previously unknown in medicine, such as direct-mail ads, coupons, and radio spots. In Flint, Michigan, St. Joseph's Hospital sought to attract prospective parents with a low-cost obstetrical package promoted as "A bundle of joy . . . a bundle of money"; the campaign increased the number of babies born at the hospital from 1,200 to 1,650 per year. A Las Vegas hospital offered patients who would come on weekends (typically slow times for admission) a chance to win a free cruise for two, raising the hospital's utilization rates by 60 percent in eighteen months. Even in New York City, hospitals enticed customers with incentives ranging from key chains to coupons for $25 off a visit to the emergency room.[32]

This aggressive advertising aimed to disrupt existing patterns of hospital referrals, which had long remained under physicians' control. As market research showed, the vast majority of patients simply followed their physicians' recommendations when choosing hospitals. The new-style promotions sought to persuade patients either to pressure their doctors to use particular hospitals or to choose the hospital first and rely on its affiliated physicians. The for-profit corporations' creation of integrated networks and willingness to spend unprecedented amounts on promoting them forced their nonprofit rivals to do the same. Following the same model, nonprofit hospitals began to widen their referral base by setting up walk-in clinics and diagnostic centers and then referring patients who needed further treatment to their own cadre of medical specialists.[33]

This promotional culture fed back into the "medical arms race" that had begun in the Cold War years. In densely populated areas, hospitals and clinic groups felt intense pressure not only to acquire the expensive specialist talent and equipment necessary to offer the latest in diagnosis and treatment but also to advertise that they had done so. Medical marketing campaigns frequently played up prowess on the cutting edge of high-tech care, from diagnostic imaging to transplant surgery. While few patients might be in the market for kidney transplants, the fact that a particular hospital stood ready to perform them seemed to guarantee similarly high standards for more common treatments. Attempting very difficult procedures could in fact be a calculated way to attract easier and more profitable forms of business. Such suspicions were raised in 1984 by Humana's highly publicized sponsorship of an Indiana businessman's artificial heart implant, which critics portrayed as a blatant attempt to promote the company's cardiac services.[34] As for-profit and nonprofit providers battled for market share, investing in and advertising the latest in cutting-edge technologies and procedures seemed essential for medical survival. Much as pharmaceutical companies hoped to develop blockbuster drugs, hospitals were eager to develop profitable procedures around which marketing campaigns could be built.

Still, in comparison to contemporary beer and fast-food advertisements, hospital and clinic promotions remained relatively conservative in the 1980s and 1990s. Fearful of mudslinging that might further undercut consumer trust in the medical profession, health care providers avoided direct attacks on competitors. As a consequence, medical ads tended to sound alike, with each facility presenting itself as the best, most convenient, and most patient-friendly in town. In addition, as a *New York Times* analysis found, hospitals and clinics jockeyed to be first or unique in some respect—the first hospital in the country to perform a 3-D laparoscopic surgery, with doctors "wearing the special glasses to give them depth perception"; the only hospital on Long Island to perform endoscopic ultrasound; the first comprehensive specialty lipid/cholesterol clinic in Queens; and the first hospital in the United States "to put low-sodium Chinese food on the menu."[35] And unlike prescription drug promotions, no hospital equivalent of the FDA policed these claims for veracity or forced retractions of false claims.

Although they felt compelled to advertise, many hospital administrators and staff physicians felt profoundly ambivalent about what one referred to as the "Wild West" atmosphere created by the new competition. Money spent on marketing was often wasted, given that insurers rather than patients usually determined the choice of hospital. Complained a Connecticut hospital executive in 1994, "I could advertise until I was blue in the face," but if a particular managed-care company had decided not to use his hospital's services, "then I'm wasting my time." Other observers lamented that money spent on advertising was money not invested in institutional services that would directly improve patient care. "It's diverting millions of dollars from the bedside," noted the acting medical director of Long Island Jewish Medical Center, and "I'm not sure about how ethical it is to do that."[36]

Although advertising professionals viewed marketing much more positively, even they worried that its excesses would hurt the credibility not just
of a particular institution but also of the health care system in general. At the
1991 meeting of the Academy for Health Services Marketing, Lawrence J.
Nelson, a bioethicist and lawyer, reminded his audience, "You're not selling tires." In the marketing of "traditional products," he noted, "buyers and
sellers are independent, equal, and self-interested." In contrast, "health care
patients are vulnerable and dependent; they're subjects, not objects, and can't
negotiate." Thus, doctors and hospitals had to hold to a higher standard of
fiduciary obligation that made certain kinds of ads unethical: a hospital that
lacked a neonatal center should not promote itself as a "safe place" to have a
baby; "satisfied customers" should not be actors; a facility should not claim
to have the most advanced technology when it did not; a hospital should
not run "emotional ads" that played on "pain of childlessness or the fear of
breast cancer"; and a physician-referral service should reveal how its doctors
were selected. But while Nelson urged his audience to take the high road in
health care advertising, he noted that to date there had been no prosecutions
for unethical health care ads that might act as a deterrent to do otherwise.[37]

The more aggressive advertising of medical services all but guaranteed that
people coming for treatment would have even higher expectations of their
physician and hospital care. The old restraints on medical advertising had
reflected a belief in the interchangeability of medical assets: a rigorous system
of medical education, coupled with a strong system of hospital accreditation,
ensured that all patients could get the best of care no matter what doctor or
facility they used. In reality, differences in quality had always existed, but
medical institutions had little incentive to call patient-consumers' attention to
them. With the corporate remodeling of medicine, however, big budgets for
advertising and marketing encouraged institutions to imply that their doctors
and facilities were far superior to others and to stress that a critical element
of consumer choice involved seeking out the "best" facility.

Thus the disruptive onset of managed medicine was intensified by a rising
volume of advertising that explicitly sought to unsettle the traditional doctor-
patient relationship. That advertising celebrated the merits of consumer
choice without necessarily being able to deliver on its promises. Previously
able to maintain some separation from the commercialism of mainstream
advertising, physicians were now dragged, for the most part against their will,
into an advertising cycle characterized by heightened expectations and keen
disappointments. Far from being a neutral aid to rational decision making,
the new medical marketing and advertising multiplied the confusing and

misleading claims that patient-consumers had to evaluate to find the care they wanted.

Private Practice in an Age of Managerial Medicine

With its managerial methods and aggressive advertising, the corporate invasion of medicine greatly unsettled private practice. Both admirers and critics of the so-called new competition used the language of retail to describe the results: as media accounts announced, American health care was becoming a "patients' market" where physicians competed to "keep patients happy" by practicing a more consumer-friendly brand of "shopping mall medicine." Yet it was also quite clear that this competition centered only on certain groups of patient-shoppers—those with generous insurance plans. Medical groups and hospitals under pressure to improve their bottom lines had no incentive to expand or improve services to poor people. As a hospital consultant admitted during a 1985 forum on economic trends, "I don't see the marketplace doing anything for the poor." In more sarcastic detail, the *New England Journal of Medicine*'s "corporate version" of the Hippocratic Oath included the line, "Into whatever clinics I may enter, I will come for the benefit of the insured, keeping myself far from all except capitated care for the underprivileged, especially if they are not covered by the group contract."[38]

Many physicians found this new version of market competition no less horrifying than the 1970s demands for "medical power to the people." According to the *New York Times*, there was deep concern that "the gentlemanly atmosphere that once reigned in the profession" had been "replaced with what many doctors call a savage competition for patients." Yet even as they decried it, physicians electing to stay in practice had to come to terms with the new economic climate. As Thomas M. Heric wrote in a 1991 text, *The Business of Medicine*, "Regrettably, you must stuff the nostalgic Norman Rockwell pictures back into the drawer and take a hard look at some of the facts that will directly affect how you will practice medicine." To survive, physicians had to learn how to negotiate a more competitive medical landscape in which patients could choose among urgent care centers and hospital outpatient services as well as old-style doctors' offices.[39]

The increased competition lent new urgency to old warnings that physicians needed to do a better job as service providers. In a 1984 speech, the president of the District of Columbia Medical Society, John Lynch, told listeners that a recent visit to his own doctor had given him new insight into the "profession's declining public image." While waiting a very long time in the reception area, he overheard the office staff discussing specific patients, their medications, and other personal information in what was a blatant "breach of confidentiality." Lynch concluded that doctors should not only lament such failures as a poor reflection on their professionalism but also realize that "in these days of increasing numbers of physicians and doctor-shopping, it could have untoward effects on the physician's practice."[40]

These pressures fell particularly hard on a profession that had yet to find a satisfactory replacement for the old-fashioned family doctor. By the late 1970s, specialization had become so widespread that even doctors who wanted a more general practice had to take some kind of specialty training. The old concept of the general practitioner was replaced by the "primary care physician," an umbrella term applied to specialists in general internal medicine, pediatrics, and after 1969, family medicine. Yet physicians in these fields saw their incomes decline steadily as a consequence of reimbursement rates that favored procedure-based specialties. Even while paying lip service to the importance of the primary care physician as gatekeeper, both public and private insurers remained willing to pay more for doctors to perform expensive diagnostic tests or treatments than to spend time talking to patients or coordinating their care. As one doctor observed in 1982, "Why not gastroscope . . . every patient at five hundred dollars for fifteen minutes' work, when an hour's time devoted to listening to and examining a patient will only bring in eighty-five dollars at best?"[41]

Regardless of specialty, most physicians faced growing pressures to make their practices appealing to a more demanding kind of patient-customer. As the 1988 edition of the *Encyclopedia of Practice and Financial Management* summarized, "Patients are becoming more difficult to please" and "more willing than ever before to go elsewhere." As a consequence, "medical practice is becoming increasingly competitive, and the competitor with the most to lose is the one who's least prepared for the melee: the private, office-based physician." Doctors needed to accept that the historical distinction between a store and a doctor's office was crumbling. The old myth that people "don't shop for medical care" was simply "not true"; doctors had better provide "a well-situated, well-planned, well-equipped" office or watch patients go elsewhere.[42]

Even as the push for managed medicine figured prominently in such warnings, the specific advice to physicians about how to court doctor-shoppers echoed Cold War prescriptions about how to run the "doctor's showroom." As in the 1950s, the basics of good practice management outlined in the 1980s and 1990s emphasized the right location, ample parking, a well-designed office space, an efficiently run appointment system, short waiting times, respect for patient privacy, and friendly office staff. Choosing the right place to open one's practice remained vital. Noted Gene Balliett in his 1978 book on practice management, the days when doctors could simply head to the nearest middle-class suburb and expect to set up a successful practice had passed; nowadays physicians needed to do market research to find a good prospect. As had been the case since the 1920s, promising locations were assumed to be in expanding suburban areas and upscale urban districts rather than poor inner-city neighborhoods or sparsely populated rural areas.[43]

Once a good community had been found, the practitioner's next task was to find attractive office space in a high-traffic area, preferably with plenty of parking. While doctors' buildings remained popular, many physicians relocated into the new mini-malls being promoted by real estate developers. In California, long a trendsetter in this regard, mini-malls became hospitable locations not only for regular physicians but also for their holistic competitors. In 1988, the Westside Granville Plaza opened in a wealthy section of Los Angeles with tenants that included restaurants, a photocopy shop, a surgical clinic, and a chiropractor's office. In suburban areas across the country, strip malls offered a similar combination of medical and retail outlets.[44]

Whether in a strip mall or a doctors' building, the overall design and layout of doctors' offices changed relatively little. A patient transported from the "modern" doctor's office of the Cold War era to its post-1980 counterpart would have felt in familiar surroundings. Color schemes and furniture styles changed, but as the floor plans provided in the 1991 guide *The Business of Medicine* show, the basic organization of the waiting room, business areas, examination rooms, and consultation area remained the same. The most noticeable change in office specifications was the effort to makes space more accessible for people in wheelchairs via entrance ramps and door clearances.[45]

But while the physical appearance of private physicians' offices remained largely static, their modes of operation did not, in part due to growing competition from for-profit clinics. The success of Humana's MedFirst chain inspired many competitors, including clinics operated by nonprofit hospitals and others run by freestanding companies such as Urgent Care Centers of America and AmeriCARE, both founded by physicians. Aimed at "white-collar, middle Americans who don't have time to wait," as the physician president of Urgent Care Centers of America explained, the new clinics sought to take advantage of patient dissatisfaction with long waits and short hours at regular physicians' offices.[46]

To compete with the new "docs in the box," physicians with nearby private practices felt compelled to match amenities such as expanded hours and easier means of payment. One Oklahoma City physician started keeping his office open until nine o'clock two nights a week so that "the mothers don't miss work and the kids don't miss school." He also furnished his office "like a living room" to make it more comfortable and welcoming. "People are doctor-shopping," he said, and "you just have to compete." Likewise, the willingness of for-profit clinics to accept credit card payments induced other physicians' offices to do the same. When credit card payments had initially been proposed in the 1960s, the District of Columbia Medical Society had opposed the idea as not "in the best interests of the doctor-patient relationship," feeling it "smacks of third-party medicine." But two decades later, the demands of patient convenience trumped such resistance, and doctors' offices began to install credit card machines.[47] One consequence of this competitive pressure was the abandonment of solo practices in favor of group practices, which enabled physicians to share the burden of longer office hours and equipment costs. Between 1965 and 1991, the percentage of physicians in private practice with other physicians increased from 10 to 33 percent; by the early 2000s, it had risen to two-thirds.[48]

In addition to longer hours and easier payments, physicians faced enormous pressure to provide patients access to the latest in medical technology. As the medical arms race continued to heat up, and hospital and clinic advertising campaigns emphasized the latest innovations in diagnostic scanning and cardiac care, doctors in private practice needed to assure patients that their care remained up-to-date. Some leased or bought the diagnostic equipment they used most frequently rather than send patients elsewhere. Others sent routine lab work to a centralized lab (often owned by another doctor) for processing rather than do it in-house. Some responded by creating facilities that both prescribed and provided imaging services, a phenomenon that would soon become a focal point of cost-related concerns. Whether doctors chose to own equipment or delegate services, competition forced them to maintain access to the latest in medical technologies. This pressure became another factor forcing physicians to join some sort of managed-care network, either an independent practice association or a preferred-provider organization, in order to gain such access.[49]

On the business side, physicians struggled to manage the growing burden of filing insurance claims. As the 1978 edition of Marian G. Cooper and Miriam Bredow's *The Medical Assistant* noted, "When payment to the doctor involves an insurance claim, there is more clerical work than when patient pays a bill directly"; thus, "along with the popularity of health insurance has come a sizable growth in paperwork in most doctors' offices." The handbook included samples of six different forms and reports with which medical assistants had to be familiar, including those for Medicare, Medicaid, and CHAMPUS, a new plan for veterans and their families. To reduce that burden, large insurers began to use a universal reimbursement form first developed by a joint initiative of the Health Insurance Council and the AMA in 1964 and revised in 1975. They also adopted the coding system developed for Medicare and Medicaid to streamline the recording of diagnoses and procedures.[50]

As managed-care plans proliferated, an already complex system of paperwork became even harder to administer. Yet physicians had no choice but to figure it out because insurance reimbursements had come to constitute the chief source of their income. In 1970, third-party payments were involved in only about 30 percent of all medical services, with patients paying for the rest directly out of pocket; by 1990, those numbers had reversed, with third-party payments involved in 75 percent of all medical care delivered in the United States. Quickly filing claims and receiving payment thus became essential to private practitioners' economic survival.[51]

The growing centrality of third-party payments helped bring about the digitization of patient records. For-profit HMOs and hospital management corporations early on saw the advantages of using computers both to share medical records and to expedite billing and fee collection, and nonprofit competitors soon followed their lead. Just as forward-looking doctors of the 1950s had invested in electric typewriters and copiers for their offices, their 1980s counterparts began to buy computer systems and software packages. Advertisements for equipment explicitly aimed at doctors appeared in both medical journals and computer magazines in the 1980s. In 1983, *Computer World* featured an article about a "comprehensive medical practice system" capable of managing clinical records, third-party claims processing, and patient billing information. The cost? $9,500. Private companies such as HBO that had developed hospital systems for data management scaled them down for use by private practitioners. As an alternative to buying computer systems that rapidly became obsolete, many physicians began in the 1990s to outsource the filing and tracking of insurance claims to national claims clearinghouses.[52]

This investment in claims processing reflected the growing importance of the patient's insurance status as an initial determinant of care. To be sure, physicians had long been concerned with figuring out which patients were likely to pay their bills. But as third-party reimbursement became more pervasive, assessing individual patient-consumers' personal finances became far less important than determining the extent of their insurance coverage. Cooper and Bredow's textbook on office management advised, "One of the first pieces of information the medical assistant should ask of a patient is whether he or she carries health insurance and if so what kind"; to that end, the assistant should ask to see the patient's insurance company identification card.[53] Verifying insurance became an increasingly important prelude to the doctor-patient encounter. In addition to questions about the difference between Blue Shield's "usual charge" and Medicare's "customary charge," office assistants started having to explain the copays and deductibles associated with the growing array of managed-care plans. What had initially been a relatively modest part of the medical assistant's job mushroomed into a full-time occupation. As a 1981 manual on medical office management noted of insurance, "Patients ask many questions and expect the assistant to know the answers."[54]

On the positive side, the spread of managed-care principles replaced the unpredictability of the old-style fee setting, in which doctors varied charges depending on their perception of patients' economic circumstances. But as third parties took charge of payments, the locus of conflict became more bureaucratic and impersonal. In 1957, when Benny Hooper's parents had questioned the physician's fee, Dr. Kris could cancel the debt. Three or four decades later, it would have been harder for a doctor to do so without wading through a mass of insurer red tape. Under managed-care methods, the setting of prices became far removed from the control of individual doctors and patients. Large insurers, public and private, negotiated with medical groups and hospitals for lower fees, with limited input from either providers or consumers. From the patient's standpoint, the end result was an insurer-dominated system that made even less sense than the old-style doctor-controlled billing.

Under the expansion of managed care, individual physicians also lost much of their control over the reimbursement process. Whereas earlier efforts to standardize fees, such as the California Medical Association's Relative Value Scale in the 1950s, had originated with physicians, third-party payers bent on cost containment now dominated the process. But doctors faced a challenge in distancing themselves from patient discontent over insurance. As was the case with the pharmaceutical industry and its prescription drugs, physicians found their fate entangled with that of an industry over which they had limited control.

In his 1978 book on practice management, Gene Balliett, a physician columnist for the *Medical World News*, acknowledged the blowback physicians were experiencing as a result of patient discontent over insurance policies.

He suggested a strategy of response that essentially turned the blame back on the patient and the insurer: "When a patient buys a policy from an insurer, you're no more a party to the deal than you are when a patient buys a basket of groceries at the supermarket." Companies were now selling policies using misleading advertising that made it sound as if the patient would never have to pay another medical bill. A physician should explain to patients who had failed to read the fine print that he or she was not the "bad guy in the deal" and that *they* had been fooled: "If the patient bought lousy insurance, put yourself on his side by telling him so." Today's doctor, Balliett suggested, had to educate his patients about the real world of health insurance, helping them to understand that "the quality of coverage varies widely" and that "your policy may be better or worse than most." He suggested that doctors develop standard patient leaflets that explained how insurance plans worked and that concluded with the statement that the patient was responsible for the charge regardless of insurance coverage.[55]

In essence, Balliett invoked a kind of medical consumerism that physicians had long espoused: patients bore responsibility for making smart choices, and if they failed to do so, they deserved the consequences. In earlier times, that logic had been applied to medical nostrums and quack treatments; now it was applied to buying a bad insurance plan. If a patient had unsatisfactory coverage, it was his or her fault, not the doctor's doing. But this "let the buyer of insurance beware" approach made less sense as the insurance landscape changed in the late twentieth century. The employees presented with insurance plans selected by their employers and the elderly people becoming eligible for Medicare on their sixty-fifth birthdays did not get to shop for their insurance plan. When patients became unhappy with their contracts—Why didn't Medicare cover mammograms? Why did Cigna deny claims for a preexisting illness?—they really could not be blamed for making poor individual choices.

By the late 1980s, physician advice givers had begun to advocate a tactic very different from Balliett's: suggesting that in the brave new world of insurance constraints, doctor and patient should work together to circumvent third-party insurers' policies. Faced with restrictive reimbursement regimes, doctors and patients could find common cause in getting around them, adopting an us-versus-them mentality with the insurer as "them." In his 1986 commentary on corporate medicine, Connecticut physician Lee Sataline wrote, "I am learning 'double speak,'" or "telling the truth 'on the slant,' as Emily Dickinson described it," to get patients' claims honored. As Sataline explained, "to reduce overburdening of the clerical mind," Medicare had created the DRGs, but physicians still had the power to choose the product code that unlocked the desired treatment and its reimbursement. To get the system to pay, doctors could diagnose a bad cold as bronchitis or order a mammogram for a cystic breast condition.[56]

Sataline's description of physician doublespeak pointed to one reason that the new managed-care methods did not reduce costs as much as their advocates had hoped: providers learned to game the system so that patients would get the care they wanted and needed while physicians received favorable rates of reimbursement: Medicare paid more for treating bronchitis than for a bad cold. For every measure designed to substitute a more cost-effective treatment for a more expensive one, three even more expensive options seemed to emerge. The corporate Hippocratic Oath captured that dynamic: "I will not use the knife unless I am a surgeon, but I will try to learn some form of endoscopy." As another analyst noted in 1990, "medical costs are like shifting sands—they don't disappear, they just move from one area to another."[57]

To counter those trends, insurance companies had to practice more stringent forms of utilization review—that is, refuse to conflate bad colds with bronchitis or to allow mammograms to monitor cystic breast disease. But when insurers tried to respond in this way, they encountered an enormous backlash from angry patients and doctors alike. Meanwhile, the logistics of reimbursement continued to militate against what many patients most wanted and needed—time to talk to their doctor. For all the emphasis on teaching doctors to communicate more effectively, insurance practices gave physicians little incentive to do so. As a pediatrician told a *New York Times* reporter in 1988, "No matter what we say about preventive care, we pay for procedures." As a result, he noted, "an orthopedist can earn more in an hour than I can earn in a week." Such disparities only increased the long-term trend away from primary care practice and toward medical specialization, making it even harder for patients to find a trustworthy personal physician to coordinate overall care.[58]

Dazed and Confused

Even before the heightened corporate presence in health care, Americans had found it hard to find doctors they trusted, to evaluate the quality of their care, and to understand how charges were figured. Now as an approach shaped increasingly by Wall Street and Madison Avenue came to dominate medicine, patient-consumers found themselves even more "dazed and confused" by their medical choices, as a hospital executive put it in 1989. Contemporary press coverage of the changes in medicine demonstrated an ambivalent sense of opportunity and anxiety. Over the course of the 1980s, a growing chorus of commentators began to question whether from the consumers' standpoint, the latest version of free enterprise medicine was an improvement over the old.[59]

By forcing doctors and hospitals to compete, the new market orientation seemed as if it should work in the empowered patients' favor. Since the 1920s, Americans had been told that getting good medical care depended on making a good choice of physician. With doctors and hospitals now being forced to compete more openly with each other, presumably this kind of strategic doctor choice would be even easier. As Susan Dentzer wrote in *Newsweek* in 1984, Americans were gaining greater freedom to "shop around" to get the best possible care at the lowest possible price.[60] Actively seeking out physicians who provided the most desirable services would have salutary effects not just for individual patients but for the whole medical system. In this positive view of doctor-shopping, informed patient choice would reward good care and encourage its proliferation.

Some encouragement to believe that this kind of doctor-shopping would work could be found in the successes of patient advocates, especially those focused on specific diseases and procedures. Breast cancer activism was a case in point. In 1975, when activist Rose Kushner had presented the case for an end to radical mastectomies at the annual meeting of the Society of Medical Oncologists, she had been booed off the podium. But breast cancer advocates had not given up the fight and had created a call center where patients could get information about alternative treatments and the doctors willing to perform them. In the face of that movement, physicians gradually modified their insistence on the radical mastectomy as the only option. Thus five years after the *Washington Post* published Kushner's first article about her experiences, it reported positively on the story of a freelance political journalist, only twenty-eight years old when her cancer was diagnosed, who exercised her right to get more information. After "some careful investigation," which she referred to as "doctor-shopping," she found a doctor willing and able to treat her without a radical mastectomy.[61] In this fashion, empowered patients not only obtained care more satisfying to them as individuals but helped to improve medical treatment for all women with breast cancer. In this context, doctor-shopping seemed laudable.

Along similar lines, newspapers and magazines echoed the message found in books such as Donald M. Vickery and James F. Fries's *Take Care of Yourself* that all patients had not only the right but an obligation to adopt their role as watchdogs. In that role, Americans should not hesitate to ask for second opinions, especially if they suspected that a diagnosis was mistaken. Carol Gino, a registered nurse, made the case for the second opinion in a 1986 story about her mother, who had hurt her arm in a fall. The emergency room doctor took an X-ray and declared that the injury was a sprain. Still in pain a week later, mother and daughter sought a second opinion, whereupon a different doctor reread the X-ray and found a broken bone. Gino concluded, "I believe that in any important diagnosis, you should always seek a second opinion. That's not doctor-shopping, it's not denial of illness, it's good common sense."[62]

But as Gino's words suggested, "doctor-shopping" still carried many negative associations. Physicians continued to use the term to refer to drug addicts seeking prescriptions for narcotics. It also got applied to hypochondriacs who went from doctor to doctor seeking treatment for imaginary illnesses. Thus in a 1989 article, Karlyn Barker equated "doctor-shoppers" with what were known colloquially as "thick file patients"—that is, people who spent so much time going to the doctor that they had acquired very fat records. As she put it, "Often, if one doctor tells them the good news—that nothing is wrong—they will go to another doctor, and another, searching for a physician who can find the problem." In this view, increasing patients' ability to doctor-shop simply enabled neurotic individuals to waste not only their own money but also physicians' time.[63]

Blaming neurotic patients for making doctors practice bad medicine was not new: the same argument had been used to explain why so much unnecessary surgery was performed in the 1950s. But in the changed policy climate of the 1980s, these concerns took on greater significance. Having supposedly gained a more active role in their treatment, patients now bore more of the blame for unwise use of medical resources. Patients who went to doctors for trivial complaints or patronized incompetent providers were helping to drive up medical costs for everyone. While some patients were being blamed for failing to live up to their weighty responsibilities by doctor-shopping too often and for the wrong reasons, others were criticized for remaining too passive and failing to fulfill their watchdog duties.

In an insightful 1985 article, Victor Cohn, the *Washington Post's* longtime medical correspondent, described the problems presented by the new expectations of doctor-shopping. Some patients remained reluctant to issue "a pink slip for Dr. Wrong," offering his own experience as a case in point. For all his years of writing about medicine, Cohn found it difficult to confront a physician with whom he was dissatisfied and instead just left his practice without explaining why, a decision he regretted. People felt guilty about changing physicians or despaired of finding anyone better, but the physicians interviewed in the article seemed more comfortable with the idea of patients shopping around. One family practice physician said, "I tell patients it's fine . . . you don't have to give a reason to change doctors." According to this doctor, "part of what we value in our medical care system" is the idea that "you can see anyone you want and don't owe anyone an explanation." But as Cohn pointed out, insurance plans were changing in ways that made seeing "anyone you want" more difficult. His comments underlined an important reason that the new systems of cost control made patients nervous. For decades, they had been told that being willing to switch doctors was critical to escaping bad medical care; thus insurance plans that limited that choice were inevitably suspect.[64]

The debate over good versus bad doctor-shopping had strong class and race overtones. "Doctor-shopping" might be envisioned as a positive strategy when used by an "educated" consumer, such as women looking for new breast cancer options or people challenging incorrect diagnoses, but viewed with suspicion when practiced by poorer, less-educated people. While Americans resisted measures that restricted their right to pick their doctor, many of them were more than willing to deny that right to people enrolled in Medicaid. By the late 1970s, restricting Medicaid patients' right to choose a physician had become a popular political issue: Ed Koch, for example, won the New York City mayoral election in 1978 on a platform that included a pledge to reduce Medicaid costs by requiring patients to "enroll with one physician of their choice" to be changed "only at specific intervals or for cause." Similarly, the public health chief of Washington, D.C., promised in 1983 that the city's 120,000 patients on Medicaid "should be 'locked in' to one doctor of their choice" to prevent prescription drug abuse.[65]

Studies of Medicaid patients suggested that they were no more likely to doctor-shop to get prescription drugs than were patients with private insurance, but the perception of poorer people as potential drug abusers proved hard to shake. While affluent white patients might be viewed as switching physicians primarily to get better care, the possibility that Medicaid patients, too, might be trying to escape long wait times, disrespectful doctors, or questionable diagnoses was ignored. Likewise, affluent patients were not discouraged from using their insurance to go "from physician to physician" and receive "a variety of treatments without coordinating any of them," as a critic of the Medicaid restrictions noted.[66]

As pressures to reduce costs escalated, the drive to "encourage" Medicaid patients to enroll in managed-care programs accelerated, especially after the

1981 passage of legislation that transformed federal medical assistance into a block-grant program that gave states less money and more leeway to experiment with managed-care plans. Some Medicaid HMOs assigned each patient to a single doctor as case manager, thereby reducing costs and improving quality. Other plans gave patients lists of doctors who met criteria for quality and cost-effectiveness. But the element of coercion was troubling: patients were being forced to give up providers they liked because they were not "approved." As National Public Radio reporter Joanne Silberner noted in 1994, some Medicaid recipients complained about "not having a free choice of doctors, having to go to a hospital that's far from home, not getting all the tests they think they need."[67] As limits on doctor choice began to affect Americans with private insurance plans, they too would sour on the whole concept of managed care.

New and Improved Shoppers' Guides

These questions of choice and coercion increased the pressure on policymakers to pay more attention to issues of quality. From its earliest days, doubters of managerial medicine had predicted it would unduly prioritize cost control over effectiveness. Its advocates realized that if limits were to be put on physician and patient choices, they needed to be justifiable by metrics other than simply saving money. By implementing more quality-control measures, health care reformers hoped to achieve the holy trinity of improved quality, reduced costs, and expanded access to care.

Policymakers' efforts to enhance quality control built on the growing sophistication of health services research. The expansion of third-party payments for health care had created a massive database of information ripe for analytic review. Government agencies collected this information as part of their fiduciary duty to taxpayers; private entities did the same for their investors. According to an article in *Modern Health Care*, "information flow" helped "to boost cash flow." Data initially collected for fiscal purposes could be reanalyzed for other purposes, such as tracking patterns and outcomes of treatment.[68] While these kinds of data were not initially meant to be shared with the public, medical consumerists had already begun to see the potential benefits of forcing public agencies to do so; Herb Denenberg's hospital "buyer's guide" did exactly that by disclosing information about both charges and mortality rates.

On a more ambitious scale, Public Citizen's Health Research Group aspired to do the same with the biggest such database in the country: that compiled by HCFA, the government body charged with overseeing Medicare and Medicaid. Starting in 1973, the Health Research Group petitioned Congress and filed lawsuits in an attempt to win the release of that information, but without success. As demands for greater transparency grew in the wake of Watergate, so did the calls for sharing data. By 1981, the prestigious Institute of Medicine (IOM) endorsed the public disclosure of hospital mortality data to "enhance consumer choice" and provide medical institutions with "public accountability."[69]

This viewpoint gained traction during the Reagan administration. In 1986, the secretary of the Department of Health and Human Services, Otis Bowen, appointed William Roper, described in the *Washington Post* as "a public health officer with a strong belief in medical accountability," to head HCFA. Both Roper and his boss were political conservatives as well as physicians, so the idea of accountability appealed to them. Roper ordered his staff to prepare a preliminary study that compared the mortality rates at 142 hospitals. Believing that the data would be too difficult for the average person to interpret, he had no intention of making the report public. But after learning of its existence, the *New York Times* announced its intention to sue for its release under the Freedom of Information Act. In December 1987, at the advice of HCFA's legal counsel, Roper agreed to release the report.[70]

The HCFA report received extensive coverage in the news media, with particular emphasis on the local hospitals that received bad grades. Critics immediately pointed out the data's flaws—the same flaws that had made HCFA officials reluctant to release the report. The analysis did not correct for the seriousness of patients' illnesses: sicker patients were more likely to die, so a hospital that treated more extremely ill people would have higher mortality rates. Despite these caveats, the data release was hailed as a "revolutionary first step in giving consumers an objective measure of the quality of care in individual hospitals," as the *Washington Post* reported. According to Jack Christy of the Public Policy Institute of the AARP, the report had "finally cracked the reticence, the guild protective mentality" that had denied the public such useful information.[71]

This new kind of public accountability posed a challenge to hospital advertising and marketing departments. At the Academy for Health Services Marketing's 1988 annual meeting, two market researchers stressed the need to use mortality data "professionally, ethically, and properly" to avoid further heightening consumer distrust of medical institutions. Given that "the health care industry is already distrusted and reeling under attack from consumer groups, employers and Congress," outcomes data should be used carefully "to avoid the scenario of hospitals racing against each other, on a muddy track, in an endless mortality data derby where nobody can emerge as a winner." The researchers advocated more "subtle" use of data: negative outcomes could be used internally to encourage improvement, while positive data should be emphasized in public statements and marketing efforts.[72]

As HCFA officials as well as the health care division of the American Marketing Association pondered how to spin data disclosures, yet another contender for the role of "honest broker" of information emerged from the ranks of the mass media. In 1990, *U.S. News and World Report* began to publish a special consumers' guide to hospitals, seeking to duplicate its earlier success in producing college and law school rankings. The newsmagazine's editors explained that hospitals were "prodigious data generators," yet with the exception of HCFA's mortality rates (which were of debatable value), none of that information was in a form that consumers could truly use: "Since no medical authority—or anyone else, for that matter—had ever devised yardsticks for rating hospitals that are both useful and statistically valid, *U.S. News* had to create its own." Realizing that hospital departments varied enormously, staff decided to focus on twelve different specialties, "from AIDS to urology."[73]

To develop the ratings, the *U.S. News* staff asked almost 1,500 physicians to fill out a confidential form listing the top ten hospitals in their area. In essence, the magazine polled experts for the purpose of sharing their responses with the public. This approach differed from that used to compile *U.S. News's* law school rankings in that there was no attempt to develop a rigid numerical ranking, just a list of the best institutions in no hierarchical order. The survey results were used to determine the best fifty-seven hospitals in the United States. The authors emphasized that the results "should not imply that other hospitals cannot deliver excellent care" or that these hospitals were perfect, but the list represented an excellent starting point to "find the very best care possible if serious illness strikes."[74]

The magazine also offered useful advice about how to assess the markers of quality care, suggesting, for example, that "people who need surgery should ask a surgeon about volume" and noting that new treatments for kidney stones required a "lithotripter, an expensive machine that hammers the stone with ultrasonic blows." Subsequent reports continued in the same tradition. The magazine's 1991 hospital issue included an overview of the year's developments in consumer health information, among them plans by the Joint Commission on Accreditation of Healthcare Organizations to measure the quality of medical specialties as well as Blue Cross/Blue Shield's decision to steer patients to selected organ transplant centers. The issue also reported on HCFA's efforts to develop more sophisticated versions of its hospital mortality data. Finally, *U.S. News* covered states' efforts to provide consumers with better decision-making tools.[75]

Having found a winning formula, *U.S. News* stuck with it. Its annual hospital issue effectively combined the solidity of numbers—survey results and ratings—with suggestions about quality indicators patients should look for and questions they should ask. In effect, the magazine positioned itself as a dependable, honest broker of information. Declared the magazine's staff, "Despite the growing information from both sides of the hospital bed on the quality of care, the *U.S. News* survey is the only broad assessment available." Its hospital rankings came to constitute news themselves: each year, local newspapers reported which of the area's hospitals had made it into the newsmagazine's ratings. Some local news outlets began to copy the formula themselves: *Philadelphia Magazine*, for one, began to produce a hospital issue profiling local health care facilities in greater depth.[76]

Lists of the best hospitals were soon followed by lists of the best doctors. Large samples of practicing physicians were asked to name the best specialists in their communities, and the results were distilled into lists of the individuals most frequently named by their peers. By the early 1990s, two companies competed for the market in guides to New York City's "top doctors," one developed by computer software analyst Richard Topp, the other by physician John Connolly. The latter proved more successful, in part because in 1997 *New York* magazine started to publish an abridged version of the list each year. Other cities and magazines followed suit, creating similar guides to the best doctors in the area.[77]

Perhaps inevitably, the idea of publicizing the best doctors led to its opposite: creating a list of doctors whom patients would do well to avoid. But even in an era of greater transparency, the disclosure of negative information about doctors ran into significant roadblocks. Starting in the 1970s, the AMA and many state medical boards had begun to keep master files of problematic physicians, but the contents of those files were not shared with anyone, even the profession's own credentialing bodies. As a consequence, doctors convicted of malpractice who lost their medical licenses in one state could simply move to another locality and resume practicing. As the number of medical malpractice suits rose in the 1970s and 1980s, consumer groups increasingly criticized this reticence. Some commentators portrayed the rise in malpractice suits as a symptom of overeager lawyers and irresponsible patients filing frivolous lawsuits to take advantage of juries' sympathy and insurers' deep pockets. But in reality, policymakers had very little reliable data on the extent and outcome of medical negligence and impairment and thus no way to determine whether it was unusual or common.[78]

In 1986, believing that better cost control required more quality assurance, congressional conservatives and liberals acted to address that lack by passing the Health Care Quality Improvement Act. The law created a National Practitioner Data Bank and required that malpractice insurance companies, state licensing boards, and other organizations report cases of negligence and incompetence, but it exempted the new data bank from the terms of the Freedom of Information Act, limiting its use to hospitals, state licensing authorities, and professional societies. Public Citizen's Health Research Group immediately challenged that limitation in court, but the restrictions on access were upheld, on the grounds that the physicians' right to privacy trumped the public's right to know. Public Citizen managed to win a seat on the data bank's governing board and to gain access to its files, which it used to publish its own list of problem doctors.[79]

With a vastly more sophisticated kind of health sciences research at their command, policy experts envisioned a path toward progress that not only used the fruits of big-data-driven research to demand more accountability from physician and hospital providers but also taught patient-consumers to use the same data, thereby reinforcing that accountability. In this optimistic scenario, patients would have a new set of empirical weapons to be deployed in support of the larger goals of national reform. It was an appealing concept in line with the general faith that all consumers' problems could be solved if only they had more and better information.

But as would quickly become evident, turning big data findings into usable tools for consumer decision making would prove no easy task. In 1994, when the federal government released results from a large-scale analysis of patient satisfaction surveys collected as part of its Hospital Consumer Assessment of Healthcare Providers and Systems initiative, even supporters of the principle of data sharing admitted that the information was not easy to use. As one nurse executive put it, "There's a lot to maneuver; I think it's going to take the average consumer a little while to understand it." Ten years later, policy experts would be making exactly the same point. Physicians as well as patient-consumers had trouble understanding and acting on the new kinds of evidence.[80]

A pattern thus emerged in the late 1980s that would repeat many times in the years to come: appealing to new standards of public accountability, patient-consumers would gradually receive access to data formerly thought suitable only for experts to see and interpret. The data were intended to enhance patient-consumers' ability to find and reward providers who practiced more "accountable" medicine. But the data would prove both hard to analyze and use and subject to creative spinning by hospital marketing departments and magazines eager to sell the latest guides to the "best hospital" and "best doctor." In the end, making patients better quality-control agents proved far harder than anticipated.

Like Walking on Shifting Sand

The proliferation of rankings and report cards in the 1990s testified to the continued faith that more and better information would enable patients to make better medical choices. Yet the emphasis on training all patients to be better doctor-shoppers ran counter to trends in the insurance industry that sought to limit patients' ability to choose doctors and treatments. Over the 1980s, a growing number of Americans enrolled in managed-care plans that determined which physicians could be seen and what treatments they could get. Thus at precisely the same time that the patients were presumed to be exercising more freedom of choice in the medical marketplace, their insurance plans often limited their choices in hidden and not-so-hidden ways. Trying to sort out the new world of HMOs and preferred-provider organizations was "like walking on shifting sand," as Sue Berkman described it in her 1997 book, *The HMO Survival Guide*.[81]

Within a relatively short time, the majority of American workers came to be enrolled in insurance plans that used some type of managed-care strategy to hold down costs. As of 1988, 73 percent of workers were covered by conventional insurance plans, compared to only 27 percent in either HMOs (16 percent) or preferred-provider plans (11 percent). By 1998, those statistics had changed dramatically: only 10 percent of employees had traditional plans, with the rest covered by some kind of managed-care plan, in the form of an HMO (28 percent), a preferred-provider plan (39 percent), or a hybrid of the two known as a point-of-service plan (24 percent). But compared to physicians, who were aware of the new insurance strategies early on, the enrollees themselves were often oblivious to the huge transformation under way in the insurance industry. Their lack of awareness reflected the fact that employers, not workers, determined the shape of the plans being offered. As insurance expert Jon Gabel and colleagues wrote in 1987, the move to managed-care plans was a "purchasers' revolution" in which employers acted on behalf of their employees but with their own fiscal ends foremost. As managed-care principles and plans spread in the 1990s, they did so not by creating an open network of providers competing to win patients by the quality or efficiency of their service but rather by locking in an employer with one insurance company. When employees were offered choices, they were usually among insurance "products" offered by the same company, which had little interest in competing against itself. Not only did employees have limited choices regarding plan provisions, but if they found the arrangement unsatisfying, they might have difficulty opting out.[82]

To some extent, these limitations were offset by an appealing feature of many managed-care plans: they covered more services than did the old-style major medical plans. Aimed at subsidizing care delivered in a hospital, the old plans created incentives for doctors to treat patients in the most expensive setting. By encouraging employees to utilize care delivered in the doctor's office, managed-care plans sought to encourage enrollees to get treated sooner and at a lower cost. But that greater access often came at a higher price, in the form of rising premiums, bigger deductibles, and substantial copays. Some plans required subscribers to get preapproval before visiting specialists; others offered no coverage for vaccinations, mammograms, and other preventive services.[83]

People who were self-employed or who worked for companies that did not offer insurance found themselves in even worse straits, with no options other than purchasing individual plans that were extremely expensive and routinely refused to cover preexisting conditions. Unable or unwilling to pay prohibitive prices for limited coverage, many workers under the age of sixty-five opted to forgo insurance entirely. In 1994, around 14 percent of all Americans had no medical insurance, a number that peaked at 16.7 percent in 2009. With health care personnel routinely requiring insurance cards at check-in, people who lacked insurance had difficulty obtaining treatment.[84]

So instead of lowering prices so that more patients could afford good care, the new competition in health insurance worked far more unevenly and unpleasantly in the late 1980s and 1990s. Insurers competed by trying to enroll the healthiest patients, a process referred to as "creaming" or "cherry picking." Doctors and hospitals engaged in their own strategizing, expanding the provision of medical services that provided the best return on investment, such as cardiac procedures and joint replacements, and cutting back on the kinds of care that were less lucrative, such as treating people with serious mental illnesses or caring for people with HIV/AIDS. Declining federal reimbursement rates for Medicare and Medicaid compelled hospitals and clinics to be less generous in providing free or very low cost care. For all these reasons, people with limited incomes and serious health problems faced increasingly high barriers to care.[85]

Even people with insurance found themselves frustrated by the highly complex, bureaucratized, and fragmented system. On one level, the problem resulted from the voluminous but confusing amount of paperwork involved in any visit to a physician. A 1995 article in the *Washington Post* described the dread with which one woman approached opening her mail and sorting through the medical bills for her aging parents: "I was absolutely and totally overwhelmed," she told the reporter. If younger people could make little sense of Medicare forms that stated "This is not a bill" but also showed the amount owed, how could older, frailer seniors possibly figure out what to do? As the *Washington Post* noted, a new service industry had emerged to handle insurance claims, with companies such as Medical Bill Management and Medical Bill Minder springing up to handle the "blizzard" of forms—for a fee. But families with limited income had little choice but to try to manage the bills themselves.[86]

Even more distressing were insurance company denials of claims. While the industry insisted that such instances were rare and likely resulted from patient-consumer negligence, press coverage of such cases suggested otherwise. A 1991 article in *U.S. News and World Report* noted that while the national political debate was primarily focused on the uninsured, private insurance companies were "also drawing increasing fire for stingily refusing to cover some expenses for the majority of Americans enrolled in private health plans." The piece explained, "In the name of 'managed care' and 'utilization review'—buzzwords for the way insurers monitor the procedures doctors perform, insurers and employers routinely deny coverage for medical care deemed experimental, unproven, unnecessary or inappropriate." The result was growing conflict between medical providers and insurers. As the head of an association of cancer care centers complained, "Insurers are using the experimental label more and more as an excuse not to pay for well-accepted treatments, and patients are suffering because of it." But insurance companies defended their policies, saying they were "only trying to protect patients from unnecessary medicine and improve the overall quality of care." Meanwhile, consumers affected by these decisions were starting to join the battle, and the article ended with a list of resources they could use to do so.[87]

By the early 1990s, the unpleasant side effects of the health care revolution, including the impact of more competition, third-party intervention, and medical marketing and advertising, began to emerge as a hot political issue.

During the 1992 presidential election, health care became a central issue. Republican incumbent George H. W. Bush favored the Reagan-era changes, and his Democratic challenger, Bill Clinton, criticized them. The extensive policy and press discussion of the subject highlighted a growing divide between conservative and moderate approaches to the insurance problem.[88]

Clinton won the election, and polling done in 1993 showed that two-thirds of Americans backed reforming the health insurance system. Clinton created the President's Task Force on Health Care, officially headed by First Lady Hillary Clinton but run in practice by longtime Clinton associate Ira Magaziner. He set up more than thirty working groups with a total of more than 500 members, most of them from within the federal government. The arrangement generated enormous political and legal resistance. One physician group sued over the task force's closed-door meetings; representatives of the private insurance industry protested that they had no role in deliberations.[89] Unveiled in September 1993, the task force's plan called for the creation of a national network of regional health alliances that would offer consumers at least three types of insurance: traditional fee-for-service, HMOs, and preferred-provider plans. All types of insurance were required to be open to everyone, regardless of prior medical conditions, and had to include certain services. Coverage would be financed primarily by subscriber premiums, with the possibility of additional funding coming from tax breaks, savings from Medicare and Medicaid cost containment, and other sources.[90]

While the plan initially seemed to have substantial support, it soon foundered as a consequence of opposition from multiple directions. Some influential Democrats still strongly preferred the single-payer model—that is, a national health system run by the government—and viewed the Clinton plan as making too many concessions to the corporatist model of managed care. Republican strategists questioned the existence of a health care crisis and instead reframed the problem as an "entitlement" crisis. In their view, Americans had become too dependent on third-party generosity from the government and their employers and needed to face up to the true costs of medical care. Conservatives preferred what became known as "consumer-driven" health care: giving everyone a lump sum to buy insurance and letting them bargain to get what they wanted.[91]

Media coverage of the Clinton plan reinforced its kinship with managed-care measures that had become increasingly unpopular. Given the uncertainties of the changing medical economy, the idea of further limiting consumers' ability to doctor-shop had limited appeal, perhaps because people still had strong attachments to their personal physicians, perhaps because of the long-running assumption that the power to switch doctors was essential. Middle-class Americans accepted the idea of forcing poor people into Medicaid HMOs but rejected that fate for themselves.

The celebrated "Harry and Louise" advertisements played to those fears. Paid for by the Health Insurance Association of America, a trade association representing smaller health insurance companies that feared being put out of business by the Clinton exchanges, the 1993–94 TV commercials featured a middle-class couple at their kitchen table, contemplating the possibility of federally imposed limits on their insurance coverage. As Louise comments sadly, "Having choices we don't like is no choice at all." Not surprisingly, given the ads' sponsors, the campaign portrayed the federal government, not the insurance industry, as the patient-consumer's enemy. In fact, relatively few Americans saw the Harry and Louise ads firsthand: they ran only on cable and targeted the New York City and Washington, D.C., areas, as well as the hometowns of key legislators, a strategy meant to maximize their political impact. The strategy worked; the ads were mentioned over 700 times in newspaper coverage of the insurance debate as a reflection of consumer fears about the Clinton plan.[92]

The perception that the Clinton plan would force many more Americans into managed-care plans or HMOs doomed the proposal. After months of bitter wrangling, Senate majority leader George Mitchell declared the legislation dead in September 1994. But in the wake of its defeat, managed-care plans made important course corrections: the harshest features were softened, and efforts to emphasize higher quality achieved new prominence.

Although the national-level reform had failed, the uproar over managed care ushered in far greater regulation and oversight of plans at the state level, where insurance regulation had traditionally been located. To protect patient-consumers from denial of care and other abuses, many states passed laws regulating the insurance plans' methods and mandating that they set up complaint and grievance procedures. The federal National Committee for Quality Assurance sought to develop voluntary standards for accrediting managed-care plans that would correct their worst flaws and improve public trust. The uproar also caused many managed-care organizations to relax the most stringent limits on patients' and physicians' options. By the early 2000s, some commentators began to declare managed care dead. More accurately, however, insurance companies had realized that the goals of cost containment had to be aligned more closely with those of quality: constraints aimed solely at saving money would fail, but those that saved money and promised better care might succeed. Thus the managed-care crisis fed back into the long-standing quest for higher medical standards.[93]

For physicians intent on wresting back some control over their therapeutic decision making, the managed-care controversy reinforced the importance of the idea that only doctors should set standards for doctors. Various medical groups began to develop clinical guidelines designed to encourage best practices for the treatment of specific illnesses. In 1990, the IOM issued a report promoting such guidelines but also critiquing their growing volume. In 1993, British physician Archie Cochrane created the Cochrane Collaboration, in which groups conducted exacting metareviews to determine evidence-based best practices. Such guidelines would enable physicians to make quality and outcome more important as measures of what care would be reimbursed.[94]

Along the same lines, the failure of national reform stimulated even more attention to the ways health sciences research could encourage "changing the system from within," in the words of journalist Michael Millenson. Extending the emphasis on accountability evident in the disclosure of the HCFA mortality data and the creation of the National Practitioner Data Bank, a variety of private and public groups, among them the NIH and the IOM, undertook efforts to improve institutional quality control. Created by Congress in 1989, the Agency for Healthcare Research and Quality survived the partisan battles of the Clinton administration and became a funding source and clearinghouse for health services research. By the late 1990s, policy experts shifted to what appeared to be a more winnable battle: as Millenson wrote, "While much public discussion focuses on the plight of the uninsured or the intricacies of managed care, the dangerous gap between 'best care' and everyday care has been ignored." To address that gap called for a "revolution of accountability for results." At the brink of a new century, Millenson optimistically concluded, "Information Age medicine lies within our grasp."[95]

In this vision of Information Age medicine, informed consumers retained an important role as useful allies whose cooperation was essential to the hard work of voluntary reform. Patients as watchdogs needed to be educated to learn what medical best practices were and to demand them from their physicians; laypersons could be taught to use decision aids to compare the performance of various health insurance plans. But the limits of that watchdog model remained evident.

Far from being a victory for enlightened medical consumerism, the managed-care "crisis" of the 1990s exposed the contradictory trends and views of the preceding two decades: the greater attention to consumer choice and preference clashed with managerial methods that limited both. Although the Harry and Louise ads succeeded by portraying middle-class patient-consumers as innocent victims of ineffective governance, other more negative views emerged of their role in creating the health care crisis. Policy experts could blame consumers for being manipulated by political sloganeering and attack ads. Or they could be lambasted for refusing to understand the urgent need for cost control. Perhaps inevitably, the enthusiasm for consumer empowerment as a new and powerful policy tool faded as its limits in fomenting deep change became all too apparent.

From the patients' perspective, the new spirit of "shopping mall medicine" created additional shopping hazards while failing to correct many of the old ones. What resulted from the ferment of the 1980s was not a well-run medical department store but a confusing and frustrating health care bazaar. Despite the tangible gains on specific issues—for example, clinics that had longer hours and allowed patients to pay with their credit cards, and better information about hospital mortality rates—other troubles emerged. The new market medicine reinforced the long-standing tendency to promote high-cost treatments regardless of their efficacy; it was the 1980s version of the old slogan, "Give the lady what she wants"—that is, doctors honored paying patients' requests for whatever expensive products and procedures they wanted. The route to profitability remained increasing the amount of care. In short, the transformation of the medical economy accentuated rather than slowed the trends toward high costs and lack of coordination.

At the same time, the new "age of accountability" trained a powerful spotlight on the system's defects: fragmentation and inefficiency were accompanied by uneven quality and medical errors. Interpreting massive new bodies of data about both therapeutic practice and spending patterns, researchers documented enormous room for improvement. Committed to more evidence-based medicine and cost-effective health care, they produced a steady stream of studies aimed at encouraging these goals. In the face of institutional fragmentation and inertia, translating their findings into formats that consumers could use to make better choices seemed like a necessary and laudable quest. With the assistance of newspaper journalists eager and willing to file Freedom of Information Act requests, the barriers against data release began to weaken. Along with the disclosure of more information came a predictable cycle of criticism that repeated over and over again in the years to come: data would be disclosed but would be found incomplete and hard to interpret and hence misleading to consumers. These criticisms would reinforce the idea that if only better information could be compiled and made available, consumers would benefit. But turning data into usable "decision aids" for individual patient-consumers proved extremely difficult. If the therapeutic and technical complexity of medical decision making proved hard for doctors and policy experts to comprehend, consumers felt even more "dazed and confused."

By virtue of becoming more prominent players, however limited their actual influence, patient-consumers became deeply implicated in policymakers' medical blame game. Even as the image of the dazed and confused consumer remained relevant, the "new consumerism" became a convenient whipping boy for the continued problems of the health care economy. Having been promoted as watchdogs against high costs and bad quality, patient-consumers now found themselves blamed individually and collectively for their failures to get good care. That blame game encompassed not only the procedures and tests that doctors ordered in medical offices and hospital suites but also the expanding array of drugs they prescribed. The same trends transforming the doctor's office affected the drugstore as well. The rise of the big box drugstore brought its own set of complications to the shopping problems faced by late-twentieth-century patients. No matter how much new information they received, the challenge of making informed choices remained daunting.

{ELEVEN}

Medicine-Chest Roulette

In May 1988, shortly before embarking on its hospital rating venture, *U.S. News and World Report* carried a sobering article about the nation's drug supply. But instead of focusing on illegal drugs such as heroin and cocaine, author Steve Findlay directed his readers' attention to America's "other drug problem"—the careless use of prescription medicines in what he dubbed "medicine-chest roulette." Accutane, a new drug for treating severe acne, illustrated his point. Thanks to the Reagan administration's efforts to reduce regulatory red tape, the FDA had fast-tracked the drug through the approval process. Then despite the maker's warnings that pregnant women should not take the drug, doctors had prescribed it to them, resulting in an estimated 1,300 babies born with birth defects, some of them very serious. While especially horrific, the Accutane tragedy was by no means unique. As Findlay reported, an estimated 6 million Americans reported adverse drug reactions each year. While most problems were transitory, some 500,000 people required hospitalization, and between 60,000 and 140,000 died from the adverse reactions.[1]

Pharmaceutical companies could not be blamed for this situation, Findlay argued, because they met their legal obligation to disclose drugs' known side effects to physicians and pharmacists. Rather, the problem lay in the fact that neither group passed on this vital information to their patients. A recent FDA survey found that 70 percent of patients had not been instructed about how to take their prescription drugs properly or what potential side effects to watch for. The same survey discovered that only 3 percent of patients felt entitled to ask their doctors or pharmacists for that information. To escape the dangers of medicine-chest roulette, patients needed to become more educated consumers. To that end, Findlay provided his readers with a checklist of questions to ask their doctors as well as a bibliography of reference books to consult about prescription medicines.[2]

Findlay's warnings arrived at a time when the drugstore was in turmoil. Like the doctor's office, the retail drug trade was strongly affected by both medical consumerism and the growing antiregulatory mood in national politics. Unlike the doctor's office, its turmoil did not reflect the sudden arrival of for-profit companies or intense competition; corporations had long been involved in both making and selling drugs, and pharmaceuticals had a well-deserved reputation for being fiercely competitive. But even in an economic sector long used to combat, post-1970 developments introduced an unprecedented degree of instability.

After almost two decades of tightening up drug regulation, the political climate changed dramatically with Ronald Reagan's 1980 election. Reagan had campaigned on a promise to reduce government red tape. As he claimed in a standard stump speech, "Free enterprise is becoming far less free in the name of something called consumerism." In the view of Reagan and his fellow conservatives, Americans were now such smart shoppers that they no longer needed the protections against the marketplace designed for an earlier, more naive generation. As James C. Miller III, Reagan's appointee to head the FTC, explained while announcing that his agency would stop enforcing 1970s truth-in-advertising rules, "Consumers are not as gullible as most regulators think they are." Virginia Knauer, the Reagan White House's consumer spokesperson, agreed: "Consumers are very sophisticated, and by making their own choices in the free marketplace, they become the regulators."[3]

Not everyone agreed that less regulation represented a gain for American consumers. As the director of Consumers Union put it, the Reagan administration's approach threatened to take the United States "back into the age of 'let the buyer beware,' or maybe even 'let the buyer be milked.'" But those critical voices were swamped by conservatives' enthusiasm for easing regulatory burdens on the pharmaceutical industry. Claiming to act on behalf of consumers' best interests, legislators and business leaders dismantled constraints on the sale and promotion of prescription drugs laid down in the Progressive era. As a result, drugstores lost their monopoly on the right to sell prescription drugs; both supermarkets and the new big box stores such as Walmart were permitted to set up prescription departments. Perhaps most dramatically, the same "advertising is information" argument used to overturn the ban on physician advertising imposed by the AMA led to a new generation of prescription drug promotions aimed directly at patient-consumers.[4]

All these changes were made with the promise that Americans could now shop for their drugs with greater confidence and convenience. But as the drugstore and its product lines changed, it soon became apparent that with new freedoms came greater risks as well. Under intense competition to maintain their profitability, pharmaceutical companies worked to find new blockbuster drugs to promote aggressively to both physicians and consumers. At the same time, the pharmaceutical industry—as well as many physicians— continued to resist mandatory leaflet programs, preferring instead to shift the obligation of asking questions to the patient. The aggressive advertising of new drugs, the growing extent of polypharmacy, and the loopholes of regulation converged to heighten the dangers involved in medicine-chest roulette. More than twenty-five years after passage of the Kefauver-Harris Amendment, the "news you could use" about prescription drugs, as *U.S. News* tagged its article, consisted of some surprisingly familiar advice: Be careful what you bring home from the drugstore.

Consumers on the Fast Track

Like the makeover of the doctor's office, the late-twentieth-century refashioning of the drugstore built on reforms put in place during the 1960s and 1970s. A conviction that both prescription and over-the-counter drugs were now safer and more carefully regulated led to a weakening of the drugstores' dominance in their sales. In the name of better serving a health-conscious America, large supermarket chains and a new kind of discount "big box" store typified by Sam Walton's Walmart began to challenge the drugstores' hold on prescription drug sales. As *Marketing News* reported in 1986, "Today's consumer is on a fast track, and retail store formats are changing with the times." The result was a fundamental alteration in the way Americans shopped for their medicines.[5]

Without necessarily intending to do so, the consumer drug reforms adopted in the 1960s contributed to the dismantling of the drugstores' traditional market protections. Both the FDA and the FTC conducted sweeping product reviews and regulatory overhauls designed to guarantee that drug products were safe, effective, and responsibly advertised. By the late 1970s, the FDA could proudly report that its Drug Efficacy Study Implementation and over-the-counter drug reviews had removed dangerous and ineffective products from the marketplace. Both the FDA and the FTC had also tightened up their surveillance of drug promotion and advertising, adopting stricter guidelines that remained in force even after growing industry resistance put a damper on regulatory activism. These changes helped to undercut the old assumption that medicines could be sold safely only in drugstores. Given that all drugs, over-the-counter as well as prescription products, had been vetted by the FDA, and that consumer drug advertising was now held to higher standards, it seemed safe to sell all these items in other stores. Citing

American consumers' rising health consciousness and desire for convenience, retailers who had long sought to challenge the drugstore's exclusive hold on prescription medicines finally began to succeed.

Predictably, given the two industries' long rivalry, supermarkets moved first to challenge the drugstore's dominance in the sale of prescription drugs. Starting in the 1960s, large supermarket chains such as Pathmark, Giant Food, and Kroger began to look to circumvent state pharmacy laws by buying and relocating drugstores next door to their supermarkets. Kroger, for example, began to operate in tandem with the Super X chain of drugstores. State pharmacy boards tried to block supermarket interlopers, but as the legislative and juridical mood turned more favorable toward both consumerism and competition, the boards lost ground. Traditional restrictions on how and where consumers could buy drugs, including prescription medications, crumbled during the 1960s. By 1970, according to the supermarket trade association, more than half of all prescriptions were being filled at supermarket pharmacies. Over the next two decades, the restrictions softened even further, so that pharmacy departments no longer needed to be housed separately but became part of the store's footprint.[6]

Along with supermarkets, drugstores gained another significant rival in the 1970s in the form of discount big box stores. The pioneers here were Sam Walton's Arkansas-based Walmart and S. S. Kresge's Michigan-based Kmart, which in the 1960s began to open big stores that lowered prices and raised the volume of sales on an expanding range of goods, including food, household items, and health and beauty products. As inflation sent more women into the workforce during the late 1960s and early 1970s, the appeal of discounted one-stop shopping increased rapidly. By 1990, the two chains had more than 3,300 stores nationwide and had inspired the growth of other "combo stores."[7]

Both the discount big box and the expanding supermarket chains sought to cut into the drugstore's sales of prescription drugs, along with over-the-counter medicines and health and beauty aids. Being able to fill prescriptions helped to boost other product categories. One supermarket manager noted that after adding prescription drugs to the store's lines, all the health and beauty sales increased and "suddenly, there was more restocking of shelves and less dusting of product."[8] Busy Americans intent on one-stop shopping at low prices could choose to buy all those products at a big box store rather than a drugstore.

Thus retail pharmacy, long an industry subject to fierce competition, became even more so, as drugstores lost their treasured hold over prescription drug sales. As fast-tracked consumers began to patronize supermarkets and big box stores, retail drugstores saw significant losses across all categories of goods. Explained the editor of *Drug Store News*, "There are just too many avenues consumers can use to get their hands on largely similar merchandise." Perhaps most painful was the end to their monopoly on the sale of prescription medicines. By the early 1990s, 22 percent of the nation's 30,300 supermarkets, 50 percent of its Kmarts, and 69 percent of its Walmarts had pharmacy departments.[9]

But after an initial period of dismay similar to that felt in medicine, drugstores regrouped and found new ways to remain both popular and profitable. They redoubled their efforts to combine convenience with service and played to their historic association with pharmacy as a means to attract a particular kind of health-conscious consumer. Responding to the unsettled state of medicine, including the advent of managed care, drugstores sought to portray themselves "as being in the healthcare and customer service sectors, rather than as purveyors of merchandise."[10] By freshening up their image as the neighborhood corner store, drugstores managed not only to survive but to prosper in an uncertain retail climate.

In reinventing themselves, retail drugstores adapted rather than abandoned their existing retail footprint. The big chains continued to seek out prime locations on busy corners, relied on familiar logos to draw the eye, and made their stores more accessible by adding drive-through windows. Drugstores also expanded their square footage: by the 1980s, a regular store averaged 7,500 square feet and a "super drugstore" 25,000 square feet, still smaller than the big box or combination store's 40,000 square feet. (Today's Walgreens stores average about 14,500 square feet.) While expanding their footprint, stores maintained their traditional arrangement of goods, with the prescription counter at the back and convenience goods at the front of the store. As one marketing analyst noted, people were so familiar with the drugstore's layout that when shopping there, "they can almost do it blindfolded."[11]

By staying smaller than a big supermarket or Walmart store and sticking to the same basic layout, drugstores aimed to make shopping easier. At the same time, their comparatively smaller size required them to be more strategic about what goods they stocked. In the face of growing competition, chains refocused their attention on what management analysts described as their "core" categories: prescriptions, over-the-counter medications, toiletries, and cosmetics. By offering what one industry analyst described as "superior assortments, convenience and prices," chain drugstores remained both popular with shoppers and profitable for investors.[12]

That refined focus started with the prescription counter. As a 1989 report on CVS Pharmacy noted, "The prescription drug business still remains the heart and soul of chain drug stores"; prescriptions accounted for 30 percent of CVS stores' sales volume, up from 25 percent in 1983. Even as supermarket pharmacies cut into their totals, chain drugstores continued to dominate the prescription-filling business, providing 41 percent of all prescriptions as of 1990, a share that has subsequently remained more or less stable. This success was helped by the fact that both the number of prescriptions and their price rose steadily during the 1980s. Surprisingly, from the retail druggists' stand-point, the growing popularity of generic drugs, old drugs that had come out of patent protection and now were cheaper, tended to work in their favor: even with lower prices, generics offered drugstores a better profit margin—50–80 percent compared to only 20–40 percent for brand-name drugs.[13]

In competing for the prescription trade, drugstores played up their long experience in providing that service while also trying to improve it. Stores sought to upgrade their tracking of customers' prescribing histories and to offer in-store drug counseling. As more people came to be covered under managed-care insurance plans with drug benefits, pharmacy department staff helped them deal with pharmacy benefit managers. To promote better ser-vice, large chain drugstores were early adopters of electronic technologies that facilitated the exchange of therapeutic and claims information. Among the first retail chains to explore the use of the Internet as a patient education tool was the Drug Emporium, a large deep-discount drug chain headquartered in Columbus, Ohio.[14]

Similarly, drugstores played to their long experience in selling over-the-counter medications, now even more popular as part of the late-twentieth-century interest in health promotion. As *Marketing News* declared in 1980, the American people had gone on a "self-medication kick": "It was physicians who were commanded 'heal thyself,' but increasingly patients are taking up the challenge, bypassing the doctor, and relying on themselves for treatment, particularly for common or minor ailments." Taking advantage of drug prod-ucts' enhanced reputation as safe and well labeled, thanks to the FDA review, drugstores concentrated on offering a bigger selection of packaged medical goods and health supplies than supermarkets carried. Drugstores also sought to attract more health-conscious shoppers by expanding shelf space to in-clude vitamins, herbal remedies, and natural foods.[15]

While seeking to draw "activated" patient-consumers with a strong interest in health, drugstores continued to offer a wide variety of nonhealth goods designed to satisfy the one-stop shopper, often depicted as a working wife and mother. As a 1984 study of more than 12,000 drugstore users concluded,

"The prime shopper is working, has less time to shop, and is spending less time shopping." At the same time, market research continued to show that most consumers did not make up their minds about what to buy until they were actually in the drugstore's aisles and that one-third of all purchases made there were unplanned. Even this busy shopper could be swayed by the right kind of in-store appeal. Thus stores devoted considerable effort not only to making sure they stocked the right mix of conveniences but also to the marketing methods necessary to draw shoppers' attention to those items. Observed an industry executive, "Retailers who put 'pizzazz' in their stores can expect much higher sales."[16]

Like their promotional store forebears, late-twentieth-century drugstores excelled at bringing "pizzazz" to their aisles, from eye-catching displays of the latest cosmetics to coupon-dispensing machines and shopping carts equipped with video displays. Led by the Connecticut firm Actmedia, specialized marketing companies sprang up to help drugstores do a better job with in-store promotions. One popular innovation was POP Radio, where for a hefty fee (as much as $1,000 per outlet) a store could get an audio system that played specially taped cassettes, complete with a disc jockey who combined music and entertainment with product promotions. Introduced in 1985, POP Radio could be found in 7,000 drugstores by 1988 and had begun to move into supermarkets.[17]

While working hard to leverage their traditional strengths in medicine and health products, drugstores paid attention to other profitable sectors as well. The big chains upgraded their cosmetic counters and hired more staff to provide beauty advice; stocked more groceries so that shoppers could buy a gallon of milk or a box of cereal; and expanded their lines of stationery and seasonal items such as Halloween candy and Easter baskets. Particularly profitable was the move into the photo-finishing business; drugstore chains set up easy-to-find and well-stocked counters at the front of the store where customers could purchase film and other camera goods as well as leave their film for processing. Thus the new corner store was reinvented to suit the late-twentieth-century consumer. Enthused the *Drug Store News* in 1997 about the Long's chain in California, stores prospered by making the one-stop-shopping experience more fun: depending on a manager's interests, local stores might feature local wines, sporting goods, art supplies, fresh produce, or recently baked bread, along with an extensive array of vitamins and a pharmacy staff very knowledgeable about the state's many managed-care plans.[18]

Faced with an end to their monopoly on selling prescription drugs, drugstores not only survived but flourished by refocusing on the product lines that had long served them well. Kroger and Walmart might have opened prescription departments, but their drugstore rivals competed effectively by offering higher levels of professional service and better rapport with doctors and patients. Despite strong competition from general retailers, drugstores found a profitable mix of their old standbys—prescriptions, packaged medical goods, and health-related products—and supplemented it with new services such as photo developing. In so doing, drugstore operators drew on their long experience with retail competition and the effective use of advertising and marketing. These efforts attracted comparatively little fanfare, unlike the new advertising by hospitals and medical groups. POP Radio and electronic dispensing of coupons hardly seemed as radical as offering discounts in the maternity ward or advertising hernia operations with a 1-800 telephone number.

This competitive environment favored large national chains, which were backed by investment capital and could take advantage of their purchasing power, over the independents, which continued to disappear, as they either went out of business or got bought by a chain. The chains prospered by following big box principles, leveraging economies of scale, careful choice of product line, and relentless advertising to their advantage. By doing so, they could still compete effectively to provide the combination of convenience, thriftiness, and self-indulgence that late-twentieth-century shoppers expected. According to a 1997 *Drug Store News* editorial, the secret to success was to "make the consumer king."[19]

In Search of the Blockbuster

Drugstores' fates remained closely tied to a pharmaceutical industry that was itself in the midst of profound change. For all the investment in film-developing kiosks and greeting-card selections, the drugstore's heart and soul remained its medical goods. By the late 1980s, Americans were spending around $35 billion on prescription medicines and $10 billion on over-the-counter drugs each year.[20] While continuing to show high profits, the companies that made those products found themselves embroiled in fierce controversies over their ways of doing business. Thus, beneath the surface of the cheerful corner store, with its comforting mix of products, lay a more complicated terrain of issues warranting patient-consumer concern.

Like the medical profession, the pharmaceutical industry faced heightened demands for cost-effectiveness, quality control, and consumer protection. On the one hand, its prospects in a postindustrial economy seemed excellent; pharmaceuticals exemplified the concept of a "sunrise industry" able to generate high-paying jobs and provide investors with profitable returns. In a health-obsessed era, its product lines seemed guaranteed to flourish. But like doctors' offices and drugstores, pharmaceutical companies also felt the pressure of growing competition.[21]

Pressure from both consumer advocates and retail outlets eager to take business away from drugstores led to a wave of legislation requiring that prescription drug prices be posted for consumers' use and allowing the substitution of lower-priced generic drugs for their expensive brand-name counterparts. In the 1970s, consumer advocates had started to push states to repeal long-standing regulations forbidding the posting or advertising of prescription drug prices. Noted *Consumer Reports* in 1970, bans on revealing drug prices had been passed "ostensibly on medical and ethical grounds but more likely at the urging of competition-shy drug interests." As prescription drug prices continued to rise, congressional Democrats, chief among them Wisconsin Democratic senator Gaylord Nelson, decried the price-fixing going on in the pharmaceutical industry. Making price information more freely available to patient-consumers seemed one logical way to induce competition and therefore lower prices.[22]

Starting in the late 1960s, a few department store pharmacy departments and drugstore chains began to challenge state laws against posting prices, hoping to win more customers in the process. In one well-publicized case in the early 1970s, the Osco drugstore chain decided to post its drug prices after market research showed consumers to be "overwhelmingly in favor" of the idea. As a company representative told *Consumer Reports*, patient-consumers "felt it was useful information that they were entitled to have"; "after all, every other product in your store is priced so that you can see it." Osco soon found itself in court, sued by state boards of pharmacy in Illinois, Wisconsin, and North Dakota for violating the rules against price advertising. But reflecting the same trend in judicial thinking that led to the removal of the AMA's ban on physician advertising, the higher courts in those states sided with Osco, striking down the drug price bans as an unconstitutional restraint of free speech. In addition, the Justice Department urged state legislators to repeal laws preventing the posting of drug prices. Over the 1970s, drugstores throughout the country came to comply with state and federal requirements that prescription drug prices be posted.[23]

The same pressures helped the fledgling generic drug industry establish its products as a safe and thrifty alternative to expensive prescription medications. The generic industry grew rapidly in the 1970s as many important drugs introduced shortly after World War II lost their patent protection, meaning that any manufacturer could make the drug and sell it without its brand name at greatly reduced prices. The rise of generics coincided with the FDA's Drug Efficacy Study Implementation, which suggested that any drug that remained on the market was both safe and efficacious. Not surprisingly, many pharmaceutical companies resisted generics, arguing that they did not really replicate the quality of their brand-name equivalents and encouraging physicians not to prescribe them.[24]

But the generic option gained strong support among consumers and consumerist groups. For Americans accustomed to hearing that brand names and their advertising campaigns added to a product's cost without necessarily improving its quality, the switch to generics made sense, particularly during the economic downturn of the 1970s. Chain drugstores had long featured proprietary brands of pain relievers and antacids at lower prices, so it seemed logical that the same principle could apply to prescription drugs. In a 1975 article, "How to Pay Less for Prescription Drugs," *Consumer Reports* provided a lengthy lesson on how pharmaceutical companies priced their products and concluded, "Apparently, most prescription dollars are not going for the medication *in* the bottle but for the name *on* it." Likewise, writing to the FTC in support of a model law intended to make generics more accessible, a Medicare recipient described the current situation as "just keeping us consumers in the dark while our savings and income are siphoned right out of our pockets for drugs we need." If in fact the two prescription products were virtually identical, there seemed no reason not to choose the more economical version.[25]

By the mid-1970s, generic alternatives now existed for more than half of the drugs used by American patients, and consumerists pushed for making their use easier. In the face of state pharmacy boards' opposition to generics, consumerists lobbied state legislatures to pass "drug product selection" laws that allowed such substitutions as long as patients were informed. By the late 1970s, all but ten states, mostly in the South and the West, had passed some kind of generic-friendly product selection law, although few were as strong as consumerists wanted.[26] Still, many physicians remained reluctant to use the lower-cost products, out of concern that they were less safe and reliable than their name-brand counterparts, a suspicion encouraged by pharmaceutical companies.

To counter that perception, deregulators and consumer advocates boosted the FDA's ability to evaluate new generic products. In 1984, over intense opposition from the pharmaceutical industry, Congress passed the Drug Price Competition and Patent Term Restoration Act, known as the Hatch-Waxman

Act, which set up an improved process for FDA approval of generic drugs. Generic drug applications subsequently jumped dramatically, and the percentage of generics prescribed steadily rose. Yet concerns about their quality persisted, especially after a late 1980s scandal in which generic companies were caught falsifying test results and bribing FDA officials to get their products approved.[27]

Meanwhile, with patents on old drugs expiring and business lost to generic competitors, pharmaceutical companies needed to discover and patent profitable new drugs. For all the generic competition, the patent-protection system created during the Cold War era still made the introduction and promotion of new brand-name medicines potentially very lucrative. In the language of the 1980s, companies sought "blockbuster" drugs—those that would generate more than $1 billion in sales each year. Two such blockbuster prizes were fluoxetine, better known by its brand name, Prozac, and blood pressure drugs such as captopril (Capoten).[28] Yet finding the next blockbuster drug was by no means easy; for every great success, there were many expensive failures. Drug manufacturers also complained that the FDA's rigorous new drug review process put American companies at a competitive disadvantage relative to their European counterparts.

Ronald Reagan came to office in 1980 promising to reduce this "drug lag," but his administration's budget cuts resulted in staff layoffs that only worsened the problem. In addition, as the AIDS epidemic spread, activists demanded quicker action on drugs that might slow its deadly progress. The Reagan administration responded by encouraging the FDA to create a fast-track system to speed up approvals for promising new drugs.[29] Consumerist critics warned that fast-tracking ran the risk that drugs would be out on the market before their full potential for harm had become clear. While the trade-off of safety for efficacy might make sense with new treatments for a deadly infection such as HIV/AIDS, it seemed more irresponsible for less serious conditions.

The Accutane tragedy brought these issues to the fore, not only forcing the FDA to rethink its fast-tracking process but also adding new intensity to the long-running battle over how much information patient-consumers were entitled to receive about their prescription drugs. Accutane was among the first new drugs fast-tracked under Reagan's "deregulation" scheme when it came on the market in 1982. Though it carried warnings to physicians that it should not be prescribed for pregnant women because it had caused birth defects in laboratory animals, the FDA had no formal system in place to monitor how new drugs were actually being prescribed or what side effects they caused. But by April 1988, the agency had received enough informal reports about Accutane to convene a panel to look into them.[30]

The following month the panel reported back that it had found substantial evidence that physicians had not heeded the FDA warnings about prescribing the drug to pregnant women. They were able to document 62 cases of babies with severe mental retardation and birth defects as a result. Internal staff estimates suggested that the total might be anywhere from 900 to 1,300 cases overall. In response to the report, Accutane's maker argued that it had fulfilled its obligation by warning that the drug should not be taken by pregnant women. But that defense was weakened by the fact that the company's warnings had been given only to doctors and pharmacists. In the absence of evidence that the women had been properly warned of the drug's risks, a wave of personal injury lawsuits followed.

The Accutane case drew attention to the consequences of another high-profile action taken by the Reagan administration: the termination of the FDA's patient information program. In 1979, after five years of debate, the FDA had finally committed to requiring mandatory patient information leaflets for certain classes of high-risk drugs. As described in its final rules for the leaflets, published in September 1980, the agency planned to conduct a three-year pilot program of inserts for ten drug classes that seemed especially prone to problems. They included such widely prescribed medications as the antibiotic ampicillin, the painkiller Darvon, the tranquilizer Valium, the morning-sickness drug Benectin, and the ulcer drug Tagamet—a total of about 300 drug products for which some 120 million prescriptions (about 16 percent of the total) were written annually in the United States. In a concession to physician sensibilities, the pilot program included an opt-out clause: doctors could request that the leaflet not be provided to individual patients whom they deemed unlikely to benefit from the information.[31]

Had the FDA plan been followed, a drug like Accutane would likely have been flagged as needing a mandatory leaflet because of its potential risks to pregnant women. But soon after Reagan's election, the new FDA commissioner, Arthur Hull Hayes, announced the administration's intention to reduce the regulatory burdens on the pharmaceutical industry, and among the first to go would be the mandatory leaflet program. In the *Federal Register* announcement of the termination in 1982, the FDA acknowledged that its decision ran counter to consumer sentiment: "Most individual consumers and consumer organizations expressed opposition to the proposal to revoke the [patient package insert] regulation based on their belief that patients have a right to know about the prescription drugs they are taking, and that health professionals currently fail to provide this information." The FDA agreed with that principle but expressed its belief that "private sector programs," not the government, bore responsibility for providing that information. The private sector had already shown a commendable willingness and ability to do so. Commercial books were now available, many at a "reasonable price," to provide patients with drug-related information. The AMA, the AARP, and the American Society of Hospital Pharmacists had all begun to develop patient-friendly leaflets. To criticisms that this voluntary system would be chaotic, the FDA emphasized instead the benefits to be obtained from competition: with many different private groups developing such materials, messages would be not only more plentiful but also better tailored to reach specific audiences.[32]

In short, the new FDA leaders announced that the private information marketplace was sufficiently strong to fulfill the need for patient counseling about prescription medications. The agency's decision to terminate the mandatory program was deliberately timed to coincide with the 1982 formation of the National Council on Patient Information and Education (NCPIE), a not-for-profit group initially funded by a pharmaceutical company, Ciba-Geigy. Headed by former Democratic congressman Paul G. Rogers, NCPIE brought together representatives from the pharmaceutical industry, retail pharmacy, the medical profession, and consumer groups to improve the quality and quantity of drug-related information provided to American patients. NCPIE was formed explicitly to prove the point that an informational free market could educate Americans about their prescription drugs without any help from the FDA. When asked about the FDA's leaflets, Rogers argued that they "would do little to stimulate the needed dialogue" between doctors and patients, quipping, "Besides, the print is so small on those things."[33]

As a better alternative, NCPIE promoted public awareness campaigns aimed at getting patient-consumers to learn more about how to use their prescription medications. The group acknowledged that doctors and pharmacists had a responsibility to provide patients this information but noted that many people, particularly the elderly, were not taking the initiative to ask for it. To solve the problem, patient-consumers had to become more responsible for getting their information needs met. "Go ahead, ask your doctor or pharmacist," began one NCPIE brochure. In that spirit, the group distributed a card with five questions that seniors should ask their caregivers, including the name of the drug; what it was supposed to do; how and when to take it; what foods, drugs, and activities to avoid while taking it; and what side effects to watch out for. Rogers explained, "We hope our question-asking campaign will close the huge gap that exists between what patients say they are receiving and what health professionals say they are communicating about prescription drugs."[34]

Similar to the NCPIE campaign, the AARP, the AMA, the National Association of Retail Druggists, and other groups sponsored a range of outreach campaigns that acknowledged doctors' and pharmacists' duties but highlighted patients' responsibility to seek out information rather than wait to receive it. If patients failed to ask questions and then had problems, they were considered "noncompliant." Adverse effects from prescription drug use could be attributed to patients' failure to take advantage of the many information sources now available to them.[35]

This "before you take it, talk about it" approach attracted considerable criticism. In an interview with the *Washington Post*, Jere Goyan, the former head of the FDA and dean of the School of Pharmacy at the University of California, San Francisco, complained, "If we believe patients are entitled to more information, then we ought to require that they get it." *Washington Post* health writer Victor Cohn agreed, "I don't think it will help much to tell an ill or infirm patient, 'you can go to the library and read about this.'" Surgeon General C. Everett Koop worried that the whole burden of responsibility was falling on the patient. But the overall tenor of the 1980s was perhaps best summed up by the physician who noted, "Noncompliance is simply one of the prices to be paid for free will."[36]

As the Accutane tragedy revealed, the "price of free will" could be very steep. The voluntary system of drug information created in the 1980s did not work as well as conservatives hoped. In 1991, when the FDA reviewed the leaflet initiative, they found it had been of limited success for precisely the reasons that consumer groups had predicted. A voluntary program left to doctor and patient discretion was not working. Surveys suggested that only 32 percent of patients received any kind of written information about their drug. The leaflets varied widely in format and comprehensiveness: some consisted of a few bullet points, while others offered several pages of information. Many were written in a technical language that most patients could not understand. Acknowledging these problems, the Clinton administration decided in 1995 once again to consider having the FDA mandate leaflets for drugs with "serious and significant side effects." But the idea again generated stiff resistance, leading the agency to settle for more authority to set "performance standards" for the private production of leaflets.[37]

The DTCA Revolution

The advent of direct-to-consumer advertising (DTCA) of prescription drugs brought even more controversy into the late-twentieth-century drug field. During the same years that patient leaflets were under debate, pharmaceutical companies began to advertise the "doctors' drugs" directly to consumers in ways they had never done before. Ironically, much as consumers' interests were invoked in striking down the AMA's ban on physician advertising, they were used also to justify a vast expansion in prescription drug promotions to the public.

The absence of DTCA of prescription drugs prior to the late 1970s reflected not a legal ban but a voluntary decision on the part of drug manufacturers. Nothing in the federal laws passed in 1938 or 1962 explicitly prohibited companies from promoting prescription drugs to patients, but as they well knew, physicians were deeply opposed to the practice. In addition, after the FDA assumed oversight of prescription drug advertising in 1962, as required by the Kefauver-Harris Amendment, its more stringent guidelines seemed to make advertising to consumers virtually impossible. Those guidelines required that ads be accompanied by a separate section, known as the "brief summary," conveying essential information about effectiveness, contraindications, and side effects. Belying their name, those sections were rarely brief. In early cable television drug ads broadcast to physicians, scrolling the brief summary could take as much as ten minutes of broadcast time. As FDA official Kenneth Feather later noted, "No one is going to pay for ten minutes of time to run a brief summary" during a prime-time TV show. If meeting the FDA criteria for ads aimed at professionals posed such problems, doing the same for promotions aimed at consumers seemed nearly impossible.[38]

But in the 1970s, these problems started to seem more surmountable. The same juridical doctrine used to overturn the AMA's ban on physician advertising—that advertising conveyed valuable information to consumers—could be used to argue for comparable forms of drug promotion. In addition, the FTC had shown that tighter regulation of over-the-counter drug advertising, long the focal point of consumerist criticism, was in fact possible. While the FTC ceased forceful prosecution under the unfairness doctrine, its guidelines regarding substantiation and comparison remained in force, ensuring that claims made for pain relievers and stomach soothers would be reasonably accurate. Over-the-counter drug advertising had become so much tamer that ads could mock their former selves: a famous 1984 advertisement for Vicks Formula 44 cough syrup had soap opera actors declare, "I'm not a doctor but I play one on TV." If the advertising for Geritol and Bufferin could be rehabilitated, why not try advertising prescription drugs as well?[39]

With the election of the probusiness, antiregulation Reagan in 1980, this prospect seemed even more likely. In the spring of 1982, his appointee to head the FDA, Arthur H. Hayes, gave a speech to pharmaceutical company executives that seemed to suggest that the agency might be rethinking its opposition to DTCA. Although he later denied having intended to send that signal, Hayes's remarks attracted considerable attention from representatives of pharmaceutical companies, physician groups, and consumer organizations.[40] Some pharmaceutical executives strongly supported the idea of DTCA as a logical extension of the new medical consumerism, which had created a seemingly insatiable appetite for information about new drugs. Others in the industry expressed caution about advertising to consumers, fearing that physicians—who still bore sole responsibility for writing prescriptions—would resent the consumer pressure that such advertising might unleash.

This fear had merit: surveys done in the early 1980s by *American Druggist* and the *AMA News* found that 69 percent of pharmacists and 64 percent of physicians opposed DTCA, compared to only 7 percent who favored it. But ignoring physician opposition to DTCA posed less of a risk now that the once-formidable power of organized medicine appeared to be on the decline. By professing their devotion to medical consumerism, pharmaceutical companies could justify this break with medical tradition. A few companies thus began cautiously to test the DTCA waters.[41]

The British pharmaceutical firm Boots was the first to dip in a toe with a February 1982 print ad campaign stressing cost and effectiveness, issues of traditional interest to patient-consumers. The Boots ads offered seniors a rebate on Rufen, one of its arthritis drugs, and promoted ibuprofen, then still a prescription drug, as cheaper yet as effective as other brands. Boots followed up the print promotion with ads on a local Tampa, Florida, television station, also with FDA approval. As the U.S. president of Boots, John Bryer, explained at a meeting of the Pharmaceutical Advertising Council, the company chose to advertise only drugs that doctors and patients were already familiar with. "We would never have considered doing something like this, going in a direct way to the consumer, if we were talking about a new drug entity." To promote a new drug with which doctors had no familiarity "would be a dangerous thing to do." But, as he acknowledged, "we know we are breaking new ground" by "trying to establish rapport with the consumer." "Ads will give information, yes, but they will also carry a silvery punch, which is to sell the product."[42]

In the wake of Boots's venture, other companies began to try out the "silvery punch" for new products that they felt represented major breakthroughs in treatment. For example, Merck Sharp and Dohme ran ads in magazines widely read by older Americans suggesting that patients ask their doctors about the company's new Pneumovax vaccine against bacterial pneumonia. Similarly, in 1983, the Peoples Drug Store chain took out full-page ads for Zovirax, a new ointment that helped heal genital herpes. As a story in the *Washington Post* noted, "For long-suffering herpes victims facing frequent flareups of an incurable disease that most people are too embarrassed to talk about, the availability of a new treatment was encouraging news."[43]

The spread of cable TV multiplied the debate regarding the new direct-to-consumer ads. Cable was quickly changing the broadcast industry by allowing far more diverse television fare than the three main networks offered. In an era of increasing awareness of market segmentation, cable networks could better target viewers with particular interests in terms of both programming and advertising. Cable executives also proved more willing than their broadcast counterparts to defy old rules about what was in good taste to show on television. Thus cable networks began to experiment with "more liberal guidelines regarding drinking, sex and other pastimes," in the words of one business journalist, broadcasting ads that broke long-standing taboos by featuring live women wearing lingerie and couples drinking wine in suggestive scenarios. Cable's "liberalization" soon came to include drug advertising to consumers as well.[44]

In 1983 the Cable Health Network, which specialized in health programming for laypeople, decided to run *Physician's Journal Club*, a weekly show aimed at physicians hosted by Dr. Art Ulene. The network obtained FDA permission to show prescription drug ads eight times per hour during the show, with both parties aware that there would be no way to prevent non-physicians from watching. Beginning in June 1983, therefore, lay viewers in an estimated 10 million American homes could see exactly the same drug ads as the target audience of physicians. According to Lloyd Milstein, acting director of the FDA's Division of Drug Advertising and Labeling, "a certain amount of eavesdropping by laymen" was inevitable, but the ads were so technical that there was little likelihood the general public could understand them.[45]

As these new forms of advertising began to appear in print and on television, they attracted fierce criticism from organized consumer groups. Echoing arguments made since the 1930s, they rejected the premise that advertising presented information useful to American patient-consumers. In March 1983, the FDA responded to these complaints by holding a "consumer exchange" at which advocates could air their concerns. Participants in the exchange pointed out the disturbing contrast between the FDA's recent abandonment of its patient package insert program and its softening stance toward DTCA. As Fred Wegner of the AARP stated, "It is incredible to some of us [that] the FDA is not developing methods of assuring widespread patient drug information from non-industry sources but is considering permitting the industry to extend its product promotions to consumers themselves." Consumer advocates spoke favorably only of advertisements that provided price comparisons and made clear their resolve to pressure their allies in Congress, such as Democrats Henry Waxman of California and John Dingell of Michigan, to resist any further FDA softening toward the ads.[46]

The FDA's subsequent decision to allow ads on Cable Health Network prompted another round of outrage. Observed Ann Everett of the Consumer Federation of America, "This is already a pill-popping society. We don't need to encourage that." Speaking on behalf of the AARP, Judy Brown noted that pharmaceutical companies already spent three times more on advertising and promotion than they did on research. "Ads by nature are meant to increase sales," she stated, and "direct-to-consumer ads would create a demand for a product not based on need." Brown's group, representing the elderly Americans who were the largest consumers of prescription drugs, sent a mass mailing to every one of its 14 million members expressing the organization's opposition to the idea. Dingell announced his intention to have his powerful house subcommittee look into the DTCA issue, and by the early fall of 1983, it had emerged as "one of the hottest issues to confront the FDA in years," as Roger Miller, the editor of the *FDA Consumer* magazine, noted.[47]

At the time the controversy began, the FDA guidelines on advertising adopted in 1968 seemed to be working reasonably well. The agency's disciplinary tools—requiring companies that ran misleading ads to write doctors confessing their errors or run corrective ads to avoid seizures of their product—kept drug advertising fairly tame in its claims. To resolve problems more peaceably and reduce the need for corrective letters, the FDA instituted an informal process of prescreening promotional campaigns.[48] The more aggressive appeals used in DTCA threatened to upset this hard-won balance. FDA staffers conducting prescreening reviews began to see advertising strategies that made them uncomfortable. Whereas advertising that stressed symptoms relieved or improved formulations could be seen as a valuable form of consumer information, these ads invoked irrational desires that seemed inappropriate in the promotion of a prescription drug.

Among those bothered by the new ads was the head of the FDA, Arthur

Hayes. The son of a former president of CBS radio, Hayes was more familiar with the advertising industry than most physicians were, and this experience made him particularly wary about the impact of DTCA. When agency staff showed him Ciba-Geigy's proposed ad for a new antihypertensive drug, Hayes decided it was time to slow down and reconsider the FDA position. The "Delores ad" highlighted the fact that unlike many antihypertensive drugs, this one did not cause impotence. Set in a health-club-type atmosphere, the ad featured a middle-aged man explaining to a friend that he was taking the new drug and that it did not interfere with his active lifestyle. Then "up to him walks this very lovely young lady"—presumably Delores—"dressed in a bathing suit or a tennis outfit . . . that made her obvious charms noticeable," who turned out to be his new wife. The "hidden message," recalled an FDA official, was clear: the drug would not keep the man from satisfying his attractive and much younger wife. The ad caused Hayes to "hit the ceiling": in his view, such "sexist, frivolous" advertising would "trivialize the importance and the dangerous nature of prescription drugs."[49]

Hayes left the agency in September 1983, yet another in a tradition of short-tenured commissioners, but his reservations bore results. On September 2, 1983, the FDA issued a policy statement requesting that companies observe a voluntary moratorium on DTCA of prescription drugs "to allow time for dialogue among consumers, health professionals, and industry" on its value. Under the oversight of Deputy Commissioner Mark Novitch, the agency began researching how its guidelines, in particular the "brief summary" requirement, could be adapted to consumer advertising. The FDA review culminated in a much-publicized June 1984 meeting during which representatives from consumer groups, pharmaceutical companies, and professional groups discussed the pros and cons of DTCA.[50]

None of this feedback suggested that advertising prescription drugs to consumers would be either easy or popular. After the FDA completed a series of mock prescription ads, Novitch announced that "serious concerns" remained about how well the "fair balance" requirement could be made to work in direct-to-consumer ads. "The primary purpose of advertisements is, by definition, to sell products," he stated. While that fact did "not make advertisements bad," it did "cast them in a limited role as vehicles for conveying a broad spectrum of patient information." For their part, consumer groups, physicians, and pharmacists continued to oppose any increase in prescription drug advertising to consumers. A 1982 Newsweek article, "Ads over the Doctor's Head," captured medical professionals' unease with the practice, which they feared would increase pressure from patients to be given prescriptions for drugs that might not be appropriate. According to Robert H. Moser, executive vice president of the American College of Physicians, "It could add to the whole idea that if you're smart enough to find the right doctor, he'll be smart enough to give you the right pill to solve all your problems." One AMA survey found that more than 60 percent of physicians and pharmacists opposed DTCA, while fewer than 8 percent approved it.[51]

Perhaps more surprising was the extent of industry opposition to the idea. While some companies were eager to press ahead with DTCA of prescription drugs, on the grounds that it represented a valuable form of consumer information, other industry leaders expressed deep reservations about it. At one level, the worries reflected concerns about cost and competition; the added burden of expensive ad campaigns to consumers could make an already intensely competitive field even more so. But leaders also worried about the potential to tarnish the industry's image. At the June 1984 symposium on DTCA of prescription drugs, industry worries were on full display. Polled using new computer technology, 70 percent of the pharmaceutical industry representatives in attendance disagreed with the statement that DTCA was a good idea, although 54 percent said that they would employ it if their competitors did.[52]

A speech by Upjohn's Lawrence C. Hoff at the symposium enumerated the reasons for industry caution. First, he noted, DTCA would be very expensive and might drain resources away from research and development. But he also said, "I see this kind of advertising—be it on television, over the radio or in the pages of our newspapers or magazines—as detrimental to our industry, and perhaps more importantly, as a potentially disruptive element in our medical delivery system as a whole." His conclusion echoed what consumer groups were saying: "There is a vast difference between education and promotion." But during the question-and-answer period, Hoff made clear that if other companies started to advertise to consumers, Upjohn would be forced to do the same: "All of us have to be ready in case the whole dam breaks."[53]

FDA surveys of public opinion suggested decidedly mixed views of DTCA. In focus groups convened to discuss the new advertising, 50 percent of participants opposed any form of prescription drug advertising to consumers, while only 20 percent thought it was a good idea and another 30 percent thought it might be allowable only if kept under very tight control. Opinion polling found similar divisions; a telephone survey done on behalf of the AMA found two-thirds of respondents opposed to television advertising of prescription drugs. But in 1985, over the near-unanimous opposition voiced by consumer advocacy groups, strong reservations expressed by physicians, and significant concerns among pharmaceutical company representatives, the FDA decided to lift the moratorium and let DTCA resume. The FDA affirmed that it would develop no new guidelines to regulate DTCA in particular but would use the same standards for all ads, regardless of their intended audience.[54]

Unlike the statement regarding the leaflet program, which noted the opposition to its termination and explained the reasons for ignoring it, the federal notice regarding the DTCA position provided no summary of the debates surrounding it. According to a House subcommittee, the Reagan White House had pressured FDA staff to rewrite the announcement to delete the statement that "the majority ... of the affected groups does not favor advertising Rx drugs directly to consumers at this time" and thought the disadvantages of doing so far outweighed the advantages. By lifting the moratorium, the administration signaled its strong support for the "belief in the freedom to advertise," in line with a larger trend in conservative thinking to portray advertising as a form of commercial free speech that needed vigorous protection.[55]

After 1985, pharmaceutical companies began to expand their advertising to consumers, moving cautiously at first, concerned about the cost as well as the product liability issues involved. Moreover, meeting the FDA guidelines represented a challenge: as a 1989 *New York Times* article noted, the consumer equivalent of the brief summary "could result in a five-minute commercial, or print so tiny that a magnifying glass would be necessary to read it." While Lexis Pharmaceuticals decided to try the full ad with the required warnings for its contraceptive pills, none of the big pharmaceutical companies followed its lead. Instead, they experimented with ads that did not mention drugs by name and thus under FDA guidelines did not have to discuss the side effects. According to the *New York Times*, "It is a loophole through which pharmaceutical companies and their ad and public relations agencies have been driving fleets of proverbial trucks."[56]

Television networks, however, greatly appreciated this loophole, since advertising revenues had been declining and pharmaceutical companies appeared to offer good prospects for a new source of income. Consumers consequently started to see an ad in which "a little pink stomach with legs and a smile talks about treating ulcers," paid for by the makers of the ulcer medication Tagamet; another spot in which "a 30-ish fellow walks along a beach with his dog, philosophizing about baldness and ways to fight it," paid for by the makers of Rogaine, a treatment for baldness; and one depicting a daughter joyfully telling her mother that "finally, there is an antihistamine that will not put her to sleep," paid for by the makers of Seldane. None of the ads mentioned the product's name; the tag line simply said, "This message brought to you by" and gave the name of the drugmaker, along with the suggestion that patient-consumers talk to their physicians about new treatments. Some companies also began to use celebrity endorsements for their prescription products. Instead of running ads for its new arthritis drug in what was already a highly competitive advertising market, Ciba-Geigy paid baseball great Mickey Mantle to promote Voltaren on talk shows. While the move infuriated many physicians, it did not constitute a form of advertising that the FDA felt it could regulate.[57]

Between 1987 and 1996, pharmaceutical company spending on prescription drug advertising increased from $35 million per year to $790 million. By the mid-1990s, three different types of ads had become common in both print and broadcast sources. The most detailed was the product claim ad, which mentioned the drug by name as well as its indications for use, thus requiring detailed disclosures of possible risks and limitations of efficacy. Product claim ads tended to appear only in print because the "brief summary" took too long for a television ad. In contrast, reminder ads could mention the name of the drug and describe its appearance (a purple pill) but said nothing about why it might be prescribed—only that patients should "ask the doctor." As FDA staffer Kenneth Feather explained, "They can't say what it's for, because that triggers the brief summary information." He continued, "As long as you don't make any representations about what the drug is used for or its dosage, you can say a lot of things in that ad, and they do." Finally, "help-seeking ads"—a new kind of institutional advertising—simply described a problem and suggested that patients see their doctors about it.[58]

Even with its rapid increase, advertising to consumers still constituted only about 19 percent of pharmaceutical promotional spending; the rest remained directed at physicians. But precisely because they were new, the DTCA campaigns attracted enormous attention. Along with continued complaints about both the side effects and high prices of prescription drugs, DTCA became a focal point for criticism. As the volume of ads increased, they inspired fierce denunciations from both medical and consumer groups. In the early 1990s, the AMA, the American College of Physicians, and the American Academy of Family Physicians all went on record as opposing DTCA. Calls for its abolition or restriction met with strong resistance from the pharmaceutical industry, which portrayed such measures as an infringement of corporate free speech. Gradually the debate shifted from whether DTCA should be permitted to what effects it was having and how it could be made more balanced.[59]

In the 1990s, the FDA began to tackle the problems posed by the new advertising campaigns. Those efforts were spearheaded by David Kessler, the FDA commissioner appointed by President George H. W. Bush in 1990. A pediatrician and a lawyer, Kessler came to the position with a deep interest in the advertising and promotion of both food and drugs. Under his guidance, the FDA began gradually to tighten up on its scrutiny of drug advertising. Kessler's approach made him more popular with Democrats than Republicans, and after Bill Clinton's election in 1992, he asked Kessler to stay on as FDA commissioner. Accepting that DTCA was here to stay, the FDA decided the best way to protect consumers was by developing clearer standards for it. To that end, the agency created guidelines, first published in 1997 and finalized in 1999, that gave drug companies more latitude to describe medications and the conditions they relieved so long as they provided a brief summary of their major side effects. By setting out clearer standards for TV ads, a FDA official explained, "we hope to end the uncertainty which has plagued both consumers and industry about the use of this medium."[60]

In the wake of that decision, pharmaceutical companies quickly scaled up their spending on prime-time DTCA, which reached $4.2 billion per year by 2005, eleven times as much as had been spent in 1995. In business terms, DTCA was spectacularly successful: the sales of advertised drugs skyrocketed. Marketing surveys in the early 2000s found that one in five people who saw a prescription drug ad went to the physician to ask for it; half walked out of the office with prescription in hand. An analysis by IMS Management Consulting, the acknowledged authority on drug trends, concluded that the return on investment for the forty-nine drug brands promoted to consumers between 1998 and 2003 had been "nearly unprecedented in terms of the positive sales response generated."[61]

By the early 2000s, drug advertisements had become a mainstay of the American advertising industry. In 2001, the New York ad industry's Effie awards, which recognized creative achievement in the industry, added a category for prescription products, recognizing the ad campaigns for Flovent, Tamiflu, and other medical products. At the same time, however, popular culture frequently began to mock the prescription drug ads flooding both cable and network television. Between 1998 and 2002, *The Tonight Show's* Jay Leno allegedly told 944 Viagra jokes, Whoopi Goldberg made a joke about drug ads while presenting an Oscar, and even Homer Simpson made fun of them. Hayes's concerns about the "Delores ad" nearly two decades earlier seemed to have been borne out by the relentless lampooning of the new drug ads, particularly those concerning erectile dysfunction. In an atmosphere of growing concern over the overuse and expense of prescription drugs, the new visibility of DTCA became a focal point for criticism.[62]

There Can Only Be Safe Patients

The dismantling of long-standing limitations on where prescription drugs could be sold and how they could be advertised had many unsettling consequences for patients and doctors. Trying to refashion the delivery of drug information in the image of a more activated patient proved surprisingly difficult. Because of their perceived status as "unavoidably unsafe," prescription drugs seemed to demand a higher standard of risk disclosure than other kinds of commodities. Invoking the automobile analogy, Feather wryly observed that "ads for Ford don't have brief summaries that give the repair rate, the breakdown rate, [or] the number of people killed in accidents." Yet while drug ads did have to convey that sort of information, the question remained whether the intended audience was doctors or patients. For all the emphasis on educating consumers to make better medical choices, substantive limits remained on the "official" information that patients had a right to get. In the end, as Joe Graedon, author of the syndicated "People's Pharmacy" column, concluded, "There are no absolutely safe drugs. There can only be safe patients: those who are informed and concerned enough to ask the right questions."[63]

The outcome of the 1980s battles over what patient-consumers had a right to know represented a defeat for medical consumerists on two counts: the death of the federally mandated patient information leaflet and the expansion of DTCA to include prescription medications. Paradoxically, resistance to sharing information with patients about their prescription medications went hand in hand with the weakening of traditional barriers on drug advertising directed at them. The argument that American consumers wanted more information to make better choices failed in relation to the mandated patient information leaflet but succeeded in the softening of restrictions on DTCA. Once again, consumer advocates asked for more information but instead got more advertising. Rather than a clearly delineated system of patient education, what emerged was a confusing system of information distribution that imposed new burdens of responsibility for being well-informed on patients without offering them a clearly marked path to achieving that condition. Thus, along with the responsibility of doctor-shopping, patients now had to learn how to decipher prescription drug ads and read their fine print.

The controversies surrounding pharmaceutical company promotional methods as well as drug safety increased pressure on the FDA to increase its level of "pharmacovigilance." Expanded efforts to monitor new drugs after they had been approved and become commonly used constituted one effort in that direction. For years, drug reformers had suggested the need for better postmarket surveillance, especially in the United States, where the means of influencing physician behavior were so diffuse. In 1993, the FDA began to facilitate that surveillance by creating MedWatch, a voluntary system to enable hospitals and health care professionals, including nurses and pharmacists as well as physicians, to report adverse events potentially related to prescription drugs or medical devices.[64]

The changing prescription drug market also encouraged the proliferation and refinement of consumer-oriented guides to prescription drugs. As had long been the case, publishers and journalists sought to provide patient-consumers the latest in "news you can use" about their prescription drug choices. So along with guides to good and bad doctors came a new generation of books devoted to discerning the good from the bad prescription drugs, now increasingly with sections on how to assess the heavy advertising being done by pharmaceutical companies.

In the tradition of Arthur Kallet and F. J. Schlink's *100,000,000 Guinea Pigs* and the Consumers Union's *Medicine Show*, consumer guides to the pitfalls of buying medicine remained one of the most durable of health publishing trends. In addition to a list of doctors to avoid, Public Citizen's Health Research Group published books aimed at helping patients monitor their doctors' prescribing habits, starting with *Pills That Don't Work* (1980) and followed by *Worst Pills, Best Pills: The Older Adult's Guide to Avoiding Drug-Induced Death or Illness* (1988). Both titles were best sellers and went through multiple editions. With the expansion of the Internet, online resources about prescription drugs—and eventually advertising for them—would be one of the main reasons that patient-consumers would venture onto the World Wide Web.[65]

The new burdens of being a "safe patient" compounded the already unsettled state of doctor-patient relationships. For almost forty years, policy and practice had reinforced, for good and ill, the concept of the physician as the patient's learned intermediary: a trusted figure who would serve as the layperson's guide to the powerful yet potentially dangerous world of the doctors' drugs. Largely as a consequence of patient complaints that doctors were doing a poor job in their role as consumer advocates, patients' right to a more informed level of consent had gained considerable ground during the 1970s. But over the next two decades, that right seemed to falter for seemingly contradictory reasons: on the one hand, the belief that physicians should remain in charge of the information flow, and on the other, the idea that advertising directed at patients would help make them better decision makers.

One side effect of these paradoxical developments was a flurry of legal cases questioning the learned intermediary doctrine—that is, the principle that drug companies needed only to warn doctors, not patients, of their products' risks because the former would guide the latter's choices and use of medications. In an era when so much was changing in medicine, the advent of DTCA seemed particularly ominous to lawyers specializing in medical malpractice and liability law. Observed an attorney involved in rewriting the guidelines for product liability, the basis of the learned intermediary doctrine would seem to be "seriously undercut when drugs such as Lipitor, Rogaine, Viagra, and Celebrex are huckstered to the public, as if they were M & M candies."[66]

In a landmark 1999 decision, *Perez v. Wyeth Laboratories*, the New Jersey Supreme Court articulated those issues in relation to the contraceptive device Norplant, which Wyeth had advertised heavily over the preceding decade. In a widely quoted opinion, the court summed up just how unsettled the medical landscape had become: the old medico-legal order had been based on the principle that "doctor knows best" at a time when pharmaceutical companies advertised their products only to physicians. Now, the court noted, "with rare and wonderful exceptions, the 'Norman Rockwell' image of the family doctor no longer exists." In modern times, "informed consent requires a patient-based decision rather than the paternalistic approach of the 1970s." Thus whether to take a drug was "not exclusively a matter for medical judgment."[67]

At the same time, because "managed care has reduced the time allotted per patient, physicians have considerably less time to inform patients of the risks and benefits of a drug." The opinion cited a recent FDA survey that found that only a third of patients had heard from their physicians about the potentially dangerous side effects of drugs being prescribed. Having spent $1.3 billion on advertising in 1998, the court noted, "drug manufacturers can hardly be said to 'lack effective means to communicate directly with patients.'" In light of all those developments, the court argued, it was time to rethink the traditional approach to product liability in the medical field.[68]

As the court concluded, "Consumer-directed advertising of pharmaceuticals thus belies each of the premises on which the learned intermediary doctrine rests." The fact that companies were advertising their products to the public "suggests that consumers are active participants in their health care decisions, invalidating the concept that it is the doctor, not the patient, who decides whether a drug or device should be used." Likewise, it was "illogical" to argue against direct warnings to consumers on the grounds that they would "undermine the patient-physician relationship, when, by its very nature, consumer-directed advertising encroaches on that relationship by encouraging consumers to ask for advertised products by name." DTCA also "effectively rebuts the notion that prescription drugs and devices and their potential adverse effects are too complex to be effectively communicated to lay consumers." For all these reasons, the court decided, "the common law duty to warn the ultimate consumer should apply."[69]

But the New Jersey Supreme Court's analysis of the unsettled state of American medicine did not herald a major change in product liability law. Although other courts followed this lead in a few cases, the learned intermediary controversy led to a different outcome: drug companies became more careful about acknowledging side effects in their advertising. By including the consumer equivalent of the brief warning in the form of a list of side effects and an urging to "consult with your doctor," drugmakers could continue advertising heavily without giving up the learned intermediary protection.[70]

Over the last quarter of the twentieth century, the drugstore underwent a sweeping renovation. Although it lost its prized exclusivity over the delivery of prescription medicines, the corner store managed effectively to position itself as a favored choice of the health-conscious consumer. Borrowing tactics from its big box competition, it carved out a profitable retail space for itself: like a retail Goldilocks, the drugstore got bigger but not too big. Retaining its familiar layout, it continued to appeal to the twin themes of self-care and convenience: the pharmacy at the back with its emphasis on professional service, the photo lab in the front, and in between an array of goods from pain relievers and vitamins to local wines and Halloween candy. Replicating in strip malls and city blocks all over the country, drugstores continued their long tradition of serving the looking-glass self.

Yet for all their success in realigning their mission with the mood of the late-twentieth-century shopper, drugstores could not escape the problems surrounding their most expensive and iconic product line, prescription drugs. Whether purchased in drugstores, supermarkets, or big box stores, the doctors' drugs remained a peculiarly complicated commodity. Their price, safety, and effectiveness continued to be a source of debate. In the end, the definition of what constituted good information for consumers and how they should get it remained highly unsettled. With the coming of the Internet and the expansion of DTCA in the late 1990s, that uncertainty would multiply many times over. No matter how much new information patient-consumers got, the challenge of making good choices remained daunting. For all the changes in the drugstore and the doctor's office, the challenge remained difficult: Americans could get good medicine at fair prices only by shopping for it very, very carefully, sorting through a welter of confusing information to do so.

The Barbarians Are at the Gate

In October 2007, Zagat Survey, well known for its popular restaurant and hotel guides, announced a new venture: a doctor guide to be developed in collaboration with WellPoint, a managed-care company that was now the nation's largest health-benefits firm. Following the format used in its other guides, Zagat's began to collect information about WellPoint patients' satisfaction with their doctors and use the data to rank practitioners on four criteria—trust, communication, availability, and office environment. Company executives hailed the advent of such "peer-to-peer" evaluations as "the missing piece of information needed to engage consumers." Enthused company cofounder Nina Zagat, "With this tool, WellPoint is helping to give consumers the power to make smart decisions about selecting doctors based on other people's experiences."[1]

Zagat's new venture prompted a range of reactions from the amused to the skeptical. "Would you like dessert with your diagnosis?," mused one newspaper article, while another noted the convenience of being able to "pick up the 'burgundy bible' to find the best restaurant in town, and then search a similar guide to find a gastroenterologist to treat the possible stomach ache afterwards." Many physicians found the prospect far less pleasing. James King, president of the American Academy of Family Physicians, warned that "choosing a physician only according to consumer ratings can deprive patients of high-quality medical care, particularly if those ratings are based on unrecognized and unvoiced anger or unjustified allegiance." But the logic underlying the guide seemed hard to resist. As Harvard physician Arnold M. Epstein wrote, "If Zagat's can rate Chinese restaurants and Greek tavernas, and *Consumer Reports* can rate skateboards and digital cameras, why can't we rate doctors?"[2]

Zagat's entry into the doctor guide business is but one example of efforts to make health care more consumer-friendly that would have been hard to imagine even a few years ago: coupons for prescription drugs, lotteries for in vitro fertilization treatments, smartphone apps to measure blood pressure or blood sugar. Armed with cellphones and wireless connections, American patient-consumers seem ready and able to take charge of their medical care. And as did previous generations of "new breed" patients, their demands are causing considerable trepidation within the medical profession. "The barbarians are at the gate," quipped physician Pauline Chen, describing how her fellow health providers felt about the prospect that patients would gain easier access to their medical records.[3]

Along with these unsettling prospects, the language of retail has made dramatic inroads into contemporary discussions of patient care. Whereas in past decades, physicians saw their work as a world apart from the car dealership or the department store, now they are not so sure; some even suggest that the medical profession needs to learn how other service industries work. In that spirit, urologist Robert Dowling reflected on what happened when his car broke down on an out-of-town business trip. With help from his hometown service representative, Dowling easily identified a nearby dealership that quickly and expertly repaired his SUV. Had this scenario involved a medical condition, he wondered what would have happened. Would his primary care physician have been as quick to respond as the service representative, as willing and able to find him a competent local doctor and to share his medical files? The answer, alas, was no. "While medical care is arguably different than automobile maintenance," Dowling suggested, "we could take a few lessons from the service industry." In a statement that would have appalled Morris Fishbein and his contemporaries, Dowling concluded that in an "age of consumer-driven health care," the medical profession needed to do a better job of "treating patients like customers."[4]

Perhaps even more startling is the advice delivered by hospital administrator Fred Lee in his very successful 2004 book, *If Disney Ran Your Hospital: 9 ½ Things You Would Do Differently*. Working at the Orlando, Florida, hospital that cares for Disney employees, Lee decided to spend some time at the theme park learning about the company's management philosophy. The experience transformed his approach to health care. "Disney World is not a service, it's an experience," Lee realized; by approaching hospital stays in the same way, staff could greatly enhance patients' experiences of care. To that end, the book presented a set of Disneyesque principles, among them "make courtesy more important than efficiency" and "close the gap between knowing and doing," aimed at making patients more satisfied with their stays. Widely read and reviewed in industry circles, the book launched Lee on a successful career as a motivational speaker.[5]

To say that the patient-as-customer model has gained advocates in American medicine does not mean that it has become universally popular, as evident in the lively exchange about Lee's book on the industry website *Hospital Impact*. As one person wrote, "A hospital is not a luxury resort, an operating room is not a ride, a surgeon is not a cute tour guide in a uniform," and more importantly, "nobody dies if they can't afford to go to Disney World." Another commentator suggested that Lee "is obviously someone who has not seen a patient's butt, dealt first hand with unreasonable and obnoxious family members interfering with lifesaving care and whose reality is based behind a desk far far away from the bedside." A third joked, "One thing Disney and hospitals DO have in common: overcharging for EVERYTHING!"[6]

Other bloggers, however, noted the important differences between hospitals and theme parks but applauded Lee's message that hospitals needed to develop more patient-centered policies. A twenty-year veteran of nursing who described herself as "familiar with the butt" wrote, "It's about having patients/clients and their families leave the hospital knowing their needs were met in an exceptionally professional and caring manner whether the client leaves the hospital by car or by hearse." Another brought in the automobile analogy, noting that after a tour of a Toyota factory, he had concluded "they treat their cars better than we treat our patients." "Sure, a hospital isn't a resort, a vacation, a getaway, but it is a customer service industry ... like it or not."[7]

The debate over Lee's book reveals the extent to which older distinctions between professionalism and commercialism have all but disappeared in American medicine today. That trend reflects the profession's growing engagement with (or some might say entrapment by) the dynamics of modern consumer culture. A half century ago, American doctors would have scoffed at the idea of emulating the auto industry or Disney World. But thanks to the economic upheavals of the late twentieth century, the profession's ability to deflect questions about the quality of care delivered to its end users, also known as patient-consumers, steadily eroded, leaving physicians less power to resist third-party demands that they become more "consumer-driven" or "patient-centered." The arguments for change present a strange mix of ethics and economics: as professionals, all doctors have a sacred duty to give their best to all their patients; as economic competitors, they must do better by their "customers" or lose them to other providers. Medicine's traditional ethos to "do no harm" has been recast in the language of consumer satisfaction.

Were we to believe everything we hear, we might be tempted to conclude that after decades of battling, those who champion the core values of critical medical consumerism—patients' rights to be safe, to be informed, to make choices, and to be heard—have finally won the war. In fact, it is hard to find any stakeholders involved in health care today who would dare to declare themselves opposed to those rights. Whereas during the Cold War, someone who advanced a more consultative approach between patient and physician might have been labeled at best a neurotic and at worst a communist, that position has become the early twentieth-first-century version of medicine, motherhood, and apple pie. But should we declare the remaking of patients into empowered consumers to be both complete and successful? Are patients better off today than they were fifty years ago, when medical consumerism was considered heretical among both physicians and policymakers? Does the deepening embrace of the rhetoric surrounding the patient as consumer reflect dramatic improvements in the overall experience of health care delivery? The answer is not at all clear.

On the one hand, it is essential to recognize the positive achievements of medical consumerism—the "glass half full" part of the story. If they could behold the twenty-first-century scene, consumerist critics of the past such as T. Swann Harding, Katharine Kellock, Walton Hamilton, and Richard Carter would surely see much to celebrate. In many important respects, decades of persistent complaining have paid off; the concept of the "educated consumer" helped to legitimate an expanded role for the patient as partner. The principles and practices of critical consumerism framed and advanced the rights to safety, choice, information, and respect so clearly articulated in the 1973 Patients' Bill of Rights. If we put on our rose-colored spectacles, we can find much to support the argument that the U.S. health care system has become far more responsive to patient-consumers.

Achieving a more patient-centered health care system has become a guiding principle of American health care policy. That effort has been led by physicians dedicated to improving the quality of care that they deliver. But reform has also expanded to include the idea of patient "engagement" or "activation": providing information and building skills that allow patients to make better decisions in both economic and therapeutic domains. Patient collaboration is now viewed as essential to achieving the "triple aims" of reform: better health, better health care, and more sustainable health care spending. With the more off-putting "supermarket" aspects of consumerism downplayed, the quest for patient engagement has attracted wide support from leading professional groups. As a 2013 issue of *Health Affairs* noted, patient engagement has become the "holy grail" and "blockbuster drug" of twenty-first-century health care reform. One contributor noted that searching the Internet for the term "patient engagement" resulted in 36 million hits, impressive testimony to the wide circulation of the concept.[8]

Particularly influential in this regard has been the work of the IOM, the medical division of the National Academy of Sciences and arguably the most prestigious source of policy leadership in the United States. Starting with its 1999 report, *To Err Is Human,* which documented high rates of medical error, the IOM has sponsored a series of very influential studies about the quality lapses that beset American health care. To correct these failures, the IOM has helped lead a national effort to foster a more patient-centered standard of care, which it defines as "providing care that is respectful of and responsive to individual patient preferences, needs, and values, and ensuring that patient values guide all clinical decisions."[9]

Along with the IOM, many groups have taken up the cause of doing better by American patients. The quality initiative has fostered collaborations among nonprofit groups, such as the IOM, the Joint Commission on Hospital Accreditation, and the AMA's Physician Consortium for Performance Improvement, as well as federal agencies, including the NIH, the Agency for Healthcare Research and Quality, and the Centers for Medicare and Medicaid Services. Many professional societies have adopted the principles of evidence-based, patient-centered medicine and developed clinical practice guidelines to achieve them. Almost 2,700 such documents are now available through the National Guideline Clearinghouse.[10]

In search of new ways to fix old problems, advocates of patient-centered care are making creative use of information technologies. With substantial contributions from the federal government, American hospitals have adopted electronic systems of medical record keeping that promise to improve communication among multiple caregivers and thus reduce both medical error and duplication of effort. Giving patients access to their electronic medical records could facilitate care in times of emergency, as Dowling suggested in his reflections on his car trouble. Proponents have advanced many ways that information technology can be used in the service of health reform's "triple aims," including clinical decision aids, guided electronic disease management, and telemonitoring systems. As more physicians and patients become comfortable with these supports, they will increase patients' capacity for health "connectivity," a development that could yield enormous benefits.[11]

Physician educators and professional societies have been front and center in efforts to refashion medicine around a more patient-centered model of care. While often a painful process, the battering that the medical profession has taken in the past half century has made it more open to constructive change. In place of the Cold War arrogance that many medical consumerists found so off-putting, physicians have adopted a willingness to acknowledge the ways in which the system does not work well. Young physicians are trained to practice evidence-based medicine and to follow clinical practice guidelines that reflect it. Their education also includes hefty doses of bioethics designed to make doctors aware of their moral, social, and legal duties as their patients' "trusted intermediary."[12]

Likewise, the profession as a whole has worked to limit the commercial influences on both research studies and treatment decision making. Medical journals and conferences now require authors and presenters to disclose potential conflicts of interest arising from funding received from pharmaceutical or medical device companies. Over the past decade and a half, physician groups as well as the Justice Department have pushed for limits on the kind and amount of gifts and services that pharmaceutical companies can offer physicians. Some academic medical centers, including Columbia and Stanford, have moved to ban all pharmaceutical promotional activities on their campuses. Physician groups such as No Free Lunch and the National Physicians' Alliance work to promote what the latter group refers to as the "unbranded doctor network" to restore physician independence in the face of growing corporate influence. In 2006, pharmaceutical companies responded to physician concerns by agreeing to a set of voluntary guidelines "to ensure their medicines are marketed in a manner that benefits patients and enhances the practice of medicine."[13]

Primary care physicians are trying to address the long-term fragmentation of patient care by aggressively promoting the concept of a "medical home"— that is, "a model or philosophy of primary care that is patient-centered, comprehensive, team-based, coordinated, accessible, and focused on quality and safety." Harkening back to the "good" HMO model, this approach weds old-fashioned values of communication and teamwork with new information technologies and evidence-based guidelines. In 2007, the four organizations representing primary care physicians adopted the Joint Principles of the Patient-Centered Medical Home, and the model is being promoted by the Mayo Clinic, the Cleveland Clinic, and academic health centers throughout the country.[14]

Even in practices where the "medical home" concept has not yet arrived, the look and feel have become more patient-friendly, starting with waiting areas that feature flat-screen televisions and aquariums. Once in the examining room, patients are more likely to find doctors willing to answer questions, to share decision making, and to tolerate and even encourage patients to try yoga, meditation, fish oil supplements, and other complementary treatments. While billing and insurance coverage remain contentious issues, physicians as well as their office staffs have shouldered the burden of making a balky system work, often spending hours on the phone with pharmacy benefit managers and insurance companies to get patients the care they need. Meanwhile, Americans have a variety of options for quick medical care. Walk-in or "immediate care" clinics have become a familiar sight in many neighborhoods. So-called retail clinics housed in Walgreens and Walmart stores now offer services such as flu shots and blood pressure screening.[15]

If a visit to the doctor's office eventually leads to a hospital stay, most people find an institution trying to be more patient-friendly. As Fred Lee's success suggests, many hospitals clearly take "the patient is a valued customer" philosophy far more seriously than they did a half century ago. While still a far cry from Disney World, the "white labyrinths" of old have warmed up and opened up, from the better signage (follow the yellow lines to admitting) to the provision of a patient ombudsman (file your complaint here). The legacy of the 1970s patients' revolt is evident in the blizzard of forms attendant on every stage of care: the privacy statements mandated by the Health Insurance Portability and Accountability Act of 1996, the informed-consent forms before treatment, the written instruction sheets for aftercare, and last but not least, the billing paperwork. In place of the original 1973 Patients' Bill of Rights, the AHA now distributes a "plain-language" brochure, *The Patient Care Partnership*, aimed at promoting a collaborative approach to care.

The twenty-first-century drugstore has also been much improved. Compared to their 1930s predecessors, stores carry a far wider range of effective medicines. Stronger drug regulation has removed many ineffective and unsafe products from their shelves; those medicines that remain have more detailed and accurate labels and instructions for use. Thanks to consumer pressure, it is far easier to shop for cheaper prescriptions, especially since the coming of the Internet. Many states now sponsor websites that allow consumers to see what local drugstores charge for common medications. The easing of restrictions on generic products has enabled doctors and patients to find less expensive alternatives for their drugs. As of 2012, almost 80 percent of all prescriptions filled in the United States are for generic drugs. And after years of hearing complaints that Medicare did not cover the cost of prescription medications, Congress finally passed the 2003 Medicare Modernization Act, the first major expansion of Medicare benefits since the program's creation in 1965.[16]

The oldest and arguably still the most important guardian of patient-consumers' welfare, the FDA has seen its powers continue to expand. In response to concerns about the agency's workload, Congress passed the 1992

Prescription Drug User Fee Act requiring that pharmaceutical companies contribute to the cost of reviewing new drug applications. The agency has used these funds to hire more staff and thus narrow the lag between U.S. and European drug approvals: of the thirty-five new drugs introduced in 2011, the FDA approved twenty-four of them before European officials did so. Meanwhile, the creation of MedWatch, which facilitates reporting of adverse drug events, has strengthened the agency's postmarket surveillance of drug safety; since its founding in 1993, it has led to removal of twenty-six drugs from the market. Recognizing the value of patients as watchdogs, the FDA in 2013 decided to open up MedWatch so that they also could report adverse drug events, and officials have begun discussing the creation of a similar national monitoring system for medical mistakes.[17]

Although critics have failed to end DTCA of prescription drugs, their efforts have resulted in voluntary changes by the pharmaceutical industry. Since its 2006 apex at $5.4 billion, spending on ads targeted at consumers has declined to $3 billion in 2012. The pharmaceutical industry has adopted comprehensive guidelines to ensure that its consumer advertising remains ethical and educational, and it has shown caution in using social media to avoid further backlash against its methods. In 2010, the FDA upgraded its old Division of Drug Marketing, Advertising, and Communication to become the Office of Prescription Drug Promotion, "a level-up that will mean more authority and resources for promotion oversight at the agency," as an industry periodical noted. The FDA continues to work with the pharmaceutical industry to make labeling information more readable, and after years of fighting over the concept, patient information leaflets now accompany most prescriptions filled in the United States.[18]

As patient-consumers visit the doctor's office and the drugstore, they can make use of an ever expanding array of information sources to guide their choices. Consumer-oriented ratings and rankings continue to flourish. While U.S. News and World Report ceased publication as a magazine in 2010, it continues to issue its lucrative guides, including the annual hospital survey. U.S. News competes with a burgeoning array of competitors that promise the inside scoop on the best and the worst of all things medical, including hospitals, physicians, and prescription drugs. The now old-style report card based on expert opinion has been supplemented by peer-to-peer evaluations. Building on the success of similar surveys devoted to ranking university professors, doctor-rating websites have expanded very quickly. WellPoint's decision to collaborate with Zagat testifies to the growing trend toward the ratings game. A for-profit managed-care company spun off from Blue Cross/Blue Shield of California, WellPoint is the second-largest health insurer in the country, covering one in nine Americans.[19]

Not only does health-related information continue to circulate via print media, broadcast television, cable television, and radio, but it has also taken on dramatic new mobility thanks to the growing reach of and access to the Internet. In 2012, according to the Pew Research Center, 72 percent of all Internet users had looked online for health information in the past year. Thirty-five percent of adults reported having tried to diagnose themselves or a family member using information retrieved online. Twenty percent had looked at online reviews and rankings of providers and treatments, and 16 percent had attempted to connect with people who had similar health concerns.[20]

The Web's connectivity has facilitated more interactive means of digital communication. Many doctors and patients now use email to exchange information; some practices are developing online clinical modules that allow patients to get quick and easy treatment of simple health problems such as sinus infections or conjunctivitis. Also important are the ways that the more interactive Web facilitates the sharing of peer-to-peer experiences and advice. Blogging, tweeting, networking through Facebook and similar sites, and other forms of social media have vastly increased the sharing of information among laypeople. Patient-consumers can go online to visit websites that provide patient reviews of individual doctors and hospitals. In a 2012 survey, 59 percent of respondents reported that online ratings were "somewhat" or "very important" in the choice of physician. As of October 2014, 64 percent of American adults owned smartphones and thus had easy access to digital communications, and the sharing of health information will only likely accelerate.[21]

Along with all these innovations, major changes have taken place in another product line essential to the "American way" of health care—the insurance policy. In 2003, President George W. Bush signed into law the Medicare Prescription Drug, Improvement, and Modernization Act, which included a provision enabling Americans to try a new-style insurance plan long promoted by conservatives, the health savings account. Under this plan, employers and employees give up the tax exemption on their insurance premiums; in return, the individual employee gets a tax-free fund to pay for routine medical expenses, plus a high-deductible insurance plan for use in case of more serious illness. As of 2015, an estimated 15.5 million Americans have signed up for some version of the health savings account. Conservatives promote these plans as a superior form of consumer-driven health care that allows personal choice while holding down medical costs.[22]

An even more dramatic change came in 2010 with passage of the Patient Protection and Affordable Care Act (ACA), which set minimum standards for what plans needed to cover and required all Americans to have health insurance coverage or pay fines. The act mandated an end to insurance companies' practice of refusing to insure people for preexisting conditions. To make it easier for the approximately 50 million Americans without insurance to acquire it, the law mandated the creation of insurance exchanges offering a variety of plans, grouped into platinum, bronze, silver, and gold categories based on price and coverage. As long as they met the minimum requirements set by the law, health savings accounts were included among the offerings. The only kind of plan Americans could not choose was a public option on the model of Medicare, although the law did allow states to apply for funds to purchase private insurance for low-income people.[23]

While the creation of insurance exchanges received the most public attention, the ACA, colloquially known as Obamacare, also included a number of other measures long sought by health care reformers. The law created new fiscal incentives for physician groups and hospitals to focus on providing more integrated, higher-quality, cost-effective care and strengthened the mechanisms for detecting and punishing Medicare and Medicaid fraud. The ACA also allocated funding for the creation of the Patient-Centered Outcomes Research Institute to study the relative effectiveness of different treatments.[24]

For all its imperfections, the ACA represented a significant step toward the long-term goals of improving access to both care and quality. After a wave of legal challenges, the U.S. Supreme Court held the ACA as constitutional in June 2012; that November, Barack Obama won reelection against Republican Mitt Romney, who had campaigned on the promise immediately to repeal the law if elected. Government ineptitude and conservative resistance meant that implementation of the insurance exchanges beginning in the fall of 2013 was rocky indeed, but by the fall of 2014, the number of uninsured Americans had declined to 13.4 percent, a substantial drop from the 17 percent rate in 2013. In June 2015, Obamacare survived yet another serious court challenge—this time to the constitutionality of tax subsidies—to remain the law of the land. The longer it stays in force, the more likely it is that the ACA will never be repealed.[25]

In August 2014, the Centers for Medicare and Medicaid issued a report showing that since 2009, the rate of increase in health care spending had slowed substantially. In spite of the backlash against managed care during the 1990s and the subsequent abandonment of many overt forms of cost control, persistent efforts to make all the parties to health care spending—doctors, hospitals, insurance companies, patients, pharmaceutical companies, and medical device makers—more aware of the need to hold down expenditures seem finally to be showing some results. The exact reasons for the decline are up for debate; it may largely be a result of the recession that began in 2008. But the increase between 2009 and 2012 is the smallest since the government began tracking these data in 1960, and the first time since 1997 that the rate of increase in health care spending was less than the rate of growth in the nation's economy.[26]

In short, the atmosphere in 2015 is very different from the one that existed in 1965. Far from insisting that American medicine is beyond reproach, medicine's leaders now accept the premise that from the patient's viewpoint, there remains great room for improvement. Not only physicians but also policy experts, government leaders, hospital administrators, and pharmaceutical company executives talk the talk about honoring the need for patient engagement in economic and therapeutic decision making. It would be virtually impossible to find an opinion leader in the medical field today who would disagree with what counted as a radical principle in 1938—Hugh Cabot's insistence that the "patient, now known as the consumer" has the "right to a very large word in what is done and in how it is done" in the world of medicine.[27]

Particularly striking have been the changes in the medical profession: physicians now project a collective degree of humility far from the persona of the "little tin god" that so aggravated the pre-1960 generation. Doctors now work willingly and enthusiastically with patient-consumer groups in ways that would have been unlikely fifty or even twenty years ago. Morris Fishbein and his peers could hardly have imagined the day would come when the American Board of Internal Medicine Foundation would partner with *Consumer Reports* in "Choosing Wisely," a joint educational initiative to reduce unneeded tests and scans.[28]

Overall, Americans enjoy a higher quality of health over a longer life span that did their grandparents. Reflecting on that accomplishment, economist David M. Cutler, a former adviser to President Obama, has repeated an observation first made back in the 1920s: medicine costs more today because it is worth more. In 1950, medical spending was only about $500 a person per year; today, it is $5,000. But as Cutler notes, few of us would want to get that $4,500 back in exchange for care only at the 1950s standard. Like many health policy leaders, Cutler believes that if the nation persists in what he terms the "quality cure," the system's worst tendencies can be tamed. By combining "information technology, realigned payment systems, and value-focused organizations," it is possible to bend the cost curve down and the quality cure up and thereby bring "a better system within our reach."[29]

If you like happy endings, stop reading here.

Taking off the rose-colored glasses reveals a very different picture, one that seems to suggest that the more things change, the more they stay the same. Despite sincere efforts to address them, many long-standing patient complaints remain unresolved. The overblown promise of the "new and improved," the misleading conflation of advertising and information, the entrenched barriers to coordination of care, the limited political clout of consumer groups, and the toxic effects of income inequality continue to pose formidable obstacles to the goal of improving patient care.

Defining and enforcing standards of quality control remains both technically challenging and politically fraught. It is one thing to propose an evidence-based approach to the treatment of a specific condition and quite another to put it into practice, particularly in light of the fast-moving nature of medical innovation. In the decentralized U.S. medical culture, new drugs, devices, and procedures come rapidly into use before either their efficacy or their cost-effectiveness relative to older treatments can be fully assessed. While comparative effectiveness studies are a laudable goal, they require considerable time and funding; while waiting for results, advocates of the new—and frequently more expensive—course of care can and do argue passionately for its worth to patients. Medical innovators draft clinical practice guidelines to promote the change, lobby specialist groups to endorse them, then pressure reluctant insurers to cover the treatment, on the grounds that the failure to do so deprives patients of a much better, possibly lifesaving measure. A 2011 report from the IOM about such guidelines raised concerns about "limitations in the scientific evidence base on which [clinical practice guidelines] rely; a lack of transparency of development groups' methodologies; conflict of interest among guideline development group members and funders; and questions regarding how to reconcile conflicting guidelines." Then even after some authoritative medical body recommends a specific course of treatment, many physicians may not follow it. In some cases, doctors are simply too busy treating patients to keep up with the latest evidence-based studies; in other cases, they ignore the guidelines because they do not accord with personal clinical experience.[30]

Much as the landmark 1954 survey of North Carolina did a half century ago, a 2003 study published in the *New England Journal of Medicine* provided a sobering view of the size of the gap between knowing and doing. Based on a sample of 13,000 Americans living in twelve different areas of the country and including preventive, acute, and chronic care, the study concluded that only 55 percent of patients received the care recommended for their particular diagnoses. For all the effort put into promoting evidence-based medicine, the gap has not narrowed substantially since 2003. In its 2012 report, *Best Care at Lower Cost*, IOM president Harvey V. Fineberg concluded that despite efforts at reform, the "U.S. health care system continues to fall far short of its potential." In short, "the nation has yet to see the broad improvements in safety, accessibility, quality, or efficiency that the American people need and deserve."[31]

Moreover, Americans pay more for their flawed medical services than do citizens of other developed countries. The tacit assumption that high price is a sign of superior quality has repeatedly been challenged by comparative studies of health spending in relation to outcomes. Simply put, although the United States spends 2.5 times more on health care than other industrialized nations, it does not get care that is 2.5 times better. While the United States ranks first in the cost of prescription drug medications and the number of diagnostic scans afforded its people, its performance on other benchmarks suggests care of only "middling or highly uneven quality," according to a 2011 report issued by the Commonwealth Fund. That report concluded, "The U.S. health system is not delivering superior results despite being more expensive."[32]

The higher prices that Americans pay for their care continue to complicate the long-term goals of insurance reform. Ironically, people without insurance are usually charged higher prices than those with it, which makes it all the more unlikely that they can afford it. As of 2013, 27 percent of the uninsured had incomes below poverty level; 61 percent of uninsured adults said that they lacked coverage because they could not afford it. While the ACA was passed to reduce this inequality, some conservative states have refused to take advantage of the funds it provides for Medicaid expansion, an action that disproportionately hurts the poor. Even many Americans who have coverage may be underinsured, in that should they face a serious illness, they could not pay all their medical bills. At the other extreme, the "broken" system continues to provide abundant if not necessarily errorless care to the very wealthy. Recent years have seen a trend toward so-called concierge or retainer medicine, in which patients pay an annual fee in exchange for easy access to the doctor, who can then escape the constraints of third-party interference.[33]

Bending the cost curve downward while improving the quality of care has proven to be very challenging. Economic pressures have encouraged a wave of mergers among hospital and provider groups that may work to reduce competition and raise prices. The incentives to engage in the medical arms race—to outdo one's rivals by investing in the latest expensive medical technology—remain formidable. Of course, not every medical innovation has proven more expensive than its predecessor; for example, early detection and treatment of heart attack and stroke clearly save money. Yet overall, the effort put into making a particular treatment more effective may well encourage providing more of it; as the cost of a particular procedure drops, more people have it done. Thus cost savings from early intervention in a cardiac event are offset by the higher number of cardiac bypass procedures performed. Better treatment protocols and economic pressures produced a marked decline in the average hospital stay, from 7.35 days in 1980 to 4.6 days in 2009. But the cost of care delivered rose from $6,600 per stay in 1997 to $9,200 per stay in 2009.[34]

The advice to doctors back in the 1980s to put down the scalpel and pick up the scope remains just as relevant today. As cost controls were imposed on "unnecessary surgery" and the like, many providers adapted by investing in the latest in diagnostic equipment and using it as often as possible. The uptick in screenings benefits not only hospitals but also diagnostic centers, which are often owned by physicians. Providers frequently justify expensive testing as a response to medical consumerism and the rising number of malpractice suits it has brought. Practicing "defensive medicine" requires the ordering of additional tests, procedures, and visits as a protection against litigation. Studies of technology use have questioned this connection, showing that with the exception of a few specialties such as obstetrics, most doctors practice aggressively "primarily because they believe such procedures to be medically indicated, not primarily because of concerns about liability," as an influential 1994 report concluded. Nevertheless, many experts agree that a surfeit of scanning and screening contributes to misdirected and sometimes unnecessary medical care.[35]

Experts also agree that in spite of efforts to alter them, prevailing reimbursement practices still provide many incentives for providers to deliver more—and more expensive—services. American medical care remains a "package of services," to use Michael Marks Davis's phrase, the component parts of which can be broken out and priced with an eye on the bottom line. Despite efforts at reform such as Medicare's Resource-Based Relative-Value Scale, reimbursement schemes continue to favor specialists over generalists, and procedure-based care over its less invasive counterparts. Time spent simply talking to the patient, no matter how important it may be to patient education and cooperation, is still not valued highly as part of the doctor's package of services. Meanwhile, despite persistent efforts to revitalize primary care medicine, the shift from generalist to specialist has continued to accelerate. As of 2010, less than one-third of the doctors involved in full-time patient care had been trained in one of the specialties now associated with the physician-generalist—that is, family medicine, general internal medicine, or pediatrics.[36]

Here lies one of the U.S. health care system's most striking failures at giving patient-consumers what they want. Since the 1920s, Americans have consistently complained about the difficulty of finding primary care physicians who are willing to spend time talking to them. Just as consistently, the medical profession has concurred that to get good care, patients need broadly trained doctor-advisers to offer guidance through the ever-increasing complexities of preventive health care and disease management. Yet the advice so long given to American patients—find a good general practitioner and stick with him or her—has never been harder to follow.[37]

The reasons for this unhappy situation are not hard to fathom. While all physicians' incomes have fallen since the mid-1990s, those of internists and family physicians have declined the most. Young people may start medical school wanting to practice a more holistic, personal style of medicine, only to discover the many inducements to follow a different path—a higher income, a more manageable workload, and a better overall quality of life. Those who stay the course and become generalists face growing pressures to see more patients to pay off loans and run offices. In order to give good care, a doctor's "panel" of patients should be less than 1,800; the average U.S. primary care physician currently has 2,300. Clinics that specialize in treating Medicaid recipients—the poorest of patients—may see 3,000 patients per doctor. While practicing primary care can still be highly rewarding, too many doctors become stuck in isolated, unstimulating settings where burnout comes easily. Meanwhile, patients suffer from the sensation that "the doctor will see you—if you're quick," as journalist Shannon Brownlee has put it. A 2010 survey found that only 27 percent of U.S. adults reported being able to "easily contact their primary care physician by telephone, obtain care or advice after hours, and schedule timely office visits." Fifty percent of those interviewed reported that their doctor visits were too short to allow them fully to understand the treatment being recommended.[38]

If it succeeds, the medical home movement could help to correct these long-term problems. But at present, this style of practice is still limited primarily to academic medical centers and large group health providers. Its spread may be slowed by the growth of retail medicine—that is, small clinics associated with supermarkets and big box stores that provide flu shots and other traditional staples of private office practice. Almost 36 percent of Americans now live within a ten-minute drive of a retail clinic; far fewer have such close proximity to a medical home.[39] The inducements that drugstores, supermarkets, and big box stores now have to augment their services with simple but lucrative medical procedures may yet further undermine the economic viability of primary care medicine.

Without a strong system of primary care physicians coordinating the flow, fragmented and expensive care from multiple specialists remains all too common. Responding to the medical arms race and a reimbursement system that pays more for complexity than simplicity, physicians have many reasons, therapeutic as well as fiscal, simply to assume that their patients' best interests are served by adopting the latest in new technologies, procedures, and drugs. As a result, many of them continue to push back against both evidence-based guidelines and third-party insurance limits, insisting, with some legitimacy, that they are doing so at their patients' request. Patient demands for the latest and best of every medical treatment regardless of its evidence-based pedigree fuel a "do everything" approach.[40]

In such a medical culture, seeing complex medical problems in a more holistic context can be very difficult. Studies of how care is delivered in the United States repeatedly identify specialization and fragmentation as barriers both to improving quality and to holding down cost. As a recent analysis of Medicare showed, a seriously ill person may be under the care of as many as fourteen doctors at a time, with no one provider devoting much effort or time to coordinating all of that care. These problems frequently show the expanding range of medical treatments that involve what Zachary D. Goldberger and Angela Fagerlin call ICDs—Incredibly Complex Decisions.[41] Given that fewer and fewer patients have a single physician they regard as coordinator of their medical care, serious muddles can result. The patient must then decide, Do I listen first to my cardiologist or to my urologist or to my gynecologist?

The tilt toward specialist care has also exacerbated the long-standing problems that surround the safety of the products and services that doctors recommend. Unlike other areas of consumption, medical care remains deeply informed by the physician's role as the patient's learned intermediary. Whereas consumers can buy many kinds of expensive and possibly dangerous goods on their own—sports cars, rifles, and drones come to mind—they cannot obtain a prescription drug, an MRI, or a hip implant without a doctor's blessing. For all the trend toward consumerism, patients' access to the most expensive and powerful medical goods remains firmly mediated by medical authority.

Although medical goods and services have come under increasing regulation as a means to guarantee their safety, they remain in that category of "unavoidably unsafe" products. Yet since the 1906 Pure Food and Drugs Act, Americans have consistently tended to overestimate how well the power of regulation works to protect them. The more powerful the drug or procedure, the more disclosure of risks has fallen on physicians, who then have the unenviable task of deciding how much of that knowledge to share with their patients. As medicine has become more complex and dependent on new drugs and procedures, the extent of corporate influence on how doctors go about selecting them has become a huge source of concern.[42]

Initially focused primarily on prescription drugs, those worries have expanded since the 1970s to include medical devices designed to assist or replace failing body parts. Once uncommon, surgeries and procedures involving these technologies have become commonplace. Between 1993 and 2008, more than 4.2 million Americans had cardiac defibrillators implanted. Hip and knee replacements are now the second-most-common operation in the United States, performed on 750,000 Americans in 2005 and expected to rise to 4.5 million people by 2030. These devices not only improve patients' quality of life but also represent challenges in terms of regulating the device manufacturers' influence over physicians' use of them. In health care parlance, such devices are referred to as physician preference items, suggesting just how much the doctor's choice matters.[43]

Vouching for the safety, efficacy, and value of medical devices has come to be an important part of the doctor's role as the patient's trusted intermediary. But the FDA's regulatory powers over those devices, first defined in 1976 and subsequently revised in 1990, have not achieved the same level of rigor as its oversight of new drugs. While many of the more than 1,700 devices on the market today work fine, those that do not have exposed patients to painful and even life-threatening conditions. In 2005, Guidant's faulty cardiac defibrillator, implanted in 50,000 Americans, had to be recalled because of the risk of unexpected shocks; in 2010, DePuy Orthopaedics voluntarily recalled 93,000 metal-on-metal hip implants whose failure was exposing some patients to toxic metal debris. Because they are used in high-volume procedures, such product failures often involve huge numbers of people: during one three-month period in 2012, recalls applied to more than 123 million individual devices.[44]

If in comparison to medical devices, the FDA's oversight of prescription drugs seems more dependable, it has by no means eliminated consumers' worries about the safety of their medications. Although a powerful force within medicine, the FDA still struggles to perform too many tasks with too little funding while enduring an acid bath of criticism: industry representatives complain it does too much while consumer advocates say it does too little. With much of the evidence for a product's effectiveness now paid for by the company that makes it, the objectivity of the new drug review process seems uncertain. Meanwhile, anticipating post-approval problems is difficult: drugs that seem safe and reliable in clinical trials turn out to have unexpected side effects that only become apparent after widespread use, or drugs are prescribed for conditions other than the ones intended (off-label use).[45]

The risks of medicine-chest roulette are far from diminished. Between 1995 and 2005, the number of adverse reactions reported to the FDA tripled. In a 2008 survey of 1,000 Americans, *Consumer Reports* found that one in six people had suffered a medication side effect serious enough to warrant a trip to the doctor or hospital, but only a third were aware that they could report side effects directly to the FDA. While life-threatening side effects may be rare, well-publicized exceptions have occurred: troubled teenagers who committed suicide after taking antidepressants, women on hormone replacement therapy who developed breast cancer, and arthritis patients who suffered heart attacks after taking Cox 2 pain medications. The reality remains that in 2012 no more than in 1962, the FDA cannot truly guarantee that powerful prescription drugs are risk-free.[46]

These risks are compounded by the trend toward polypharmacy. In a 2008 report, the Centers for Disease Control and Prevention estimated that 11 percent of all Americans and 40 percent of people over the age of sixty took five or more medications. With each drug added to the mix, the possibilities for interactions multiply. In some cases, the interactions among multiple drugs are simply unknown; in other cases, despite black box warnings to physicians and pharmacists, patients still receive drugs that are known to be dangerous in combination with each other. The risks are especially high among elderly Americans, due to the greater number of drugs they take, but are rising among young people as they experiment with what they find in the family medicine cabinet. Commenting on the fact that deaths from prescription drug mishaps now outnumber traffic fatalities, a member of the Los Angeles Sheriff's Department told a reporter in 2011, "People feel they are safer with prescription drugs because you get them from a pharmacy and they are prescribed by a doctor."[47]

Medicine-chest roulette has been complicated by the growing use of dietary supplements and herbal products that are not subject to FDA scrutiny. As the potential for combining prescription drugs and supplements multiplies, doctors and pharmacists are hard-pressed to keep up with the possible hazards, much less apprise patients of them. In 2011, *Consumer Reports* published the results of an undercover shoppers' investigation that suggested the potential problems that might result: people posing as patients went to twenty pharmacies armed with prescriptions for Lipitor and instructions to ask about taking it along with red rice yeast, a popular dietary supplement known to increase the risk of side effects when combined with Lipitor. In twelve cases, pharmacists gave the wrong advice, including one who reported that his wife was taking the two together.[48]

In the context of recurrent recalls and media coverage of them, the tensions between the imperative to trust in one's physician and the need to play consumer watchdog have unsettled an already fragile doctor-patient relationship. The doctor's responsibility to promote evidence-based medicine has evolved in tandem with the duty of the intelligent patient to recognize good care when it is offered. But while this approach to shared decision making sounds very sensible, in practice it is extremely hard to execute, in large part because experts disagree so frequently about what best practices actually are. To give but one example, after decades of recommending that all women over forty should have annual mammograms, the U.S. Preventive Services Task Force recommended in 2009 that except in cases of high genetic risk, women could wait until fifty and then be screened every other year. Other experts, including some who wanted to showcase their "new and improved" mammogram devices, decried the advice as unscientific and dangerous. Expert opinion remains divided over the question, leaving women no choice but to "sort through the thicket of apparently irreconcilable opinions," as one journalist concluded.[49]

All these patterns—the continual flow of new products and services, the incentives for ever-more-expensive packages of care, the difficulties involved in evaluating value and safety, and physicians' inability to agree on their own standards—have contributed to the need for more and better information about medical choices. The complexity and uncertainty surrounding medical care have created a persistent demand for "insider advice" on how to get good medical care. Since the 1970s, giving patients more information has been one of the few types of reform on which both liberals and conservatives could agree. But like the faith in smart shopping, the power of information alone to protect patient-consumers has proven illusory.

In part, the limits of the "information Rx" as practiced in the United States reflect its paradoxical relationship with modern advertising. Along with their request for more family doctors, Americans' wish to be spared more health-related advertising and marketing has been consistently ignored over the past century. When consumer advocates in the 1930s and again in the 1970s demanded better information about medical choices, more advertising was definitely *not* what they had in mind. Instead, the lifting of traditional bans on physician and prescription drug advertising came at the initiative of a very different group of actors: regulators and jurists who sought to remove the medical profession's "shawl of privilege" and make it more responsive to market factors.

The FTC and the Justice Department challenged long-standing bans on medical advertising in hopes of encouraging advertising that would stress objective information about prices, credentials, and office hours—that is, data that would help consumers shop more wisely and thus pressure medical providers to improve their efficiency. But the advertising that emerged as part of the corporate makeover of medicine focused not on price but on raising expectations, many of them unrealistic, about the unique and miraculous services that particular doctors, hospitals, and drugmakers had to offer. At the same time, the peculiarly American legal doctrine that corporations have the same constitutional rights as individuals means that advertising and marketing efforts have been protected as a form of commercial free speech.

These developments have worked to make medicine and health care one of the fastest-growing areas of American advertising since the 1980s. A 2012 survey by *Medical Marketing and Media* compiled a list of more than 130 firms that handle health-related accounts. The list includes not only branches of industry giants such as DDB, McCann, Ogilvy, and Saatchi and Saatchi but also many boutique firms that specialize in particular areas of medicine and pharmaceuticals. Yet while it has become a vital and highly visible part of the industry, the upsurge in medical advertising and marketing has hardly helped promote the "triple aims" of better health, better health care, and more sustainable health care spending.[50]

Similarly, the pharmaceutical industry's efforts to make DTCA of prescription drugs more palatable have not succeeded in diminishing concerns about the practice. While there is little evidence that such advertising is a prime driver of high drug prices, in-depth studies of the ads' content and reception have not supported their claim to be a balanced, high-quality form of patient education. To avoid lawsuits, pharmaceutical companies have adopted voluntary guidelines to make ads more informative, but questions remain about whether these efforts amount to a good-faith effort at informed consent. For example, a recent study of ads for the treatment of erectile dysfunction aired after the new 2006 guidelines went into force found a "consistent pattern of noncompliance" with the industry's own ethical principles, and a recent study published in *Psychological Science* suggested that required warnings may have unintended results, causing listeners to forget the information but retain a sense of trust in the product because the risks are so extensively detailed.[51]

Drug companies have paid a reputational price by ignoring patient-consumers' strong dislike of drug advertising. Since the medicine show took to the radio airways back in the 1930s, Americans have expressed little love for the advertising ballyhoo surrounding over-the-counter products; by adopting the same measures to promote prescription drugs, pharmaceutical companies have transferred that dislike to them. A 2007 survey by Pricewaterhouse-Coopers showed that industry representatives regard direct-to-consumer ads much more favorably than does the public and concluded ominously, "The disconnect is contributing to the decline in the industry's reputation and causing the U.S. industry's messages about its value to society to fail in the court of public opinion." Meanwhile, the long-term side effects of DTCA as a source of patient expectations and pressure on physician prescribing patterns remain a matter of concern.[52]

Despite efforts to contain their influence, pharmaceutical company promotions still play a major role in shaping American doctors' treatment choices. As of 2012, some 72,000 pharmaceutical sales representatives visited doctors to promote products, often providing meals and gifts to sweeten the pitch. Although continuing medical education programs have become better firewalled against industry-paid speakers, many physicians still receive fees to give promotional talks to fellow doctors at restaurants and other private venues. In short, the incentives for physicians to be persuasive vendors rather than cautious consumerists remain significant. The amount spent on promotions to physicians—$24 billion in 2012—far outweighs the funding available for more neutral forms of medical education or comparative drug evaluations.[53]

While attracting less policy attention to date, growing investments by hospitals, physician groups, and medical clinics in marketing and advertising campaigns have also had unsettling results. Ironically, at the same time physicians are being asked to resist pharmaceutical company blandishments, they are asked to support the medical branding efforts of their local hospitals. In response to competition and demands for accountability, hospitals, clinics, and physician practices continue to merge into fewer but larger networks.

Such consolidation potentially reduces price competition as well as increases spending on advertising and marketing, as the conglomerates feel the need to fend off rivals. In some cases, the sense of competition may enhance concern with patient well-being and satisfaction; however, it can also multiply the number of repetitive and misleading ads. Lamented one physician blogger, those ads commonly feature da Vinci robotic surgery, promote orthopedic procedures with tired formulas such as "it will get you back in the game," and describe their care as "state of the art, leading edge or cutting edge." In answer to her question "Can we put the hospital marketing genie back in the bottle?," the answer seems to be a resounding no.[54]

The proliferation of medical advertising for prescription drugs, hospitals, and physicians has only heightened the need for more objective information of the sort that both physician reformers and medical consumerists have long sought. Both public and private groups have tried to oblige by producing a wide array of tools that can be used to make better decisions about every aspect of medical care, including the choice of doctor, insurance plan, and specific therapeutic modalities from prescription drugs to cancer treatments. Yet the construction and use of rankings and ratings remain mired in controversy and difficulty.

In theory, institutions and individuals are supposed to use performance measures as a goad to do better; for example, public reporting of hospitals' rates of serious infection or providers' rates of success with a particular procedure will create a positive pressure for them to improve in those areas. Some studies suggest that this phenomenon is indeed happening. But others suggest that some providers and hospitals are gaming the system simply to look better, a tendency long noted in our modern audit culture. For example, researchers noted in 2005 that since New York State had begun publicly to report on physicians' performance, almost 80 percent of cardiologists surveyed reported that they avoided treating critically ill patients because they feared that bad outcomes would affect their scorecards. A more comprehensive review published that same year in the *Journal of the American Medical Association* warned of the same problem.[55]

Meanwhile, Americans find many of the new information databases aimed at helping them make better decisions hard to use. A 2004 survey of consumers done by the Kaiser Family Foundation and the Agency for Healthcare Research and Quality found that only 19 percent had used the comparative quality ratings provided by government agencies, employers, consumer groups, or the media. The majority continued to rely on personal recommendations from family and friends when picking physicians, hospitals, or health plans.

Recognizing these problems, researchers are now working hard to convert quality measurements into information that consumers can use more easily. But the gap between what a journalist dubbed "smart data" and "foolish choices" continues to yawn. A 2012 policy brief warned that "many consumers are at risk of information overload" and concluded that "much remains to be done to make public reports accessible, understandable, and relevant."[56]

The proliferation of patient-oriented report cards and decision guides has itself become a source of confusion. Patient-consumers now require guides to the guides: the Medical Library Association's consumer health section provides a "top 100 list" of "health websites you can trust" to help consumers distinguish between good and bad information sources. Its list of criteria testifies to just how complicated this process has become: websites are judged on their "credibility, sponsorship/authorship, content, audience, currency, disclosure, purpose, links, design, interactivity, and caveats." To be well informed, consumers now have to devote even more time to verifying the quality of the information sources being offered them. This style of information seeking tends to favor Americans of higher income and educational levels who have the time and ability to use databases to compare physicians or hospitals. A 2011 study found that the consumers most likely to use websites that compare hospital performance were "white, college educated, and over age 45."[57]

Nor has the proliferation of web-based sources helped to create a reliable information highway. As savvy users know, the Internet offers a great many infomercials disguised as objective information. "If you're seeking answers on the Internet instead of from a health-care professional, you're 'swimming in shark-infested waters,'" one of Consumer Reports's medical advisers recently warned. "Brand drugmakers have so much money and are so smart that it is very difficult to find information online that they do not influence heavily." Thus he concluded, "Unless you are very careful and already well informed, you should assume that whatever you read on the Internet is coming from a drug company."[58]

Advocates of more informed patient choices are struggling with how to create better alternatives—what one terms the "If you build it, will they come?" problem. Designing information sources that convey complex data while being easy for consumers to navigate has proven difficult. According to a 2013 study, when patients were presented with new decision aids, some expressed interest in the information but did not know how to use such data, others were unaware that such variations in price and quality existed and saw little use in studying them, and still others were put off by the "lackluster" presentation. Whatever the reasons, the study concluded, "These results are disappointing in light of decades of effort and investment in the measurement and public reporting of health care quality data."[59]

Similar problems have dogged the introduction of decision aids targeted at therapeutic decision making. In an effort to engage patients more fully, researchers have worked to develop better brochures, videos, and websites. Some studies suggest that providing this kind of information can help patients feel far more skilled and confident about their treatment choices. But significant barriers to their effective use still remain, especially among vulnerable populations: the elderly; low-income, minimally educated families; and recent immigrants. In other words, the shopping model still works best for affluent, middle-class, college-educated Americans.[60]

Particularly sobering have been assessments of Americans' "health literacy"—that is, the extent to which people possess the reading and mathematical skills needed to use the decision-making tools being developed for them. A 2006 study by the National Center for Education Statistics based on a diverse sample of more than 19,000 people pointed to significant unevenness in the distribution of those abilities. Only 12 percent of the respondents were "proficient" in their skills, while 53 percent were "intermediate," 22 percent were "basic," and 14 percent were "below basic." That study also found that respondents who were white, better-educated, more affluent, and native English speakers tended to score better on measures of health literacy.[61]

These findings point to a persistent scaling-up problem. In the 1930s, when people such as Katharine Kellock and T. Swann Harding articulated the ideal of the educated patient-consumer, they did not present it as a universal aspiration; rather, they thought of themselves as speaking for the great majority of Americans who were neither very rich nor very poor.[62] During the early 1970s, that idea of the educated consumer was democratized and invigorated as one that could be claimed by all Americans—welfare mothers, corporate lawyers, farmers, mental patients. That more universalistic conception suited the political and economic interests of stakeholders primarily interested in cutting costs. But after forty years of concerted effort, the difficulties of preparing the entire American population to shoulder the heavy responsibilities of being "watchbirds" have become abundantly clear. Attempting to universalize the "intelligent patient" model highlights the fact that today, just as in 1935, people vary enormously both in how much responsibility for medical information collection and fact-checking they want and how well-equipped they are to do that work.

Trying to create a nation of sophisticated doctor-shoppers based on a middle-class model of entitlement has also made clear how extremely varied their preferences are. The more Americans converted to the cause of medical consumerism, the more apparent have become the limits of any one single model of a choosy consumer. As Kaiser Permanente executive Kathy Swenson noted during a 1998 roundtable, choice means different things to different consumers: for some, it means, "My doctor must be in the network," while for others it becomes "a proxy for quality," a desire that they could exit care "if they are concerned about quality." Among Kaiser Permanente's patient base, research revealed no single consumer orientation but rather eight or nine distinct groups. Thus, she concluded, "One cookbook approach to healthcare coverage and access often does not satisfy all consumers"; insurers had to realize that "they cannot be all things to all people."[63]

Much as advertisers "discovered" market segmentation in the 1970s, policy advocates today are struggling to develop more flexible models of patient engagement. But while market segmentation may seem more benign in the choice of cereals or cellphones, it seems harder to acknowledge and accommodate in medical care. The realization that not all patient-consumers want the same thing from their doctors or their health plans easily slides into disparagement of those variations that follow familiar patterns of discrimination. Given the white, middle-class origins of the concept of the intelligent patient, it is hardly surprising that in today's medicine, elderly, uneducated, poor, and immigrant patients are viewed as more difficult to "engage" or "activate" than their affluent counterparts. Gender biases also persist: when commentators describe the overentitled patient making bad decisions, the examples are often female, from the 1950s woman who "loved to be operated on" to the twenty-first-century woman who kept "doctor-shopping" until she got a colonoscopy.[64]

The other side of the change equation—that is, convincing physicians that engaging and activating patients is a desirable goal—has encountered its own roadblocks. When asked if they think patient-centered medicine is a good idea, physicians today will readily assent. At the same time, many of them fail to use the new patient decision aids in their practices. The problem, according to one study, was "overworked physicians, insufficient provider training, and inadequate clinical information systems." At a time when doctors are already overloaded with paperwork aimed at making them more accountable not only to their practice groups but to third-party payers, the time and energy to take on the task of mastering the latest in patient-centered decision aids can be hard to muster.[65]

Underlying some of that physician resistance may also be persistent reluctance to view the patient as worthy partner. For all the distance the profession has put between its authoritarian, paternalistic past and its patient-centered, consultative present, physician doubts remain about the ability of even "educated" patients to be good decision makers. Although they may downplay their views, physicians who prefer a more old-fashioned paternalism or authoritarian approach have by no means disappeared. A recent focus group study found that patients looking for more consultative doctors still had trouble finding them. "Many participants," the study noted, "reported that they did not feel respected or heard because their physician was often authoritarian, rather than authoritative." In a statement that might just as well have been written in the 1950s, the study observed, "Although participants recognized the expertise of physicians, they also felt that the authoritarian stereotype was often perpetuated by physicians themselves." Even patients who in objective terms would rate as "proficient" in their health literacy hesitated to challenge a doctor's judgment for fear of retribution. Like journalist Victor Cohn back in 1985, they feared being labeled "difficult" and thus having even more trouble finding good care. That dilemma provided the premise for a *Seinfeld* episode in which Elaine got labeled as difficult and then could not find a doctor willing to treat her.[66]

Of course, these conflicts reflect the fact that some patients are indeed difficult, unreasonable, and obnoxious. If doctors do not rate haloes and wings, as 1950s observers put it, neither do patients.[67] Now as in the past, personality differences and individual preferences continue to shape the doctor-patient interaction. As the recent focus group study found, some patients preferred more authoritative physicians, while others did not. But recognizing those differences remains even harder to do in contemporary medicine, given the policy investment in promoting watchdog patients as the key to health care reform.

All of these unresolved tensions carry over into the heated debates regarding who should bear the rising costs of medical care. In the wake of the managed-care controversy, many policy experts concluded that the American public had little interest in curbing the cost of medical care. This disinterest reflected their being shielded from the real costs of their care by the deep pockets of third-party payers, in particular employers and the federal government. Policymakers are now intent on making patients more cost-conscious on the assumption that it will make them more willing to shoulder their fair share of the price. But as this history has shown, patients who start to think about how medical costs are determined and what they are worth may not be more resigned to a bigger bill. Much as the itemized bill in the

1950s opened the way for complaints about overcharging, pressuring today's patient-consumers to look more closely at their insurance premiums or their hospital charges may make for less rather than more cooperation.

Such was the experience of Massachusetts health reporter Martha Bebinger, who in 2012 decided to try her hand at being "an engaged, savvy patient." After a bout of migraines, her physician suggested she have an MRI. Aware that she would be required to contribute only a $25 copay, she set out to discover what her plan would be billed for the scan. One hospital bounced her from radiology to billing and never called her with the promised estimate. A second told her the rate for an uninsured patient ($5,315) but was unable to provide information about the charge for a patient with insurance. She then called an independent lab that specialized in MRIs and learned that the test would run between $2,000 and $3,600 but that her plan would be billed either $600 or $1,200, depending on whether an injectable dye was used. She returned to the first hospital, the one recommended by her doctor, and had the test done, assuming it would be somewhere between $600 and $5,300. Her final bill totaled almost $7,500, in part because the hospital ran the scan twice, for reasons that were never explained. As Bebinger concluded, "This is all incredibly confusing and about as far from the transparent process that is supposed to help us 'shop' for care as you can get."[68]

Far from restoring faith in the rationality of the marketplace, excursions such as Bebinger's venture into the seemingly chaotic world of medicine often reinforce the long U.S. tradition of seeing medicine as an unprincipled "bazaar" operated according to "pushcart peddler" principles, to combine phrases used by Richard Carter in 1958 and the *Health in America* documentary in 1970. Historically, medical and lay critics alike have expressed concerns about the "doctor's dilemma," unnecessary or hip-pocket operations, and price collusion in both medicine and the pharmaceutical industry. More recently, the expert portrayals of a dysfunctional American health care system provide considerable evidence that the high prices Americans pay are not a measure of their quality. Focusing more attention on the business of medicine does not seem calculated immediately to soften public suspicions.[69]

At a time when national experts routinely describe the U.S. health care system as riddled with inefficiency, waste, and substandard care, citizens might well wonder what their care *is* worth. How is that price set, and who profits? Encouraging patient-consumers to investigate medical costs may well lead them to studies such as "It's the Prices, Stupid," which document the consistently higher prices that Americans pay for their care compared to their counterparts in other developed nations. Or they may find similar studies showing that Americans pay up to a third more for many of their prescription drugs than do Canadians or Europeans. When told that pharmaceutical companies explain this price differential as essential to their research and development budgets, patient-consumers might well wonder how much of those budgets goes to finance prescription drug detailing to physicians and advertising to consumers via television and the Internet.[70]

A 2010 study of patient-consumers' views of cost-conscious medical decision making suggests the depth of suspicions about the real motives behind health care reform. Participants from across the social spectrum were asked to consider various hypothetical scenarios in which quality was balanced against price. The results suggested forms of economic reasoning not likely to favor cost controls. Most participants assumed that the most expensive care was the best care, and three-quarters objected to the idea of cost containment. For some, the reasons were simple and self-centered: "I don't care about everybody else. I care about myself." Other participants equated cost control with the interests of politicians and insurance companies: "We're all against the government, or our insurance at work." Hence choosing the most expensive treatment becomes an attempt "to screw the man, if you will." Still others argued that they had been paying premiums and thus deserved to get the best care back: "We feel like we've been gouged for all these years." At the same time, "Many participants espoused the belief that medical decisions should be 'pure'—that is, patients and physicians should not think about money when making decisions about health."[71]

In light of the history told in this book, these seemingly contradictory viewpoints seem less illogical. On the one hand, they reflect a mind-set encouraged by the culture of medicine, a faith in "new and improved" care that is almost invariably more expensive than the old. Americans have long been conditioned to assume that expensive is good when it comes to medicine. The fear expressed in the 1938 *Ladies' Home Journal* survey—"cheap pay would bring cheap care"—remains alive and well.[72] Understandably, patient-consumers seeking the most consequential of medical care—the repair of a failing heart, a cancer cure, the reversal of infertility—want the best care, not the most economical care. No one goes looking for a bargain-basement neurosurgeon or oncologist. Even for more common procedures, the prevailing assumption remains that the more expensive procedure will have better results.

On the other hand, American patient-consumers have a deep-seated fear of the profit motive as it operates in health care. Patients have been inclined to see medicine that was too businesslike—whether the individual-entrepreneur model of the 1920s or the managed-medicine model of the 1990s—as a serious threat to their well-being. As a result, calls for health policy reforms justified by any kind of market-based claims are likely to arouse suspicion. Unlike economists, most patient-consumers regard more market-minded medicine as a threat, not an opportunity. They tend to assume, with good reason, that the health care system works to benefit providers, employers, and insurers more than patients. And they are aware that when it comes to legislation and regulation, those who stand to profit have more lobbying power than patients do.

Thus, the synergisms between medical consumerism and "new and improved" medicine are doomed to repeat a cycle of enthusiasm and disappointment. That sense of "one step forward, two steps back" reflects the tensions between the two directives that have shaped the American health care system: to make medicine profitable and to make it better serve patients. There can be no doubt which is the prime directive: the American system favors innovations that make money for those who invest in them. The system is hardwired to sustain the "new and improved" credo. As much as all the parties involved insist that the goal of better serving patients is paramount, the truth is that the need to make money from medical care remains a more powerful incentive. Innovations that reduce costs thus are never likely to be adopted as quickly or easily as those that increase them. And where the two directives conflict, the push for profits will likely triumph.

Critics may complain that the health care system is "broken," but in fact the majority of companies engaged in its delivery continue to post very healthy profit margins. The exception is the medical profession: many physicians have found their incomes falling. But for most other players, the system is not broken but rather works quite well to do what it is designed to do—provide a good return on investment. Therein lies the appeal of the new and improved in medicine. Ironically, in advertising circles, the phrase "new and improved" has come to signify a lame attempt "to give the impression of radical improvement in the quality or performance of a product which might not actually be there."[73] Yet in medicine, the linked assumptions that new is always better than old and that more is always better than less persist because they facilitate lucrative ways of doing business. Those assumptions will likely continue to flourish as long as they serve the interests of important stakeholders such as pharmaceutical companies, medical device makers, insurance companies, and hospital corporations. Reflecting the effective capitalist enterprises that they are, health care industries have shown remarkable facility in adapting to external regulation: stakeholders have learned not only to tolerate "consumer protection" but to turn it to their own advantage.

As long as so many of its moving parts remain profitable, this complex system is not going to change easily. Critics may be right when they warn that the graying of the baby boomers makes the present course unsustainable. The health care system will go bankrupt or be fixed. Yet until that doomsday scenario arrives, change will remain difficult. Since the Great Depression, the health care industry has acquired a reputation for being recession-proof. It is no coincidence that health care stocks now dominate our retirement plans: they are dependable investments.

At the heart of that success has been a shrewd assessment of health as a commodity that Americans value. Along with the other elements of the American dream—the fine home, the new car, the stylish clothes—free enterprise medicine has promised to make buying health as predictable as choosing a refrigerator or an automobile. The mantra of "new and improved" has shaped the American health care system for more than a century. The same methods used to promote consumption in general have been creatively adapted to health: the newspaper chronicles of medical breakthroughs, the flood of advertising evoking a life of good health, free of disease, free of pain, free of worry. But in the end, this approach to medical care inevitably oversells the virtues of newness and abundance.

Market actors have repeatedly and skillfully turned medical consumerism to their own purposes. In their study of guidelines for DTCA, Denis G. Arnold and James L. Oakley used the term "deceptive blocking strategy" to describe how companies may appear to adopt a supportive position as a means to ward off undesired political or regulatory action. That same concept can be applied to other aspects of patient protection, from informed consent forms to product labels to patient information leaflets. As long as the possible risks are mentioned, the end user must assume responsibility for anything bad that happens. Expressing a concern for patient-consumers serves primarily as a means to deflect criticism and responsibility. It is, to borrow Arnold and Oakley's terms, a "ruse" and "smokescreen."[74]

Although there are 260 million of them, patients do not exercise an organized force commensurate with their numbers. Since Oscar Ewing first dreamed up the idea in 1952, the idea of an American Patients Association, a large, powerful group dedicated solely to promoting the well-being of all American patients, has never become reality. That said, the cause of patient empowerment has produced many a David group willing to go after Goliath.

Now as in the past, small groups can have an impact disproportionate to their overall budgets. As a recent study done by Community Catalyst showed, nonprofit organizations in every state continue to work to voice the needs and concerns of patient-consumers, including those most vulnerable to the downsides of managed medicine. Nonprofit groups such as Health Care for All and Healthy Families USA attempt to bring those perspectives to bear on important debates about health care. Many private foundations, among them the Kaiser Permanente Foundation, the Robert Wood Johnson Foundation, and the Commonwealth Fund, seek to do the same. But for all their value, these groups tend to have less clout than their for-profit counterparts.

The David-versus-Goliath problem is perhaps nowhere better illustrated than in the realm of information outreach. The funds available to a pharmaceutical company to promote a particular drug far outweigh the budget of the Patient-Centered Outcomes Research Institute. Private for-profit enterprises can have their pick of the best advertising and marketing firms in the world; they can use their years of experience in crafting accessible, comprehensible, and attention-getting campaigns. While they are easy to mock, direct-to-consumer ads reach many more people than a public service message on the same subject. Given the fierce pushback from industry against efforts to restrict corporate free speech, the messages disseminated by these ads will remain hard to control or counteract.

The celebration of patient empowerment to be found in marketing materials, along with images of Disney World and Acura dealerships, must be put in this larger and more depressing context. In some ways, the movement of medical consumerism from the margins to the mainstream of policy debates has compounded the problems patients face. While patient initiatives and activism have secured the expansion of some valuable kinds of choices and safeguards, they have been offset by growing demands for cost containment and "market discipline" that have limited the autonomy of both individual physicians and patients. Expectations of doctor-patient partnership have been complicated not only by persistent asymmetries in their knowledge and power bases but also by contradictory pressures to limit costs while securing the best—and usually most expensive—treatments. While the idea of the patient as watchdog has produced positive change, it has been no match for the powerful economic forces that have shaped American medicine for more a century. The ability of individual patient-consumers to reshape and redirect the dysfunctional characteristics of our health care system has been greatly overestimated. To invoke René Dubos's image of the U.S. health care system as a glamorous but off-course ocean liner, patient-consumers alone cannot fix its "defective compass and an absurdly small rudder."[75]

While encouraging much-needed attention to cost, quality, and safety, the 2015 version of medical consumerism has flaws that mirror the medical culture in which it operates. Medical consumerism tends to direct attention to discrete products (insurance plans, prescription drugs) and procedures (mammograms, cardiac bypass procedures) rather than global outcomes; its skills work better to study the trees than to see the forest. Moreover, medical consumerism tends to get stuck with a menu of choices that patients have had a limited role in developing. The available products and procedures are developed and promoted by stakeholders with their own interests. Although the major stakeholders in the health care economy today are more consumer conscious than they used to be, they are still committed primarily to selling their particular products or services and exercise their considerable political and financial clout to that end.

Past efforts to practice consumerism in the doctor's office and the drugstore give us very little reason to anticipate that the latest version of doctor-shopping will magically solve all the problems in the health care system. Faced with the messy reality of a dysfunctional health care system, it is tempting to revert to an oversimplified cast of heroes and villains and to replace the old-style doctor-bashing with new-style patient-blaming. The United States has a long tradition of blaming ignorant, irrational patient-consumers for the failures of American medicine. Patients' irrationality provides a simple explanation for why the system remains broken: they refuse to believe in the truths revealed by "real" science or "real" economics; they resist paying what services are "really" worth; they seek the "wrong" service (Botox, breast implants) and ignore the prudent action (smoking cessation, healthy diet). While this line of argument is by no means novel, it carries new weight at a time when "everyone agrees" that patients are now empowered to get whatever they want. In the new era of collaborative medicine, patient-consumers have no place to hide.

In fact, "consumerism" provides an easy target for frustrated physicians, policymakers, and politicians, especially because the term is used interchangeably for both critical consumerism and its noncritical counterparts of the "keeping up with the medical Joneses" type. In the past as well as the present, that term has meant many different things to many different people. In one context, it means critical consumerism of the watchdog variety; in another, the impetus to "give the lady what she wants." Making "consumerism" of either sort the sole explanation for what is wrong with the U.S. health care system makes no more sense than assuming that all physicians or all managed-care companies are heroic or villainous. This history attests to the fact that the advocates of "critical consumerism"—the argument that patients deserve to be as informed as possible, to be involved as partners in their own care, to be treated as whole human beings, and to be protected from price gouging—have played an important role in advancing the "triple aims" of health reform. So why has the late-twentieth-century embrace of the activated patient not done more good?

While useful in some ways, the skills of medical consumerism are no match for the complexities of human disease, medical science, and entrepreneurial capitalism. Making medicine more like the rest of consumer culture has not improved patient care nearly as much as expected. That should come as no surprise, given the fundamental flaws that exist in consumer culture as a whole. At a time when automobile manufacturers are having to recall millions of vehicles due to potential safety problems and Disney World has come under fire for planning to hire immigrant workers to run its online services, the idea that medicine will excel by emulating such "consumer friendly" industries rightly inspires skepticism. Moreover, the goal of making medicine more like other businesses repeatedly founders on the reality already recognized by 1933: medical care "cannot be bought and sold like a box of soap."[76] No amount of marketization or consumerification can offset the "shopping problems" that patients face when making choices about their doctors and their medicines. Thus the belief that Americans can cheerfully shop their way out of the current health care mess is and has always been an illusion. Reshaping the economic and therapeutic expectations of some 220 million Americans is not going to be easy, and anyone who suggests otherwise is seriously deluded.

So in the face of all this messiness, should we give up on the idea of empowering patients as individuals and as an interest group? Absolutely not. In pointing out the problems that consumerist practices have faced in the past and still face today, I intend not to discredit the cause but to inject it with a needed dose of realism. Even if the ideal of a more broadly engaged patient-consumer does not provide a magic wand to fix a broken system, it is still a worthwhile goal to pursue. A growing body of research suggests that enhancing shared decision making between doctor and patient can indeed improve the quality of care while bending the cost curve down. When done with skill and compassion, engaging patients in their own care can help build rather than tear down trust in their medical team. So while no magic cure-all, fostering patient engagement and shared decision making represents a sound investment for a better health care future.

What does the history told here suggest about how to go forward? The successes and failures of past efforts to turn patients into partners suggest the following modest conclusions. First, strategies that focus only on very narrowly defined economic choices of insurance policies are not likely to succeed. What is needed is a far more inclusive set of principles and practices to facilitate patient-citizen input at every level of policymaking and planning: a harkening back to the unrealized aspirations of the 1970s of the sort Rachel Grob and Mark Schlesinger have argued for so eloquently in their 2011 "Principles for Engaging Patients in U.S. Health Care and Policy." Second, the reforms most likely to succeed are those that build on the strong connections that still exist between doctors and patients. For all their frustrations with the health care system, Americans maintain a deep respect for medicine in general and for individual doctors in particular. A 2009 Gallup poll found that 73 percent of those surveyed felt that doctors were far better guides to health care policy than were members of Congress, health insurance administrators, or pharmaceutical company executives. Patient-consumers are thus likely to respond positively to the reforms that physicians lead and support. This reservoir of respect makes it all the more important that the medical profession fulfill its duties as the patient-consumers' trusted intermediary by firewalling its scientific and ethical standards against the corrosive forces of commercialism.[77]

If history be a reliable guide, that commercialism will be no easy foe to vanquish. In recognizing that fact, we need to pay more attention to the problems of scaling up the skills of patient vigilance. The concept of the watchdog patient was the product of often unconscious (and perhaps now fast disappearing) patterns of middle-class privilege: a high degree of education, access to affordable insurance, and not-so-subtle racial and gender prejudices. Revamping that concept means taking seriously the values and preferences of the many Americans who do not fit the old model of the "intelligent" consumer. Of all the challenges ahead, this one may be the hardest to resolve. But the goal of helping all Americans feel more engaged with and empowered regarding their medical care is so important that we must persevere.

While perhaps not as powerful or unbiased a tool as we might prefer, medical consumerism remains a useful mind-set for approaching the challenges that lie ahead. As long as the current system prevails—and no end appears to be in sight—protecting oneself and one's family requires critical consumerism. Perhaps the most surprising aspect of this history is how relevant the consumerist solutions put forth in the past remain. Despite the many changes that have taken place in the past twenty or even fifty years, the advice given to people wanting to find good medical care in 1930 remains remarkably useful in 2015. Now, as then, verify your doctor's credentials, read the labels on your medicine bottles, consider the pros and cons of every procedure, and seek an insider's knowledge concerning every medical decision. Before trusting any expert, make sure he or she is worth trusting. Be skeptical about the forces of commercialism at work beneath the surface of the modern medical miracle. Adopted with a keen sense of their limitations, the skills of the modern medical consumer are still well worth acquiring. In short, as F. J. Schlink wrote in 1936, "We will get good medical service only insofar as those who need it are critically informed and as expert as laymen can be toward it."[78]

NOTES

This is a very long book. To keep its size manageable, I have had to give up the historian's preferred habit of citing multiple primary sources to back up every argument and settle only for the handful that I quote. Likewise, I am sparing in my citations and historiographic commentary on the secondary literature. What has been written about the topics I cover here could fill a good-sized library. Although I depend heavily on those prior studies, I can highlight only a few that I found most useful. The best I can do is to give the interested reader a place to start in exploring the wealth of primary and secondary sources that touch on this topic.

Abbreviations

CR Records • Consumers' Research Inc. Records, Special Collections, Alexander Library, Rutgers University, New Brunswick, New Jersey

Davis Collection • Michael M. Davis Collection, Malloch Rare Book Room, New York Academy of Medicine Library, New York

FDA Records • Records of the Food and Drug Administration, Record Group 88, National Archives, College Park, Maryland

Harding Papers • T. Swann Harding Papers, MSS24885, Library of Congress, Manuscript Division, Washington, D.C.

House Committee Hearings • U.S. Congress, House, Committee on Interstate and Foreign Commerce, Hearings on Federal Food, Drug, and Cosmetic Act, 82nd Cong., 1st sess., May 1–5, 1951

JWT Archives • J. Walter Thompson Company Archives, David M. Rubenstein Rare Book and Manuscript Library, Duke University, Durham, North Carolina

NYT • *New York Times*

WP • *Washington Post*

Preface

1. Tara Parker-Pope, "Plenty of Blame in a Health System 'Designed to Fail,'" *NYT*, May 8, 2012.

Introduction

1. Scalise, "Patient Satisfaction."

2. Tara Parker-Pope, "Plenty of Blame in a Health System 'Designed to Fail,'" *NYT*, May 8, 2012.

3. For a good example of this kind of argument, see Frist, "Connected Health."

4. On the history of Henderson's famous quote, see Rothstein, "When Did a Random Patient Benefit?" On the concept of the golden age as well as historians' critiques of it, see Burnham, "American Medicine's Golden Age"; Brandt and Gardner, "Golden Age." My fellow historians of medicine have long been skeptical of the "golden age" myth. For two insightful studies of the doctor-patient relationship that challenge the myth of the totally passive patient in the pre-1960 era, see Crenner, *Private Practice*, esp. chap. 7; Lerner, "Beyond Informed Consent."

5. Whorton, *Nature Cures*.

6. Ray Lyman Wilbur, foreword to Falk, Rorem, and Ring, *Costs of Medical Care*, v; Clark, *How to Budget Health*, 27 (industry rankings).

7. "Consumerism"; "Text of Kennedy's Message to Congress on Protections for Consumers," *NYT*, March 16, 1962; Cohen, *Consumers' Republic*; Glickman, *Buying Power*. Consumer advocates are sometimes referred to as "consumerists," a usage I adopt in this book. What I am calling medical consumerism is a direct antecedent of today's policy model of the engaged, activated patient. But for reasons this history helps explain, the term "consumerism" is so laden with negative baggage that it tends to get downplayed in policy discussions. For a very insightful discussion of this issue, see Rachel Grob, "Heart of Patient-Centered Care."

8. On "the shopping problem," see Dranove, *Economic Evolution*, chap. 1.

9. "Consumerism."

10. Cohen, *Consumers' Republic*, 261.

11. Lee Sataline, "A Physician Learns the 'Double Speak' of Insurance Forms," *NYT*, September 14, 1986; Ellen Goodman, "We've Become Health Care Consumers—And We're Getting Indigestion," *Boston Globe*, June 17, 1999.

12. This argument has been inspired by Audre Lorde's famous statement that "the Master's tools will never dismantle the Master's house" (Lorde, *Sister Outsider*, 110).

13. Bredow, *Handbook* (1943), 43.

14. Ewing devised the idea after the defeat of Harry S. Truman's health insurance plan (see Chap. 5). Cron came up with the idea in 1970 (see Chap. 8). As far as I know, Cron had no knowledge of Ewing's proposal.

15. On astroturfing, see Walker, *Grassroots for Hire*.

16. Tannenbaum and Branden, *Patient's Dilemma*, ix.

17. Sontag, *Illness as Metaphor*, 3; for a recent overview of scholarship on patient activism, see Epstein, "Patient Groups and Health Movements."

18. Farquhar, *American Way of Life*. I also focus on licit rather than illicit drugs, although their histories are inseparable, as shown by Courtwright, *Forces of Habit*.

19. Jenner and Wallis, "Medical Marketplace." The pioneering work on this topic was Porter, *Health for Sale*. For an overview of recent work on twentieth-century medical consumerism and patients' rights, see Mold and Reubi, *Assembling Health Rights*. Great Britain and the United States make for an especially interesting comparison. See Mold, "Making the Patient-Consumer"; Mold, "Repositioning the Patient."

20. Robert and Donna Trussell, "Chaos Theory: Everybody, Let's Play Health Care," http://www.politicsdaily.com/2009/11/12/chaos-theory-everybody-lets-play-health-care/ (accessed July 1, 2015).

Chapter One

1. Young, *Pure Food*, 22.
2. Okun, *Fair Play*.
3. [Tennent], *Every Man His Own Doctor*. There is no surviving copy of the first edition. My description of early medical traditions in this chapter relies on Abel, *Hearts of Wisdom*; Beier, *Health Culture*; Breslaw, *Lotions, Potions*; Lamar Riley Murphy, *Enter the Physician*; Risse, Numbers, and Leavitt, *Medicine without Doctors*; Shryock, *Medicine and Society*; Ulrich, *Midwife's Tale*. I also draw heavily on the portrayal of medicine and popular medicine in Rosenberg, "Therapeutic Revolution"; Rosenberg, "Book in the Sickroom"; Rosenberg, "Medical Text and Social Context"; Rosenberg, "John Gunn."
4. Beier, *Health Culture*, 12.
5. Strasser, "Historical Herbal."
6. On Ballard, see Ulrich, *Midwife's Tale*; on Randolph, see Beier, *Health Culture*, 12; on Binah, see Fett, *Working Cures*, 124.
7. My account here relies on Kett, *Formation*; Rothstein, *American Physicians*; Shryock, *Medical Licensing*.
8. Rosenberg, "Practice of Medicine"; Leavitt, "'Worrying Profession.'"
9. As an example of persistence, muckraking journalist Mark Sullivan, born in 1874 on a farm outside West Chester, Pennsylvania, recalled that his thrifty mother collected herbs such as pennyroyal and St. John's wort to treat her ten children, preferring those remedies to the Hood's Sarsaparilla and Ayer's Cherry Pectoral advertised in the almanac that the local store owner gave them every year (*Education of an American*, 13).
10. On home medical texts, see Rosenberg, "Medical Text"; Rosenberg, "John Gunn"; Rosenberg, "Book in the Sickroom." On early patent medicines and their advertising, see Young, *Toadstool Millionaires*, esp. chap. 3. On newspapers, see John, *Spreading the News*, esp. chap. 2, where de Tocqueville's reaction is mentioned on 41.
11. Shryock, *Medical Licensing*; Whorton, *Nature Cures*.
12. On proprietary medical schools, see Ludmerer, *Learning to Heal*. On physicians as patent medicine entrepreneurs, see Young, *Toadstool Millionaires*. On physicians' views regarding monopoly and patenting, see Gabriel, *Medical Monopoly*.
13. Rosen, *Fees and Fee Bills*. For a colorful account of a rural office practice, see Hertzler, *Horse and Buggy Doctor*.
14. Pusey, "Old Time Country Doctor," 584. See also Rosenberg, "Practice of Medicine"; Rosenberg, "Therapeutic Revolution"; Leavitt, "'Worrying Profession.'"
15. Hertzler, *Horse and Buggy Doctor*, 112. On patient interactions with physicians, see Sheila M. Rothman, *Living in the Shadow*; Morantz-Sanchez, *Conduct Unbecoming a Woman*.
16. Walton Hamilton, "Ancient Maxim," 1180.
17. Mohr, *Doctors and the Law*; De Ville, *Medical Malpractice*. Both the old common law tradition and the newer contractual approach emphasized the importance of consent to treatment. For an overview of nineteenth-century concepts of informed consent, see Pernick, "Patient's Role."
18. "Opinion of the Court," *Thomas v. Winchester*, Court of Appeals of New York,

1952, http://www.courts.state.ny.us/reporter/archives/thomas_winchester.htm (accessed July 1, 2015). On the history of poisons, see Bartrip, "'Pennurth of Arsenic'"; Deborah Blum, *Poisoner's Handbook*.

19. Shryock, *Medical Licensing*, 54–55. See also the very useful summary of medical licensing legislation in Rothstein, *American Physicians*, appendix II.

20. Naomi Rogers, *Alternative Path*; Whorton, *Nature Cures*.

21. There is a huge literature on the reorganization of medicine in this period. Good overviews are provided by Starr, *Social Transformation*; Rosen and Rosenberg, *Structure*. On health insurance, see Beatrix Hoffman, *Wages of Sickness*; Numbers, *Almost Persuaded*. On the reform of medical education, see Ludmerer, *Learning to Heal*; on the AMA, see Burrow, *Organized Medicine*; on medicine's ethical codes, see Robert B. Baker et al., *American Medical Ethics Revolution*. For case studies of the changing dynamics of private medical practice, see Crenner, *Private Practice*; Schafer, *Business*.

22. Cathell, *Book*, 122, 123.

23. Stout, "Alagazam," 26 ("pioneers of novelties"); Young, *Toadstool Millionaires*; Lears, *Fables of Abundance*.

24. Young, *Toadstool Millionaires*.

25. Alcohol remains widely used in medicines but at lower concentrations than existed in most old proprietary remedies. Well into the twentieth century, pharmacy textbooks contained lengthy discussions of how to improve the taste of medicines in order to make them more appealing to patients. See, for example, "Making Medicines Taste Better"; Potter and Scott, *Therapeutics*, esp. 538.

26. On the testimonial, see Young, *Toadstool Millionaires*, 187–89.

27. On patent medicine's pioneering use of outdoor advertising, see ibid., 119–24. On the history of mail order and the development of a national consumption culture, see Strasser, *Satisfaction Guaranteed*. On the history of the U.S. Postal Service, see John, *Spreading the News*.

28. Quoted in Young, *Toadstool Millionaires*, 101.

29. On the Progressive era concept of "the consumer," see Glickman, *Buying Power*, esp. 155–62.

30. On the impact of the 1906 law, see Young, *Pure Food*. A third standard-setter joined the United States Pharmacopeia and the National Formulary in 1905, when the American Medical Association set up the Council on Pharmacy and Chemistry to evaluate new drugs; that group subsequently began to issue a guide to "new and nonofficial remedies."

31. "Poison Squad Escapes Federal Food Experts," *NYT*, May 22, 1904. See also Carol Lewis, "Poison Squad." The Division of Chemistry of the U.S. Department of Agriculture was founded in 1862, renamed the Bureau of Chemistry in 1901 and then the Food, Drug, and Insecticide Administration in 1927, and finally shortened to the Food and Drug Administration in 1930.

32. Goodwin, *Pure Food, Drink, and Drug Crusaders*; Bok, *Americanization*, esp. chap. 30; Krabbendam, *Model Man*, esp. chap. 4.

33. Adams, *Great American Fraud*, 84; Cassedy, "Muckraking and Medicine."

34. Young, *Pure Food*.

35. Adams, *Great American Fraud*, 68.

36. Young, *Pure Food*, 253.

37. Ibid., 187–89; "Killing Public Health Legislation," 795.

38. Young, *Medical Messiahs*, 35–37.

39. Griffenhagen and Bogard, *History of Drug Containers*, 89–90.

40. *United States v. Johnson*, 221 U.S. 488 (1911). Justice Holmes was the son of Oliver Wendell Holmes, who had once consigned all of medical therapeutics to the bottom of the ocean.

41. On the Sherley Amendment, see Young, *Medical Messiahs*, 49–51, 59–65.

42. "A Directory of the Habit-Forming Drugs," *The Survey*, June 18, 1910; "National Fight on Baby-Killers," *The Survey*, October 1, 1910. On the impact of the 1906 law, see Young, *Medical Messiahs*, esp. chap. 3, and Hilts, *Protecting America's Health*, esp. chap. 4. For an interesting before-and-after comparison of ads, see Cramp, "Therapeutic Thaumaturgy," 425.

43. On the Harrison Act, see Courtwright, *Dark Paradise*, esp. 100–109. The required label is shown in Griffenhagen and Bogard, *History of Drug Containers*, 90. On doctors and Prohibition, see Gage, "Just What the Doctor Ordered," and Okrent, *Last Call*, esp. 195–97.

44. Not surprisingly, companics that were disadvantaged by Wiley's rulings protested to the secretary of agriculture. For a critical view of Wiley, see Coppin and High, *Politics of Purity*; for a more sympathetic view, see Junod, review of *Politics of Purity*.

45. U.S. Census, 1920. For an overview of consumer culture in these decades, see Blaszczyk, *American Consumer Society*.

46. Matt, *Keeping up with the Joneses*.

47. Hansen, *Picturing Medical Progress*, esp. pts. 2 and 3.

48. Silent film summaries taken from the American Film Institute database www .afi.com/members/catalog. For overviews of the highly diverse and often negative portrayals of physicians in both silent and sound films, see Spears, *Hollywood*, 314–32; Dans, *Doctors in the Movies*.

49. Ephraim, *Take Care of Yourself*; Cooley, *Human Nature*, 179–85. On the post–World War I ideal of positive health, see Toon, "Managing the Conduct."

50. Lynd and Lynd, *Middletown*, 438.

51. Morgan, "Hearts in the Breaking," 182.

52. Galdston, "Pathogenicity of Progress." On the demographic debates, see Alter and Carmichael, "Classifying the Dead." On the changing disease order, I draw here on Tomes, "Reshuffling the Cards." During bad years for respiratory infections, cancer would slip from second to third among death rates.

53. White, "Heart Disease," 952; Saltzstein, "Cancer," 219.

54. "We Die Differently Now," 26. The "we die differently now" was an updated version of a very old argument. See Porter, "Diseases of Civilization."

55. Boas, "Heart Diseases," 313–14; "Clues to Cancer," 20; George Gray Ward, "What You Should Know," 822.

56. Wallace R. Boren, "Mental Lunch Counters for Consumers," *J. Walter Thompson Bulletin* 13 (May 1930): 24, 26, 27.

57. Loren A. Schuler, "Talk Given by Mr. Loren A. Schuler, Editor of the *Ladies' Home Journal*," May 26, 1930, Staff Meeting Minutes, box 8, JWT Archives.

58. Morrill Goddard, "Talk Given at Monday Evening Meeting," March 17, 1930, Staff Meeting Minutes, box 5, JWT Archives.

59. Walter C. Alvarez to T. Swann Harding, January 7, 1928, Harding Papers.

60. Morrill Goddard, "Talk Given at Monday Evening Meeting," March 17, 1930, Staff Meeting Minutes, box 5, JWT Archives; "How to Tell," 3.

61. Armstrong, "Health Facts."

62. "If, by Rudyard Zilch," 27.

Chapter Two

1. Rinehart, "High Cost," 92, 94, 39.

2. Damrau, "Has the Doctor," 44.

3. Mason, "Business of Doctoring," 739.

4. Cabot, *Doctor's Bill*, 51–52; Ludmerer, *Learning to Heal*, 60; Schafer, *Business*, 166.

5. Pusey, "Medical Education and Medical Service," 1505. On the Flexner Report, see Starr, *Social Transformation*, 118–27; Bonner, *Iconoclast*.

6. Burrow, *Organized Medicine*.

7. Hertzler, *Horse and Buggy Doctor*, 58.

8. Rosenberg, *Care of Strangers*; Rosemary Stevens, *In Sickness and in Wealth*.

9. Sinai et al., *Survey*, 25.

10. Cabot, *Doctor's Bill*, 115–16; Rosemary Stevens, *American Medicine*, 181. For an insightful look at the growing trend toward specialism in Philadelphia, see Schafer, *Business*.

11. On the origins of fee splitting, see Rosemary Stevens, *American Medicine*, 83–84, 91.

12. For a comparative overview of specialism, see Weisz, *Divide and Conquer*.

13. Parson, *In the Doctor's Office*, 51.

14. "Practice-Building Offices," 59–60.

15. Rinehart, "High Cost," 92.

16. See Shumsky, Bohland, and Knox, "Separating Doctors' Homes," 1051.

17. Baketel, "Come Early," 35.

18. Leven, *Incomes of Physicians*, 42.

19. Harry H. Moore, *American Medicine*, 519; Cabot, *Doctor's Bill*, 35–39; Hertzler, *Horse and Buggy Doctor*, 130.

20. Schafer, *Business*.

21. Falk, Rorem, and Ring, *Costs of Medical Care*, 388, 399.

22. Hertzler, *Horse and Buggy Doctor*, 35. For an excellent discussion of the class and racial segregation inherent in the interwar clustering of physician's offices, see Schafer, *Business*.

23. "Doctor's Wife Speaks Up," 350.

24. Baketel, "Come Early," 35; Bicknell, "Making the Office Attractive," 17.

25. Veteran Patient, "Some Dressing Rooms," 19, 21.

26. "Well-Equipped Office," 22; "Modern Office Equipment," 27.

27. "Doctor's Wife Speaks Up," 349. For an insightful look at how these trends transformed the doctor's office, see Crenner, *Private Practice*.

28. Advertisements in *Medical Economics* and the *New York State Journal of Medicine*, late 1920s. Physicians understandably took great pride in the new equipment they acquired, as evident in the photographs in Apple, *Illustrated Catalogue*, such as image 685, "X-ray Equipment in Dr. Lehnhoff's Office; Nebraska, c. 1910," 39; image 1676, "Dr. Beshoar amid X-ray and Other Equipment in His Office; Trinidad, Colo., 1900," 80. The Library of Congress's Prints and Photographs Online Catalog includes many photographs of doctors' offices that document the variety of equipment and decors to be found there (http://www.loc.gov/pictures/; accessed July 1, 2015).

29. *Medical Economics* 2 (March 1925): 26, and 3 (April 1926): 29.

30. It is difficult to generalize about exactly what medical students were taught about how to take a patient history before 1940. But American medical education in these decades was heavily influenced by the example of William Osler, who emphasized the importance of physical diagnosis as the foundation of medical practice. On Osler and his influence, see Bliss, *William Osler*. For a perceptive account of the methods used by one exceptionally thorough practitioner, see Crenner, *Private Practice*.

31. Michael Marks Davis, *America Organizes Medicine*, 9. In his survey of surgical procedures done between 1928 and 1931, Selwyn D. Collins found that 30 percent were done in the office or clinic ("Frequency of Surgical Procedures," 617).

32. See Dale Smith, "Appendicitis." On changing therapeutics, see also Gerald Grob, "Rise of Peptic Ulcer"; Gerald Grob, "Rise and Decline." On the introduction of insulin, see Feudtner, *Bittersweet*.

33. Peebles, *Survey*, 145; *Medical Economics* 5, no. 1 (October 1927): 47.

34. Selwyn D. Collins, "Frequency of Surgical Procedures," 617.

35. Pringle, "Aesculapius," 364. On focal infection, see Gerald Grob, "Rise and Decline," 387–90; Gerald Grob, "Rise of Peptic Ulcer."

36. Musgrave, "Who Is Your Doctor?," 233, 234.

37. On the variability of doctors' training, see Harry H. Moore, *American Medicine*, 518–20. Moore discussed this problem in relation to rural practitioners, but there is no reason to think it did not apply to urban doctors as well.

38. Rowell, "How to Get Your Money's Worth," 76; "Doctor's Wife Speaks Up," 348.

39. Ruth Henderson, "Rather Worse," 32.

40. Falk, Rorem, and Ring, *Costs of Medical Care*, 221.

41. Rinehart, "High Cost," 96; Albright, "High Cost," 591; Lloyd Morris, "Mammon, M.D.," 614, 617.

42. Mason, "Business of Doctoring," 739.

43. "Doctor's Wife Speaks Up," 350.

44. Rowell, "How to Get Your Money's Worth," 77.

45. Wingate M. Johnson, "Family Doctor Speaks His Mind," 55.

46. Merle Farmer Murphy, "Flivver System in Medicine," *Independent*, April 25, 1925; Ruth Henderson, "Rather Worse," 52; Swackhamer, *Choice and Change*, 12–13.

47. Albright, "High Cost," 593; Donald B. Armstrong, "See Your Doctor," 393.

48. Doctors such as Baker encouraged the public to criticize organized medicine. As Baker told his radio listeners, "Let [doctors] know that you are not boobs, that you are people with intelligence, and won't stand for any underhanded dirty tricks." Medical professionalism was not altruistic but rather another manifestation of the "doctors'

trust," resisting anything that would "flatten out their purses" (Juhnke, *Quacks and Crusaders*, 50, 52).

49. Peebles, *Survey*, 46; Rinehart, "High Cost," 39.

50. Woolley, *Physicians' Systems*, 7.

51. Baketel, "Chorus Grows."

52. Brewer's article originally appeared in 1926 and was reprinted in the appendix of Harry H. Moore, *American Medicine*, 556–58, quotes on 556, 557; Mason, "Business of Doctoring," 738, 739.

53. Woolley, *Physicians' Systems*, 90.

54. Brewer, reprinted in Harry H. Moore, *American Medicine*, 556; Michael Marks Davis, *Paying Your Sickness Bills*, 7.

55. Linsly R. Williams, "Your Doctor's Bill," 28; Harry H. Moore, *American Medicine*, 554.

56. Pringle, "Aesculapius," 366; Michael Davis, "Blunderbuss,"438.

57. "Why the Doc's Bills Aren't Paid," 65; Linsly R. Williams, "Your Doctor's Bill," 21.

58. Eleanor Roosevelt to Missy LeHand, January 8, 1936, framed and on display at the Franklin D. Roosevelt Presidential Library and Museum, Hyde Park, New York. Their son had seen the doctor eleven times for treatment of hemorrhoids.

59. Sinai et al., *Survey*, 202.

60. Falk, Rorem, and Ring, *Costs of Medical Care*, 520.

61. Donald B. Armstrong, "See Your Doctor," 388; undated, handwritten note, likely written by either F. J. Schlink or Eleanor Loeb, box 439, file 21, CR Records. In addition to Kallet's experience, the note also reported that many physicians kept recommending mercurochrome despite its ineffectiveness and that some even prescribed the use of radium water, one of the most dangerous patent medicines of the 1930s.

62. Peña, *Body Electric*; Juhnke, *Quacks and Crusaders*; Watkins, *Estrogen Elixir*; Lloyd Morris, "Mammon, M.D."

63. Dale Smith, "Appendicitis," 424; Harding, "How Scientific Are Our Doctors?," 348.

64. Damrau, "Has the Doctor," 47.

65. Albright, "High Cost," 592, 593.

66. Joseph Collins, "Doctor Looks at Doctors," 350.

67. Harry H. Moore, *American Medicine*, 555.

68. Foster, "Medicine's Right to Control," 588–89.

69. On the CCMC, see Starr, *Social Transformation*, 261–66. On larger currents of economic thinking in medicine, see Daniel M. Fox, "From Reform to Relativism."

70. Ray Lyman Wilbur, foreword to Falk, Rorem, and Ring, *Costs of Medical Care*, vi. On the impact of the cultural lag theory on the CCMC work, see Perkins, "Economic Organization."

71. Falk, Rorem, and Ring, *Costs of Medical Care*, 384, 385, 520.

72. Ibid., 527.

73. Committee on the Costs of Medical Care, *Medical Care*, 103–44 (majority recommendations), 151–83 (first minority report), 184–88 (second minority report), 189–201 (two personal dissents).

74. Fishbein, "Committee on the Costs of Medical Care," 1952.

75. Rubinow, "In Defense of Socialized Medicine," 509.

76. Michael Marks Davis, *Paying Your Sickness Bills*, 54.

Chapter Three

1. LeBlanc, "Medicine Show," 235, 237.

2. "Restrained Suburban Drugstore," 140.

3. Gathercoal, *Prescription Ingredient Survey*, 6.

4. Rorem and Fischelis, *Costs of Medicines*, 153.

5. "500 Corner Drugstores," 73; Levinson, *Great A&P*; Leach, *Land of Desire*.

6. Bacon, *America's Corner Store*, 27–28. My account of Walgreen's career here is taken largely from Bacon.

7. By 1932, four years of pharmacy training had become the norm; see Sonnedecker, *Kremers and Urdang's History*, 240.

8. Bacon, *America's Corner Store*, 34. On the low status of community pharmacy, see Elenbaas and Worthen, "Transformation of a Profession."

9. Bacon, *America's Corner Store*, 29–30, 38–39.

10. Ibid., 85; Nolen and Maynard, *Drug Store Management*, 160.

11. "500 Corner Drugstores," 71; *Sales Management*, April 23, 1932, 100. On the growth of chains, see Lebhar, *Chain Stores in America*. For a case study of the antichain movement, see Levinson, *Great A&P*, esp. 112–24, 151–66, 195–205.

12. "Unique Survey," 88. On the Rexall Company, see Mickey C. Smith, *Rexall Story*. For a good overview of the different kinds of drugstores, see Nolen and Maynard, *Drug Store Management*. On black-owned drugstores, see Harmon, "Negro as a Local Business Man," 142; Weems, *Desegregating the Dollar*, 9.

13. Nolen and Maynard, *Drug Store Management*, 3, 5; Falk, Rorem, and Ring, *Costs of Medical Care*, 367, 368.

14. On state regulation of pharmacies, see Sonnedecker, *Kremers and Urdang's History*, esp. chap. 13. On the proprietary exemption, see Fletcher, *Market Restraints*, 98–99. Rorem and Fischelis, *Costs of Medicines*, 246–48, provides a summary of state laws regarding the sale of proprietary medicines outside drugstores.

15. Whereas the 1905 edition of Remington's classic pharmacy text did not have a chapter on pharmacy and the law, the 1936 version had two sections, one on commercial law and the other on laws relating to public health; see Remington, *Practice of Pharmacy*; Cook and LaWall, *Remington's Practice of Pharmacy*, 1343–70. The increased attention to regulation of drugs is also evident in Rorem and Fischelis, *Costs of Medicines*, esp. chap. 11.

16. For an overview of prescription sales, see Rorem and Fischelis, *Costs of Medicines*, 58–69.

17. Gathercoal, *Prescription Ingredient Survey*, 6; Nolen and Maynard, *Drug Store Management*, 280, 85.

18. Nolen and Maynard, *Drug Store Management*, 268.

19. "500 Corner Drugstores," 77.

20. "Drug Chain Concentrates Prescription Business in Centrally Located Stores," *Printers' Ink*, June 3, 1920, 125; De Leslie Jones, "Drugstore Has Become a Convenience

Store," esp. 76. A few stores even carried refrigerators and automobile tires, but this trend did not catch on in large urban stores. As Jones notes, drugstores in smaller cities with fewer retail stores tended to have more eclectic merchandise.

21. De Leslie Jones, "Drugstore Has Become a Convenience Store," 74, 76.

22. "500 Corner Drugstores," 73.

23. LeBlanc, "Medicine Show," 237.

24. On aspirin, see Mann and Plummer, *Aspirin Wars*; on Ehrlich and salvarsan, see Brandt, *No Magic Bullet*; on Banting and insulin, see Bliss, *Discovery of Insulin*.

25. Liebenau, *Medical Science and Medical Industry*. For changes in patent law that undergirded these developments, see Gabriel, *Medical Monopoly*.

26. Rorem and Fischelis, *Costs of Medicines*, 113.

27. For contemporary overviews of the industry, see Cramp, "Debunking Drugs," and Rorem and Fischelis, *Costs of Medicines*, chap. 7.

28. Cramp, "Debunking Drugs," 346. On Parke, Davis's institutional advertising, see Duffin and Li, "Great Moments." On the move of ethical companies into the proprietary trade, see "Representatives' Meeting," May 21, 1929, box 1, Staff Meeting Minutes, JWT Archives.

29. "Whoever Shouts the Loudest"; Rorty, *Our Master's Voice*, 21 (statistics on ad agencies).

30. Hettinger, "Broadcasting Advertising Trends," 307.

31. Sizemore and Sizemore, interview; Strout, "Radio Nostrum Racket," 66.

32. Lederer, *Crazy English*, 43; "Representatives' Meeting," April 3, 1929, box 1, Staff Meeting Minutes, JWT Archives. On the problems posed by commercial advertising on the radio, see Flynn, "Radio." On the medicine show traditions that shaped radio, see Strasser, "Sponsorship and Snake Oil"; Ann Anderson, *Snake Oil*; Armstrong and Armstrong, *Great American Medicine Show*, chap. 18; McNamara, *Step Right Up*.

33. "Representatives' Meeting," April 3, 1929, box 1, Staff Meeting Minutes, JWT Archives; Walsh, "Medicine Men," 686.

34. "Special Procedure," 117–22.

35. *Annual Report*, 209, 210; Young, *Medical Messiahs*, chap. 6.

36. William Legler, "The Use of the Negative Copy Appeal," Staff Meeting Minutes, September 1, 1931, box 4, JWT Archives.

37. Harriet Anderson, "The End of the Era of Humbug," *J. Walter Thompson News Bulletin* 100 (July 1923): 12; William Legler, "The Use of the Negative Copy Appeal," Staff Meeting Minutes, September 1, 1931, box 4, JWT Archives.

38. *J. Walter Thompson News Bulletin* 130 (May 1927): 4.

39. For a 1929 defense of puffery, see Mildred Holmes, "Bunk," *J. Walter Thompson News Bulletin* 139 (August 1929): 1–4. Forty years later, another JWT executive expressed a similar sentiment: "We might even hope to make the reader feel better just from seeing our ad!" (H. J. Barnum Jr., Creative Forum Paper 14, March 1967, box 55, JWT Archives).

40. "'Patent Medicine' Business," 1018.

41. William Legler, "The Use of the Negative Copy Appeal," Staff Meeting Minutes, September 1, 1931, box 4, JWT Archives.

42. Tomes, *Gospel of Germs*.

43. "How to Combat the 7 Most Common Ailments of Mankind," Sal Hepatica, 1928, temporary box 1; "Do You Pay for Every Brilliant Hour with a Dull Day?" Sal Hepatica, *Liberty Magazine*, 1927, temporary box 1; "Bodyguards," Phillips' Milk of Magnesia, *Ladies' Home Journal*, March 1933, box 23, all in Competitive Advertisements Collection, JWT Archives.

44. Walter Alvarez to T. Swann Harding, January 30, 1928, Harding Papers; "500 Corner Drugstores," 72.

45. Peebles, *Survey*.

46. Rorem and Fischelis, *Costs of Medicines*, 18, 23; Rorty, *American Medicine Mobilizes*, 175.

47. K. E. Miller, "Public Health Aspects," 884, 885.

48. Austin Smith, "Doctors Say . . . ," 658–59; Campion, *AMA and U.S. Health Policy*, 115–16, 469–77. The AMA seal program ended as a consequence of fears that the AMA would be sued for injuries sustained by use of physical therapy devices carrying the official seal (474–76).

49. Listerine ads in Competitive Advertisements Collection, JWT Archives; "Chemical Laboratory." Listerine continued heavily to feature scientific themes; for example, "The Germ Nobody Knows" (1934) presented a lengthy discussion of scientific efforts to isolate the cold virus.

50. Pierce, *Gringo Gaucho*, 273–80.

51. Kay, *Dying to Be Beautiful*, 145 (n. 108). Consumers' Research founder F. J. Schlink sent a copy of one of Pusey's Camay ads to Cramp, asking, "Does it not give you some concern that a former President, AMA, the Editor-in-Chief of 'Archives of Dermatology,' an outstanding authority in general, should be, while setting forth what is formally the truth, responsible for a very considerable misleading of the public mind?" Cramp responded with one sentence: "I'll say I've noticed it, and I feel much worse about it than even you can!" (F. J. Schlink to Arthur Cramp, September 9, 1929, Arthur Cramp to F. J. Schlink, September 12, 1929, both in box 440, F 24, CR Records).

52. William Kimball, "Scientific Approach to Copy Ideas," Staff Meeting Minutes, November 25, 1930, box 3, folder 2, JWT Archives; Strout, "Radio Nostrum Racket," 66.

53. Peebles, *Survey*, 141.

54. Fowler, *Fowler's Publicity*, 430, 431.

55. Hoyt, *Practical Therapeutics*, 206, 207.

56. Peebles, *Survey*, 30.

57. Cramp, "Debunking Drugs," 347; Gathercoal, *Prescription Ingredient Survey*, 24; for a table summarizing the different studies, see 21.

58. Cramp, "Debunking Drugs," 346, 354.

59. Harding, "How Scientific Are Our Doctors?," 348. One entrepreneur who started a mail order business selling high-quality drugs and vitamins to discerning customers was Jerome W. Ephraim. As evident from correspondence in the Harding Papers, Harding was among Ephraim's customers.

60. Bacon, *America's Corner Store*, 65.

61. Gerrish, *Prescription Writing*, 16–17.

62. The discussion of Latin was unchanged between the 1905 and 1936; compare Remington, *Practice of Pharmacy*, 1086, and Cook and LaWall, *Remington's Practice of*

Pharmacy, 1578. On the *signa*, see Griffenhagen and Bogard, *History of Drug Containers*, 48.

63. Potter and Scott, *Therapeutics*, 542.

64. Cook and LaWall, *Remington's Practice of Pharmacy*, 1599.

65. Remington, *Practice of Pharmacy*, 1141. The same wording appears in the 1936 version (Cook and LaWall, *Remington's Practice of Pharmacy*, 1597).

66. On price competition in the 1930s, see Alderson, "Trends in Distribution." Rorem and Fischelis observed that "there has been no general outcry" about spending on medicinal drugs (*Costs of Medicines*, 217).

67. Bacon, *America's Corner Store*, 39–40.

68. On the increasing efforts to guard against accidental poisoning, see Marion Moser Jones and Benrubi, "Poison Politics."

69. Nolen and Maynard, *Drug Store Management*, 264–65.

70. Stuart Chase and Schlink, "Consumers in Wonderland," 349.

71. Ibid., 134, 144.

72. Cramp, "Therapeutic Thaumaturgy," 423.

73. Perry, "Weak Spots," 25. See also Strout, "Radio Nostrum Racket."

74. "Advertisers' Ten Commandments," 6; "Ballyhoo Institute," 26; Rorty, *Our Master's Voice*, 382.

75. Rorty, *Our Master's Voice*, 383.

76. Stuart Chase and Schlink, "Consumers in Wonderland."

Chapter Four

1. Kellock, "Shopping," 16, 17, 20.

2. Ibid, 20.

3. Rorty, *American Medicine Mobilizes*, 307; Kallet and Schlink, *100,000,000 Guinea Pigs*.

4. F. J. Schlink to W. D. Sutliff, January 3, 1936, box 437, folder 16, CR Records.

5. As Cohen argues, the New Deal "broker state" began to cultivate the "citizen consumer" as a political interest group to counterbalance the private business influences thought responsible for the Great Depression (*Consumer's Republic*, esp. part 1).

6. Rorty, *American Medicine Mobilizes*, 33; Horowitz, *Morality of Spending*, 30–37, 72–73.

7. See Apple, "Liberal Arts or Vocational Training?"; Goldstein, *Creating Consumers*, esp. chap. 2.

8. Stuart Chase and Schlink, *Your Money's Worth*, 2, 264.

9. Ibid., 267.

10. On the early history of Consumers' Research, see Gregory L. Williams, Descriptive Summary, CR Records. The historical overview provided in this inventory is extremely useful.

11. Silber, *Test and Protest*; Mayer, *Consumer Movement*, 21.

12. See Glickman, *Buying Power*, chaps. 5 and 6.

13. On the shared history of Consumers' Research and Consumers Union, see Glickman, *Buying Power*, chap. 6; Williams, Descriptive Summary, CR Records. On the

differences between the two organizations, see Norman D. Katz, "Consumers Union," esp. 120; Alkon, "Late Twentieth-Century Consumer Advocacy," 39. As Alkon shows, the more leftist Consumers Union was far more willing to take on the issue of medical authority than was the more conservative Consumers' Research.

14. Cohen, *Consumers' Republic*, 28–31.

15. Ephraim, *Take Care of Yourself*, 4. The annual editions of the *Readers' Guide to Periodical Literature* document the expanding print interest in health and medical issues.

16. Best-seller list issued jointly by *Bowker's Annual* and *Publishers' Weekly*, http:// people.lis.illinois.edu/~unsworth/courses/bestsellers/best30.cgi (accessed July 1, 2015); Kallet and Schlink, *100,000,000 Guinea Pigs*, vii. The book sold an estimated 250,000 copies; see Gregory L. Williams, Descriptive Summary, CR Records. Data on public library purchases comes from the Main Street Public Library Database. Four of the five small-town libraries whose circulation records were used to create the database had copies of Kallet and Schlink.

17. Kallet and Schlink, *100,000,000 Guinea Pigs*, 116.

18. Ibid., 176.

19. Ibid., 77.

20. Ibid., viii.

21. Ibid., 302–3.

22. Edward Davis to President Franklin D. Roosevelt, June 6, 1933, Mrs. E. M. Winters to Mrs. Eleanor Roosevelt, October 21, 1933, both in General Correspondence, 1919–1937, 1933 015-121, box 307, FDA Records.

23. Kyrk, "100,000,000 Guinea Pigs," 352, 353; W. G. Campbell to Simon E. Sobeloff, January [illegible], 1933, General Correspondence, 1919–1937, 1933 015-121, box 307, FDA Records.

24. Charles O. Jackson, *Food and Drug Legislation*, 6–20; Silber, *Test and Protest*; Kay, *Dying to Be Beautiful*.

25. Lamb, *American Chamber of Horrors*, 81–82.

26. Ibid., viii, 109.

27. Robins, *Copeland's Cure*, 192–93, 200. Charles O. Jackson describes Tugwell as "a liberal of the far left type" (*Food and Drug Legislation*, 35).

28. Pease, *Responsibilities of American Advertising*, 121–25, quote on 123; Charles O. Jackson, *Food and Drug Legislation*, esp. 137.

29. My account of the Elixir tragedy relies on Lesch, *First Miracle Drugs*, esp. 177–80, and Charles O. Jackson, *Food and Drug Legislation*, esp. chap. 7.

30. Ballentine, "Taste of Raspberries."

31. Ibid.

32. Charles O. Jackson, *Food and Drug Legislation*, 37, 87, 137.

33. Baldwin and Kirlin, "Consumers Appraise"; Handler, "Control of False Advertising," 105, 110.

34. Ephraim, *Take Care of Yourself*, 4.

35. Fishbein, *Morris Fishbein*, 188.

36. Hamilton quoted in Cabot, *Doctor's Bill*, 58–59.

37. Kallet and Schlink, *100,000,000 Guinea Pigs*, 158.

38. Harding, "Metamorphosis," 446.

39. Kallet and Schlink, *100,000,000 Guinea Pigs*, 141.

40. F. J. Schlink to L. B. Ross, September 12, 1932, box 440, folder 21, CR Records; Harding, *Fads, Frauds, and Physicians*, 172, 175–76.

41. Harding, *Fads, Frauds, and Physicians*, 252. Johns Hopkins surgeon Bertram Bernheim discussed fee splitting at length in his 1939 book, *Medicine*.

42. Kellock, "Shopping."

43. Ibid., 16, 21. My discussion of this article is also based on material in box 437, CR Records.

44. See Harry H. Moore, *American Medicine*; Falk, Rorem, and Ring, *Costs of Medical Care*.

45. M. C. Phillips to K. A. Kellock, December 2, 1935, Dr. J. A. Ruetenik to Consumers' Research, March 28, 1937, both in box 437, folder 14, CR Records; Dr. T. L. Hyde to Consumers' Research, September 29, 1935, box 437, folder 15, CR Records. Approximately forty physicians wrote in about the piece, many at considerable length. I found very few letters from laypeople in the file, and those who wrote in did so to object to Kellock's clearly stated disdain for "cultists."

46. Harding's article was published as an appendix to Harry H. Moore's *American Medicine*. This comment came in a review of Moore's book that noted that he was not a doctor and portrayed the inclusion of Harding's article as a sign of Moore's very poor judgment; see "Book Notices."

47. Ross, "Issue of Health," 581.

48. For a very pro-Kingsbury version of the Milk Bottle Wars, see Rorty, *American Medicine Mobilizes*, 116–30. For information on Borden's prescription products, see Borden, *Company History*, http://www.fundinguniverse.com/company-histories/Borden-Inc-company-History.html (accessed July 1, 2015). On the infant food industry, see Apple, *Mothers and Medicine*.

49. F. J. Schlink to W. D. Sutliff, January 3, 1936, box 437, folder 16, CR Records; Rorty, *American Medicine Mobilizes*.

50. Patricia Spain Ward, "In Recognition"; Schnabel, "Esther Everett Lape."

51. The form letter Lape sent out to recruit participants is reproduced in American Foundation, *American Medicine*, 2:1296.

52. Ibid., 1:195, 185.

53. Ibid., 51, 10, 44.

54. Ibid., 52.

55. "Nationalized Doctors?," 26, 28.

56. "National Policy on Health Asked by 430 Doctors," *NYT*, November 7, 1937. On the committee, see Lundberg, "John P. Peters."

57. Reed, review, 612; Bernheim, *Medicine*, 235–38. Bernheim was one of the original committee members.

58. Fishbein, *Morris Fishbein*, 205, 206–7.

59. "Medical Democracy," *NYT*, November 7, 1937.

60. Weisz, "Epidemiology"; Rorty, *American Medicine Mobilizes*, 16.

61. Igo, *Averaged American*; Pringle, "What Do the Women of America Think?"

62. Pringle, "What Do the Women of America Think?," 14.

63. Ibid., 14, 15.

64. "American Doctor's Dilemma," *Book-of-the-Month Club News*, June 1939, in scrapbook, Bertram M. Bernheim Collection, Alan Mason Chesney Medical Archives of the Johns Hopkins Medical Institutions, Baltimore.

65. "American Medical Association Dissected," 168.

66. Bernheim, *Medicine*, 39.

67. Patricia Spain Ward, "United States versus American Medical Association."

68. Rorty, *American Medicine Mobilizes*.

69. Ibid., 34, 32, 33.

70. On medical ambivalence about the national health insurance crusade, see Engel, *Doctors and Reformers*.

71. Rorty, *American Medicine Mobilizes*, 307.

72. Aaron, *Good Health and Bad Medicine*, viii.

73. Olga Owens, "Socialized MDs," *Boston Transcript*, undated review of *Medicine at the Crossroads*, in scrapbook, Bertram M. Bernheim Collection, Alan Mason Chesney Medical Archives of the Johns Hopkins Medical Institutions, Baltimore; "*Liberty* and Ethics," 15.

74. George D. Eaton to T. Swann Harding, September 12, 1928, Harding Papers.

75. Walter Alvarez to T. Swann Harding, December 2, November 22, 1930, February 19, 1931, Harding Papers.

76. George D. Eaton to T. Swann Harding, September 12, 1928, Harding Papers.

77. Harding, *Fads, Frauds, and Physicians*, 17.

78. Ephraim, *Take Care of Yourself*, 279.

Chapter Five

1. "U.S. Medicine in Transition," 156, 157, 158.

2. Berge, "Justice and the Future," 8, 14, 15; Carter, *Doctor Business*, 21. Carter attributes the term "fourth necessity" to Alan Gregg of the Rockefeller Foundation (26–27).

3. For a clear, concise discussion of the conflicting viewpoints, see Bud, "Antibiotics, Big Business, and Consumers."

4. *NYT*, November 7, 1937.

5. "Drive to Conquer 5 Diseases Asked," *NYT*, June 2, 1958; Harden, *Short History*; Rosemary Stevens, *In Sickness and in Wealth*, esp. 216–24.

6. On the AMA's shift in position on hospital insurance, see Starr, *Social Transformation*, esp. 280–86. I use the term "private" rather than "voluntary" because it is more consistent with current usage.

7. American Foundation, *American Medicine*, 2:1023.

8. Cunningham and Cunningham, *Blues*.

9. Starr, *Social Transformation*, 300; Herman Somers and Somers, *Doctors, Patients, and Health Insurance*, 11 (statistic). See also Beatrix Hoffman, *Health Care for Some*, chap. 5.

10. The traditional view that employer medical insurance was an "accidental" result of World War II decision making has been persuasively challenged by Jost, *Health Care at Risk*, esp. chap. 5. See also Dobbin, "Origins of Private Social Insurance."

11. Patricia Spain Ward, "United States versus American Medical Association," 144.

12. Poen, *Harry S. Truman*; Blumenthal and Morone, *Heart of Power*, chap. 2.

13. Raymond Rich Associates, "Report on Public Relations to The Trustees of the American Medical Association, May 24, 1947," and Albert Hamilton, "Memorandum: Resignation Raymond Rich Associates Public Relations Council," July 3, 1947, both in box 58, Davis Collection; Campion, *AMA and U.S. Health Policy*, 123–25, 143–46.

14. Whitaker quoted in Lepore, "Lie Factory," 57.

15. See Lepore, "Lie Factory"; Blumenthal and Morone, *Heart of Power*, 90–94; Warner, "Aesthetic Grounding." The administrator of the Federal Security Agency from 1947 to 1953, Ewing headed Truman's informal insurance working group. In his 1969 oral history, he said of the AMA's campaign, "Their main appeal was to tell about how much political influence the country doctor had with his patients." The bill's defeat made Ewing realize "that if we were ever going to get any program through, Medicare or anything of the like, there had to be support of an organization that had real political power," hence he "toyed with the idea of organizing the American Patients' Association." A certificate of incorporation and bylaws for the association were drawn up in 1954; the incorporators included prominent labor lawyers and philanthropists as well as the public health leaders C. E. A. Winslow and Haven Emerson. But the organization failed to go forward. Instead, Aimee Forand and the Council of Senior Citizens would spearhead the grassroots movement that led to the passage of Medicare. See American Patients' Association folder, Oscar Ewing Papers, Harry S. Truman Library and Museum, Independence, Missouri; Ewing, interview, esp. 192–94.

16. Jennifer Klein, *For All These Rights*, esp. chap. 6; Thomasson, "Importance of Group Coverage."

17. Thomasson, "Importance of Group Coverage." See also Thomasson, "From Sickness to Health."

18. Herman Somers and Somers, *Doctors, Patients, and Health Insurance*, 226, 254–55, 547.

19. *Newsweek*, October 6, 1952, 99.

20. David Rothman, "Public Presentation."

21. Beatrix Hoffman, *Health Care for Some*, esp. 105–13; Beatrix Hoffman, "Restraining the Health Care Consumer."

22. Herman Somers and Somers, *Doctors, Patients, and Health Insurance*, esp. 281–85, 383–87.

23. President's Commission, *Building America's Health*, 5:66.

24. Ibid.

25. Bud, *Penicillin*, esp. chap. 2; Younkin, "Making the Market."

26. Wendell Berge, "Science and Monopoly," *Free World*, March 1944, reprint in box 35, Speeches and Articles, March–June 1944, Wendell Berge Papers, MSS12468, Manuscript Division, Library of Congress, Washington, D.C. My account here is based on the clippings collected in Scrapbook, Berge Papers.

27. As one admirer wrote upon hearing of Berge's resignation, it was plain to see that with Roosevelt's death "there died also (& how untimely!) his struggle for economic and political equality" (Paul Standard to Wendell Berge, February 16, 1947, box 43, Berge Papers).

28. Bud, *Penicillin*, esp. 106; Temin, *Taking Your Medicine*, 66. For the history of drug patenting, see Gabriel, *Medical Monopoly*.

29. Temin, *Taking Your Medicine*, esp. 66–67. For two recent comprehensive overviews of the pharmaceutical industry in this era, see Carpenter, *Reputation and Power*, esp. chaps. 2 and 3; Tobbell, *Pills, Power, and Policy*.

30. Temin, *Taking Your Medicine*, 67–82; Kitch, "Patent System." For a good overview of patent law as applied to pharmaceuticals, see Schacht and Thomas, "Patent Law."

31. Greene, "Attention to 'Details.'"

32. Nevis Cool to Lamar Howe, November 7, 1952, General Subject Files, 1955, box 1994, FDA Records; Swann, "FDA and the Practice of Pharmacy."

33. House Committee Hearings, 41.

34. Swann, "FDA and the Practice of Pharmacy," 61. See also Rasmussen, *On Speed*, esp. chap. 4.

35. House Committee Hearings, 63–64, 45.

36. Marks, "Revisiting 'The Origins of Compulsory Drug Prescriptions,'" esp. 111; Swann, "1941 Sulfathiazole Disaster."

37. *U.S. v. Jordan James Sullivan (Sullivan's Pharmacy)*, 332 U.S. 696–97. For background on this case, see Young, *Medical Messiahs*, 269–71.

38. House Committee Hearings, 59.

39. Frates, "Durham-Humphrey Bill," 88; House Committee Hearings, 61–62.

40. See Frates, "Durham-Humphrey Bill"; Swann, "FDA and the Practice of Pharmacy," 67.

41. House Committee Hearings, 45, 46. On the variant labeling of drugs, see 64–67.

42. Ibid., 118–42.

43. Ibid., 37.

44. Ibid., 107–8.

45. Nevis Cool to Lamar Howe, November 7, 1952, General Subject Files, 1955, box 1994, FDA Records.

46. "Sale of Dangerous Drugs," 292; *NYT*, February 6, 1952; Frates, "Durham-Humphrey Bill," 88.

47. Wallace F. Janssen to George Larrick et al., December 2, 1958, General Subject Files, 1958, 500.67, box 2532, FDA Records. Janssen was preparing a draft talk to be given to a Missouri medical meeting by Congressman James C. Davis, who had asked for material "that spells out the philosophy of Durham-Humphrey."

48. As an FDA official noted in 1951, the term "over-the-counter" "has come into quite general use in the trade to denote any drug subject to the Federal Food, Drug, and Cosmetic Act which is not legally restricted to prescription sale, regardless of how the particular product is promoted or advertised" (Nevis E. Cool to Stanley Wolder, August 27, 1952, General Subject Files, 1955, box 1994, FDA Records).

49. President's Commission, *Building America's Health*, 5:211–12.

50. "Legion Avoids AF Fight," 298; Brickman, "'Medical McCarthyism,'" 388; Glickman, *Buying Power*, 258–59.

51. *Kiplinger's Washington Newsletter*, 1955, General Correspondence, 3.82, box 1900, FDA Records; Langford, "Medical Care," 1053.

52. Kobler, "Why Mac Isn't Dead," 28. On representations of medical progress, see Hansen, *Picturing Medical Progress*, esp. chap. 9.

53. Turow, *Playing Doctor*; Spears, "The Doctor on the Screen," in *Hollywood*, 314–32.

54. For an early postwar argument that American health and health care compared poorly to other nations, see Malmberg, *140 Million Patients*. On post–World War II developments in the United States and Great Britain, see Daniel M. Fox, *Health Policies, Health Politics*.

55. President's Commission, *Building America's Health*, esp. vol. 5; Koos, *Health of Regionville*. Regionville was a pseudonym for a small town near Rochester, New York.

56. Thomas, *Deluxe Jim Crow*; Love, *One Blood*. On the larger attention to civil rights as a Cold War problem, see Dudziak, *Cold War Civil Rights*.

57. In 1955, physician-demographer Thomas McKeown published an article suggesting that the mortality transition resulted primarily from improvements in overall living standards, particularly better nutrition. Although little noticed in the 1950s, McKeown's work became influential in the late 1970s and 1980s. Subsequent research has challenged much of his argument, but most scholars still accept his point "that curative medical measures played little role in mortality decline prior to the mid-20th century" (Colgrove, "McKeown Thesis," 728).

58. Brandt, *Cigarette Century*; Oppenheimer, "Becoming the Framingham Study"; Mark Jackson, *Age of Stress*; Nate Hazeltine, "Easy Life Called Root of Man's Ills," *WP*, November 7, 1951.

59. American Foundation, *American Medicine*, 1:53. On the emergence of the risk factor concept, see Rothstein, *Public Health*.

60. Whorton, *Nature Cures*, esp. chap. 10; Gevitz, *D.O.'s*.

61. Rodale, *Health Finder*, 5, 659.

62. Jarvis, *Folk Medicine*, frontispiece; "Dr. Jarvis's Great Switchel Revival"; "Dr. D. C. Jarvis, Author of 'Folk Medicine,' Dead," *NYT*, August 19, 1966.

63. Cousins, *Modern Man*, 18–19.

64. See also Gilbert, *Men in the Middle*.

65. Horowitz, *Vance Packard*.

66. "Norman Rockwell Visits a Family Doctor," 31; W. Eugene Smith, "Country Doctor," 126.

67. Mintz, *Therapeutic Nightmare*.

Chapter Six

1. McCandlish Phillips, "Doctor Cancels $1,500 Bill for Hoopers at Medical Group's Urging," *NYT*, June 23, 1957; "Doctor at Rescue 'Upset' by Ordeal," *NYT*, May 19, 1957.

2. "Parents of Boy Rescued in Well Get Bill for $1,500 from Doctor," *NYT*, June 21, 1957; McCandlish Phillips, "Hooper Boy's Doctor Criticized on Big Fee," *NYT*, June 22, 1957; McCandlish Phillips, "Doctor Cancels $1,500 Bill for Hoopers at Medical Group's Urging," *NYT*, June 23, 1957.

3. Carter, *Doctor Business*, 17.

4. Maurer, "M.D.'s Are Off Their Pedestal"; Greenberg, "Decline of the Healing Art," 134.

5. Alan Gregg, "We Must Not Lag in Medical Research," *NYT*, August 7, 1949.

6. George Weisz, *Medical Mandarins* (where the term describes the French Academy of Medicine). The *Oxford English Dictionary* notes the first use of the term "biomedicine" in 1922. See "Biomedicine, n.," OED Online, March 2015, Oxford University Press. http://www.oed.com.proxy.library.stonybrook.edu/view/Entry/240676?redirected From=biomedicine& (accessed July 1, 2015). The term's use expanded in both Europe and the United States after World War II; see Quirke and Gaudillière, "Era of Biomedicine."

7. Ludmerer, *Time to Heal*.

8. Rosemary Stevens, *American Medicine*, 181.

9. Bush, "As We May Think." Statistics come from "Introduction and History," 3. The phrase "information explosion" gained widespread use after its use in Toffler, *Future Shock*. On the increasing importance of annual review volumes, see Mather, "Scientist's Bookshelf," 311–12. On the role of drug detailers, see Greene, "Attention to 'Details.'"

10. Herman Somers and Somers, *Doctors, Patients, and Health Insurance*, 204, 206, 208.

11. Mari Edwards, "Shopping Center Practice," 103, 105; Lowell, "Choosing a Location," 181, 182.

12. Lowell, "Choosing a Location," 190; Haskell, "No Parking Problem Here," 132. Mussolini never built his garage, but Dr. Callison did; see Haskell, "No Parking Problem Here," 134.

13. "The House-Call Habit," *Time*, September 15, 1961. For an interesting discussion of transportation and the shift to office practice, see Starr, *Social Transformation*, 65–71. Although Starr describes the late 1800s, his argument extends to the post–World War II period as well.

14. Lois Hoffman, "Well-Planned Office," 119.

15. Ibid., 121.

16. Lindsey, "How to Have a Well-Run Appointment System," 140, 141, 142.

17. Bredow, *Medical Assistant*, 20, 21. The medical assistant was only one of a number of women's occupations of this era centered on personal service. See Barry, *Femininity in Flight*.

18. Owens, "Health Questionnaires," 135; *Cornell Medical Index: A Brief History*, http://library.med.cornell.edu/About/cornellmedindex.html (accessed July 1, 2015).

19. My description of office-based practices is based on Peterson et al., *Analytical Study*.

20. Bredow, *Medical Assistant*, 309, 328, 351; *Medical Economics* 28 (April 1951): 182.

21. See Bredow, *Medical Assistant*; Bredow, *Handbook* (1959).

22. The various editions of the Bredow handbook provide a good sense of the growing sophistication of office forms and equipment. Bredow, *Handbook* (1943) featured Histacount forms and Remington Rand's "visible filing" system. Bredow, *Handbook* (1959), 62, mentions the Colwell Company's willingness to customize forms for individual doctors. Bredow, *Medical Secretarial Procedures* (1966), 62, mentions copiers.

23. Michael Marks Davis, *Medical Care for Tomorrow*, 12.

24. Schafer, *Business*, esp. 161–62.

25. Greer Williams, "How to Choose Your Doctor," 431.

26. Peterson et al., *Analytical Study*, 18, 20. Based on their performance, doctors were

divided into five categories; the 44 percent figure represents the sum of the two low-est categories. Scores for the 30 percent in category three, portrayed as the "average" doctor, were significantly lower than those for the top 8 percent.

27. Walter Alvarez, "Dr. Alvarez's 'Danger Signals,'" *New York Herald Tribune*, May 20, 1953; Means, "Evolution," 727. See also Walter Alvarez, "How to Find a Family Doctor in Any Locality," *New York Herald Tribune*, March 14, 1955. In many respects, this "take care of yourself" health philosophy recycled themes that had long been part of tradi-tional health advice dating back to ancient times. See, for example, Rosenberg, *Right Living*. But it also dovetailed with a broader 1950s craze for do-it-yourself activities, from home remodeling to building high-fidelity stereo systems. A Richwood, West Virginia, newspaper editor wrote a spoof of the do-it-yourself articles so popular in the 1950s in which he explained how readers could perform appendectomies on themselves: "You can save yourselves upward of $200 in hospital costs and doctor's fees by doing the job yourself . . . with some items right from your own kitchen." Much to his surprise, many of his readers did not realize that the article was a joke, and he was overwhelmed with requests for further information. See "Layman Told How."

28. Greer Williams, "How to Choose Your Doctor," 431.

29. Ibid., 432.

30. Ibid.; "How to Pick a Doctor," 29; Rosemary Stevens, *American Medicine*, 181. Membership in the American Academy of General Practice required doctors to do 150 hours of continuing education every three years.

31. "How to Pick a Doctor," 30–31.

32. Greer Williams, "How to Choose a Doctor," 432; "How to Pick a Doctor," 31.

33. "How to Pick a Doctor," 27.

34. Odin W. Anderson and Lerner, *Measuring Health Levels*, 36; Richard Rutter, "Billions for Service," *NYT*, June 7, 1956.

35. See Cohen, *Consumers' Republic*, esp. 133–51.

36. American Medical Association, *County Medical Public Relations Manual*, 2.

37. "How to Pick a Doctor," 31.

38. Menges, "They Settle Doctor-Patient Disputes," 185; "Study Reveals Too Few Grievance Committees," 278; American Medical Association, Council on Medical Service, *Nationwide Survey*, 5, 6, 7, 12, 13, 14, 15, 16. By 1954, almost 700 American cit-ies had emergency call services operated by county medical societies ("How to Pick a Doctor," 31).

39. John Newton Baker, *Your Public Relations Are Showing*, 166.

40. Garbarino, "Price Behavior and Productivity," 3.

41. Bredow, *Handbook* (1943), 77. All of the editions of Bredow's book published from 1943 to 1959 contain this sentence about doctors finding economics distasteful. On 1950s status anxiety, see Mills, *White Collar*.

42. Herman Somers and Somers, *Doctors, Patients, and Health Insurance*, 10.

43. Ibid., 58.

44. Edith Asbury, "Hospital Strife over Costs Aired," *NYT*, September 23, 1955.

45. "Report to the Board of Trustees of the American Medical Association of the Committee on Medical Practices, November 1954," 17, box 57, Davis Collection; Mari Edwards, "Set Your Surgical Fees."

46. "Report to the Board of Trustees of the American Medical Association of the Committee on Medical Practices, November 1954," box 57, Davis Collection.

47. Baketel, "Fee Control"; "Our Name Is Mud," 79; "Time to Get That Step Fixed," 63.

48. Croatman, "With These Forms," 137; "Be Wise: Itemize," 69.

49. Walters, "Show Them What They're Paying For," 59, 203.

50. "Use of, and Satisfaction with, C.M.A. Relative Value Studies." On the development of the International Classification of Diseases coding system, see World Health Organization, *History of the Development of the ICD*, http://www.who.int/classifications /icd/en/HistoryOfICD.pdf. Accessed July 1, 2015 (accessed July 1, 2015).

51. "72% of U.S. Population Has Health Insurance," *NYT*, June 26, 1960; Bredow, *Handbook* (1943), 80–81; Bredow, *Handbook* (1959), chap. 7.

52. Bredow, *Handbook* (1959), 110–11; Bredow, *Medical Secretarial Procedures*, 176–77.

53. "Needless Surgery," 48, 49, 53; "Maj Gen Paul R. Hawley." The American College of Surgeons, along with the AMA and the AHA, oversaw the powerful Joint Committee on Hospital Accreditation. Hawley elaborated on the concept of the medical audit in Hawley, "Evaluation."

54. "Needless Surgery," 48.

55. Ibid., 55.

56. "Doctors to Weigh Censure of Critic," *NYT*, June 3, 1953. When he appeared before the committee, Hawley reported that he had no idea the interview would be published in full. At any rate, Hawley had let his AMA membership lapse, so the organization could not have expelled him.

57. "Too Many Wrong Ideas." The press coverage of Hawley was largely favorable, as was the treatment of him in Carter, *Doctor Business*, 119–20.

58. "Report to the Board of Trustees of the American Medical Association of the Committee on Medical Practices, November 1954," box 57, Davis Collection. Like the Rich Report discussed in Chapter 5, the AMA trustees found the Committee on Medical Practices' final report so negative that they did not want to distribute it. Some members of the organization's House of Delegates objected, so the report was distributed; but no new action resulted. This would be the AMA's last formal discussion of the fee-splitting problem.

59. Greer Williams, "Unjustified Surgery," 36, 39.

60. Ibid.; Lois Mattox Miller, "Hysterectomy"; "Is This Hysterectomy Really Necessary?"

61. Nate Haseltine, "Doctors Told They Abuse, Overuse Drugs and Blood," *WP*, November 2, 1954; Leonard Engel, "Doctor's Dilemma: How to Keep Up," *NYT*, June 7, 1959.

62. See Gerald Grob, "Rise and Decline"; Gerald Grob, "Rise of Peptic Ulcer."

63. Wylie, "Doctors' Conspiracy" (emphasis in original). Hawley had read this article and referred to it in his interview with *U.S. News* ("Needless Surgery," 53).

64. American Medical Association, *What Americans Think*, 6, 7, 8, 9, 3.

65. Ibid., 11, 64–65, 67.

66. Koos, *Health of Regionville*, 75; Koos, "'Metropolis,'" 1552. Unlike earlier surveys, Koos used a random sample of subjects across a wide socioeconomic spectrum and compared the responses of upper-, middle-, and lower-income interviewees. Although

the data collected came from the late 1940s in the case of Regionville and the mid-1950s for Rochester, the findings continued to be cited as representative for many years; the Regionville study was reprinted in 1967.

67. Koos, *Health of Regionville*, 55, 77, 146, 147.

68. The structuralist-functionalist approach championed by Parsons and, later, Robert Merton assumed that the asymmetry in knowledge and experience between doctor and patient inevitably forced the latter to be subservient to the former. Yet starting in the 1930s, there had been hints of the idea that mature democracy required a more egalitarian exchange between educated doctor and educated patient, especially in the arena of child guidance and family counseling. Rogers began to develop the principles of what he termed "client-centered" therapy in the 1930s and published a major exposition of the approach in 1946. See Carl R. Rogers, "Significant Aspects."

69. Finding aid, Ernest Dichter Papers, Accession 2407, Manuscripts and Archives Department, Hagley Museum and Library, Wilmington, Delaware.

70. Dichter, *Psychological Study*, 4.

71. Ibid., 7, 11.

72. "Report to the Board of Trustees of the American Medical Association of the Committee on Medical Practices, November 1954," box 57, Davis Collection.

73. Ibid.

74. Richard H. Blum, *Management*, xiv.

75. Bess Furman, "Doctors Urged to Discuss Fees," *NYT*, March 28, 1958.

76. Geiger, "Patient as a Human Being."

77. Szasz and Hollender, "Contribution." In the first two models, the doctor decided for the patient, with no input from the latter; the assumption was that "the patient does not possess the knowledge to dispute the physician's word." In contrast, in the third model, the physician did not "profess to know exactly what is best for the patient" but rather searched for that goal with the patient in the belief that "the patient's own experiences furnish indispensable information for eventual agreement, under otherwise favorable circumstances, as to what 'health' might be for him" (589).

78. Richard H. Blum, *Management*, 83.

79. Perrin, "He Thinks You Mishandle Patients," 39–40.

80. "Why M.D.s Have a Tough Time."

81. Charles Miller, "How to Help," 76; "Most Fees Are Modest," 83. For the chart, see "What Americans Spend." It was reproduced in the letters section a few months later with information that reprints were now for sale; see *Medical Economics* 32 (October 1955): 48.

82. Maurer, "M.D.'s Are Off Their Pedestal," 138; Wallace, "How Prosperous Should You Look?," 283.

83. Greenberg, "Decline of the Healing Art," 132.

84. Ibid., 132, 133, 134.

85. Dubos, "Beyond Traditional Medicine," 166. The October 1960 issue of *Harper's* is the earliest I have found the word "crisis" used to describe the state of American medicine.

86. Sanders, *Crisis*; "No Medical Crisis Yet, Official Says," *WP*, October 3, 1960. On the response to the issue, see "As *Harper's* Readers See It."

87. Sam Dawson, "Per Capita Health Cost Up 359% since 1929," *WP*, December 5, 1959; "42% Rise Reported in Medical Costs," *NYT*, February 15, 1960; "U.S. Is Found Spending More for Gum Than Medical Study," *NYT*, July 15, 1957; "Tobacco-Liquor Outlay Tops Medical Spending," *NYT*, March 3, 1958. On the controversy over whether the Consumer Price Index inflated medical costs, see "Doctors Fees Disputed," *NYT*, May 7, 1958; Austin C. Wehrwein, "A.M.A. Denies Rise in Medical Costs," *NYT*, October 28, 1960.

88. "7 Ways to Cut Your Medical Costs," *WP*, June 28, 1960; Bankers Life ad, *WP*, May 25, 1959; Blue Cross/Blue Shield ad, *WP*, September 26, 1960.

89. Eve Edstrom, "Most Aged Persons Eager to Pay Own Way for Medicine If They Can," *WP*, April 17, 1960.

90. "Physicians Warned on Hospital Costs," *NYT*, April 24, 1960. For Plumb's series, see Robert K. Plumb, "Medicine Faces Challenge," *NYT*, January 7, 1957; Robert K. Plumb, "Plans Insure 70% of Medical Bills," *NYT*, January 8, 1957; Robert K. Plumb, "Group Practice Divides Doctors," *NYT*, January 9, 1957; Robert K. Plumb, "Health Experts War over Ethics," *NYT*, January 10, 1957; Robert K. Plumb, "U.S. Studies Gaps in Medical Plans," *NYT*, January 11, 1957. For a contemporary overview of private health insurance, see Odin W. Anderson and Feldman, *Family Medical Costs*.

91. The 4 percent figure appears in Robert K. Plumb, "Plans Insure 70% of Medical Bills," *NYT*, January 8, 1957.

92. "HIP on Staten Island," *NYT*, July 27, 1960. For a contemporary study of the HIP program, see Freidson, *Patients' Views*.

Chapter Seven

1. Harris, *Real Voice*, 3–4; "A Big Pill to Swallow," *Life*, February 15, 1960, 99.

2. Cohen, *Consumers' Republic*, esp. chap. 3; statistics on 121.

3. Higgins, "Drugstore Products," 61–62.

4. "Postwar Project," 114–15; "Restrained Suburban Drugstore," 140.

5. Bacon, *America's Corner Store*, 159. For an illustrated history of drugstores that shows these changes, see Mobley, *Prescription for Success*, esp. chaps. 4 and 5.

6. "Grocer Horns In," 160; "Advertising and Marketing News," *NYT*, August 15, 1952; "Self Service Reaches the Drugstore," 43; "Still, They Call It a Drugstore," *NYT*, March 18, 1956; "Allen Funt's Candid Camera," 78.

7. Albert Gray, "Who Should Sell Vitamins?," 28. See also Apple, *Vitamania*, 54–65.

8. Fletcher, *Market Restraints*, esp. chap.5; "State Regulation of Drugs."

9. Ratcliff, "Aspirin"; Harry Henderson, "Original Miracle Drug"; Drotning, "Aspirin Can Be Deadly"; Bliss, "Don't Be an Ass." On the FDA warning label, see "FDA's Aspirin Ruling." On aspirin's history, see Mann and Plummer, *Aspirin Wars*.

10. "State Regulation of Drugs," 553. For the restrictionist argument, see Herzog, "Twixt Supermarket and Courts."

11. "State Regulation of Drugs," 559. See also Fletcher, *Market Restraints*, chaps. 5 and 6.

12. "Allen Funt's Candid Camera," 78.

13. Bacon, *America's Corner Store*, 153, 154.

14. "Where Are All the Salesclerks?," 119; U.S. Census, 1960, http://www.census.gov/hhes/socdemo/education/data/cps/1960/cp60pcs1–37/cp60pcs1–37.pdf (accessed July 1, 2015); Creighton, *Pretenders*. Although Creighton described consumer education in high schools as widespread, she did not think it was very good.

15. Bacon, *America's Corner Store*, 152–53, 154–56; Higgins, "Drugstore Products," 61–62; "Where Are All the Salesclerks?," 119. In the drug trade, the definition of a "self-service" store was one where counter service was limited to the prescription department, the soda fountain, and the tobacco department.

16. Bacon, *America's Corner Store*, 157–58, 158; "Self Service Reaches the Drugstore," 43.

17. "Self Service Reaches the Drugstore," 43–44; "Still, They Call It a Drugstore," 151; Bacon, *America's Corner Store*, 161; "Every Customer a Clerk," 54.

18. "Where Are All the Salesclerks?," 119.

19. "McKesson's 'American Look,'" 113; Swan, "New Packages"; "Still, They Call It a Drugstore," 151.

20. "Sponsors of Primetime Television," *The Classic TV Archive*, http://ctva.biz/CTVA_Sponsors.htm (accessed July 1, 2015); Sivulka, *Soap, Sex, and Cigarettes*, 230–31.

21. Poltrack, *Television Marketing*, 78; Weiss, "New Slant," esp. 38.

22. "Renowned yet Unknown, Voice Actor Dick Beals Dies at Age 85," *Tulsa (Oklahoma) World*, June 2, 2012.

23. Charisse, "'Solid Dose,'" chap. 4.

24. "FTC Urged to Study 'White Coat' Drug Ads," *NYT*, February 3, 1959; William M. Blair, "TV Men Prodded on Self-Policing," *NYT*, November 20, 1959; Lawrence Laurent, "New Ruling Calls Off All Those 'Dr. Kildares,'" *WP*, January 3, 1959; "The 'Doctors' on TV," *NYT*, July 26, 1958.

25. Steiner, *People Look at Television*, 218; Leslie H. Farber, "Ours Is the Addicted Society," *NYT*, December 11, 1966.

26. For a contemporary view of the U.S. pharmaceutical industry's rise to dominance, see Mahoney, *Merchants of Life*.

27. Bacon, *America's Corner Store*, 92; J. M. Hiebert, "Medicine Sales in Drugstores Seen at $2 Billion," *Oil, Paint, and Drug Recorder*, September 24, 1956, 5.

28. Although national newspapers noted the passage of the Durham-Humphrey Amendments in 1951, the coverage included little discussion of the reform's implications for patient-consumers. Only in the late 1950s, as the controversy grew over high prices, did these changes start to get popular attention.

29. Irvin Kerlan to R. T. Stermont, Secretary, Council on Pharmacy and Chemistry, AMA, November 14, 1952, General Subject Files, 1955, box 1994, FDA Records.

30. Aware that not all patients were easily able to read, pharmacists also devised symbols to designate how medicine should be taken. See Griffenhagen and Bogard, *History of Drug Containers*, 35.

31. Remington, Cook, and Martin, *Remington's Practice of Pharmacy*, 1230; M. L. Takowitz to Henry Heinie, November 26, 1952, General Subject Files, 1955, box 1994, FDA Records; Remington, Cook, and Martin, *Practice of Pharmacy*, 1424.

32. Remington and Cook, *Practice of Pharmacy*, 1149.

33. N. Cook to Mrs. Joseph Dabes, May 22, 1953, and John L. Harvey to Hon. William H. Ayres, August 29, 1952, General Subject Files, 1955, box 1994, FDA Records.

34. For a summary of the consumer consultants' work, see Carla S. Williams, Director, to John L. Harvey, Deputy Commissioner, November 6, 1962. According to the January 17, 1955, press release announcing the committee's formation, its fourteen members had been "selected for their interest in civic affairs and broad knowledge of consumer and industry problems." Both documents are in Records of the Consumer Advisory Committee, 1950–1969, box 1, FDA Records.

35. Older plant-based remedies could also pose this danger; for example, foxglove and the digitalis distilled from it could be toxic if too much was ingested. Although the 1937 Elixir Sulfanilamide tragedy resulted from the solvent rather than the drug, the incident still reinforced the idea that strong drugs were dangerous drugs.

36. *Oxford English Dictionary*, 2nd ed. (1989).

37. "Penicillin Danger Cited," *NYT*, May 8, 1953; Nate Haseltine, "72 Deaths Laid to Penicillin Use," *WP*, October 4, 1957.

38. Hilts, *Protecting America's Health*, 108–16.

39. Harris, *Real Voice*, 14; William Laurence, "Congress on Rheumatic Diseases Told of Results with New Anti-Arthritis Drugs," *NYT*, June 7, 1959; Roueché, "Ten Feet Tall," 48.

40. Tone, *Age of Anxiety*; Herzberg, *Happy Pills*.

41. The range and severity of side effects associated with the new antipsychotic drugs became evident as their use increased in the second half of the 1950s. See, for example, Lynn and Friedhoff, "Patient on a Tranquilizing Regimen." For an insightful analysis of the debate over psychoactive drugs, see Klerman, "Psychotropic Drugs."

42. "Any Medicine," 74; Maxine Davis, "Self-Diagnosis," 184.

43. Austin Smith, "Health of the Nation," 212; "Threat to Industry," 12. The 1929 figure appears in Rorem and Fischelis, *Costs of Medicines*, 220.

44. Greene, "Attention to 'Details.'"

45. Dowling, "Twixt the Cup," 659, 660.

46. Greene, "Attention to 'Details,'" 272; Harris, *Real Voice*, 92. The postwar growth in prescription drugs accelerated a blurring of boundaries between the ethical and proprietary sectors of the pharmaceutical industry that had begun before World War II. See Dowling, *Medicines for Man*, esp. pp. 80–86; Silverman and Lee, *Pills, Profits, and Politics*, esp. 207–11. For a contemporary view of these developments, see "Drug Industry's Ethical-Proprietary Line Is Blurring," *Oil, Paint, and Drug Reporter*, September 3, 1956, 5.

47. "Threat to Industry," *Printers' Ink*, December 25, 1959, 12.

48. Austin Smith, "Health of the Nation," 215.

49. See Tobbell, *Pills, Power, and Policy*, esp. chap. 3; Greene and Herzberg, "Hidden in Plain Sight." Many corporations adopted this kind of corporate image building. See Marchand, *Creating the Corporate Soul*. On the fact that no law forbids direct-to-consumer advertising of prescription drugs, see "Statement of Nancy Ostrove, Deputy Director of Division of Drug Marketing, Advertising, and Communications, before the Senate Subcommittee on Consumer Affairs, Foreign Commerce, and Tourism," July 24, 2001, http://www.hhs.gov/asl/testify/t010724.html.C. (accessed July 1, 2015).

50. "Report from Pfizer," *NYT*, March 31, 1957, sec. 10. On the Parke, Davis series, see Duffin and Li, "Great Moments." The ads featuring the man returning to work and the child taking the ballet lesson can be found in Parke, Davis & Company, Competitive Ads, box 13 (1957), JWT Archives.

51. "Drugs: Less Than Wonderful."

52. For a good discussion of the changing congressional climate, see Tobbell, *Pills, Power, and Policy*. As discussed in Chapter 5, New Dealers such as Berge became concerned about the pharmaceutical industry's trend toward cartelization. Those concerns reemerged during the Kefauver investigations. See Bud, "Antibiotics, Big Business, and Consumers."

53. My account here is drawn from Harris, *Real Voice*. Walton Hamilton did not live to see the results of the investigation that his sore throat had launched; he died in October 1958, just short of his seventy-seventh birthday. See *WP*, October 28, 1958.

54. On Magnuson's role in the FTC investigation, see "Price Fixing Reported in New 'Miracle' Drugs," *NYT*, June 9, 1956, 28; Bess Furman, "Drug Price Case Gets Under Way," *NYT*, September 28, 1958, 59. On the 1963 ruling, see Robert C. Toth, "U.S. Agency Rules 6 Companies Rig Antibiotic Prices," *NYT*, August 11, 1963, 1.

55. Scroop, "Faded Passion?"

56. My narrative of the Kefauver hearings relies chiefly on McFadyen, "Estes Kefauver"; Tobbell, *Pills, Power, and Policy*; Carpenter, *Reputation and Power*.

57. U.S. Senate, Committee on the Judiciary, *Administered Prices*; "Drug Hearings," 1299–1300.

58. A Proquest search of historical newspapers between 1958 and 1963 turned up over 400 articles on the Kefauver hearings. The *Readers' Guide to Periodical Literature* also shows a high volume of magazine articles about the hearings.

59. George E. Sokolsky, "These Days: The Drug Industry," *WP*, July 21, 1961.

60. McFadyen, "FDA's Regulation and Control."

61. Packard's three best sellers were *Hidden Persuaders* (1957), *The Status Seekers* (1959), and *The Waste Makers* (1960). The concept of "planned obsolescence" appeared in *Waste Makers*. Horowitz, *Vance Packard*, argues that Packard's work profoundly influenced 1960s social criticism.

62. "Drugs: Less Than Wonderful," 70, 72.

63. Silverman and Lee, *Pills, Profits, and Politics*, 40; Louis Lasagna testimony, June 27, 1961, in U.S. Senate, Committee on the Judiciary, *Administered Prices*, 170.

64. Klerman, "Drugs and Social Values"; Mickey C. Smith, *Small Comfort*, esp. 4–7; Metzl, *Prozac on the Couch*; Speaker, "From 'Happiness Pills'"; Watkins, *Estrogen Elixir*, esp. chap. 2.

65. May, "Selling Drugs," 1; Haskell J. Weinstein testimony, June 27, 1961, in U.S. Senate, Committee on the Judiciary, *Administered Prices*, 174. May suffered professionally for his critical stance toward the pharmaceutical industry (Mintz, *Therapeutic Nightmare*, 182–84). I thank Ernest Hook for bringing this point to my attention.

66. The term "learned intermediary" was first used in a 1966 liability suit concerning the drug chloroquine phosphate. For an overview of its history, see Paytash, "Learned Intermediary Doctrine." There is a huge legal literature on the learned intermediary doctrine. For a good introduction to its complexity, see Ferguson, "Liability." The

legal concept itself may have been articulated as early as a 1948 case, *Marcus v. Specific Pharmaceuticals, Inc.*; see Cooner, "Intersection." For a 1964 characterization of physicians as a specialized subset of consumers, see Bauer, "Risk Handling."

67. Robinson, "Don't Be Your Own Doctor," 155; "Drug Hearings," 1300. See also U.S. Senate, Committee on the Judiciary, *Administered Prices*, 160.

68. Lavieties, "Information on Drugs," 488; "Evaluating New Drugs," 48. Kallet founded the *Medical Letter* after being fired as Consumers Union's director in 1957. Norman D. Katz recounts that Kallet had been so scarred by his experiences with the House Committee on Un-American Activities that other Consumers Union members felt the need for stronger leadership and replaced him with Dexter Masters; see Katz, "Consumers Union," 330–31. Aaron was still listed as the organization's medical adviser in 1961.

69. Mintz, *Therapeutic Nightmare*, 566–67. Mintz (165n) states that in 1963, the *Medical Letter* had 25,000 subscribers. Carpenter, *Reputation and Power*, 328, notes that by 1977, it had more than 100,000 subscribers in the United States and Canada. In its early years, there is no internal evidence in the *Medical Letter* that its editors expected or wanted consumers to subscribe. But Consumers Union's 1961 consumer guide, *The Medicine Show*, referred to the *Medical Letter*'s findings to buttress warnings about the dangers of prolonged use of over-the-counter analgesics such as Anacin. See Consumer Reports, *Medicine Show*, 11. Consumerists might well have added a subscription to the *Medical Letter* to their lists of what to look for in a doctor.

70. For an excellent discussion of Consumers Union in this period, see Alkon, "Late Twentieth-Century Consumer Advocacy," esp. chap. 1.

71. Consumer Reports, *Medicine Show*, 1, 3, 181, 184.

72. "A Big Pill to Swallow," *Life*, February 15, 1960, 97, 102.

73. "Drug Hearings," 1299–1300.

Chapter Eight

1. Goodman, "Doctor's Image."

2. Ibid. The "prestige and scorn" quote here comes from the original study; see Gamson and Schuman, "Some Undercurrents," 464.

3. *NYT*, October 30, November 6, 1966.

4. John P. MacKenzie, "'Great Society . . . Sick Society,' Fulbright Tells American Bar," *WP*, August 9, 1967. The "sick society" phrase became an issue in the 1968 election. A Gallup poll taken that year asked, "Is US a 'sick society'"? Thirty-six percent agreed, 58 percent did not; see "Most in Poll Say U.S. Is Not 'Sick,'" *NYT*, July 3, 1968.

5. Branch, "Patient Must Prescribe," 403–9. For an excellent overview of medical politics in this period, see Wailoo, *Pain*.

6. "Text of Kennedy's Message to Congress on Protections for Consumers," *NYT*, March 16, 1962. Kennedy did not use the phrase "Consumer's Bill of Rights." That concept originated with Helen Nelson, a California consumerist who convinced the president to give the speech. See "Consumer Action: Helen Nelson (1913–2005) Will Be Greatly Missed by the Consumer Movement," http://www.consumer-action.org/press/articles/helen_nelson_1913_2005 (accessed July 1, 2015).

7. "Text of Kennedy's Message to Congress on Protections for Consumers," *NYT*, March 16, 1962. My summary of the legislative history here and in the next two paragraphs is taken from McFadyen, "Estes Kefauver"; Tobbell, *Pills, Power, and Policy*; Carpenter, *Reputation and Power*.

8. George E. Sokolsky, "These Days: The Drug Industry," *WP*, July 21, 1961. The outcome of the FTC antibiotic suit suggested just how hard drug regulation could be. Pfizer, charged with misleading the U.S. Patent Office, fought the case all the way to the Supreme Court; the FTC order took effect only after the Supreme Court refused to hear the case in 1969, and the order applied to exactly one drug. Years of legal effort thus had minimal effect. For an insightful overview of the 1962 law's mixed results, see Bud, "Antibiotics, Big Business, and Consumers."

9. Blumenthal and Morone, *Heart of Power*, 288. Reagan's speech was distributed on a record for use by the AMA's women's auxiliary, which played it at meetings with homemakers to build opposition to the proposed legislation.

10. Nate Haseltine, ". . . to Match the Achievements of Medicine . . . to the Afflictions of Our People," *WP*, January 20, 1965. As recently released tapes of Oval Office conversations make clear, Johnson and Mills together came up with the "three-layer cake" plan (Blumenthal and Morone, *Heart of Power*, 12–13). Thus the administration's original bill became Part A of Medicare, covering hospital costs for the elderly; the Republican proposal known as Bettercare became Part B of Medicare, which covered physicians' bills; and an expanded version of the AMA's proposed Eldercare became Medicaid, a cost-sharing program between state and federal governments that covered medical care for low-income Americans regardless of age.

11. Langer, "Doctors' Debate," 164; Goodman, "Doctor's Image."

12. Klarman, "Financing of Health Care," 215–16, 234.

13. Goodman, "Doctor's Image." On the broader problems of 1960s liberalism, see Matusow, *Unraveling of America*.

14. Bazell, "Health Radicals," 506–9.

15. "Women Who," 8.

16. Rorty, *American Medicine Mobilizes*, 307; Marcuse, *Essay on Liberation*. As evidence of medicine's failings, activists needed only point to recent revelations about the practice of human experimentation; see Beecher, "Ethics and Clinical Research," and Jean Heller, "Syphilis Victims in U.S. Study Went Untreated for 40 Years," *NYT*, July 26, 1972. Also in 1972, Geraldo Rivera, a reporter for WABC New York, exposed the long-term neglect and abuse suffered by mentally disabled children at the Willowbrook State School on Staten Island. See David Rothman, *Strangers at the Bedside*; David Rothman and Rothman, *Willowbrook Wars*.

17. Barbara Ehrenreich, Ehrenreich, and Health/PAC, *American Health Empire*, esp. 29–39; Illich, *Medical Nemesis*, 4, 35; Dekkers, "American Murderers' Association," 4. Health-PAC used the term "medical-industrial complex" ten years before Relman's "New Medical-Industrial Complex," which is sometimes cited as the first use of the term. For the larger evolution of the "misuse of science" theme, see Kelly Moore, *Disrupting Science*.

18. Dittmer, *Good Doctors*; Naomi Rogers, "Caution"; Chowkwanyun, "New Left and Public Health."

19. John Ehrenreich and Ehrenreich, "New Left"; Illich, *Medical Nemesis*, 4, 35. White middle-class women had participated in earlier reforms but did so in keeping with a gender inequality that often downplayed or limited their impact.

20. Haug and Sussman, "Professional Autonomy," 155.

21. Langer, "Doctors' Organization," 283; Richard D. Lyons, "The AMA Reads the Portents More Carefully," *NYT*, June 23, 1968; "Physician, Heal Thyself," *Liberation News Service*, July 17, 1969. See also Jon Nordheimer, "Protester Likens AMA to Saigon Government," *NYT*, July 16, 1969.

22. For a sympathetic account of the Lincoln Hospital takeover, see Barbara Ehrenreich, Ehrenreich, and Health/PAC, *American Health Empire*, 253–67.

23. Feldman and Windle, "NIMH Approach," 174; Lefkowitz, *Community Health Centers*, 14; Ruzek, *Women's Health Movement*, 61. For histories of the women's health movement that chronicle the rise of the feminist clinics, see, for example, Kline, *Bodies of Knowledge*; Morgen, *Into Our Own Hands*; Ruzek, *Women's Health Movement*; Weisman, *Women's Health Care*. On the Office of Economic Opportunity clinics, see Sardell, *U.S. Experiment*; Lefkowitz, *Community Health Centers*. On the Black Panther clinics, see Nelson, *Body and Soul*.

24. "Free City Directory," *Seed*, May 5, 1972, 23, Underground Newspaper Collection, reel 113, item 4.

25. See Taylor, "Free Medicine."

26. Brenner, "Free Clinic"; Bazell, "Health Radicals," 508.

27. Bazell, "Health Radicals," 508; "Anatomy," 10. On the history and significance of the self-exam, see Michelle Murphy, "Immodest Witnessing."

28. Nelson, *Body and Soul*.

29. Checkoway, *Citizens and Health Care*.

30. Bazell, "Health Radicals," 508; Geiger, "Hidden Professional Roles," 31; Levy, "Counter Geiger"; Morgen, *Into Our Own Hands*, 23.

31. See Lefkowitz, *Community Health Centers*.

32. Dittmer, *Good Doctors*, 241. In Barbara Ehrenreich, Ehrenreich, and Health/ PAC, *American Health Empire*, Health-PAC also adopted "consumer," reflecting an interest in coalition building and community outreach characteristic of the early 1970s. See Chowkwanyun, "New Left and Public Health," esp. 238; Alkon, "Late Twentieth-Century Consumer Advocacy," 128–29.

33. Among the most important pieces of legislation were the Automobile Safety Act (1966), the Freedom of Information Act (1966, revised 1974), the Fair Packaging and Labeling Act (1966), the Consumer Credit Protection Act (1968), the National Environmental Policy Act (1970), the Clean Air Act (1970), the Clean Water Act (1972), the Consumer Product Safety Act (1972), and the Magnuson-Moss Warranty Act (1975).

34. Nader, *Consumer and Corporate Accountability*, 2, 3.

35. Herrmann, "Consumerism," 58–59; Kritzer, "Ideology," 493.

36. See *A Brief History of the Center for Science in the Public Interest*, http://www .cspinet.org/history/cspihist.htm; *About Us*, http://medicalconsumers.org/about/; *A Brief History of the NWHN*, http://nwhn.org/brief-history-nwhn-0 (accessed July 1, 2015); Alkon, "Late Twentieth-Century Consumer Advocacy," esp. 121–29.

37. Nicholas Johnson, "Yes, We Can All Be Naders," *NYT*, March 21, 1971. On Nader's background, see McCarry, *Citizen Nader*, and Martin, *Nader*.

38. Nader, *Unsafe at Any Speed*, ix; McCleery, *One Life—One Physician*, 158.

39. Alkon, "Late Twentieth-Century Consumer Advocacy," chap. 2.

40. Vogl, "See Yourself," 162.

41. Edward P. Morgan, "Results Showing in Consumer Fight," *WP*, November 24, 1970.

42. Cron, "Model Consumer," 2. See also Charlotte Rosenberg, "A Militant New Consumer Group: Out to Get M.D.s?" *Medical Economics* 47 (May 11, 1970): 230–33. On Cron's later career, see "Ted Cron," *WP*, December 30, 2006. He became a speechwriter for surgeon general C. Everett Koop.

43. Pertschuk, *Giant Killers*.

44. Bishop and Hubbard, *Let the Seller Beware!*; Nadel, *Politics of Consumer Protection*; Lemov, *People's Warrior*. See also Magnuson and Carper, *Dark Side*. On the new willingness to regulate medicine, see Starr, *Social Transformation*, chap. 4.

45. Sardell, *U.S. Experiment*, argues that agency "subgovernments" became easier to destabilize as more activist groups entered the political battlefield. In addition to responding to direct pressure, agencies also started to change policies to defuse anticipated consumer discontent.

46. Kurtz, "Law of Informed Consent." For a good overview of changing product liability law in the 1950s and 1960s, see Welke, "Cowboy Suit Tragedy."

47. Starr, *Social Transformation*, 388–93. For an excellent overview of the changing terrain of law and bioethics, see David Rothman, *Strangers at the Bedside*. The learned intermediary doctrine shielded pharmaceutical companies from a direct duty to warn patient-consumers. But the overall trend of liability law put more pressure on the FDA to scrutinize new drug applications and to monitor physicians' failures to fulfill their responsibilities as learned intermediaries.

48. Schorr, *Don't Get Sick*, 6, 114, 51, 78, 77. *Health in America* was not the first mention of the phrase "health care crisis" on national television. On May 10, 1961, Dave Garroway of NBC's *Today Show* interviewed Dr. David D. Rutstein, one of the contributors to Sanders, *Crisis in American Medicine*. See "Television Highlights," *WP*, May 10, 1961.

49. Schorr, *Don't Get Sick*, 19, 214, 218–19. The documentary earned him a place on Richard Nixon's enemies list because the president felt that *Health in America* was too critical of his administration's health initiatives; see Schorr, *Staying Tuned*, 228. Schorr's views may have been influenced by his wife, Lisbeth, who was a health advocate for the American Federation of Labor.

50. For a perceptive account of the "intellectual euphoria" experienced in Health-PAC, see Chowkwanyun, "New Left and Public Health."

51. Bazell, "Health Radicals," 508.

52. My summary here is based on Beatrix Hoffman, "'Don't Scream Alone.'"

53. For the full text of the 1973 Bill of Rights, see Annas, *Rights of Hospital Patients*, 25–27.

54. Hogan, "Patient's Rights," 112.

55. Hogan, "Patient's Rights," 112. Compare Beatrix Hoffman's assessment of the document's defects in "'Don't Scream Alone'" with the more optimistic view of it in 1986 in Faden, Beauchamp, and King, *History and Theory*.

56. "Text of Kennedy's Message to Congress on Protections for Consumers," *NYT*, March 16, 1962; Countryman and Gekas, *Development and Implementation*, 1.

57. Walter Lear, "Do People Have Patients' Rights?," paper presented at the National Conference on Social Welfare, September 1974 (draft), 6, in possession of the author; Monaghan, "Whatever Happened," 109.

58. Lear, "Do People Have Patients' Rights?," 15.

59. Gaylin, "Patient's Bill of Rights," 22.

60. Monaghan, "Whatever Happened," 109, 110; Annas, *Rights of Hospital Patients*, 27; Beatrix Hoffman, "'Don't Scream Alone,'" 143.

61. Hogan, "Patient's Rights," 111.

62. *Liberation News Service*, December 14, 1969.

63. U.S. Task Force on Prescription Drugs, *Final Report*, 23–24. See also Chadduck, "'In Brief Summary'"; Feather, interview. With relatively few changes, the 1968 guidelines continue to govern drug labeling and advertising.

64. For a basic explanation of product liability law and the medical exceptions to it, see Jasper, *Law of Product Liability*, esp. chap. 9. The category of "unavoidably unsafe product" was defined in American Law Institute, *Restatement of the Law Second, Torts*, section 402a, which Jasper reprints in appendix 2, 85–98; see also 90–91.

65. Watkins, *On the Pill*; Tone, *Devices and Desires*.

66. Seaman, *Doctors' Case against the Pill*, 12.

67. Watkins, *On the Pill*, 121–28; Tone, *Devices and Desires*, 249–50. The AMA distributed only about 4 million of the longer brochures between 1970 and 1976; see Tone, *Devices and Desires*, 250.

68. For contemporary accounts of the concerns over product safety, see Magnuson and Carper, *Dark Side*; Bishop and Hubbard, *Let the Seller Beware!* See also Welke, "Cowboy Suit Tragedy."

69. David Rothman has described the prevailing ethos of research as "laissez-faire in the laboratory" (*Strangers at the Bedside*, 51). In therapeutic relationships, standards for obtaining consent to treatment were also subject to physician discretion. But as Barron Lerner and Chris Crenner have argued, those standards were not nearly as one-sided as has been assumed. Developments in the 1970s legitimated already existing trends in medicine. See Lerner, "Beyond Informed Consent"; Crenner, *Private Practice*, esp. chap. 7. Also, consent to treatment had long been a principle of American medical practice. See Pernick, "Patient's Role."

70. Beecher, "Ethics and Clinical Research"; Rothman, *Strangers at the Bedside*, esp. chap. 9. In the late 1960s, health radicals had begun to accuse the medical-industrial complex of treating patients, particularly women and people of color, in inhumane and callous ways, particularly as teaching or research material, but their charges remained vague and easily dismissed. The initial impetus for reexamining consent protocols in experimental medicine came not from radical activists but from within the research community.

71. Reverby, *Examining Tuskegee*.

72. Leslie J. Miller, "Informed Consent," 2100.

73. Ibid. My general discussion here is based on contemporary summaries, such as Leslie J. Miller's series in the *Journal of the American Medical Association*, as well as the still-valuable overview in Faden, Beauchamp, and King, *History and Theory*.

74. William Curran, foreword to Rozovsky, *Consent to Treatment*, xxxi.

75. Lerner, *Breast Cancer Wars*, esp. chaps. 7 and 8.

76. Rozovsky, *Consent to Treatment*. The appendix includes sample consent forms.

77. Luis Kutner, "Due Process of Euthanasia"; Dempsey, "Living Will"; M. L. Tina Stevens, *Bioethics in America*, esp. 109–48. Quinlan's parents argued that she would not want to be kept alive under these circumstances, and the courts agreed that her wishes should be honored.

78. Ennis, *Prisoners of Psychiatry*; Garrow, *Liberty and Sexuality*.

79. Dolan, "Book Reviews," 690. *Patients' Rights Digest* ceased publication in 1989.

80. Morgen, *Into Our Own Hands*, 82; Kline, *Bodies of Knowledge*, 14–15; Ruzek, *Women's Health Movement*, 166 n. 28.

81. The demand for medical accountability came in the wake of a larger push for political accountability and transparency manifest in the 1966 passage of the Freedom of Information Act. In 1976, in the wake of the Watergate scandal, Congress significantly strengthened that law. See Theoharis, *Culture of Secrecy*; Schudson, *Watergate in American Memory*.

82. Howard S. Shapiro, *How to Keep Them Honest*, 7; "They Are All Afraid of Herb the Horrible," *Time*, July 10, 1972, 80, 82.

83. Howard S. Shapiro, *How to Keep Them Honest*, 9–10; Pennsylvania Department of Insurance, *Shoppers' Guide*.

84. Pennsylvania Department of Insurance, *Shoppers' Guide*, 1. For the criticism Denenberg received, see Howard S. Shapiro, *How to Keep Them Honest*, 10–11. His response was, "If you do not like our Guide, publish a better one yourself" (11).

85. See Denenberg, "Shopper's Guide"; Denenberg, *Shopper's Guidebook*; *Philadelphia Inquirer*, March 20, 2010.

86. Public Citizen and the Health Research Group, *Consumer's Directory*.

87. Ibid.

88. Ibid., vii, viii, ix.

89. Ibid., xv, xviii.

90. Ibid., xix.

91. McGarrah, "It's Time Consumers Knew More," 267.

92. Reynolds, "What If You're Listed," 291–92.

93. "How to Develop a Local Directory," 685, 687. See also "How to Find a Doctor."

94. Reynolds, "What If You're Listed," 290; see also Jane E. Brody, "How Educated Patients Get Proper Health Care," *NYT*, January 30, 1976. A similar directory in northern Virginia also ran into resistance in 1973; see "HSA Puts Out U.S. Financed Doctor Directory," 12.

Chapter Nine

1. Donald L. Cooper, "Get Ready," 91, 95, 101.

2. Bazell, "Health Radicals," 509; Schorr, *Don't Get Sick*, 183.

3. Austin Smith, "Changing Health Care Scene," 102.

4. Lipset and Schneider, *Confidence Gap*, 48–49.

5. Ibid.

6. Klaw, *Great American Medicine Show*, xiii–xiv; Lander, *Defective Medicine*, 6; Aday, "Social Surveys and Health Policy," 513.

7. Haug, "Erosion," 83. For a good summary of the work that resulted from the sociological "discovery" of the patient-consumer, see Haug and Lavin, *Consumerism in Medicine*.

8. Kisch and Reeder, "Client Evaluation," 57; Kasteler et al., "Underlying Prevalence."

9. Herrmann, "Today's Young Adults," 26. Herrmann does not claim that baby boomers had received a very thorough consumer education. In her 1976 study of consumerism, Creighton echoed that assessment but noted that what Americans had received served "to arm buyers for the confrontation with sellers" (*Pretenders*, 77).

10. Herrmann, "Today's Young Adults," 25–26; Reidelbach, *Completely Mad*.

11. See Sanjek, *Gray Panthers*.

12. Nadel, *Politics of Consumer Protection*. On Watergate and its consequences, see Schudson, *Watergate in American Memory*. Reflecting the new emphasis on transparency, Congress acted to strengthen the 1966 Freedom of Information Act by passage in 1976 of the Government in the Sunshine Act.

13. Bishop and Hubbard, *Let the Seller Beware!* For overviews of the health politics of this era, see Blumenthal and Morone, *Heart of Power*, esp. 224–47; Brown, *Politics and Health Care Organization*.

14. Califano, *America's Health Care Revolution*, 145; Starr, *Social Transformation*, 398–405; Hacker, *Divided Welfare State*, 147–53.

15. Turner, "Consumer Report/FDA," 251. By 1968, most of the Drug Efficacy Study Implementation panels had completed their work, but the remainder took almost a decade to complete. At the same time industry groups tried to slow the process down, the FDA faced lawsuits from consumer groups who complained that the agency was taking too long, first in 1972 and again in 1976. In both cases, the courts agreed with the consumerists and ordered the FDA to pick up its pace. See Irvin Molotsky, "U.S. Review of Prescription Drugs Ends," *NYT*, September 16, 1984.

16. Richard D. Lyons, "FDA Asks Changes in Some Antacid Labels," *NYT*, April 5, 1973; "The Big Question: FDA's OTC Review," *American Druggist*, June 1, 1974, 21–22. On the review process, see Charles E. Edwards, "Closing the Gap." The project also had the reputation among some staff members as "kind of boring." See Schmidt, interview, 68. On the over-the-counter review, see Pray, *History*, esp. chap. 9.

17. Rados, "Medical Device"; Mintz, *At Any Cost*; Bacigal, *Limits of Litigation*.

18. See Pitofsky, "Beyond Nader."

19. Grady, "Regulating Information," 238. The FTC commissioners dismissed the case against Pfizer but upheld the validity of the Pfizer rule.

20. "Legal Developments in Marketing," 82–83.

21. Patrick E. Murphy and Wilkie, *Marketing and Advertising Regulation*, 51, 53. For two views, one largely positive, one negative, of the FTC's consumerist turn in the 1970s, see Clarkson and Muris, *Federal Trade Commission*; James C. Cooper, *Regulatory Revolution*.

22. My account of the FTC case here is based on Campion, *AMA and U.S. Health Policy*, 348–51; Avellone and Moore, "Federal Trade Commission."

23. Avellone and Moore, "Federal Trade Commission," 479; *Bates v. State Bar of Ariz.*, 433 U.S. 350 (1977).

24. Anne Ramsay Somers, *Promoting Health*, xxi.

25. Hardy, *Sick*, vii.

26. Herbert E. Klein, "See Yourself," 95; Wertheimer, "Prescription," 844–45; Rees and Young, *Consumer Health Information*, 30. Steinem suggested that doctors keep a copy of the *PDR* in their office waiting rooms, saying "it would be more useful than sitting there reading *Sports Illustrated* or whatever" (Herbert E. Klein, "See Yourself," 99).

27. *Whole Earth Catalog*, 47. The catalog's review of the *Merck Manual* warned readers that they would need a medical dictionary to understand it and that it did not include alternative treatments. But "if you want to understand what is going on when a member of your family or community is seriously ill, this volume can be helpful." Below the entry for the *Merck Manual* the catalog's creator, Stewart Brand, noted that "many prescription drugs can be obtained without a prescription and at low cost from veterinary supply houses." On the manual's history, see Lane and Berkow, "*The Merck Manual.*"

28. Rees and Young, *Consumer Health Information*, 8. The range of health-related publications is evident in the bibliographies that Rees and Young provide. See also Philbrook, *Medical Books*, which lists several hundred books, including Barbara Ehrenreich, Ehrenreich, and Health/PAC, *American Health Empire*.

29. Terry H. Anderson, *Movement and the Sixties*, xxii. I sampled several alternative press titles from 1970 to 1975 and found a great deal of health-related material. See Alternative Press Syndicate, *Underground Newspaper Collection*.

30. Arthur Frank and Frank, *People's Handbook*, 278–91; Schoenfeld, *Advice Your Family Doctor Never Gave You*, xii. On Schoenfeld's background, see Eric Berne, "Dear Doctor Hip Pocrates," *NYT*, February 16, 1969.

31. On the proliferation of women's health handbooks produced in this era, see Kline, *Bodies of Knowledge*, 166 n. 27; Ruzek, *Women's Health Movement*, 147–48.

32. Kline, *Bodies of Knowledge*, esp. chap. 1; Kathy Davis, *Making of Our Bodies, Ourselves*; Ginty, "Our Bodies."

33. Whorton, *Nature Cures*, esp. part 3.

34. Gross, *Our Roots Grow Deep*.

35. Chisari, Nakamura, and Thorup, *Consumers' Guide*, 3.

36. Ibid., 4, 12.

37. Vickery and Fries, *Take Care of Yourself* (1976). Explaining when symptoms required a doctor's visit had long been a central preoccupation of popular medical manuals. See esp. Rosenberg, "Health in the Home"; Rosenberg, "John Gunn."

38. Vickery and Fries, *Take Care of Yourself* (1976), 23.

39. Ibid., 23–24.

40. Vickery and Fries, *Take Care of Yourself* (1976), 67; Rees and Young, *Consumer Health Information*, 4; Victor Cohn, "What Patients Have a Right to Expect," *WP*, March 6, 1990.

41. Rees and Young, *Consumer Health Information*.

42. Graedon, *People's Pharmacy*, 1; *Joe and Teresa Graedon*.

43. Lawrence P. Williams, *How to Avoid Unnecessary Surgery*. "Williams" was a pseudonym, presumably adopted to protect the author from censure.

44. Rees and Young, *Consumer Health Information*, 102. On the importance of the surgical second opinion, see Denenberg, "Shopper's Guide," and McCarthy, Astor, and Tucker, *Second Opinion Handbook*. On hysterectomies as "hip-pocket surgery," see National Women's Health Network, *Hysterectomy*, 14.

45. Donald Vickery, "Foreword," in Rees and Young, *Consumer Health Information*, xi. Another sign that health consumerism had "arrived" was the appearance of college textbooks on the subject, such as Cornacchia, *Consumer Health*, and Hamilton, *Health Care Consumerism*.

46. Rees and Young, *Consumer Health Information*, 9; Eakin, Jackson, and Hannigan, "Consumer Health Information," 221.

47. Anne Ramsay Somers, *Promoting Health*, 32–33.

48. Joubert and Lasagna, "Patient Package Inserts," 507.

49. American Medical Association, *Physician Distribution*.

50. Dubbed the medical profession's version of *Cosmopolitan*, *Medical Economics* emulated many features of a popular magazine rather than a professional journal. Like *Time* and *Fortune*, it was printed on coated paper; like *Reader's Digest*, it carried cartoons. But most important, *Medical Economics* provided physicians with a lively mix of articles about personal and professional issues.

51. Halberstam, "When Women's Lib Marches," 129, 137, 140. The journal sent Halberstam's article out for comment to several women doctors, one of whom wrote back, "I hope you do not publish this drivel" (141).

52. Herbert E. Klein, "See Yourself."

53. Vogl, "See Yourself"; Halberstam, "Doctor-Friend Talks Back," 71, 72, 73.

54. Halberstam, "Doctor-Friend Talks Back," 72, 73. Nader had been a Harvard classmate of Halberstam's brother, journalist David Halberstam. In spite of—or perhaps because of—that personal connection, the tone of Michael Halberstam's commentary was very personal.

55. Lipkin, *Care of Patients*; Cassell, *Healer's Art*, 131.

56. Ludmerer, *Time to Heal*, esp. chaps. 11 and 13; Lee Jacobs, "Interview"; M. L. Tina Stevens, *Bioethics in America*. The new orientation toward patients was particularly noticeable in textbook discussions of how to take a patient history. Guckian, *Clinical Interview*, began by reprinting the 1972 Patients' Bill of Rights.

57. "Book Review," 544; Cousins, "Anatomy of an Illness."

58. Cousins, "Anatomy of an Illness," 1458–59. See also Ingelfinger, "Listen."

59. Cousins, *Anatomy of an Illness*, 53.

60. I base these observations on Norman Cousins Papers, Department of Special Collections, Charles E. Young Research Library, University of California at Los Angeles.

61. Cousins, *Anatomy of an Illness*, 122.

62. Richard Selzer, letter to the editor, *Commentary* 70 (August 1980): 12–13; Richard D. Smith and Marvin Epstein, letter to the editor, *Commentary* 70 (August 1980): 15. These letters were in response to Ruderman, "Placebo," a withering critique of Cousins's book.

63. Rees and Young, *Consumer Health Information*, 6.

64. DeFriese et al., "From Activated Patient." On the growing interest in the problem of patient compliance, see Lerner, "From Careless Consumptives to Recalcitrant Patients."

65. Phillips, *In the Name of the Patient*. The National Society for Patient Representation and Consumer Affairs was founded in 1971; by 1995, more than half of the nation's 3,300 hospitals had some kind of patient representation program. See Phillips, *In the Name of the Patient*, xi.

66. Sehnert, "A Course for Activated Patients," 42; Sehnert and Eisenberg, *How to Be Your Own Doctor*.

67. Mullen, "(Already) Activated Patient," 282; DeFriese et al., "From Activated Patient."

68. Donabedian, "Evaluating the Quality"; Reverby, "Stealing the Golden Eggs." As Reverby wrote, Codman's "end results system" reflected what he described as "the common sense notion that every hospital should follow every patient it treats, long enough to determine whether or not the treatment has been successful, and then to inquire, if not, why not, with a view to preventing a similar failure in the future" (158). Along with Florence Nightingale, Codman is frequently cast as a pioneer of quality assessment. See, for example, Badger, "Patient Care Report Cards." For a good overview of the quality assessment movement's development in the late twentieth century, see Millenson, *Demanding Medical Excellence*.

69. Lavin and Busek, "What Makes Americans So Operation-Happy?"

70. Bunker, "Surgical Manpower"; Bunker, Barnes, and Mosteller, *Costs, Risks, and Benefits*.

71. McCarthy and Widmer, "Effects of Screening"; Millenson, *Demanding Medical Excellence*, 43–49; Mechanic, "General Medical Practice." McCarthy later coauthored a "guide for medical self-defense." See McCarthy, Astor, and Tucker, *Second Opinion Handbook*.

72. Leape, "Unnecessary Surgery."

73. Lavin and Busek, "What Makes Americans So Operation-Happy?," 73, 71, 70.

74. Greer Williams, "Unjustified Surgery," 39; Ingelfinger, "Listen."

75. The petition is summarized in Regier, "Drug Labeling."

76. Schmidt, interview, 60; Kruger, "Patient Package Inserts," 19; Herzberg, *Happy Pills*, 122–49.

77. Hecht, "Developing Drug Information," 17. See also Rowe, "Patient Package Inserts." The proposal to extend the leaflet requirement to all estrogen products originated from the FDA's own obstetrics and gynecology group. See also Susan V. Lawrence, "Patient Package Insert"; Watkins, *Estrogen Elixir*, esp. chap. 7; Watkins, "'Doctor, Are You Trying to Kill Me?,'" esp. 92.

78. U.S. Food and Drug Administration, "Proposed Rule," 40020–21.

79. Vincent, "Patient Package Inserts," 138.

80. Fleckenstein, "Attitudes."

81. Barclay, "Patient Package Inserts," 3; Dorsey, "Patient Package Insert," 1939, 1937.

82. Vincent, "Patient Package Inserts," 136.

83. U.S. Food and Drug Administration, "Proposed Rule," 40032; Schluster, "FDA's Experience," n. 34.

84. Rowe, "Patient Package Inserts," 114 (n. 140). Goyan was the first and to date the only pharmacist ever to head the FDA.

85. "When Patients Know What's Good for Them," 7.

86. Lander, *Defective Medicine*, 174–75.

87. Norman Dorsen and Aryeh Neier, preface to Annas, *Rights of Hospital Patients*, ix. Dorsen and Neier were the editors of the American Civil Liberties Union's handbook series in which Annas's book appeared.

88. Kotlowski, "Knowles Affair." The essay was later republished in Knowles, *Doing Better*.

89. Knowles, "Responsibility," 59–60.

90. Eakin, Jackson, and Hannigan, "Consumer Health Information," 220–21.

91. See Millenson, *Demanding Medical Excellence*.

Chapter Ten

1. Freudenheim, "Shopping-Mall Medicine," 146.

2. Ibid.

3. Ibid.

4. Fuchs, "Economics, Health, and Post-Industrial Society," 154. A search of the *NYT* database turned up the first use of the term "health care industry" on December 30, 1966: the American Hospital Supply Company was advertising for an engineer to work in the "growing health care industry." Two years later, the term appeared again in "Wall St. Is Analyzing Convalescent-Home Potential," *NYT*, March 3, 1968 (describing financiers' interest in this "comparatively new segment of the health care industry").

5. Bedrosian, "Health Care Industry," 554.

6. Ginzberg, "Monetarization"; see also Relman, "New Medical-Industrial Complex."

7. Sheila K. Johnson, "My Doctor," 8. On the Internal Revenue Service and professional corporations, see Parker and Polubinski, "Professional Associations and Corporations." By the late 1980s, the code had changed so that the tax advantages were less clear; see Farber, *Encyclopedia*, 807. I do not mean here to equate the professional corporation as a tax strategy with the business corporation as an investment tool and managerial entity. My point here is a simpler one about how the term "corporation" became so much more ubiquitous in medicine after 1970 and how that usage coincided with growing awareness of a "health care industry."

8. On the history of biomedicine, see Quirke and Gaudillière, "Era of Biomedicine." For two thoughtful accounts of its significance, see Brandt, *Cigarette Century*; Rose, *Politics of Life*.

9. Kevles, *Naked to the Bone*; Callahan, *Taming the Beloved Beast*; David S. Jones, *Broken Hearts*; Wailoo, *How Cancer Crossed the Color Line*.

10. David Rothman, *Strangers at the Bedside*; Starr, *Social Transformation*. On the larger context of postindustrial society and the kind of "consultative commonwealth" it encouraged, see Bell, *Coming of Post-Industrial Society*; Eulau, "Skill Revolution."

11. For a balanced and comprehensive overview of Medicare reform, see Mayes and Berenson, *Medicare Prospective Payment*. Scholars still disagree about which set of changes came first, Medicare reform or the private sector embrace of managed care. Mayes and Berenson make a good case for the importance of the Medicare side. In my synthesis here, I treat the two not as an either/or proposition but rather as mutually reinforcing movements toward a shared goal of cost containment.

12. Friedman, *Capitalism and Freedom*, chap. 9.

13. For a good overview of presidential policy in the Carter and Reagan administrations, see Blumenthal and Morone, *Heart of Power*, chaps. 7 and 8.

14. My discussion here relies heavily on Mayes and Berenson, *Medicare Prospective Payment*. See also Chilingerian, "Origins of DRGs."

15. Mayes, "Origins," 45, 50. See also Mayes and Berenson, *Medicare Prospective Payment*.

16. On the Resource-Based Relative-Value Scale, see Mayes and Berenson, *Medicare Prospective Payment*, esp. chap. 5. On the impact of Medicare's methods in the United States and elsewhere, see Kimberly, Pouvourville, and D'Aunno, *Globalization*.

17. Califano, *America's Health Care Revolution*, chap. 2; Abramowitz, "Black Book," 43. National companies were also looking to escape the reach of state insurance laws. Insurance regulation remained primarily a state rather than federal responsibility; during the turbulent 1970s, many state legislatures passed laws requiring employers to cover specific services such as prenatal care and treatment for mental illness and drug addiction. Large companies with employees in multiple states found this variation both expensive and confusing. Using an obscure provision in the 1974 Employee Retirement Income Security Act, national companies began to escape the more generous state-level requirements by adhering to the more minimal national standards.

18. On for-profit hospitals, see Starr, *Social Transformation*, esp. chap. 5. On the history of Humana, see David A. Jones biography, http://www.miis.edu/about/governance/board/djones/node/608. On HCA, see *Our History*, http://hcahealthcare.com/about/our-history.dot (accessed July 1, 2015).

19. Kaiser Family Foundation, *For-Profit Health Care Companies*; Relman, "New Medical-Industrial Complex."

20. Bradford H. Gray, "Rise and Decline"; Coombs, *Rise and Fall*; Cunningham and Cunningham, *Blues*, chap. 9; Bodenheimer and Grumbach, *Understanding Health Policy*, 63–67.

21. Lawrence K. Altman and Elisabeth Rosenthal, "Changes in Medicine Bring Pain to Healing Profession," *NYT*, February 18, 1990. For a good overview of the factors behind rising demands for accountability, see Gray, *Profit Motive*. See also Dranove, *Economic Evolution*.

22. Salsberg and Forte, "Trends"; "Now the Doctor Will Call You," *NYT*, February 18, 1990. See also Starr, *Social Transformation*, 421–25.

23. Julie Kosterlitz, "Organized Medicine's United Front in Washington Is Showing More Cracks," *National Journal*, January 11, 1986, 82; Roger Collier, "American Medical Association Membership Woes Continue," *Canadian Medical Association Journal*, August 9, 2011, 109; "The AMA at a Glance," *Associated Press*, June 22, 1987. On the continued force of specialization, see Rosemary Stevens, *American Medicine*.

24. "Doctors Will Reassert Their Roles in Health-Care System," *Marketing News*, April 11, 1986; Schiedermayer, "Hippocratic Oath," 62. See also Lawrence K. Altman and Elisabeth Rosenthal, "Changes in Medicine Bring Pain to Healing Profession," *NYT*, February 18, 1990.

25. Lee Sataline, "A Physician Learns the 'Double Speak' of Insurance Forms," *NYT*, September 14, 1986.

26. Linda Greenhouse, "Justices Uphold Right of Doctors to Solicit Trade," *NYT*, March 24, 1982.

27. Campion, *AMA and U.S. Health Policy*, 348–51. Campion describes the FTC lawsuit as reflecting an outdated view of the AMA as well as the agency's general tendency to overstep its regulatory bounds.

28. "Now the Doctor Will Call You," *NYT*, February 18, 1990. On directory advertising, see Reade and Ratzan, "Yellow Professionalism."

29. "Now the Doctor Will Call You," *NYT*, February 18, 1990.

30. Betsy Sharkey, "Kaiser's Image RX," *Adweek*, April 8, 1985; Tom Delaney, "Health Care Services Shop for Agency Treatment," *Adweek*, October 21, 1985. See also the special health care marketing section in *Advertising Age*, November 5, 1979.

31. Lutz, "Ask-A-Nurse's Company"; Linda Perry, "Physician Referral Service," 36; Shepard and Fell, "Marketing on the Internet."

32. N. R. Kleinfield, "A Push to Market Health Care," *NYT*, April 16, 1984; Melinda Henneberger, "Hospitals Learning the Not-Subtle Art of Self-Promotion," *NYT*, July 4, 1994.

33. See Cunningham and Cunningham, *Blues*.

34. Trafford, "As Controversy Mounts," 61.

35. Melinda Henneberger, "Hospitals Learning the Not-Subtle Art of Self-Promotion," *NYT*, July 4, 1994.

36. Ibid.

37. Lynn G. Coleman, "Marketing and Medicine Can Mix and Still Be Ethical," *Marketing News*, May 13, 1991.

38. John C. Freed, "Glut of Doctors Creating a Patient's Market," *NYT*, April 8, 1985; "Noted Expert to Advise Physicians on Keeping Patients Happy," *Business Wire*, April 17, 1989; Freudenheim, "Shopping-Mall Medicine"; Inglehart, "U.S. Health Care System," 121; Schiedermayer, "Hippocratic Oath," 62.

39. "Now the Doctor Will Call You," *NYT*, February 18, 1990; Thomas M. Heric, "Choosing Other Types of Practice," in Gitnick, Rothenberg, and Weiner, *Business of Medicine*, 106. See also Carroll and Gagnon, "Identifying Consumer Segments," 23.

40. "Editorial: From a Commentary by John J. Lynch, President of the D.C. Medical Society," *WP*, December 28, 1984.

41. Pinckney and Pinckney, *Patient's Guide*, xx–xxi. On the usage of "primary care physician," see Vickery and Fries, *Take Care of Yourself* (1989), 77.

42. Farber, *Encyclopedia*, 311, 449.

43. Balliett, *Practice Management*, 1–2

44. Sloane and Sloane, *Medicine Moves*, 159.

45. Joanne Moser, "Office Design," in Gitnick, Rothenberg, and Weiner, *Business of Medicine*, 243. See also Farber, *Encyclopedia*.

46. "Business-Minded Health Care," *NYT*, February 12, 1985. See also Sari Horwitz, "Walk-In Centers Transforming the Business of Medicine," *WP*, May 27, 1985.

47. John C. Freed, "Glut of Doctors Creating a Patient's Market," *NYT*, April 8, 1985; Nate Haseltine, "District Medical Society Rejects Proposal for Credit Card Billing," *WP*, June 30, 1963.

48. Rodwin, *Medicine, Money, and Morals*, 17; Hing and Burt, "Characteristics."

49. Gitnick, Rothenberg, and Weiner, *Business of Medicine*; Farber, *Encyclopedia*.

50. Marian G. Cooper and Bredow, *Medical Assistant*, 159; chap. 13, "Insurance for the Patient," 159–78, includes samples of various forms.

51. Lester L. Sacks, "Utilization Review," in Gitnick, Rothenberg, and Weiner, *Business of Medicine*, 67.

52. "Medical Practice System Based on MUMPS," *Computer World*, November 28, 1983, 132; Farber, *Encyclopedia*, chap. 12, "Learning to Live with a Computer," 515–67; Susan M. Ostoya, "Computerization of Medical Office Systems," in Gitnick, Rothenberg, and Weiner, *Business of Medicine*, 317–29.

53. Marian G. Cooper and Bredow, *Medical Assistant*, 166.

54. Bredow, Becklin, and Sunnarborg, *Medical Office Procedures*, 98.

55. Balliett, *Practice Management*, 75.

56. Lee Sataline, "A Physician Learns the 'Double Speak' of Insurance Forms," *NYT*, September 14, 1986.

57. Schiedermayer, "Hippocratic Oath"; Christine Woolsey, "Claims Systems Generate Savings in Work Comp Bills," *Business Insurance*, July 23, 1990.

58. Tessa Melvin, "Students Get a Taste of a Doctor's Life," *NYT*, December 25, 1988.

59. Kimmel, "How to Be Ethical," 15. Victor Cohn's coverage of health care change in the 1980s *Washington Post* was particularly insightful. See, for example, "Mastering the Medical Maze," *WP*, October 10, 1984, and "The Forgotten Patient," *WP*, February 27, 1985.

60. Susan Dentzer, "Hospitals Take the Cure," *Newsweek*, July 2, 1984, 56.

61. Sandy Rover, "Breast Sculpture: Three Women and the New Art of Post-Surgical Reconstruction," *WP*, December 14, 1980.

62. Carol Gino, "As I See It: A Second Opinion Is Common Sense," *Long Island Newsday*, January 8, 1986.

63. Karlyn Barker, "Hypochondria: Doc, I Think I've Got It," *WP*, June 6, 1989.

64. Victor Cohn, "A Pink Slip for Dr. Wrong," *WP*, March 20, 1985; Blendon and Altman, "Public Attitudes," esp. 614.

65. Lee Dembart, "A List of Mayor-Elect's Promises and Proposals during Campaign," *NYT*, November 9, 1977; Sandra Evans Teeley, "Health Chief Seeks Change in Attitudes," *WP*, May 2, 1983. Maryland added the same requirement in 1991. See Amy Goldstein, "Poor Required to Have Own Doctor under Md's New Medicaid Program," *WP*, December 10, 1991. As early as 1970, a Senate subcommittee report on rising medical costs pointed to Medicaid doctor-shopping as a cause and suggested that the government require the assignment of "a 'primary care physician' in areas where those eligible for Medicaid have gone from one doctor to another for treatment of the same condition" ("Medicare Study in Senate Seeks Urgent Reforms," *NYT*, February 9, 1970). Although costs for Medicare were also rising at that time, the report made no such suggestion for its recipients.

66. Amy Goldstein, "Poor Required to Have Own Doctor under Md's New Medicaid Program," *WP*, December 10, 1991.

67. Temkin-Greener, "Medicaid Families"; Olson, *Politics of Medicaid*, esp. 158–61.

68. Elizabeth Gardner, "Hospital Uses Information Flow to Boost Cash Flow," *Modern Health Care*, March 26, 1990, 34.

69. Victor Cohn, "Behind the Hospital Death Statistics," *WP*, December 22, 1987.

70. Ibid.; Robert Pear, "Mortality Data Released for 6,000 U.S. Hospitals," *NYT*, December 18, 1987; Matt Clark and Bob Cohn, "Sickbeds and Deathbeds," *Newsweek*, March 24, 1986, 63.

71. Victor Cohn, "Behind the Hospital Death Statistics," *WP*, December 22, 1987.

72. Allen and Roberts, "Data Driven Quality Differentiation," 170.

73. Findlay, Roberts, and Silberner, "Best Hospitals."

74. Ibid.

75. Ibid.; Podolsky, "America's Best Hospitals."

76. Podolsky, "America's Best Hospitals."

77. "Who Decides? Frequently Asked Questions about How the Best Doctors Are Chosen," *New York*, June 18, 2007; Alex Kuczynski, "Rating of Doctors Now a Business unto Itself," *NYT*, March 25, 1999.

78. Heffernan, "Health Care Quality Improvement Act."

79. Sandra G. Boodman, "What You Can't Know about Your Doctor," *WP*, September 14, 1993.

80. Sandra G. Boodman, "Report Cards for Hospitals," *WP*, December 6, 1994. See also Sandra G. Boodman, "Smart Data, Foolish Choices: Consumers Spurn New Sources of Health Quality Information," *WP*, December 19, 2000.

81. Berkman, *HMO Survival Guide*, 9.

82. Gabel et al., "Commercial Health Insurance Industry in Transition," 47; Kaiser Family Foundation, *2013 Employer Health Benefits Survey*, 9. On the disparity between the "open network" promise and the "locked in" realities of managed care, see Curtis, Kurtz, and Stepnick, *Creating Consumer Choice*. There is no consistency in the numbers given in the late 1980s and early 1990s for people enrolled in managed-care plans, which likely reflects the widespread confusion between managed care as a set of strategies and managed care as a type of organization—for example, an HMO. On the confusion surrounding the term, see Hacker and Marmor, "Misleading Language."

83. Levit, Freeland, and Waldo, "National Health Care Spending Trends," 177–80. On the use of deductibles and copays, see Hoffman, "Restraining the Health Care Consumer." For a consumer's-eye perspective on the complex options available, see Morton Hunt, "A Common-Sense Guide to Health Insurance," *NYT*, May 3, 1987.

84. Cohen et al., *Health Insurance Coverage Trends*. For a good journalistic summary of the insurance problems written at the time of the Clinton health care debate, see Eckholm, *Solving America's Health-Care Crisis*.

85. Beatrix Hoffman, *Health Care for Some*, esp. chaps. 8 and 9.

86. Mary Beth Franklin, "Buried in Bills," *WP*, December 5, 1995.

87. Findlay, "Coverage Denied," 80.

88. Blumenthal and Morone, *Heart of Power*, esp. chaps. 9 and 10.

89. See Starr, *Remedy and Reaction*.

90. Domestic Policy Council (U.S.), *President's Health Security Plan*.

91. Christopher Farley and Kevin Fedarko, "The Rise and Fall of the Political Catchphrase," *Time*, February 14, 1994, 1–4; Jost, *Health Care at Risk*.

92. Kathleen Hall Jamieson, "When Harry Met Louise," *WP*, August 15, 1994.

93. There is now a huge literature on the aftermath of the managed-care debate. For

good overviews, see Mechanic, "Rise and Fall," and the special issue on managed care, *Journal of Health Politics, Policy and Law* 24 (October 1999).

94. Institute of Medicine, Committee on Standards for Developing Trustworthy Clinical Practice Guidelines, *Clinical Practice Guidelines*; Bero and Rennie, "Cochrane Collaboration."

95. Millenson, *Demanding Medical Excellence*, xii–xiii.

Chapter Eleven

1. Findlay, "Medicine-Chest Roulette," 76; Penny Chorlton, "FDA Outpaced Firm on Acne Drug," *WP*, September 14, 1982.

2. Findlay, "Medicine-Chest Roulette."

3. Michael deCourcy Hinds, "The Rational Consumer May Be Just a Deregulator's Dream," *NYT*, November 1, 1981.

4. Ibid.

5. "'Combos' Lead in Health and Beauty Sales: Nielsen Study," *Marketing News*, August 15, 1986.

6. "Drug Pricing," 140. Kroger battled in Michigan from 1962 to 1965 before winning the right to operate its Super X stores. For an overview of the retail competition with groceries, see Fletcher, *Market Restraints*. Fletcher, an economics professor at the Wharton School, concluded from his study that "the restrictions were too numerous, too uniform, and too clearly discriminatory to be anything but economic weapons directed toward those who would disrupt the status quo of retail drug distribution" (4).

7. Lichtenstein, *Retail Revolution*; Moreton, *To Serve God*; Thomas C. Hayes, "Wal-Mart Net Jumps by 31.8%," *NYT*, February 28, 1990; Philip Wiggins, "K Mart Drops 10.2%," *NYT*, March 17, 1981.

8. *Supermarket News*, July 22, 2002.

9. Marie Griffin, "As an Era Ends, the Future Takes Form," *Drug Store News*, December 8, 1997, 6. On the competition between drugstores and supermarkets, see Faye Brookman, "Turn About Is Fair Play," *Supermarket Business*, June 1997; Deborah Circelli, "Supermarket Pharmacies Storm into Competitive Business," *Lakeland (Florida) Ledger*, November 7, 1998; and Baum, "CVS," 48, 50 (statistics on supermarkets, Walmart, and Kmart).

10. Marie Griffin, "As an Era Ends, the Future Takes Form," *Drug Store News*, December 8, 1997.

11. Albert D. Bates, "Three New Store Formats Will Soon Dominate Drug Retailing," *Marketing News*, March 7, 1980; *Frequently Asked Questions*, http://news.walgreens .com/fact-sheets/frequently-asked-questions.htm (accessed July 1, 2015); "The Power of Persuasion at the Moment of Truth," *Drug Store News*, December 8, 1997.

12. Baum, "CVS," 46. As part of an analysis of CVS's potential as an investment, this report provides an excellent overview of how drugstores responded to competition from supermarkets and big box stores.

13. Ibid., 48; Joseph Serwach, "Walgreens Growth Fuels Drugstore Wars," *Crain's Business*, October 9, 2000, 21; Baum, "CVS," 54.

14. Marie Griffin, "As an Era Ends, the Future Takes Form," *Drug Store News*, De-

cember 8, 1997; Carol Ukens, "Rx On-Line: Drug Emporium Pharmacist Counsels in Cyberspace," *Drug Topics*, December 8, 1997, 110. Unfortunately for Drug Emporium, this trendsetting use of the web did not make up for its failure to fend off Walgreens and CVS, and it declared bankruptcy in 2001.

15. "Public Goes on Strong 'Self-Medication Kick,'" *Marketing News*, June 27, 1980; Faye Brookman, "Turn About Is Fair Play," *Supermarket Business*, June 1997.

16. "Panelists Comment on Study of Drugstore Merchandising Efforts," *Marketing News*, December 7, 1984.

17. Jonathan Rabinovitz, "All About/In-Store Promotions," *NYT*, August 18, 1991; Philip H. Dougherty, "POP Radio Is a Hit with Retailers," *NYT*, January 28, 1988.

18. Faye Brookman, "Turn About Is Fair Play," *Supermarket Business*, June 1997; Allene Symons, "In It for the Long Haul with Innovation, Service," *Drug Store News*, November 3, 1997. Long's was acquired by CVS Caremark in 2008.

19. "The Power of Persuasion at the Moment of Truth," *Drug Store News*, December 8, 1997.

20. Larry Thompson, "Over-the-Counter Drugs: How Safe Are They?," *WP*, September 26, 1989.

21. Frederick M. Rowe, "Decline of Antitrust," esp. 1555–56.

22. "What's the Price of an Rx Drug?," *Consumer Reports*, May 1970, 279.

23. "Drug Pricing," 137; "Drug-Price Advertising Gathers Steam in Courts," *Consumer Reports*, March 1973; "Will Stores Begin Advertising Prices of Prescription Drugs?," *Consumer News*, November 15, 1971, abstract in *Journal of Marketing*, July 1972, 101.

24. For an excellent account of the making of the "generic consumer," see Greene, *Generic*.

25. U.S. Federal Trade Commission, *Drug Product Selection*, 101; "How to Pay Less," 49.

26. U.S. Federal Trade Commission, *Drug Product Selection*, 153, 158, 155. Most states made the choice voluntary rather than mandatory, only 16 percent required that patients be notified of the substitution, and only 6 percent required that they consent to it. Recognizing that the new substitution laws were not working as effectively as hoped, the FTC provided a model law in 1979 designed to improve their efficacy while preserving the right of physicians to prescribe name-brand drugs as "medically necessary."

27. Greene, *Generic*. One source of concern was a bribery scandal involving FDA officials in charge of generic drug approvals. See Pope, "FDA Reorganizes."

28. For the first drug-related use I found of "blockbuster," see Doug McInnis, "Herpes: Burroughs Wellcome Sees Its Treatment as a Way to Cure Profit Ills," *NYT*, June 19, 1983.

29. Michael deCourcy Hinds, "Speeding FDA Drug Review," *NYT*, September 22, 1982; Stone, "Fast Tracking." On AIDS activists and the FDA, see Epstein, *Impure Science*, esp. 278–80.

30. My account of the Accutane case here and in the next paragraph relies on Michael Abramowitz, "FDA Eyes Ban on Acne Drug," *WP*, April 23, 1988; Gina Kolata, "F.D.A. Panel Calls for Curbs on Acne Drug Linked to Birth Defects," *NYT*, April 27, 1988; Lawrence K. Altman, "Drug Inquiry Set on Birth Defects," *NYT*, May 28, 1988.

31. U.S. Food and Drug Administration, "Proposed Rule."

32. "Rules and Regulations: Prescription Drug Products; Revocation of Patient Pack-

age Insert Requirements," *Federal Register* 47 (September 7, 1982): 39147–55. Ironically, this decision came around the same time that Virginia Knauer, Reagan's consumer affairs adviser, announced in April 1981 that she would emphasize "consumer information and education" rather than regulation. Patient information leaflets apparently were considered "regulation" rather than "education" (Karen De Witt, "Reagan's Consumer Chief Notes Policy Shift," *NYT*, April 4, 1981).

33. John Wilkes, "Prescription Drugs Used Improperly, FDA Chief Says," *WP*, July 30, 1983; *PR Newswire*, April 30, 1984; see "Patient Package Inserts Could Become Necessary for MFRS to Limit Liability," *F-D-C Reports*, May 7, 1984, 11–12.

34. Molly Sinclair, "Vital Questions Should Be Asked over Drug Counter," *WP*, July 6, 1983.

35. For a contemporary view of the problem, see Louis A. Morris and Halperin, "Effects of Written Drug Information."

36. John Wilkes, "Prescription Drugs Used Improperly, FDA Chief Says," *WP*, July 30, 1983; Don Colburn, "The Pill Not Taken," *WP*, January 9, 1985; Goyan, "Fourteen Fallacies."

37. See Rowe, "Patient Package Inserts," 114–16; Schluster, "FDA's Experience." See also Watkins, "'Doctor, Are You Trying to Kill Me?'" Pharmacists ultimately gave up their opposition to distributing the patient information leaflets as new computer systems made printing and updating them easier and as the pharmacists became more "comfortable," in historian Gregory Higby's words, with their role as patient counselors (e-mail to author, February 22, 2005). In 1996 Congress passed a law giving the FDA the authority to develop these performance standards with the goal of having 95 percent of patients receive them by 2006. The actual work of developing and monitoring those performance standards was contracted out to a private organization to minimize government involvement.

38. Feather, interview, 35. See also 34–36 for a general discussion of the brief summary and the problems it posed to advertising.

39. Tom Shales, "TV Docs: Just Say Aargh!," *WP*, October 8, 1989. So well-known was the line that comics used it to skewer President Reagan ("He's not President, he just plays one on TV."). See Stephen Holden, "Reagan Becoming a Comic's Delight," *NYT*, March 9, 1987.

40. "No Consumer Rx Ad Regs or Guidelines Coming from FDA Soon," *F-D-C Reports*, February 21, 1983, 5.

41. Linda E. Demkovich, "Proceed with Caution," *National Journal*, April 23, 1983, 855.

42. Michael deCourcy Hinds, "Prescription Drug Ads: Direct Dose to Consumers," *NYT*, May 29, 1983; "Boots' *Rufen* Consumer Rebate Launch Promotion Tied to MD and Patient Familiarity with Ibuprofen," *F-D-C Reports*, February 22, 1982, 7; Matt Clark, "Ads over the Doctor's Head," *Newsweek*, March 15, 1982, 69. See also Hilary deVries, "Advertising of Prescription Drugs Meets Opposition," *Christian Science Monitor*, June 28, 1983.

43. Jerry Knight, "Peoples' Ad for Herpes Salve Fuels Debate over Drug Policy," *WP*, January 10, 1983.

44. Sandra Salmans, "Advertising: Cable TV's Liberalized Guidelines," *NYT*, June 10, 1983. On the history of cable TV, see Cohen, *Consumers' Republic*, esp. 304–6.

45. Patricia McCormack, "Doctors' Hour to Bow on Cable TV," UPI, May 17, 1983. Cable Health Network later merged with another channel to become Lifetime.

46. Linda E. Demkovich, "Proceed with Caution," *National Journal*, April 23, 1983, 855; Novitch, "Direct-to-Consumer Advertising," 310; "No Consumer Rx Ad Regs or Guidelines Coming from FDA Soon," *F-D-C Reports*, February 21, 1983, 6.

47. Hilary deVries, "Advertising of Prescription Drugs Meets Opposition," *Christian Science Monitor*, June 28, 1983; "FDA Mulls Ethical-Drug Ads," *Chemical Week*, December 7, 1983, 21. My account of the timing and specifics of the FDA debate over DTCA relies heavily on Johnstone, "Special Problems."

48. See Feather, interview, esp. 13–18.

49. Ibid. 40; "Arthur Hayes Jr.," *NYT*, March 1, 2010.

50. Johnstone, "Special Problems," 317–18. For the FDA's trial study, see Louis A. Morris and Millstein, "Drug Advertising to Consumers." The study developed eight test ads for TV and radio for a hypothetical hypertension drug and a hypothetical arthritis medication. The ads included varying amounts of information—from none to very detailed—and were shown to 1,509 subjects in four cities; the participants were then tested to see what they remembered and what formats they preferred. The study concluded that the "ads with specific risks were more informative, but subjects preferred the general risk ads. Evidently, people would prefer reassuring messages, such as 'ask your doctor about the drug,' rather than specific drug messages such as 'the drug causes gout'" (503). The study noted that it could not predict how people would react when presented with real drug ads.

51. "Prescription Drugs," *Toronto Globe and Mail*, May 23, 1984; Matt Clark, "Ads over the Doctor's Head," *Newsweek*, March 15, 1982, 69; Hilary deVries, "Advertising of Prescription Drugs Meets Opposition," *Christian Science Monitor*, June 28, 1983.

52. "Direct to Consumer RX Ad Costs for Upjohn's Top Five Drugs," *F-D-C Reports*, May 7, 1984, 10.

53. Lawrence C. Hoff, "Advertising Prescription Drugs," 573, 576; Hoff's response in the question-and-answer period appears in "Direct to Consumer RX Ad Costs for Upjohn's Top Five Drugs," *F-D-C Reports*, May 7, 1984, 10.

54. Louis A. Morris et al., "Attitudes of Consumers," 83–84; "Notices: Direct-to-Consumer Advertising of Prescription Drugs; Withdrawal of Moratorium," *Federal Register* 50 (September 9, 1985): 36677–78.

55. "Direct-to-Consumer Rx Drug Ads Will Draw Hill Hearing," *F-D-C Reports*, January 13, 1986, 8.

56. Claudia H. Deutsch, "The Brouhaha over Drug Ads," *NYT*, May 14, 1989.

57. Ibid. On the push from TV networks, see Penelope Wang, "A New Way to Push Drugs," *Newsweek*, December 30, 1985, 34. On Voltaren, see Feather, interview, 27–29.

58. Morgan, "Direct-to-Consumer Advertising"; Feather, interview, 37, 38.

59. "Miracle Drugs"; Walsh and Pyrich, "FDA Regulation of Pharmaceutical Advertising." See also "Pushing Drugs."

60. David Stout, "Drug Makers Get Leeway on TV Ads," *NYT*, August 9, 1997. See also Kessler and Pines, "Federal Regulation"; Pines, "New Challenges."

61. Wilkes, Bell, and Kravitz, "Direct-to-Consumer Prescription Drug Advertising."

62. Vares, "Viagra"; "Finally, Prescription Drugs Make It to the Effie Awards," 24. One

of Leno's Viagra jokes was "What is it with Republicans and Viagra? First Bob Dole, he was doing the ads for Viagra. Now you got Rush Limbaugh. Say what you want about Bill Clinton, but the man was always there to answer the call, ladies and gentlemen."

63. Feather, interview, 34; Findlay, "Medicine-Chest Roulette."

64. For an insightful discussion of postmarket surveillance, see Carpenter, *Reputation and Power*, 585–634.

65. Wolfe, Coley, and Public Citizen Health Research Group, *Pills That Don't Work*; Wolfe et al., *Worst Pills, Best Pills*.

66. Twerski, "Liability," 1149.

67. *Perez v. Wyeth Laboratories Inc.*, Supreme Court of New Jersey, 1999, http://caselaw.findlaw.com/nj-supreme-court/1094741.html (accessed July 1, 2015).

68. Ibid.

69. Ibid.

70. Twerski, "Liability."

Conclusion

1. "Doctors Getting Rated by Zagat," *Business Insurance*, October 29, 2007.

2. "Would You Like Dessert with Your Diagnosis?," *USA Today*, January 17, 2008; James King, "Ratings Can Mislead," *USA Today*, January 17, 2008; "Cures for an Ailing System," *Newsweek*, December 10, 2007, 78–84.

3. Pauline W. Chen, "Should Patients Read the Doctor's Notes?," *NYT*, July 27, 2010.

4. Robert A. Dowling, "Valuable Lessons for Urologists from the Auto Service Industry," *Urology Times*, July 1, 2012, 53–54.

5. Lee, "Change the Concept of Work from Service to Theater"; Lee, *If Disney Ran Your Hospital*, 27, 193. Lee's speaking fees range from $9,000 to $12,000 per talk, according to his entry on the website Innovative Healthcare Speakers, innovativehealthcarespeakers.com/speaker?id=7 (accessed July 1, 2015).

6. "What Can We Learn from Mickey Mouse?," *Hospital Impact*, April 11, 2005, http://www.hospitalimpact.org/index.php/leadership/2005/04/11/what_if_disney_ran_your hospital (accessed July 1, 2015).

7. Ibid.

8. Rachel Grob, "Heart of Patient-Centered Care." The special issue on patient engagement is *Health Affairs* 32 (February 2013).

9. Institute of Medicine, Committee on Quality of Health Care in America, *Crossing the Quality Chasm*, 6. See also Kohn, Corrigan, and Donaldson, *To Err Is Human*.

10. Millenson, *Demanding Medical Excellence. Health Affairs* provides regular reporting on the latest in quality initiatives. See for example the theme issue "Still Crossing the Quality Chasm," 30 (April 2011). The 2,700 guidelines are mentioned in Institute of Medicine, Committee on Standards for Developing Trustworthy Clinical Practice Guidelines, *Clinical Practice Guidelines*, 2.

11. Agency for Healthcare Research and Quality, *Enabling Patient-Centered Care*; Robert Pear, "New System for Patients to Report Medical Mistakes," *NYT*, September 23, 2012. See also Ricciardi et al., "National Action Plan."

12. American Society for Bioethics and Humanities, *Report.*

13. Grande, "Limiting the Influence."

14. Patient-Centered Primary Care Collaborative, *Defining the Medical Home.* See also "Patient-Centered Medical Homes"; Pollack, Gidengil, and Mehrotra, "Growth of Retail Clinics."

15. Snow, "Open for Business"; Pollack, Gidengil, and Mehrotra, "Growth of Retail Clinics." A mini-industry has grown up around the provision of television in doctors' waiting rooms. See, for example, Prentice, "Airing Your Message." Not surprisingly, waiting room amenities are linked to the need to compete for patients with good insurance coverage.

16. Katie Thomas, "Use of Generics Produces an Unusual Drop in Drug Spending," *NYT*, March 18, 2013; Tu and Corey, "State Prescription Drug Price Websites"; Oliver, Lee, and Lipton, "Political History."

17. American Pharmacists Association, "FDA's MedWatch Program Turns 20"; Grabowski and Wang, "Quantity and Quality"; Carpenter, *Reputation and Power,* esp. chap. 9.

18. Matthew Arnold, "Say So Long"; Kornfield et al., "Promotion of Prescription Drugs"; Denis G. Arnold and Oakley, "Politics and Strategy"; Greene and Kesselheim, "Pharmaceutical Marketing"; "Requirements on Content and Format of Labeling for Human Prescription Drug and Biological Products," *Federal Register* 71 (January 24, 2006): 3922–97. The 2006 effort sought to improve labeling information intended for physicians, not patients.

19. *About U.S. News and World Report,* http://www.usnews.com/info/features/about-usnews (accessed July 1, 2015); "WellPoint Patients Can Give Critiques," *Los Angeles Times,* January 12, 2008.

20. Susannah Fox and Duggan, *Health Online 2013.* See also Cline and Haynes, "Consumer Health Information Seeking."

21. Baer, "Patient-Physician E-Mail Communication"; Moeller, "Study"; Hanauer et al., "Public Awareness"; Pew Research Center, *Mobile Technology Fact Sheet.*

22. Starr, *Remedy and Reaction,* 146–58; "America's Health Insurance Plans—Health Savings Accounts and Consumer-Directed Plans," http://www.ahip.org/Issues/Health-Savings-Accounts-and-Consumer-Directed-Plans.aspx (accessed July 1, 2015).

23. For an account of the ACA that puts it in long historical perspective, see Starr, *Remedy and Reaction.* For a contemporary explanation of the law presented as a graphic book, see Gruber, *Health Care Reform.*

24. For an overview of the ACA's reform provisions, see Millenson and Macri, *Will the Affordable Care Act Move Patient-Centeredness?*

25. Sabrina Tavernise, "Number of Americans without Health Insurance Falls, Survey Shows," *NYT*, September 16, 2014.

26. Hartman et al., "National Health Spending in 2013."

27. Rorty, *American Medicine Mobilizes,* 33.

28. Millenson, *Demanding Medical Excellence.*

29. Cutler, *Quality Cure,* xvi; Cutler, *Your Money or Your Life,* xi–xii.

30. Institute of Medicine, Committee on Standards for Developing Trustworthy

Clinical Practice Guidelines, *Clinical Practice Guidelines*, xii. On the time-lag problem in cardiac care, see David S. Jones, *Broken Hearts*, esp. chap. 16. See also Kushner, "Other War."

31. Peterson et al., *Analytical Study*; McGlynn et al., "Quality of Health Care"; Mark D. Smith et al., *Best Care*, ix. See also Kohn, Corrigan, and Donaldson, *To Err Is Human*.

32. Squires, *U.S. Health System*, 11, 2.

33. Majerol, Newkirk, and Garfield, *Uninsured*; Commonwealth Fund, *Insured and Still at Risk*; Pittman, "Concierge Medicine Gains Ground."

34. Martin Tolchin, "Length of Average Hospital Stay Drops 22%," *NYT*, May 25, 1988; Jaimie Oh, "Average Inpatient Hospital Stay Shorter but More Expensive in 2009 than 1997," *Becker's Hospital Review*, December 8, 2011.

35. U.S. Office of Technology Assessment, *Defensive Medicine*, 1.

36. Michael Marks Davis, *Medical Care for Tomorrow*, 12; Agency for Healthcare Research and Quality, *Number of Practicing Primary Care Physicians*. Only 25 percent of recent medical school graduates are choosing primary care specialties, suggesting that this problem will only increase in the future. See Robert Graham Center, *Medical School Production*.

37. On the decline of primary care, see Bodenheimer, "Primary Care"; Howell, "Reflections." Howell's article is part of a special theme issue, "Reinventing Primary Care," *Health Affairs* 29 (May 2010). A thoughtful documentary on the subject is *MIA MD*.

38. Brownlee, "Doctor Will See You"; "Patient-Centered Medical Homes," 3. On the travails of primary care practice, see Timothy Hoff, *Practice under Pressure*. Long before managed care arrived, patients were complaining that physicians rushed through their visits. See for example, Goodman's 1966 lament, "Doctor's Image."

39. Pollack, Gidengil, and Mehrotra, "Growth of Retail Clinics," 999.

40. Mendelson and Carino, "Evidence-Based Medicine." See also Institute of Medicine, Committee on Standards for Developing Trustworthy Clinical Practice Guidelines, *Clinical Practice Guidelines*, 1–3.

41. Goldberger and Fagerlin, "ICDs."

42. The rise of so-called risk factor medicine has made communication between doctor and patient all the more consequential. For a broad study of risk, see Rothstein, *Public Health*. On its impact on therapeutic practice, see Greene, *Prescribing by Numbers*.

43. Nicholas Bakalar, "Infections Follow Rise in Cardiac Implants," *NYT*, August 29, 2011; Wilson et al., "Hip and Knee Implants."

44. Steve Sternberg, "Heart Devices under Scrutiny," *USA Today*, June 21, 2005; Barry Meier, "Maker Hid Data about Design Flaw in Hip Implant, Records Show," *NYT*, January 25, 2013; "Medical Device Recalls Reach Eight-Quarter High," *Medical Device Daily*, August 24, 2012. On the challenges of device regulation, see Institute of Medicine, Committee on the Public Health Effectiveness of the FDA 510(k) Clearance Process, *Medical Devices and the Public's Health*.

45. The best overview of the FDA's balancing act is Carpenter, *Reputation and Power*. On the complexities of pharmaceutical science more generally, see Avorn, *Powerful Medicines*.

46. Sandroff, "Got Side Effects?" On the extent of adverse drug events in hospital and

ambulatory care, see Kanjanarat et al., "Nature of Preventable Adverse Drug Events"; Gurwitz et al., "Incidence and Preventability."

47. Lisa Girion, Scott Glover, and Doug Smith, "Drug Deaths Now Outnumber Traffic Fatalities in U.S., Data Show," *Los Angeles Times*, September 17, 2011; Gu, Dillon, and Burt, "Prescription Drug Use."

48. "How Much Does Your Druggist Know?"

49. Knox, "Breast Cancer."

50. James Chase, "100 Agencies."

51. Denis G. Arnold and Oakley, "Politics and Strategy"; Steinhart, Carmon, and Trope, "Warnings." For a good overview of the divergent views, see "Should Prescription Drug Ads Be Reined In?"

52. "Consumers and Pharma Companies."

53. Pew Charitable Trusts, *Persuading the Prescribers*.

54. Conroy, "Can We Put the Hospital Marketing Genie Back in the Bottle?"

55. Narins et al., "Influence of Public Reporting"; Werner and Asch, "Unintended Consequences." For a positive view of rankings, see Hibbard, Stockard, and Tusler, "Hospital Performance Reports." On the gaming problem in the law, see Espeland and Sauder, "Rankings and Reactivity."

56. Kaiser Family Foundation, *Five Years*; "Smart Data, Foolish Choices: Consumers Spurn New Sources of Health Quality Information," *WP*, December 19, 2000; "Health Policy Brief."

57. Medical Library Association, Consumer and Patient Health Information Section, *Top 100 Health Websites*; "Health Policy Brief."

58. "Best Drugstores: 2011."

59. Yegian et al., "Engaged Patients," 238.

60. "Health Policy Brief."

61. M. Kutner et al., *Health Literacy*.

62. Harding, *Fads, Frauds, and Physicians*, 17.

63. Curtis, Kurtz, and Stepnick, *Creating Consumer Choice*, 30.

64. "Needless Surgery," 48; Tara Parker-Pope, "Plenty of Blame in a Health System 'Designed to Fail,'" *NYT*, May 8, 2012.

65. Friedberg et al., "Demonstration," 271.

66. Frosch et al., "Authoritarian Physicians"; "The Package," *Seinfeld*, aired October 17, 1996.

67. "Head Mirror or Halo?"

68. Bebinger, "How Much?"

69. Carter, *Doctor Business*, 17; Schorr, *Don't Get Sick*, 77.

70. Gerard F. Anderson et al., "It's the Prices, Stupid."

71. Sommers et al., "Focus Groups," 342–43.

72. Pringle, "What Do the Women of America Think?," 15.

73. *New and Improved*, http://tvtropes.org/pmwiki/pmwiki.php/Main/NewAnd Improved (accessed July 1, 2015).

74. Denis G. Arnold and Oakley, "Politics and Strategy." For a similar argument about informed consent, see Zussman, *Intensive Care*.

75. Dubos, "Beyond Traditional Medicine," 166.

76. Clark, *How to Budget Health*, 3. For a recent commentary in the same vein, see Paul Krugman, "Patients Are Not Consumers," *NYT*, April 22, 2011.

77. Rachel Grob and Mark Schlesinger, "Epilogue: Principles for Engaging Patients in U.S. Health Care and Policy," in *Patients as Policy Actors*, ed. Beatrix Hoffman et al., 278–91; Saad, *On Healthcare*. See also Pescosolido, Tuch, and Martin, "Profession of Medicine and the Public."

78. F. J. Schlink to W. D. Sutliff, January 3, 1936, box 437, folder 16, CR Records.

BIBLIOGRAPHY

Archival Sources

Baltimore, Maryland
   Alan Mason Chesney Medical Archives of the Johns Hopkins Medical
      Institutions
      Bertram M. Bernheim Collection
Bethesda, Maryland
   National Library of Medicine, Archives and Modern Manuscripts Collection
      Harry Filmore Dowling Papers, MS C 372
College Park, Maryland
   National Archives
      Records of the Food and Drug Administration, Record Group 88
Durham, North Carolina
   Duke University, David M. Rubenstein Rare Book and Manuscript Library
      J. Walter Thompson Company Archives
Independence, Missouri
   Harry S. Truman Library and Museum
      Oscar Ewing Papers
Los Angeles, California
   University of California, Charles E. Young Research Library, Department of
      Special Collections
      Norman Cousins Papers
   University of Southern California, Doheny Memorial Library, University
      Archives
      Joseph A. Hailer Papers
New Brunswick, New Jersey
   Rutgers University, Alexander Library, Special Collections
      Consumers' Research Inc. Records
New York, New York
   New York Academy of Medicine Library, Malloch Rare Book Room
      Michael M. Davis Collection
Washington, D.C.
   Library of Congress, Manuscript Division
      Wendell Berge Papers, MSS12468
      T. Swann Harding Papers, MSS24885

Wilmington, Delaware
  Hagley Museum and Library, Manuscripts and Archives Department
    Ernest Dichter Papers, Accession 2407
Yonkers, New York
  Consumers Union
    Consumers Union Archives

Books, Articles, Reports, Papers, Interviews, and Dissertations

"500 Corner Drugstores." *Fortune*, September 12, 1935, 71–80, 100.

Aaron, Harold. *Good Health and Bad Medicine: A Family Medical Guide.* New York: McBride, 1940.

Abel, Emily K. *Hearts of Wisdom: American Women Caring for Kin, 1850–1940.* Cambridge, Mass.: Harvard University Press, 2000.

Abramowitz, Kenneth S. "Black Book: The Future of Health-Care Delivery in America." *Bernstein Research Report,* July 12, 1985, 1–198.

Adams, Samuel Hopkins. *The Great American Fraud: Articles on the Nostrum Evil and Quacks Reprinted from Collier's Weekly.* 4th ed. Chicago: Press of the AMA, 1907.

Aday, Lu Ann. "Social Surveys and Health Policy." *Public Health Reports* 92 (November–December 1977): 508–17.

"Advertisers' Ten Commandments." *Ballyhoo* 3 (November 1932): 6.

Agency for Healthcare Research and Quality. *Enabling Patient-Centered Care through Health Information Technology: Executive Summary.* Evidence Report/Technology Assessment No. 206. June 2012. http://effectivehealthcare.ahrq .gov/ehc/products/451/1158/EvidenceReport206_Patient-Centered-Care _ExecutiveSummary_20120614.pdf. Accessed July 1, 2015.

———. *The Number of Practicing Primary Care Physicians in the United States.* October 2014. http://www.ahrq.gov/research/findings/factsheets/primary/ pcwork1/index.html. Accessed July 1, 2015.

Albright, Ida. "High Cost of Babies." *Atlantic Monthly,* May 1925, 586–94.

Alderson, Wroe. "Trends in Distribution of Drug Products." *American Marketing Journal* 2 (January 1, 1935): 53–58.

Alford, Robert. *Health Care Politics: Ideological and Interest Group Barriers to Reform.* Chicago: University of Chicago Press, 1975.

Alkon, Ava. "Late Twentieth-Century Consumer Advocacy, Pharmaceuticals, and Public Health: A Historical Study of the Public Citizen's Health Research Group (HRG)." Ph.D. diss., Columbia University, 2012.

Allen, Bruce, and Brenda Roberts. "Data Driven Quality Differentiation: Using PRO Mortality Data to Market your Hospital." In *Marketing Is Everybody's Business,* edited by Peter Sanchez. Chicago: Academy for Health Services Marketing, 1988.

"Allen Funt's Candid Camera Shows Druggists How to Sell." *Business Week,* January 5, 1952, 78.

Alter, George, and Ann Carmichael. "Classifying the Dead: Toward a History of the Registration of Causes of Death." *Journal of the History of Medicine and Allied Sciences* 54 (April 1999): 114–32.

Alternative Press Syndicate. *Underground Newspaper Collection.* Wooster, Ohio: Micro Photo Division, Bell and Howell, 1970–85.

American Foundation. *American Medicine: Expert Testimony Out of Court.* 2 vols. Edited by Esther E. Lape. New York: American Foundation, 1937.

American Law Institute. *Restatement of the Law Second, Torts.* 2nd ed. St. Paul, Minn.: American Law Institute Publishers, 1965.

American Medical Association. *County Medical Public Relations Manual.* Chicago: American Medical Association, 1955.

———. *Physician Distribution and Medical Licensure in the U.S.* Chicago: Center for Health Services Research and Development, 1975.

———. *What Americans Think of the Medical Profession: Report on a Public Opinion Survey.* Chicago: American Medical Association, 1956.

American Medical Association, Council on Medical Service. *Nationwide Survey of County Medical Society Activities.* Chicago: American Medical Association, 1955.

"The American Medical Association Dissected." *Fortune,* November 1938, 88–92, 150–68.

American Pharmacists Association. "FDA's MedWatch Program Turns 20: What's New?" http://www.pharmacist.com/fdas-medwatch-program-turns-20-whats-new. Accessed July 1, 2015.

American Society for Bioethics and Humanities. *Report of the Task Force on Ethics and Humanities Education in Undergraduate Medical Programs.* Glenview, Ill.: American Society for Bioethics and Humanities, 2009. http://www.asbh.org/uploads/files/pubs/lcmereport.pdf. Accessed July 1, 2015.

"Anatomy: Dig Yourself." *off our backs* 1 (August 31, 1971): 10.

Anderson, Ann. *Snake Oil, Hustlers, and Hambones: The American Medicine Show.* Jefferson, N.C.: McFarland, 2000.

Anderson, Gerard F., Uwe E. Reinhardt, Peter S. Hussey, and Varduhi Petrosyan. "It's the Prices, Stupid: Why the United States Is So Different from Other Countries." *Health Affairs* 22 (May–June 2003): 89–105.

Anderson, Odin W., and Jacob J. Feldman. *Family Medical Costs and Voluntary Health Insurance: A Nationwide Survey.* New York: Blakiston, 1956.

Anderson, Odin W., and Monroe Lerner. *Measuring Health Levels in the United States, 1900–1958.* New York: Health Information Foundation, 1960.

Anderson, Terry H. *The Movement and the Sixties.* New York: Oxford University Press, 1996.

Annas, George J. *The Rights of Hospital Patients: The Basic ACLU Guide to a Hospital Patient's Rights.* New York: Discus, 1975.

———. *Some Choice: Law, Medicine, and the Market.* New York: Oxford University Press, 1998.

Annual Report of the Federal Trade Commission, 1931. Washington, D.C.: U.S. Government Printing Office, 1931.

"Any Medicine Can Hurt Some People." *Science Digest* 32 (October 1952): 74.

Apple, Rima, comp. *Illustrated Catalogue of the Slide Archives of Historical Medical Photographs at Stony Brook.* Westport, Conn.: Greenwood, 1984.

———. "Liberal Arts or Vocational Training? Home Economics for Girls." In *Rethinking Home Economics,* edited by Sarah Stage and Virginia Vincenti. Ithaca: Cornell University Press, 1997.

———. *Mothers and Medicine: A Social History of Infant Feeding.* Madison: University of Wisconsin Press, 1988.

———. *Perfect Motherhood: Science and Childrearing in America.* New Brunswick, N.J.: Rutgers University Press, 2006.

———. *Vitamania: Vitamins in American Culture.* New Brunswick, N.J.: Rutgers University Press, 1996.

Armstrong, David, and Elizabeth Metzger Armstrong. *The Great American Medicine Show.* New York: Prentice Hall, 1991.

Armstrong, Donald B. "Health Facts—What to Tell." *American Journal of Public Health* 32 (March 1932): 271–80.

———. "See Your Doctor." *The Survey* 58 (July 1, 1927): 386–88.

Arnold, Denis G., and James L. Oakley. "The Politics and Strategy of Industry Self-Regulation: The Pharmaceutical Industry's Principles for Ethical Direct-to-Consumer Advertising as a Deceptive Blocking Strategy." *Journal of Health Politics, Policy, and Law* 38 (June 2013): 505–44.

Arnold, Matthew. "Say So Long to DDMAC as FDA's OPDP Levels Up." *Medical Marketing Media,* September 19, 2011. http://www.mmm-online.com/say-so-long-to-ddmac-as-fdas-opdp-levels-up/article/212320/. Accessed July 1, 2015.

"As *Harper's* Readers See It: A Roundup of Comments." *Harper's,* January 1961, 76–82.

Avellone, Joseph C., and Francis D. Moore. "The Federal Trade Commission Enters a New Arena: Health Services." *New England Journal of Medicine* 299 (August 31, 1978): 478–83.

Avorn, Jerry. *Powerful Medicines: The Benefits, Risks, and Costs of Prescription Drugs.* New York: Knopf, 2004.

Bacigal, Ronald J. *The Limits of Litigation: The Dalkon Shield Controversy.* Durham, N.C.: Carolina Academic Press, 1990.

Bacon, John U. *America's Corner Store: Walgreens' Prescription for Success.* Hoboken, N.J.: Wiley, 2004.

Badger, Kathy A. "Patient Care Report Cards: An Analysis." *Outcomes Management for Nursing Practice* 2 (January–March 1998): 29–36.

Baer, David. "Patient-Physician E-Mail Communication: The Kaiser Permanente Experience." *Journal of Oncology Practice* 7 (July 2011): 230–33.

Baker, John Newton. *Your Public Relations Are Showing.* New York: Twayne, 1958.

Baker, Robert B., Arthur L. Caplan, Linda L. Emanuel, and Stephen Latham. *The American Medical Ethics Revolution.* Baltimore: Johns Hopkins University Press, 1999.

Baketel, H. Sheridan. "The Chorus Grows." *Medical Economics* 5 (December 1927): 28–29.

———. "Come Early for Tea." *Medical Economics* 5 (November 1927): 34–35.

———. "Fee Control Coming." *Medical Economics* 27 (February 1950): 45–46.

Baldwin, Louise G., and Florence Kirlin. "Consumers Appraise the Food, Drug, and Cosmetic Act." *Law and Contemporary Problems* 6 (Winter 1939): 144–50.

Ballentine, Carol. "Taste of Raspberries, Taste of Death: The 1937 Elixir Sulfanilamide Incident." *FDA Consumer Magazine*, June 1981. http://www.fda.gov/AboutFDA/WhatWeDo/History/ProductRegulation/SulfanilamideDisaster/. Accessed July 1, 2015.

Balliett, Gene. *Practice Management*. New York: Medical World News, 1978.

"Ballyhoo Institute and Medical Center." *Ballyhoo* 3 (November 1932): 26.

Barclay, William R. "Patient Package Inserts: A Symposium." *Transactions and Studies of the College of Physicians of Philadelphia* 45 (July 1977): 2–3.

Barry, Kathleen M. *Femininity in Flight: A History of Flight Attendants*. Durham, N.C.: Duke University Press, 2007.

Bartrip, Peter. "A 'Pennurth of Arsenic for Rat Poison': The Arsenic Act, 1851 and the Prevention of Secret Poisoning." *Medical History* 36 (1992): 53–69.

Bauer, Raymond A. "Risk Handling in Drug Adoption: The Role of Company Preference." In *Understanding Consumer Behavior*, edited by Martin Grossack. Boston: Christopher, 1964.

Baum, Richard N. "CVS." *Black Book—Bernstein Research Notes*, August 28, 1989, 39–59.

Bazell, Robert J. "Health Radicals: Crusade to Shift Medical Power to the People." *Science* 173 (August 6, 1971): 506–9.

Bebinger, Martha. "How Much for an MRI? $500? $1500? A Reporter Struggles to Find Out." *Kaiser Health News*, December 9, 2012. http://www.kaiserhealthnews.org/stories/2012/december/09/mri-cost-price-comparison-health-insurance.aspx. Accessed July 1, 2015.

Bedrosian, John C. "The Health Care Industry." *Vital Speeches of the Day* 47 (July 1981): 554–57.

Beecher, Henry K. "Ethics and Clinical Research." *New England Journal of Medicine* 274 (June 16, 1966): 1354–60.

Beier, Lucinda McCray. *Health Culture in the Heartland, 1880–1980: An Oral History*. Urbana: University of Illinois Press, 2009.

Bell, Daniel. *The Coming of Post-Industrial Society: A Venture in Social Forecasting*. New York: Basic Books, 1973.

Bellah, Robert N. *Habits of the Heart: Individualism and Commitment in American Life*. Berkeley: University of California Press, 2008.

Belsky, Martin S. and Leonard Gross. *How to Choose and Use Your Doctor: The Smart Patient's Way to a Longer, Healthier Life*. Greenwich, Conn.: Fawcett Publications, 1975.

Berge, Wendell. "Justice and the Future of Medicine." *Public Health Reports* 60 (January 5, 1945): 1–16.

Berkman, Sue. *The HMO Survival Guide: Save Money, Play by the Rules, and Get the Best Care*. New York: Villard, 1997.

Bernabeo, Elizabeth, and Eric S. Holmboe. "Patients, Providers, and Systems Need to Acquire a Specific Set of Competencies to Achieve Truly Patient-Centered Care." *Health Affairs* 32 (February 2013): 250–58.

Bernheim, Bertram M. *Medicine at the Crossroads*. New York: Morrow, 1939.

Bero, L., and D. Rennie. "The Cochrane Collaboration: Preparing, Maintaining, and Disseminating Systematic Reviews of the Effects of Health Care." *Journal of the American Medical Association* 274 (December 27, 1995): 1935–38.

"Best Drugstores: 2011." *Consumer Reports*, May 2011, 24–29.

"Be Wise: Itemize." *Medical Economics* 29 (April 1952): 69.

Bicknell, D. M. "Making the Office Attractive." *Medical Economics* 3 (April 1926): 17–20.

Bishop, James, and Henry W. Hubbard. *Let the Seller Beware!* Washington, D.C.: National Press, 1969.

Blaszczyk, Regina Lee. *American Consumer Society, 1865–2005: From Hearth to HDTV*. Wheeling, Ill.: Harlan Davidson, 2009.

Blendon, Robert J., and Drew E. Altman. "Public Attitudes about Health-Care Costs: A Lesson in National Schizophrenia." *New England Journal of Medicine* 311 (August 30, 1984): 613–16.

Bliss, Michael. *The Discovery of Insulin*. Chicago: University of Chicago Press, 1982.

———. *William Osler: A Life in Medicine*. Oxford: Oxford University Press, 2007.

Bliss, Roger W. "Don't Be an Ass about Aspirin." *Reader's Digest*, July 1957, 67–69.

Blum, Deborah. *The Poisoner's Handbook: Murder and the Birth of Forensic Medicine in Jazz Age New York*. New York: Penguin, 2010.

Blum, Richard H. *The Management of the Doctor-Patient Relationship*. New York: McGraw-Hill, 1960.

Blumenthal, David, and James A. Morone. *The Heart of Power: Health and Politics in the Oval Office*. Berkeley: University of California Press, 2009.

Boas, Ernst P. "Heart Diseases of Middle Life." *Hygeia* 13 (April 1935): 312–14.

Bodenheimer, Thomas. "Primary Care—Will It Survive?" *New England Journal of Medicine* 355 (August 31, 2006): 861–64.

Bodenheimer, Thomas, and Kevin Grumbach. *Understanding Health Policy*. 6th ed. New York: McGraw-Hill Medical, 2012.

Bok, Edward William. *The Americanization of Edward Bok: The Autobiography of a Dutch Boy Fifty Years After*. New York: Scribner's, 1922.

Bonner, Thomas. *Iconoclast: Abraham Flexner and a Life in Learning*. Baltimore: Johns Hopkins University Press, 2002.

"Book Notices." *Journal of the American Medical Association* 90 (March 3, 1928): 716.

"Book Review: The Silent World of Doctor and Patient." *New England Journal of Medicine* 311 (August 23, 1984): 544–45.

Boston Women's Health Book Collective. *Our Bodies, Ourselves*. 40th anniv. ed. New York: Simon and Schuster, 2011.

Branch, C. H. Hardin. "The Patient Must Prescribe for the Physician." *Mental Hygiene* 53 (July 1969): 403–9.

Brandt, Allan M. *The Cigarette Century: The Rise, Fall, and Deadly Persistence of the Product That Defined America*. New York: Basic Books, 2007.

———. *No Magic Bullet: A Social History of Venereal Disease in the United States since 1880*. Expanded ed. New York: Oxford University Press, 1987.

Brandt, Allan M., and Martha Gardner. "Antagonism and Accommodation:

Interpreting the Relationship between Public Health and Medicine in the United States during the Twentieth Century." *American Journal of Public Health* 90 (May 2000): 707–15.

———. "The Golden Age of Medicine." In *Medicine in the Twentieth Century*, edited by Roger Cooter and John Pickstone. Amsterdam: Harwood Academic, 2000.

Bredow, Miriam. *Handbook for the Medical Secretary*. New York: McGraw-Hill, 1943.

———. *Handbook for the Medical Secretary*. 4th ed. New York: Gregg Division, McGraw-Hill, 1959.

———. *The Medical Assistant: A Guidebook for the Nurse, Secretary, and Technician in the Doctor's Office*. New York: Blakiston Division, McGraw-Hill, 1958.

———. *Medical Secretarial Procedures*. 5th ed. New York: Gregg Division, McGraw-Hill, 1966.

Bredow, Miriam, Karonne J. Becklin, and Edith M. Sunnarborg. *Medical Office Procedures*. 2nd ed. New York: McGraw-Hill, 1981.

Brenner, Joseph. "A Free Clinic for Street People." *New York Times Sunday Magazine*, October 11, 1970.

Breslaw, Elaine G. *Lotions, Potions, Pills, and Magic: Health Care in Early America*. New York: New York University Press, 2014.

Brickman, Jane P. "'Medical McCarthyism': The Physicians Forum and the Cold War." *Journal of the History of Medicine and Allied Sciences* 49 (July 1994): 380–418.

Brown, Lawrence D. *Politics and Health Care Organization: HMOs as Federal Policy*. Washington, D.C.: Brookings Institution, 1983.

Brownlee, Shannon. "Doctor Will See You—If You're Quick." *Newsweek*, April 30, 2012, 46–50.

Bud, Robert. "Antibiotics, Big Business, and Consumers: The Context of Government Investigations into the Postwar American Drug Industry." *Technology and Culture* 46 (April 2005): 329–49.

———. *Penicillin: Triumph and Tragedy*. New York: Oxford University Press, 2007.

Bunker, John P. "Surgical Manpower: A Comparison of Operations and Surgeons in the United States and in England and Wales." *New England Journal of Medicine* 282 (January 15, 1970): 135–44.

Bunker, John P., Benjamin A. Barnes, and Frederick Mosteller. *Costs, Risks, and Benefits of Surgery*. New York: Oxford University Press, 1977.

Burnham, John C. "American Medicine's Golden Age: What Happened to It?" *Science* 215 (March 19, 1982): 1474–79.

———. *How Superstition Won and Science Lost: Popularizing Science and Health in the United States*. New Brunswick, N.J.: Rutgers University Press, 1987.

Burrow, James Gordon. *Organized Medicine in the Progressive Era: The Move toward Monopoly*. Baltimore: Johns Hopkins University Press, 1977.

Bush, Vannevar. "As We May Think." *Atlantic Monthly* 176 (July 1945): 101–8.

Cabot, Hugh. *The Doctor's Bill*. New York: Columbia University Press, 1935.

Califano, Joseph A. *America's Health Care Revolution: Who Lives? Who Dies? Who Pays?* New York: Random House, 1986.

Callahan, Daniel. *Taming the Beloved Beast: How Medical Technology Costs Are Destroying Our Health Care System*. Princeton: Princeton University Press, 2009.

Campion, Frank D. *The AMA and U.S. Health Policy since 1940.* Chicago: Chicago Review Press, 1984.

Capella, Michael L., Charles R. Taylor, Randall C. Campbell, and Lance S. Longwell. "Do Pharmaceutical Marketing Activities Raise Prices?" *Journal of Public Policy and Marketing* 28 (Fall 2009): 146–61.

Carpenter, Daniel. *Reputation and Power: Organizational Image and Pharmaceutical Regulation at the FDA.* Princeton: Princeton University Press, 2010.

Carroll, Norman V., and Jean Paul Gagnon. "Identifying Consumer Segments in Health Services Markets." *Journal of Health Care Marketing* 3 (Summer 1983): 22–34.

Carter, Richard. *The Doctor Business.* Garden City, N.Y.: Doubleday, 1958.

Cassedy, James H. "Muckraking and Medicine: Samuel Hopkins Adams." *American Quarterly* 16 (Spring 1964): 85–99.

Cassell, Eric. *The Healer's Art: A New Approach to the Doctor-Patient Relationship.* Philadelphia: Lippincott, 1976.

Cathell, D. W. *Book on the Physician Himself from Graduation to Old Age.* Baltimore: Lord Baltimore, 1922.

Center for the Study of Civil Liberties and Civil Rights. *Patients' Rights Digest.* Montgomery, Ala.: Center for the Study of Civil Liberties and Civil Rights, 1977–89.

Chadduck, H. W. "'In Brief Summary': Prescription Drug Advertising, 1962–71." *FDA Papers* 6 (February 1972): 13–25.

Chambers, Jason. *Madison Avenue and the Color Line: African Americans in the Advertising Industry.* Philadelphia: University of Pennsylvania Press, 2007.

Charisse, Marc S. "'A Solid Dose of Accurate Information': America's Unfilled Drug Advertising Prescription." Ph.D. diss., University of Washington, 1992.

Chase, James. "100 Agencies: How Do You Feel?" *Medical Marketing and Media,* July 1, 2012.

Chase, Stuart. "Your Money's Worth Twenty-Five Years Later." *Consumer Reports,* February 1954, 93–95.

Chase, Stuart, and F. J. Schlink. "Consumers in Wonderland, Part III: What We Get for Our Money When We Buy from Quacks and Venders of Cure-Alls." *New Republic,* February 16, 1927, 348–51.

———. *Your Money's Worth: A Study in the Waste of the Consumer's Dollar.* New York: Macmillan, 1927.

Checkoway, Barry, ed. *Citizens and Health Care: Participation and Planning for Social Change.* New York: Pergamon, 1981.

"The Chemical Laboratory." *Journal of the American Medical Association* 96 (April 18, 1931): 1303–6.

Chilingerian, Jon. "Origins of DRGs in the United States: A Technical, Political, and Cultural Story." In *The Globalization of Managerial Innovation in Health Care,* edited by John R. Kimberly, Gérard de Pouvourville, and Thomas D'Aunno. New York: Cambridge University Press, 2008.

Chisari, Francis, Robert Nakamura, and Lorena Thorup. *Consumers' Guide to Health Care.* Boston: Little, Brown, 1976.

Chowkwanyun, Merlin. "The New Left and Public Health: The Health Policy Advisory Center, Community Organizing, and the Big Business of Health, 1967–1975." *American Journal of Public Health* 101 (February 2011): 238–49.

Clark, Evans. *How to Budget Health: Guilds for Doctors and Patients*. New York: Harper, 1933.

Clarkson, Kenneth W., and Timothy J. Muris, eds. *The Federal Trade Commission since 1970: Economic Regulation and Bureaucratic Behavior*. New York: Cambridge University Press, 1981.

Cline, R. J. W., and K. M. Haynes. "Consumer Health Information Seeking on the Internet." *Health Education Research* 16 (December 2001): 671–92.

"Clues to Cancer." *Literary Digest* 123 (April 17, 1937): 20.

Cohen, Lizabeth. *A Consumers' Republic: The Politics of Mass Consumption in Postwar America*. New York: Knopf, 2003.

———. "The New Deal State and the Making of Citizen Consumers." In *Getting and Spending: European and American Consumer Societies in the Twentieth Century*, edited by Susan Strasser. New York: Cambridge University Press, 1998.

Cohen, Robin A., Diane M. Makuc, Amy B. Bernstein, Linda T. Bilheimer, and Eve Powell-Griner. *Health Insurance Coverage Trends, 1959–2007*. National Health Statistics Reports no. 17. Hyattsville, Md.: National Center for Health Statistics, 2009.

Colgrove, James. "The McKeown Thesis: A Historical Controversy and Its Enduring Influence." *American Journal of Public Health* 92 (May 2002): 725–29.

Collins, Joseph. "A Doctor Looks at Doctors." *Harper's Monthly*, February 1927, 348–56.

Collins, Selwyn D. "The Frequency of Surgical Procedures in a General Population Group." *Milbank Memorial Fund Quarterly* 16 (April 1938): 123–44.

Committee on the Costs of Medical Care. *Medical Care for the American People*. Chicago: University of Chicago Press, 1932.

Commonwealth Fund. *Insured and Still at Risk: Number of Underinsured Adults Increased 80 Percent between 2003 and 2010*. September 8, 2011. http://www .commonwealthfund.org/publications/press-releases/2011/sep/insured-and-still-at-risk. Accessed July 1, 2015.

Community Catalyst. "Consumer Health Advocacy: A View from 16 States." http://www.communitycatalyst.org/docstore/publications/consumer_health _advocacy_a_view_from_16_states_oct06.pdf. Accessed July 1, 2015.

Conroy, Joanne. "Can We Put the Hospital Marketing Genie Back in the Bottle?" Wing of Zock. http://wingofzock.org/2013/04/02/can-we-put-the-hospital-marketing-genie-back-in-the-bottle/. Accessed July 1, 2015.

"Consumerism." In *The American Heritage Dictionary of the English Language*, edited by William Morris. New college ed. Boston: Houghton Mifflin, 1980.

Consumer Reports. *The Medicine Show: Some Plain Truths about Popular Remedies for Common Ailments*. New York: Simon and Schuster, 1961.

"Consumers and Pharma Companies Far Apart in Views of Drug Industry." *PharmaLetter*, January 22, 2007. http://www.thepharmaletter.com/article/ consumers-and-pharma-companies-far-apart-in-views-of-drug-industry-pwc-finds. Accessed July 1, 2015.

Cook, E. Fullerton, and Charles H. LaWall. *Remington's Practice of Pharmacy.* 8th ed. Philadelphia: Lippincott, 1936.

Cooley, Charles Horton. *Human Nature and the Social Order.* New York: Scribner, 1902.

Coombs, Jan Gregoire. *The Rise and Fall of HMOs: An American Health Care Revolution.* Madison: University of Wisconsin Press, 2005.

Cooner, David J. "The Intersection of Madison Avenue and the Learned Intermediary Doctrine." http://library.findlaw.com/2003/Mar/7/132622.html. Accessed July 1, 2015.

Cooper, Donald L. "Get Ready for a New Breed of Patients!" *Medical Economics* 51 (August 5, 1974): 91–102.

Cooper, James C., ed. *The Regulatory Revolution at the FTC: A Thirty-Year Perspective on Competition and Consumer Protection.* New York: Oxford University Press, 2013.

Cooper, Marian G., and Miriam Bredow. *The Medical Assistant: A Basic Text Covering Administrative, Clinical, and Assisting Functions.* New York: McGraw-Hill, 1978.

Coppin, Clayton A., and Jack C. High. *The Politics of Purity: Harvey Washington Wiley and the Origins of Federal Food Policy.* Ann Arbor: University of Michigan Press, 1999.

Cornacchia, Harold J. *Consumer Health.* St. Louis: C. V. Mosby Co., 1976.

Countryman, Kathleen M., and Alexandra B. Gekas. *Development and Implementation of a Patient's Bill of Rights in Hospitals.* Chicago: American Hospital Association, 1980.

Courtwright, David T. *Dark Paradise: A History of Opium Addiction in America.* Enl. edition. Cambridge, Mass.: Harvard University Press, 2009.

———. *Forces of Habit: Drugs and the Making of the Modern World.* Cambridge, Mass.: Harvard University Press, 2002.

Cousins, Norman. "Anatomy of an Illness (as Perceived by the Patient)." *New England Journal of Medicine* 295 (November 23, 1976): 1458–63.

———. *Anatomy of an Illness as Perceived by the Patient.* New York: Norton, 1979.

———. *Modern Man Is Obsolete.* New York: Viking, 1945.

Cramp, Arthur J. "Debunking Drugs." *American Mercury,* March 1928, 345–54.

———. "Therapeutic Thaumaturgy." *American Mercury,* December 1924, 423–30.

Creighton, Lucy Black. *Pretenders to the Throne: The Consumer Movement in the United States.* Lexington, Mass.: Lexington Books, 1976.

Crenner, Christopher. *Private Practice: In the Early Twentieth-Century Medical Office of Dr. Richard Cabot.* Baltimore: Johns Hopkins University Press, 2005.

Crile, George. *Surgery: Your Choices, Your Alternatives.* New York: Delacorte/Lawrence, 1978.

Croatman, Wallace. "With These Forms, It's Easier to Talk Fees." *Medical Economics* 30 (March 1953): 135–37.

Cron, Theodore. "The Model Consumer." *American Patient* 1 (April 10, 1970): 2.

Cunningham, Robert III, and Robert M. Cunningham Jr. *The Blues: A History of the Blue Cross and Blue Shield System.* DeKalb: Northern Illinois University Press, 1997.

Curtis, Richard, Trisha Kurtz, and Larry S. Stepnick, eds. *Creating Consumer Choice in Healthcare: Measuring and Communicating Health Plan Performance Information*. Chicago: Health Administration Press, 1998.

Cutler, David M. *The Quality Cure: How Focusing on Health Care Quality Can Save Your Life and Lower Spending Too*. Berkeley: University of California Press, 2014.

———. *Your Money or Your Life: Strong Medicine for America's Health Care System*. New York: Oxford University Press, 2004.

Damrau, Frederic. "Has the Doctor of To-Day Spoiled His Patients?" *Scribner's*, July 1927, 44–48.

Dans, Peter E. *Doctors in the Movies: Boil the Water and Just Say Aah*. Bloomington, Ill.: Medi-Ed, 2000.

Davis, Adelle. *Let's Eat Right to Keep Fit*. New York: Harcourt, Brace, 1954.

Davis, Kathy. *The Making of Our Bodies, Ourselves: How Feminism Travels across Borders*. Durham, N.C.: Duke University Press, 2007.

Davis, Maxine. "Self-Diagnosis and Self-Treatment." *Good Housekeeping*, April 1953, 182–86.

Davis, Michael Marks. *America Organizes Medicine*. New York: Harper, 1941.

———. "The Blunderbuss of Illness." *The Survey* 59 (June 1, 1928): 435–38.

———. *Medical Care for Tomorrow*. New York: Harper, 1955.

———. *Paying Your Sickness Bills*. Chicago: University of Chicago Press, 1931.

DeFriese, G. H., A. Woomert, P. A. Guild, A. B. Steckler, and T. R. Konrad. "From Activated Patient to Pacified Activist: A Study of the Self-Care Movement in the United States." *Social Science and Medicine* 29, no. 2 (1989): 195–204.

Dekkers, Onka. "American Murderers' Association." *off our backs*, July 10, 1970, 4.

Dempsey, David. "The Living Will—and the Will to Live." *New York Times Sunday Magazine*, June 23, 1974.

Denenberg, Herbert S. *The Shopper's Guidebook to Life Insurance, Health Insurance, Auto Insurance, Homeowner's Insurance, Doctors, Dentists, Lawyers, Pensions, Etc.* Washington, D.C.: Consumer News, 1974.

———. "A Shopper's Guide to Surgery." *Prevention* 25 (January 1973): 85–92.

Denney, Myron K. *Second Opinion*. New York: Grosset and Dunlap, 1979.

De Ville, Kenneth Allen. *Medical Malpractice in Nineteenth-Century America: Origins and Legacy*. New York: New York University Press, 1990.

Dichter, Ernest. *The Psychological Study of the Doctor-Patient Relationship Submitted to California Medical Association, Alameda County Medical Association, May, 1950*. San Francisco: California Medical Association, 1950.

Dittmer, John. *The Good Doctors: The Medical Committee for Human Rights and the Struggle for Social Justice in Health Care*. New York: Bloomsbury, 2009.

Dobbin, Frank R. "The Origins of Private Social Insurance: Public Policy and Fringe Benefits in America, 1920–1950." *American Journal of Sociology* 97 (March 1992): 1416–50.

"A Doctor's Wife Speaks Up." *Harper's Monthly* 164 (February 1932): 344–53.

Dolan, Andrew K. "Book Reviews: The Law of Hospital and Health Care Administration by Arthur F. Southwick; Problems in Hospital Law by David G. Warren." *Medical Care* 17 (June 1979): 690–92.

Domestic Policy Council (U.S.). *The President's Health Security Plan: The Clinton Blueprint*. New York: Times Books, 1993.

Donabedian, Avedis. "Evaluating the Quality of Medical Care." *Milbank Memorial Fund Quarterly* 44 (July 1966): 166–203.

Dorsey, Richard. "The Patient Package Insert: Is It Safe and Effective?" *Journal of the American Medical Association* 238 (October 31, 1977): 1936–39.

Dowling, Harry F. *Medicines for Man: The Development, Regulation, and Use of Prescription Drugs*. New York: Knopf, 1970.

———. "Twixt the Cup and the Lip." *Journal of the American Medical Association* 165 (October 12, 1957): 657–61.

Dranove, David. *The Economic Evolution of American Health Care: From Marcus Welby to Managed Care*. Princeton: Princeton University Press, 2009.

"Dr. Jarvis's Great Switchel Revival." *Vermont Life*, 1960. http://www.jcrows.com/vermontlife.html. Accessed July 1, 2015.

Drotning, Philip. "Aspirin Can Be Deadly." *American Mercury*, August 1944, 210–13.

"The Drug Hearings." *Science* 131 (April 29, 1960): 1299–1300.

"Drug Pricing and the RX Police State." *Consumer Reports*, March 1972, 136–40.

"The Drugs: Less Than Wonderful." *Business Week*, August 7, 1954, 70–76.

Dubos, René J. "Beyond Traditional Medicine." *Harper's*, October 1960, 166–68.

Dudziak, Mary L. *Cold War Civil Rights: Race and the Image of American Democracy*. Princeton: Princeton University Press, 2000.

Duffin, Jacalyn, and Alison Li. "Great Moments: Parke, Davis and Company and the Creation of Medical Art," *Isis* 86 (March 1995): 1–29.

Eakin, Dottie, Sara Jean Jackson, and Gale G. Hannigan. "Consumer Health Information: Libraries as Partners." *Bulletin of the Medical Library Association* 68 (April 1980): 220–29.

Eckholm, Eric. *Solving America's Health-Care Crisis: A Guide to Understanding the Greatest Threat to Your Family's Economic Security*. New York: New York Times Company, 1993.

Edwards, Charles E. "Closing the Gap: OTC Drugs." *FDA Papers* 6 (February 1972): 4–8.

Edwards, Mari. "Set Your Surgical Fees with This Scale." *Medical Economics* 32 (September 1955): 137–39, 303.

———. "Shopping Center Practice Here to Stay." *Medical Economics* 31 (September 1954): 100–112.

Ehrenreich, Barbara, John Ehrenreich, and Health/PAC. *The American Health Empire: Power, Profits, and Politics*. New York: Random House, 1970.

Ehrenreich, Barbara, and Deirdre English. *Complaints and Disorders: The Sexual Politics of Sickness*. Old Westbury, N.Y.: Feminist Press at CUNY, 1973.

Ehrenreich, John, and Barbara Ehrenreich. "The New Left: A Case Study in Professional Managerial Class Radicalism." *Radical America* 11 (May–June 1977): 7–22.

Elenbaas, Robert M., and Dennis B. Worthen. "Transformation of a Profession: An Overview of the 20th Century." *Pharmacy in History* 51, no. 4 (2009): 151–82.

Engel, Jonathan. *Doctors and Reformers: Discussion and Debate over Health Policy, 1925–1950*. Columbia: University of South Carolina Press, 2002.

Ennis, Bruce J. *Prisoners of Psychiatry: Mental Patients, Psychiatrists, and the Law.* New York: Harcourt Brace Jovanovich, 1972.

Ephraim, Jerome William. *Take Care of Yourself: A Practical Guide to Health and Beauty, Stressing the Proper Way to Use and the Prudent Way to Buy Home Remedies and Cosmetics.* New York: Simon and Schuster, 1937.

Epstein, Steven. *Impure Science: AIDS, Activism, and the Politics of Knowledge.* Berkeley: University of California Press, 1996.

———. "Patient Groups and Health Movements." In *The Handbook of Science and Technology Studies*, 3rd ed., edited by Edward J. Hackett, Olga Amsterdamska, Michael Lynch, and Judy Wajcman, 499–539. Cambridge, Mass.: MIT Press, 2008.

Espeland, Wendy N., and Michael Sauder. "Rankings and Reactivity: How Public Measures Recreate Social Worlds." *American Journal of Sociology* 113 (July 2007): 1–40.

Eulau, Heinz. "Skill Revolution and Consultative Commonwealth." *American Political Science Review* 67 (March 1973): 169–91.

"Evaluating New Drugs." *Science* 132 (July 1, 1960): 48.

"Every Customer a Clerk." *American Magazine* 156 (September 1953): 54.

Ewing, Oscar R. Interview by J. R. Fuchs, August 1, 1969. http://www.trumanlibrary .org/oralhist/ewing3.htm. Accessed July 1, 2015.

Faden, Ruth, Tom L. Beauchamp, and Nancy M. P. King. *A History and Theory of Informed Consent.* New York: Oxford University Press, 1986.

Falk, I. S., C. Rufus Rorem, and Martha D. Ring. *The Costs of Medical Care.* Chicago: University of Chicago Press, 1933.

Families USA. "Shared Decision Making: Engaging Patients to Improve Health Care." http://familiesusa.org/product/shared-decision-making-engaging-patients-improve-health-care. Accessed July 1, 2015.

Farber, Lawrence, ed. *Encyclopedia of Practice and Financial Management.* 2nd ed. 3 vols. Oradell, N.J.: Medical Economics Books, 1988.

Farquhar, John W. *The American Way of Life Need Not Be Hazardous to Your Health.* New York: Norton, 1978.

"FDA's Aspirin Ruling Made for Child Safety." *Oil, Paint and Drug Reporter* 168 (October 24, 1955): 4, 57.

Feather, Kenneth R. Interview by John Swann, Ronald T. Ottes, and Robert A. Tucker, May 7, 1997. http://www.fda.gov/downloads/AboutFDA/WhatWeDo/History/OralHistories/SelectedOralHistoryTranscripts/UCM264119.pdf. Accessed July 1, 2015.

Feldman, Saul, and Charles Windle. "The NIMH Approach." *Health Services Reports* 88 (February 1973): 174–80.

Ferguson, Pamela R. "Liability for Pharmaceutical Products: A Critique of the 'Learned Intermediary' Rule." *Oxford Journal of Legal Studies* 12 (Spring 1992): 59–82.

Fett, Sharla M. *Working Cures: Healing, Health, and Power on Southern Slave Plantations.* Chapel Hill: University of North Carolina Press, 2002.

Feudtner, Chris. *Bittersweet: Diabetes, Insulin, and the Transformation of Illness.* Chapel Hill: University of North Carolina Press, 2003.

"Finally, Prescription Drugs Make It to the Effie Awards." *Medical Marketing and Media* 37 (July 2001): 24.

Findlay, Steven. "Coverage Denied." *U.S. News and World Report*, December 9, 1991, 80–82.

———. "Medicine by the Book." *U.S. News and World Report*, July 6, 1992, 68–71.

———. "Medicine-Chest Roulette." *U.S. News and World Report*, May 9, 1988, 76–77.

Findlay, Steven, Marjory Roberts, and Joanne Silberner. "The Best Hospitals, from AIDS to Urology." *U.S. News and World Report*, April 30, 1990, 68–86.

Fishbein, Morris. "The Committee on the Costs of Medical Care." *Journal of the American Medical Association* 99 (December 3, 1932): 1950–52.

———. *Morris Fishbein, M.D.: An Autobiography.* Garden City, N.Y.: Doubleday, 1969.

Fitzgerald, F. Scott. *The Great Gatsby.* New York: Scribner's, 1925.

Fleckenstein, Lawrence. "Attitudes toward the Patient Package Insert: A Survey of Physicians and Pharmacists." *Drug Information Journal* 11 (March 1977): 23–29.

Fletcher, F. Marion. *Market Restraints in the Retail Drug Industry.* Philadelphia: University of Pennsylvania Press, 1967.

Flynn, John T. "Radio: Medicine Show." *American Scholar*, October 1938, 430–37.

Foster, William Trufont. "Medicine's Right to Control." *Survey Graphic*, December 1934, 588–89.

Fowler, Nathaniel C. *Fowler's Publicity: An Encyclopedia of Advertising and Printing.* New York: Publicity, 1897.

Fox, Daniel M. "From Reform to Relativism: A History of Economists and Health Care." *Milbank Memorial Fund Quarterly: Health and Society* 57 (July 1979): 297–336.

———. *Health Policies, Health Politics: The British and American Experience, 1911–1965.* Princeton: Princeton University Press, 1986.

Fox, Susannah, and Maeve Duggan. *Health Online 2013.* January 15, 2013. http://www.pewinternet.org/2013/01/15/health-online-2013. Accessed July 1, 2015.

Frank, Arthur, and Stuart Frank. *People's Handbook of Medical Care.* New York: Random House, 1972.

Frank, Thomas. *The Conquest of Cool: Business Culture, Counterculture, and the Rise of Hip Consumerism.* Chicago: University of Chicago Press, 1997.

Frates, George H. "Durham-Humphrey Bill Is in the Public Interest." *Hospital Progress* 34 (September 1953): 88, 104–5.

Freidson, Eliot. *Patients' Views of Medical Practice: A Study of Subscribers to a Prepaid Medical Plan in the Bronx.* New York: Sage, 1961.

———. *Profession of Medicine: A Study of the Sociology of Applied Knowledge.* New York: Dodd, Mead, 1970.

Freudenheim, Milt. "Shopping-Mall Medicine." *New York Times Sunday Magazine*, December 5, 1982.

Friedberg, Mark W., Kristin Van Busum, Richard Wexler, Megan Bowen, and Eric C. Schneider. "A Demonstration of Shared Decision Making in Primary Care Highlights Barriers to Adoption and Potential Remedies." *Health Affairs* 32 (February 2013): 268–75.

Friedman, Milton. *Capitalism and Freedom*. Chicago: University of Chicago Press, 1962.

Frist, William H. "Connected Health and the Rise of the Patient-Consumer." *Health Affairs* 33 (February 2014): 191–93.

Frosch, Dominick L., Suepattra G. May, Katharine A. S. Rendle, Caroline Tietbohl, and Glyn Elwyn. "Authoritarian Physicians and Patients' Fear of Being Labeled 'Difficult' among Key Obstacles to Shared Decision Making." *Health Affairs* 31 (May 2012): 1030–38.

Fuchs, Victor R. "Economics, Health, and Post-Industrial Society." *Milbank Memorial Fund Quarterly: Health and Society* 57 (Spring 1979): 153–82.

Furman, A. L., and Harold Hadley. *Drugstore*. New York: Macaulay, 1935.

Gabel, Jon, Steven DiCarlo, Steven Fink, and Gregory de Lissovoy. "Employer-Sponsored Health Insurance in America." *Health Affairs* 8 (Summer 1989): 116–28.

Gabel, Jon, Cindy Jajich-Toth, Karen Williams, Sarah Loughran, and Kevin Haugh. "The Commercial Health Insurance Industry in Transition." *Health Affairs* 6 (Fall 1987): 46–60.

Gabriel, Joseph M. *Medical Monopoly: Intellectual Property Rights and the Origins of the Modern Pharmaceutical Industry*. Chicago: University of Chicago Press, 2014.

Gage, Beverly. "Just What the Doctor Ordered." *Smithsonian* 36 (April 2005): 112–17.

Galdston, Iago. "The Pathogenicity of Progress: An Essay on Medical Historiography." *Medical History* 9 (April 1965): 127–32.

Galton, Lawrence. *The Patient's Guide to Successful Surgery*. New York: Hearst, 1976.

Gamson, William A., and Howard Schuman. "Some Undercurrents in the Prestige of Physicians." *American Journal of Sociology* 68 (January 1963): 463–70.

Garbarino, Joseph W. "Price Behavior and Productivity in the Medical Market." *Industrial and Labor Relations Review* 13, no. 1 (1959): 3–15.

Gardner, Martha N., and Allan M. Brandt. "'The Doctors' Choice Is America's Choice': The Physician in US Cigarette Advertisements, 1930–1953." *American Journal of Public Health* 96 (February 2006): 222–32.

Garrow, David J. *Liberty and Sexuality: The Right to Privacy and the Making of Roe v. Wade*. New York: Macmillan, 1994.

Gathercoal, Edmund Norris. *The Prescription Ingredient Survey*. Chicago: American Pharmaceutical Association, 1933.

Gaylin, Willard. "The Patient's Bill of Rights." *Saturday Review of the Sciences* 1 (February 24, 1973): 22.

Geiger, H. Jack. "Hidden Professional Roles: The Physician as Reactionary." *Social Policy* 1 (March–April 1971): 24–33.

———. "The Patient as a Human Being." *New York Times Sunday Magazine*, December 2, 1956.

Gerrish, Frederic Henry. *Prescription Writing*. Portland, Maine: Loring, Short, and Harmon, 1888.

Gevitz, Norman. *The D.O.'s: Osteopathic Medicine in America*. Baltimore: Johns Hopkins University Press, 1982.

Geyman, John P. *The Corporate Transformation of Health Care*. New York: Springer Pub. Co., 2004.

Gilbert, James. *Men in the Middle: Searching for Masculinity in the 1950s*. Chicago: University of Chicago Press, 2005.

Ginty, Molly. "Our Bodies, Ourselves Turns 35 Today." *WeNews*, May 4, 2004. http://womensenews.org/story/health/040504/our-bodies-ourselves-turns-35-today. Accessed July 1, 2015.

Ginzberg, Eli. *The Medical Triangle: Physicians, Politicians, and the Public.* Cambridge, Mass.: Harvard University Press, 1990.

————. "The Monetarization of Medical Care." *New England Journal of Medicine* 310 (May 3, 1984): 1162–65.

Gitnick, Gary, Fred Rothenberg, and July L. Weiner, eds. *The Business of Medicine*. New York: Elsevier, 1991.

Glickman, Lawrence B. *Buying Power: A History of Consumer Activism in America.* Chicago: University of Chicago Press, 2009.

Goldberger, Zachary D., and Angela Fagerlin. "ICDs—Incredibly Complex Decisions." *Archives of Internal Medicine* 172 (July 23, 2012): 1106–7.

Goldhill, David. *Catastrophic Care: How American Health Care Killed My Father—and How We Can Fix It.* New York: Knopf, 2013.

Goldstein, Carolyn M. *Creating Consumers: Home Economists in Twentieth-Century America.* Chapel Hill: University of North Carolina Press, 2012.

Goodman, Walter. "The Doctor's Image Is Sickly." *New York Times Sunday Magazine*, October 16, 1966.

Goodwin, Lorine Swainston. *The Pure Food, Drink, and Drug Crusaders, 1879–1914.* Jefferson, N.C.: McFarland, 1999.

Gordon, Colin. *Dead on Arrival: The Politics of Health Care in Twentieth-Century America.* Princeton: Princeton University Press, 2003.

Goyan, Jere E. "Fourteen Fallacies about Patient Package Inserts." *Western Journal of Medicine* 135 (June 1981): 463–68.

Grabowski, Henry G., and Y. Richard Wang. "The Quantity and Quality of Worldwide New Drug Introductions, 1982–2003." *Health Affairs* 25 (March 1, 2006): 452–60.

Grady, Mark F. "Regulating Information: Advertising Overview." In *The Federal Trade Commission: Economic Regulation and Bureaucratic Behavior*, edited by Kenneth W. Clarkson and Timothy J. Muris. New York: Cambridge University Press, 1981.

Graedon, Joe. *The People's Pharmacy: A Guide to Prescription Drugs, Home Remedies, and Over-the-Counter Medications.* New York: St. Martin's, 1976.

Grande, David. "Limiting the Influence of Pharmaceutical Industry Gifts on Physicians: Self-Regulation or Government Intervention?" *Journal of General Internal Medicine* 25 (January 2010): 79–83.

Gray, Albert. "Who Should Sell Vitamins, Druggist or Grocer?" *Advertising and Selling* 36 (October 1943): 28.

Gray, Bradford H. *The Profit Motive and Patient Care: The Changing Accountability of Doctors and Hospitals.* Cambridge, Mass.: Harvard University Press, 1991.

————. "The Rise and Decline of the HMO." In *History and Health Policy in the United States: Putting the Past Back In*, edited by Rosemary Stevens, Charles E.

Rosenberg, and Lawton R. Burns. New Brunswick, N.J.: Rutgers University Press, 2006.

Greenberg, Selig. "The Decline of the Healing Art." *Harper's*, October 1960, 132–37.

Greene, Jeremy A. "Attention to 'Details': Etiquette and the Postwar Pharmaceutical Salesman." *Social Studies of Science* 34 (April 2004): 271–92.

———. *Generic: The Unbranding of Modern Medicine*. Baltimore: Johns Hopkins University Press, 2014.

———. *Prescribing by Numbers: Drugs and the Definition of Disease*. Baltimore: Johns Hopkins University Press, 2007.

———. "What's in a Name." *Journal of the History of Medicine and Allied Sciences* 66 (October 2011): 468–506.

Greene, Jeremy A., and David L. Herzberg. "Hidden in Plain Sight: Marketing Prescription Drugs to Consumers in the Twentieth Century." *American Journal of Public Health* 100 (May 2010): 793–803.

Greene, Jeremy A., and Aaron S. Kesselheim. "Pharmaceutical Marketing and the New Social Media." *New England Journal of Medicine* 363 (November 25, 2010): 2087–89.

Griffenhagen, Charles, and Mary Bogard. *A History of Drug Containers and Their Labels*. Madison, Wis.: American Institute of the History of Pharmacy, 1999.

Grob, Gerald. "The Rise and Decline of the Tonsillectomy in Twentieth Century America." *Journal of the History of Medicine and Allied Sciences* 62 (October 2007): 383–421.

———. "The Rise of Peptic Ulcer, 1900–1950." *Perspectives on Biology and Medicine* 46 (Autumn 2003): 550–66.

Grob, Rachel. "The Heart of Patient-Centered Care." *Journal of Health Politics, Policy, and Law* 38 (April 2013): 457–65.

"Grocer Horns In on the Druggist." *Business Week*, February 16, 1952, 158–62.

Gross, Daniel. *Our Roots Grow Deep: The Story of Rodale*. Emmaus, Pa.: Rodale, 2009.

Gruber, Jonathan. *Health Care Reform: What It Is, Why It's Necessary, How It Works*. New York: Hill and Wang, 2011.

Gu, Quiping, Charles F. Dillon, and Vicki L. Burt. "Prescription Drug Use Continues to Increase: U.S. Prescription Drug Data for 2007–2008." *NCHS Data Brief*, no 42. Hyattsville, Md.: National Center for Health Statistics, 2010.

Guckian, James C., ed. *The Clinical Interview and Physical Examination*. Philadelphia: Lippincott, 1987.

Gurwitz, Jerry H., Terry S. Field, Leslie R. Harrold, Jeffrey Rothschild, Kristin Debellis, Andrew C. Seger, Cynthia Cadoret, Leslie S. Fish, Lawrence Garber, Michael Kelleher, and David W. Bates. "Incidence and Preventability of Adverse Drug Events among Older Persons in the Ambulatory Setting." *Journal of the American Medical Association* 289 (March 5, 2003): 1107–16.

Hacker, Jacob S. *The Divided Welfare State: The Battle over Public and Private Social Benefits in the United States*. New York: Cambridge University Press, 2002.

Hacker, Jacob S., and Theodore R. Marmor. "The Misleading Language of Managed Care." *Journal of Health Politics, Policy, and Law* 24 (October 1999): 1033–43.

Halberstam, Michael J. "A Doctor-Friend Talks Back to Ralph Nader." *Medical Economics* 51 (May 27, 1974): 71–73.

———. "When Women's Lib Marches into Your Examining Room." *Medical Economics* 50 (May 28, 1973): 129–41.

Halpern, Sydney. "Medical Authority and the Culture of Rights." *Journal of Health Politics, Policy, and Law* 29 (August–October 2004): 835–52.

Hamilton, Patricia A. *Health Care Consumerism.* St. Louis: Mosby, 1982.

Hamilton, Walton. "The Ancient Maxim Caveat Emptor." *Yale Law Journal* 40 (June 1931): 1133–87.

Hanauer, David A., Kai Zheng, Dianne C. Singer, Achamyeleh Gebremariam, and Matthew M. Davis. "Public Awareness, Perception, and Use of Online Physician Rating Sites." *Journal of the American Medical Association* 311 (February 19, 2014): 734–35.

Handler, Milton. "The Control of False Advertising under the Wheeler-Lea Act." *Law and Contemporary Problems* 6 (Winter 1939): 91–110.

Hansen, Bert. *Picturing Medical Progress from Pasteur to Polio: A History of Mass Media Images and Popular Attitudes in America.* New Brunswick, N.J.: Rutgers University Press, 2009.

Harden, Victoria. *A Short History of the National Institutes of Health.* http://history .nih.gov/exhibits/history/index.html. Accessed July 1, 2015.

Harding, T. Swann. *Fads, Frauds, and Physicians: Diagnosis and Treatment of the Doctors' Dilemma.* New York: MacVeagh, Dial, 1930.

———. "How Scientific Are Our Doctors?" *The Forum,* June 1929, 345–51.

———. "The Metamorphosis of the Horse Doctor." *Scientific Monthly* 34 (May 1932): 446–53.

Hardy, Robert C. *Sick: How People Feel about Being Sick and What They Think of Those Who Care for Them.* Chicago: Teach'em Inc., 1978.

Harmon, J. H., Jr. "The Negro as a Local Business Man." *Journal of Negro History* 14 (April 1929): 116–55.

Harris, Richard. *The Real Voice.* New York: Macmillan, 1964.

———. *A Sacred Trust.* New York: New American Library, 1966.

Hartman, Micah, Anne B. Martin, David Lassman, Aaron Catlin, and the National Health Expenditure Accounts Team. "National Health Spending in 2013: Growth Slows, Remains in Step with the Overall Economy." *Health Affairs* 34 (January 1, 2015): 150–60.

Haskell, Eric. "No Parking Problem Here." *Medical Economics* 32 (October 1955): 132–34.

Haug, Marie R. "The Erosion of Professional Authority." *Milbank Memorial Fund Quarterly* 54 (Winter 1976): 83–106.

Haug, Marie R., and Bebe Lavin. *Consumerism in Medicine: Challenging Physician Authority.* Beverly Hills: Sage Publications, 1983.

Haug, Marie R., and Marvin B. Sussman. "Professional Autonomy and the Revolt of the Client." *Social Problems* 17 (Fall 1969): 153–61.

Hawley, Paul. "Evaluation of the Quality of Patient Care." *American Journal of Public Health* 45 (December 1955): 1533–37.

"Head Mirror or Halo?" *Medical Economics* 32 (November 1955): 125–39.

"Health Policy Brief: Public Reporting on Quality and Costs." *Health Affairs*, March 8, 2012. http://www.healthaffairs.org/healthpolicybriefs/brief.php?brief _id=65. Accessed July 1, 2015.

Hecht, Annabel. "Developing Drug Information for Patients." *FDA Consumer* 11 (September 1977): 16–19.

Heffernan, Margot. "The Health Care Quality Improvement Act of 1986 and the National Practitioner Data Bank." *Bulletin of the Medical Library Association* 84 (April 1996): 263–69.

Henderson, Harry. "The Original Miracle Drug." *Colliers* 132 (November 27, 1953): 112–15.

Henderson, Ruth Evelyn. "Rather Worse." *The Survey* 61 (October 1, 1928): 31–32, 51–52.

Herrmann, Robert O. "Consumerism: Its Goals, Organizations, and Future." *Journal of Marketing* 34 (October 1970): 55–60.

———. "Today's Young Adults as Consumers." *Journal of Consumer Affairs* 4 (Summer 1970): 19–30.

Hertzler, Arthur E. *The Horse and Buggy Doctor*. New York: Harper, 1938.

Herzberg, David L. *Happy Pills in America: From Miltown to Prozac*. Baltimore: Johns Hopkins University Press, 2009.

Herzlinger, Regina E. *Market-Driven Health Care: Who Wins, Who Loses in the Transformation of America's Largest Service Industry*. Reading, Mass.: Addison-Wesley, 1997.

Herzog, Sol A. "Twixt Supermarket and Courts—Whither Pharmacy?" *Journal of the American Pharmaceutical Association* 14 (December 1953): 764–70.

Hettinger, Herman S. "Broadcasting Advertising Trends in 1935." *National Marketing Review*, Spring 1936, 301–15.

Hibbard, Judith, Jean Stockard, and Martin Tusler. "Hospital Performance Reports: Impact on Quality, Market Share, and Reputation." *Health Affairs* 24 (July–August 2005): 1150–60.

Higgins, Charles M. "Drugstore Products Have Come Out of Hiding." *Advertising and Selling* 35 (October 1942): 61–62.

Hilts, Philip J. *Protecting America's Health: The FDA, Business, and One Hundred Years of Regulation*. New York: Knopf, 2003.

Hing, Esther, and Catharine W. Burt. "Characteristics of Office-Based Physicians and Their Practices: United States, 2003–04." *Vital and Health Statistics*, ser. 13, *Data from the National Health Survey*, no. 164 (January 2007): 1–34.

Hoff, Lawrence C. "Advertising Prescription Drugs Direct to the Public." *Vital Speeches* 50 (July 1984): 573–76.

Hoff, Timothy. *Practice under Pressure: Primary Care Physicians and Their Medicine in the Twenty-First Century*. New Brunswick, N.J.: Rutgers University Press, 2009.

Hoffman, Beatrix. "'Don't Scream Alone': The Health Care Activism of Poor Americans in the 1970s." In *Patients as Policy Actors*, edited by Beatrix Hoffman, Nancy Tomes, Rachel Grob, and Mark Schlesinger, 132–47. New Brunswick, N.J.: Rutgers University Press, 2011.

————. *Health Care for Some: Rights and Rationing in the United States since 1930.* Chicago: University of Chicago Press, 2012.

————. "Restraining the Health Care Consumer: The History of Deductibles and Copayments in U.S. Health Insurance." *Social Science History* 30 (Winter 2006): 501–28.

————. *The Wages of Sickness: The Politics of Health Insurance in Progressive America.* Chapel Hill: University of North Carolina Press, 2001.

Hoffman, Beatrix, Nancy Tomes, Rachel Grob, and Mark Schlesinger, eds. *Patients as Policy Actors.* New Brunswick, N.J.: Rutgers University Press, 2011.

Hoffman, Lois. "Planning Paid Off in This One-Man Office." *Medical Economics* 32 (August 1955): 129–39.

————. "A Well-Planned Office for a Family Doctor." *Medical Economics* 32 (October 1955): 119–25.

Hogan, Norma Shaw. "Patient's Rights: Voluntary or Mandatory." *Hospitals* 52 (November 16, 1978): 111–16.

Horowitz, Daniel. *The Anxieties of Affluence: Critiques of American Consumer Culture, 1939–1979.* Amherst: University of Massachusetts Press, 2005.

————. *The Morality of Spending: Attitudes toward the Consumer Society in America, 1875–1940.* Baltimore: Johns Hopkins University Press, 1985.

————. *Vance Packard and American Social Criticism.* Chapel Hill: University of North Carolina Press, 1994.

Howell, Joel D. "Reflections on the Past and Future of Primary Care." *Health Affairs* 29 (May 2010): 760–65.

"How Much Does Your Druggist Know?" *Consumer Reports,* May 1, 2011. http://www.consumerreports.org/cro/2013/01/best-drugstores/index.htm. Accessed July 2, 2015.

"How to Develop a Local Directory of Doctors." *Consumer Reports,* September 1974, 685–91.

"How to Find a Doctor for Yourself." *Consumer Reports,* September 1974, 681–84.

"How to Pay Less for Prescription Drugs." *Consumer Reports,* January 1975, 48–53.

"How to Pick a Doctor." *Changing Times,* September 1954, 27–31.

"How to Tell What the Ad Pages Are Talking about in One Easy Lesson." *Ballyhoo* 3 (September 1932): 3.

Hoyt, Daniel M. *Practical Therapeutics.* St. Louis: Mosby, 1914.

"HSA Puts Out U.S. Financed Doctor Directory." *Medical World News* 21 (March 17, 1980), 12.

"If, by Rudyard Zilch." *Ballyhoo* 3 (December 1932): 27.

Igo, Sarah Elizabeth. *The Averaged American: Surveys, Citizens, and the Making of a Mass Public.* Cambridge, Mass.: Harvard University Press, 2007.

Illich, Ivan. *Medical Nemesis: The Expropriation of Health.* 1st American ed. New York: Pantheon, 1976. Reprint of 1975 London ed.

Ingelfinger, F. J. "Listen: The Patient—Once Again." *New England Journal of Medicine* 295 (December 23, 1976): 1478–79.

Inglehart, John K. "U.S. Health Care System: A Look to the 1990s." *Health Affairs* 4 (August 1985): 120–27.

Institute of Medicine, Committee on Quality of Health Care in America. *Crossing the Quality Chasm: A New Health System for the 21st Century.* Washington, D.C.: National Academy Press, 2001.

Institute of Medicine, Committee on Standards for Developing Trustworthy Clinical Practice Guidelines. *Clinical Practice Guidelines We Can Trust.* Washington, D.C.: National Academies Press, 2011.

Institute of Medicine, Committee on the Public Health Effectiveness of the FDA 510(k) Clearance Process. *Medical Devices and the Public's Health: The FDA 510(k) Clearance Process at 35 Years.* Washington, D.C.: National Academies Press, 2011.

"Introduction and History, National Library of Medicine Index Mechanization Project." *Bulletin of the Medical Library Association* 49, no. 1, pt. 2 (January 1961): 1–7.

"Is This Hysterectomy Really Necessary?" *Medical Economics* 31 (October 1953): 276–82.

Jackson, Charles O. *Food and Drug Legislation in the New Deal.* Princeton: Princeton University Press, 1970.

Jackson, Mark. *The Age of Stress: Science and the Search for Stability.* New York: Oxford University Press, 2013.

Jacobs, Lee. "Interview with Lawrence Weed, MD—The Father of the Problem-Oriented Medical Record Looks Ahead." *Permanente Journal* 13, no. 3 (2009): 84–89.

Jacobs, Meg. *Pocketbook Politics: Economic Citizenship in Twentieth-Century America.* Princeton: Princeton University Press, 2005.

Jain, S. Lochlann. *Injury: The Politics of Product Design and Safety Law in the United States.* Princeton: Princeton University Press, 2006.

Jarvis, D. C. *Folk Medicine: A Vermont Doctor's Guide to Good Health.* New York: Holt, 1958.

Jasper, Margaret C. *The Law of Product Liability.* Dobbs Ferry, N.Y.: Oceana, 2001.

Jenner, Mark S. R., and Patrick Wallis. "The Medical Marketplace." In *Medicine and the Market in England and Its Colonies, c.1450–c.1850,* edited by Mark S. R. Jenner and Patrick Wallis, 1–23. New York: Palgrave Macmillan, 2007.

Jewson, N. D. "The Disappearance of the Sick Man in Medical Cosmology." *Sociology* 10 (May 1976): 225–44.

Joe and Teresa Graedon Celebrate 25 Successful Years. September 15, 2003. http://kingfeatures.com/2003/09/joe-and-teresa-graedon-celebrate-25-successful-years-of-%E2%80%9Cthe-people%E2%80%99s-pharmacy%E2%80%9D-with-honors/. Accessed July 1, 2015.

John, Richard R. *Spreading the News: The American Postal System from Franklin to Morse.* Cambridge, Mass.: Harvard University Press, 1995.

Johnson, Sheila K. "My Doctor, the Corporation." *New York Times Magazine,* December 29, 1974.

Johnson, Wingate M. "A Family Doctor Speaks His Mind." *Harper's,* December 1928, 50–56.

Johnstone, James M. "Special Problems in Direct-to-Consumer Advertising of Prescription Drugs." *Food Drug Cosmetic Law Journal* 42 (1987): 315–22.

Jones, David S. *Broken Hearts: The Tangled History of Cardiac Care.* Baltimore: Johns Hopkins University Press, 2013.

Jones, De Leslie. "The Drugstore Has Become a Convenience Store." *Advertising and Selling*, September 7, 1927, 74, 76.

Jones, Marion Moser, and Isidore Daniel Benrubi. "Poison Politics." *American Journal of Public Health* 103 (May 2013): 801–12.

Jost, Timothy. *Health Care at Risk: A Critique of the Consumer-Driven Movement.* Durham, N.C.: Duke University Press, 2007.

Joubert, Pieter, and Louis Lasagna. "Patient Package Inserts. I. Nature, Notions and Needs." *Clinical Pharmacology and Therapeutics* 5 (November 1975): 507–13.

Juhnke, Eric S. *Quacks and Crusaders: The Fabulous Careers of John Brinkley, Norman Baker, and Harry Hoxsey.* Lawrence: University Press of Kansas, 2002.

Junod, Suzanne White. Review of *The Politics of Purity*, by Clayton Coppin and Jack High. *Business History Review* 74 (Spring 2000): 151–55.

Kaiser Family Foundation. *2013 Employer Health Benefits Survey.* August 20, 2014. http://kff.org/private-insurance/report/2013-employer-health-benefits/. Accessed July 1, 2015.

———. *Five Years after IOM Report on Medical Errors, Nearly Half of All Consumers Worry about the Safety of Their Health Care.* http://kff.org/other/poll-finding/five-years-after-iom-report-on-medical/. Accessed July 1, 2015.

———. *For-Profit Health Care Companies: Trends and Issues—Fact Sheet.* February 11, 1998. http://kff.org/health-costs/poll-finding/for-profit-health-care-companies-trends-and/. Accessed July 1, 2015.

Kallet, Arthur, and F. J. Schlink. *100,000,000 Guinea Pigs: Dangers in Everyday Foods, Drugs, and Cosmetics.* New York: Grosset and Dunlap, 1933.

Kanjanarat, P., A. G. Winterstein, T. E. Johns, R. C. Hatton, R. Gonzalez-Rothi, and R. Segal. "Nature of Preventable Adverse Drug Events in Hospitals: A Literature Review." *American Journal of Health Systems Pharmacy* 60 (September 2003): 1750–59.

Kasteler, Josephine, Robert L. Kane, Donna M. Olsen, and Constance Thetford. "Underlying Prevalence of 'Doctor-Shopping' Behavior." *Journal of Health and Social Behavior* 17 (December 1976): 328–39.

Katz, Jay. *The Silent World of Doctor and Patient.* New York: Free Press, 1984.

Katz, Norman D. "Consumers Union: The Movement and the Magazine, 1936–1957." Ph.D. diss., Rutgers University, 1977.

Kay, Gwen. *Dying to Be Beautiful: The Fight for Safe Cosmetics.* Columbus: Ohio State University Press, 2005.

Kellock, Katharine A. "Shopping for Medical Care." *Confidential Bulletin* 2 (November 1935): 16–21.

Kessler, David A., and Wayne L. Pines. "The Federal Regulation of Prescription Drug Advertising and Promotion." *Journal of the American Medical Association* 264 (December 14, 1990): 2409–15.

Kett, Joseph F. *The Formation of the American Medical Profession: The Role of Institutions, 1780–1860.* New Haven: Yale University Press, 1968.

Kevles, Bettyann. *Naked to the Bone: Medical Imaging in the Twentieth Century.* New Brunswick, N.J.: Rutgers University Press, 1996.

"Killing Public Health Legislation." *Journal of the American Medical Association* 68 (March 10, 1917): 795.

Kimberly, John R., Gérard de Pouvourville, and Thomas D'Aunno, eds. *The Globalization of Managerial Innovation in Health Care.* New York: Cambridge University Press, 2008.

Kimmel, Robert. "How to Be Ethical while Eating Your Competitor's Lunch." In *Ninth Annual Symposium for Health Care Marketing.* Chicago: Academy of Health Care Marketing, American Marketing Association, 1989.

King, Jaime, and Benjamin Moulton. "Group Health's Participation in a Shared Decision-Making Demonstration Yielded Lessons, Such as Role of Culture Change." *Health Affairs* 32 (February 2013): 294–302.

Kirk, Paul Hayden, and Eugene D. Sternberg. *Doctors' Offices and Clinics, Medical and Dental.* New York: Reinhold, 1955.

Kisch, Arnold I., and Leo J. Reeder. "Client Evaluation of Physician Performance." *Journal of Health and Social Behavior* 10 (March 1969): 51–58.

Kitch, Edmund W. "The Patent System and New Drug Applications." In *Regulating New Drugs,* edited by Richard L. Landau. Chicago: University of Chicago, 1973.

Klarman, Herbert E. "The Financing of Health Care." *Daedalus* 106 (Winter 1977): 215–34.

Klaw, Spencer. *The Great American Medicine Show: The Unhealthy State of U.S. Medical Care, and What Can Be Done about It.* New York: Viking, 1975.

Klein, Herbert E. "See Yourself as V.I.P.s See You: Gloria Steinem." *Medical Economics* 51 (April 15, 1974): 92–103.

Klein, Jennifer. *For All These Rights: Business, Labor, and the Shaping of America's Public-Private Welfare State.* Princeton: Princeton University Press, 2003.

Klerman, Gerald. "Drugs and Social Values." *International Journal of the Addictions* 5, no. 2 (1970): 313–19.

———. "Psychotropic Drugs as Therapeutic Agents." *Hastings Center Studies* 2 (January 1974): 81–93.

Kline, Wendy. *Bodies of Knowledge: Sexuality, Reproduction, and Women's Health in the Second Wave.* Chicago: University of Chicago Press, 2010.

Knowles, John H., ed. *Doing Better and Feeling Worse: Health in the United States.* New York: Norton, 1977.

———. "The Responsibility of the Individual." *Daedalus* 106 (Winter 1977): 57–80.

Knox, Richard. "Breast Cancer: What We Learned in 2012." NPR.org. http://www .npr.org/sections/health-shots/2013/01/01/167973537/breast-cancer-what-we-learned-in-2012. Accessed July 1, 2015.

Kobler, John. "Why Mac Isn't Dead." *Saturday Evening Post,* August 18, 1956, 28–29, 71–72.

Kohn, Linda T., Janet M. Corrigan, and Molla S. Donaldson, eds. *To Err Is Human: Building a Safer Health System.* Washington, D.C.: National Academy Press, 2000.

Koos, Earl Lomon. *The Health of Regionville: What the People Thought and Did about It.* New York: Columbia University Press, 1954.

———. "'Metropolis'—What City People Think of Their Medical Services." *American Journal of Public Health* 45 (December 1955): 1551–57.

Kornfield, Rachel, Julie Donohue, Ernst R. Berndt, and G. Caleb Alexander. "Promotion of Prescription Drugs to Consumers and Providers, 2001–2010." *PloS One* 8, no. 3 (2013). http://journals.plos.org/plosone/article?id=10.1371/journal.pone.0055504. Accessed July 1, 2015.

Kotlowski, Dean J. "The Knowles Affair: Nixon's Self-Inflicted Wound." *Presidential Studies Quarterly* 30 (September 2000): 443–63.

Krabbendam, Hans. *The Model Man: A Life of Edward William Bok, 1863–1930.* Amsterdam: Rodopi, 2001.

Kritzer, Herbert M. "Ideology and American Political Elites." *Public Opinion Quarterly* 42 (December 1, 1978): 484–502.

Kruger, Isaak D. "Patient Package Inserts: The Patient's Right to Know." *Bulletin of the American College of Physicians* 18 (January 1977): 18–19.

Kurtz, Sheldon F. "Law of Informed Consent: From Doctor Is Right to Patient Has Rights." *Syracuse Law Review* 50 (2000): 1243–60.

Kushner, Howard I. "The Other War on Drugs: The Pharmaceutical Industry, Evidence-Based Medicine, and Clinical Practice." *Journal of Policy History* 19, no. 1 (2007): 49–70.

Kutner, Luis. "Due Process of Euthanasia: The Living Will, a Proposal." *Indiana Law Journal* 44, no. 1 (1969): 539–54.

Kutner, M., E. Greenberg, Y. Jin, and C. Paulsen. *The Health Literacy of America's Adults: Results from the 2003 National Assessment of Adult Literacy.* Washington, D.C.: National Center for Education Statistics, 2006. http://nces.ed.gov/pubs2006/2006483.pdf. Accessed July 1, 2015.

Kyrk, Hazel. "100,000,000 Guinea Pigs: Dangers in Everyday Foods, Drugs, and Cosmetics." *Journal of Business* 6 (October 1933): 352–54.

Lamb, Ruth deForest. *American Chamber of Horrors: The Truth about Food and Drugs.* New York: Farrar and Rinehart, 1936.

Lander, Louise. *Defective Medicine: Risk, Anger, and the Malpractice Crisis.* New York: Farrar, Straus, and Giroux, 1978.

Lane, Keryn A. G., and Robert Berkow. "*The Merck Manual*: A Century of Medical Publishing and Practice." *CBE Views* 22, no. 4 (1999): 112–13.

Langer, Elinor. "The Doctors' Debate." *Science* 149 (July 9, 1965): 164–67.

———. "Doctors' Organization Faces Growing Outside Criticism." *Science* 149 (July 16, 1965): 282–83, 328.

Langford, Elizabeth A. "Medical Care in the Consumer Price Index, 1936–56." *Monthly Labor Review* 80 (September 1957): 1053–58.

Lavieties, Paul H. "Information on Drugs." *Science* 132 (August 19, 1960): 488.

Lavin, John H., and Linda C. Busek. "What Makes Americans So Operation-Happy?" *Medical Economics* 50 (January 8, 1973): 67–75.

Lawrence, Christopher, and George Weisz. *Greater Than the Parts: Holism in Biomedicine, 1920–1950.* New York: Oxford University Press, 1998.

Lawrence, Susan V. "Patient Package Insert Lands in Courts." *Bulletin of the American College of Physicians* 18 (November 1977): 7–12, 63.

"Layman Told How to Cut Out His Own Appendix." *Medical Economics* 32 (February 1955): 277–78.

Lazare, Aaron, Sherman Eisenthal, Arlene Frank, and John D. Stoeckle. "Studies on a Negotiated Approach to Patienthood." In *The Doctor-Patient Relationship in the Changing Health Scene*, edited by Eugene B. Gallagher. Washington, D.C.: U.S. Government Printing Office, 1976.

Leach, William R. *Land of Desire: Merchants, Power, and the Rise of a New American Culture*. New York: Vintage, 1994.

Leape, Lucian L. "Unnecessary Surgery." *Annual Review of Public Health* 13 (1992): 363–83.

Lears, T. J. Jackson. *Fables of Abundance: A Cultural History of Advertising in America*. New York: Basic Books, 1994.

Leavitt, Judith Walzer. *Make Room for Daddy: The Journey from Waiting Room to Birthing Room*. Chapel Hill: University of North Carolina Press, 2009.

———. "What Do Men Have to Do with It? Fathers and Mid-Twentieth Century Childbirth." *Bulletin of the History of Medicine* 77 (Summer 2003): 235–62.

———. "'A Worrying Profession': The Domestic Environment of Medical Practice in the Mid-Nineteenth Century." *Bulletin of the History of Medicine* 69 (Spring 1995): 1–29.

Lebhar, Godfrey Montague. *Chain Stores in America, 1859–1950*. New York: Chain Store, 1952.

LeBlanc, Thomas. "The Medicine Show." *American Mercury*, June 1925, 233–37.

Lederer, Richard. *Crazy English*. Rev. ed. New York: Simon and Schuster, 2010.

Lee, Fred. "Change the Concept of Work from Service to Theater." For Your Advantage. January 7, 2008. http://www.foryouradvantage.com/fya010708.pdf. Accessed July 1, 2015.

———. *If Disney Ran Your Hospital: 9½ Things You Would Do Differently*. Bozeman, Mont.: Second River Healthcare Press, 2004.

Lefkowitz, Bonnie. *Community Health Centers: A Movement and the People Who Made It Happen*. New Brunswick, N.J.: Rutgers University Press, 2007.

"Legal Developments in Marketing: In re Bristol-Myers Company." *Journal of Marketing* 48 (Spring 1984): 82–83.

"Legion Avoids AF Fight." *Facts on File* 13 (September 10, 1953): 298.

Lemov, Michael R. *People's Warrior: John Moss and the Fight for Freedom of Information and Consumer Rights*. Teaneck, N.J.: Fairleigh Dickinson University Press, 2011.

Lepore, Jill. "The Lie Factory." *New Yorker*, September 24, 2012, 50–59.

Lerner, Barron H. "Beyond Informed Consent: Did Cancer Patients Challenge Their Physicians in the Post–World War II Era?" *Journal of the History of Medicine and Allied Sciences* 59 (October 2004): 507–21.

———. *The Breast Cancer Wars: Hope, Fear, and the Pursuit of a Cure in Twentieth-Century America*. New York: Oxford University Press, 2001.

———. "From Careless Consumptives to Recalcitrant Patients." *Social Science and Medicine* 45, no. 9 (1997): 1423–31.

———. *When Illness Goes Public: Celebrity Patients and How We Look at Medicine.* Baltimore: Johns Hopkins University Press, 2006.

Lesch, John E. *The First Miracle Drugs: How the Sulfa Drugs Transformed Medicine.* New York: Oxford University Press, 2007.

Leven, Maurice. *The Incomes of Physicians: An Economic and Statistical Analysis.* Chicago: University of Chicago Press, 1932.

Levinson, Marc. *The Great A&P and the Struggle for Small Business in America.* New York: Hill and Wang, 2011.

Levit, K. R., M. S. Freeland, and D. R. Waldo. "National Health Care Spending Trends: 1988." *Health Affairs* 9, no. 2 (1990): 171–84.

Levy, Howard. "Counter Geiger." *Social Policy* 1 (May–June 1971): 50–57.

Lewis, Carol. "The Poison Squad." *FDA Consumer Magazine*, November–December 2002. http://permanent.access.gpo.gov/lps1609/www.fda.gov/fdac/features/2002/602_squad.html. Accessed July 1, 2015.

Lewis, Sinclair. *Arrowsmith.* New York: Grosset and Dunlap, 1925.

"*Liberty* and Ethics." *Journal of the American Medical Association* 94 (April 12, 1930): 15.

Lichtenstein, Nelson. *The Retail Revolution: How Wal-Mart Created a Brave New World of Business.* New York: Metropolitan, 2009.

Liebenau, Jonathan. *Medical Science and Medical Industry: The Formation of the American Pharmaceutical Industry.* Baltimore: Johns Hopkins University Press, 1987.

Lindsey, John R. "How to Have a Well-Run Appointment System." *Medical Economics* 32 (September 1955): 140–42.

Lipkin, Mack. *Care of Patients: Concepts and Tactics.* New York: Oxford University Press, 1974.

Lipset, Seymour Martin, and William Schneider. *The Confidence Gap: Business, Labor, and Government in the Public Mind.* New York: Free Press, 1983.

Lorde, Audre. *Sister Outsider: Essays and Speeches.* Trumansburg, N.Y.: Crossing Press, 1984.

Love, Spencie. *One Blood: The Death and Resurrection of Charles R. Drew.* Chapel Hill: University of North Carolina Press, 1996.

Lowell, Paul. "Choosing a Location: The Office Site." *Medical Economics* 32 (October 1954): 181–95.

Ludmerer, Kenneth M. *Learning to Heal: The Development of American Medical Education.* New York: Basic Books, 1985.

———. *Time to Heal: American Medical Education from the Turn of the Century to the Era of Managed Care.* New York: Oxford University Press, 1999.

Lundberg, George. "John P. Peters and the Committee of 430 Physicians." *Yale Journal of Biology and Medicine* 75 (January–February 2002): 23–27.

Lutz, Sandy. "Ask-A-Nurse's Company Plans Initial Offer of Stock." *Modern Healthcare*, February 17, 1992, 20.

Lynd, Robert Staughton, and Helen Merrell Lynd. *Middletown: A Study in American Culture.* New York: Harcourt, Brace, Jovanovich, 1956.

Lynn, Frances H., and Arnold J. Friedhoff. "The Patient on a Tranquilizing Regimen." *American Journal of Nursing* 60 (February 1960): 234–40.

Magnuson, Warren G., and Jean Carper. *The Dark Side of the Marketplace: The Plight of the American Consumer.* Englewood Cliffs, N.J.: Prentice-Hall, 1968.

Mahoney, Tom. *The Merchants of Life: An Account of the American Pharmaceutical Industry.* New York: Harper, 1959.

Main Street Public Library Database, Center for Middletown Studies, Ball State University. http://cms.bsu.edu/academics/centersandinstitutes/middletown/research/middletownread/mainstreetpubliclibrarydatabase. Accessed July 1, 2015.

Majerol, Melissa, Vann Newkirk, and Rachel Garfield. *The Uninsured: A Primer— Key Facts about Health Insurance and the Uninsured in America.* http://kff.org/uninsured/report/the-uninsured-a-primer/. Accessed July 1, 2015.

"Maj Gen Paul R. Hawley, MC, USA, Dies." *Journal of the American Medical Association* 195 (January 3, 1966): 39.

"Making Medicines Taste Better." *Literary Digest* 99 (November 17, 1928): 24.

Malmberg, Carl. *140 Million Patients.* New York: Reynal and Hitchock, 1947.

Mann, Charles C., and Mark L. Plummer. *The Aspirin Wars: Money, Medicine, and 100 Years of Rampant Competition.* New York: Knopf, 1991.

Manring, Maurice. *Slave in a Box: The Strange Career of Aunt Jemima.* Charlottesville: University of Virginia Press, 1998.

Marchand, Roland. *Advertising the American Dream: Making Way for Modernity, 1920–1940.* Berkeley: University of California Press, 1985.

———. *Creating the Corporate Soul: The Rise of Public Relations and Corporate Imagery in American Big Business.* Berkeley: University of California Press, 1998.

Marcuse, Herbert. *An Essay on Liberation.* Boston: Beacon, 1969.

Marks, Harry M. *The Progress of Experiment: Science and Therapeutic Reform in the United States, 1900–1990.* New York: Cambridge University Press, 1997.

———. "Revisiting 'The Origins of Compulsory Drug Prescriptions.'" *American Journal of Public Health* 85 (January 1995): 109–15.

Martin, Justin. *Nader: Crusader, Spoiler, Icon.* Cambridge, Mass.: Perseus Publishing, 2002.

Mason, Cleon. "The Business of Doctoring." *North American Review*, December 1928, 737–42.

Mather, Kirtley F. "The Scientist's Bookshelf." *American Scientist* 42 (April 1954): 309–53.

Matt, Susan J. *Keeping Up with the Joneses: Envy in American Consumer Society, 1890– 1930.* Philadelphia: University of Pennsylvania Press, 2003.

Matusow, Allen J. *The Unraveling of America: A History of Liberalism in the 1960s.* New York: Harper and Row, 1984.

Maurer, Herrymon. "The M.D.'s Are Off Their Pedestal." *Fortune*, February 1954, 138–42, 176, 179–80, 182, 184, 186.

May, Charles. "Selling Drugs by 'Educating' Physicians." *Journal of Medical Education* 36 (January 1961): 1–23.

Mayer, Robert M. *The Consumer Movement: Guardians of the Marketplace.* Boston: Twayne, 1989.

Mayes, Rick. "The Origins, Development, and Passage of Medicare's Revolutionary

Prospective Payment System." *Journal of the History of Medicine and Allied Sciences* 62 (January 2007): 21–55.

Mayes, Rick, and Robert A. Berenson. *Medicare Prospective Payment and the Shaping of U.S. Health Care.* Baltimore: Johns Hopkins University Press, 2008.

McCarry, Charles. *Citizen Nader.* New York: Saturday Review Press, 1972.

McCarthy, Eugene G., and Geraldine W. Widmer. "Effects of Screening by Consultants on Recommended Elective Surgical Procedures." *New England Journal of Medicine* 291 (December 19, 1974): 1331–35.

McCarthy, Eugene G., Lisa Astor, and John Tucker. *The Second Opinion Handbook: A Guide for Medical Self-Defense.* New York: Nick Lyons Books, 1987.

McCleery, Robert S. *One Life—One Physician: An Inquiry into the Medical Profession's Performance in Self-Regulation: A Report to the Center for Study of Responsive Law.* Washington, D.C.: Public Affairs Press, 1971.

McFadyen, Richard E. "Estes Kefauver and the Drug Industry." Ph.D. diss., Emory University, 1973.

———. "The FDA's Regulation and Control of Antibiotics in the 1950s: The Henry Welch Scandal, Felix Marti-Ibanez, and Charles Pfizer & Co." *Bulletin of the History of Medicine* 53 (Summer 1979): 159–69.

McGarrah, Rob. "It's Time Consumers Knew More about Their Doctors." *Medical Economics*, March 4, 1974, 267–90.

McGlynn, Elizabeth A., Steven M. Asch, John Adams, Joan Keesey, Jennifer Hicks, Alison DeCristofaro, and Eve A. Kerr. "The Quality of Health Care Delivered to Adults in the United States." *New England Journal of Medicine* 348 (June 26, 2003): 2635–45.

McGovern, Charles F. *Sold American: Consumption and Citizenship, 1890–1945.* Chapel Hill: University of North Carolina Press, 2006.

"McKesson's 'American Look' Captures Customers for Druggists." *Sales Management*, November 1, 1948, 113.

McLean, Thomas, and Edward P. Richards. "Health Care's 'Thirty Years War': The Origins and Dissolution of Managed Care." *New York University Annual Survey of Law* 60 (2004): 283–328.

McNamara, Brooks. *Step Right Up.* Garden City, N.Y.: Doubleday, 1976.

Mead, Nicola, and Peter Bower. "Patient-Centredness: A Conceptual Framework and Review of the Empirical Literature." *Social Science and Medicine* 51 (October 2001): 1087–1110.

Means, J. H. "Evolution of the Doctor-Patient Relationship." *Bulletin of the New York Academy of Medicine* 29 (September 1953): 725–32.

Mechanic, David. "General Medical Practice: Some Comparisons between the Work of Primary Care Physicians in the United States and England and Wales." *Medical Care* 10 (September–October 1972): 402–20.

———. "The Rise and Fall of Managed Care." *Journal of Health and Social Behavior* 45, extra issue (2004): 76–86.

Medical Library Association, Consumer and Patient Health Information Section. *Top 100 Health Websites You Can Trust.* 2013. http://caphis.mlanet.org/consumer/index.html. Accessed July 1, 2015.

Medicine and Madison Avenue. Duke University Libraries Digital Collections. http://scriptorium.lib.duke.edu/mma/. Accessed July 1, 2015.

Mendelson, Dan, and Tanisha V. Carino. "Evidence-Based Medicine in the United States—De Rigueur or Dream Deferred?" *Health Affairs* 24 (January 1, 2005): 133–36.

Menges, Roger. "They Settle Doctor-Patient Disputes." *Medical Economics* 28 (April 1951): 60–63, 181–85.

Metzl, Jonathan. *Prozac on the Couch.* Durham, N.C.: Duke University Press, 2003.

MIA MD: A Documentary about Our Doctors. 2010. http://mia-md.com/. Accessed July 1, 2015.

Millenson, Michael M. *Demanding Medical Excellence: Doctors and Accountability in the Information Age.* Chicago: University of Chicago Press, 1997.

Millenson, Michael, and Juliana Macri. *Will the Affordable Care Act Move Patient-Centeredness to Center Stage?* March 2012. http://www.rwjf.org/en/research-publications/find-rwjf-research/2012/03/will-the-affordable-care-act-move-patient-centeredness-to-center.html. Accessed July 1, 2015.

Miller, Charles. "How to Help Your Patients Pay." *Medical Economics* 27 (November 1950): 76–78, 162.

Miller, K. E. "Public Health Aspects of Unrestrained Advertising." *American Journal of Public Health* 30 (August 1940): 880–86.

Miller, Leslie J. "Informed Consent: I." *Journal of the American Medical Association* 244 (November 7, 1980): 2100–2103.

Miller, Lois Mattox. "Hysterectomy: Medical Necessity or Surgical Racket?" *Reader's Digest,* August 1953, 82–84.

Mills, C. Wright. *White Collar: The American Middle Classes.* New York: Oxford University Press, 1951.

Mintz, Morton. *At Any Cost: Corporate Greed, Women, and the Dalkon Shield.* New York: Pantheon, 1985.

——. *The Therapeutic Nightmare.* Boston: Houghton Mifflin, 1965.

Mintzes, Barbara. "Advertising of Prescription-Only Medicines to the Public: Does Evidence of Benefit Counterbalance Harm?" *Annual Review of Public Health* 33 (April 2012): 259–77.

"Miracle Drugs or Media Drugs?" *Consumer Reports,* March 1992, 142–46.

Mobley, Jane. *Prescription for Success: The Chain Drug Story.* Kansas City: Hallmark Cards, 1990.

"Modern Office Equipment." *Medical Economics* 5 (October 1927): 27.

Moeller, Philip. "Study: More Caregivers Seeking Health Information Online." *U.S. News and World Report,* June 24, 2013. http://money.usnews.com/money/blogs/the-best-life/2013/06/24/study-more-caregivers-seeking-health-information-online. Accessed July 1, 2015.

Mohr, James C. *Doctors and the Law: Medical Jurisprudence in Nineteenth-Century America.* New York: Oxford University Press, 1993.

Mold, Alex. "Making the Patient-Consumer in Margaret Thatcher's Britain." *Historical Journal* 54 (June 2011): 509–28.

————. "Patients' Rights and the National Health Service in Britain, 1960s–1980s." *American Journal of Public Health* 102 (November 2012): 2030–38.

————. "Repositioning the Patient: Patient Organizations, Consumerism, and Autonomy in Britain during the 1960s and 1970s." *Bulletin of the History of Medicine* 87 (Summer 2013): 225–49.

Mold, Alex, and David Reubi, eds. *Assembling Health Rights in Global Perspective: Genealogies and Anthropologies.* New York: Routledge, 2013.

Monaghan, Jane. "Whatever Happened to the Patients' Bill of Rights?" *Medical Economics* 52 (August 4, 1975): 109–12.

Moore, Harry H. *American Medicine and the People's Health.* New York: Appleton, 1927.

Moore, Kelly. *Disrupting Science: Social Movements, American Scientists, and the Politics of the Military, 1945–1975.* Princeton: Princeton University Press, 2008.

Morantz-Sanchez, Regina Markell. *Conduct Unbecoming a Woman: Medicine on Trial in Turn-of-the-Century Brooklyn.* New York: Oxford University Press, 1999.

Moreton, Bethany. *To Serve God and Wal-Mart: The Making of Christian Free Enterprise.* Cambridge, Mass.: Harvard University Press, 2009.

Morgan, Herman G. "Hearts in the Breaking." *Hygeia* 12 (February 1934): 110–13, 180–82.

Morgan, Steven G. "Direct-to-Consumer Advertising and Expenditures on Prescription Drugs: A Comparison of Experiences in the United States and Canada." *Open Medicine* 1, no. 1 (2007): 1–8.

Morgen, Sandra. *Into Our Own Hands: The Women's Health Movement in the United States, 1969–1990.* New Brunswick, N.J.: Rutgers University Press, 2002.

Morris, Lloyd. "Mammon, M.D.: A Composite Portrait." *Harper's,* October 1928, 614–21.

Morris, Louis A., and J. A. Halperin. "Effects of Written Drug Information." *American Journal of Public Health* 69 (January 1979): 47–52.

Morris, Louis A., and Lloyd G. Millstein. "Drug Advertising to Consumers: Effects of Formats for Magazine and Television Advertisements." *Food Drug Cosmetic Law Journal* 39 (1984): 497–502.

Morris, Louis A., David Brinberg, Ron Klimberg, Carole Rivera, and Lloyd G. Millstein. "Attitudes of Consumers toward Direct Advertising of Prescription Drugs." *Public Health Reports* 101 (January–February 1986): 82–89.

"Most Fees Are Modest." *Medical Economics* 32 (December 1955): 83.

Mullen, Patricia Dolan. "The (Already) Activated Patient: An Alternative to Medicocentrism." *Springer Series on Health Care and Society* 4 (1980): 281–98.

Murphy, Lamar Riley. *Enter the Physician: The Transformation of Domestic Medicine, 1760–1860.* Tuscaloosa: University of Alabama Press, 1991.

Murphy, Michelle. "Immodest Witnessing: The Epistemology of Vaginal Self-Examination in the U.S. Feminist Self-Help Movement." *Feminist Studies* 30 (Spring 2004): 115–47.

Murphy, Patrick E., and William L. Wilkie, eds. *Marketing and Advertising Regulation: The Federal Trade Commission in the 1990s.* Notre Dame: University of Notre Dame, 1990.

Musgrave, William Everett. "Who Is Your Doctor? Sixteen Points on Which to Judge the Merits of a Physician." *Hygeia* 5 (May 1927): 233–34.

Nadel, Mark V. *The Politics of Consumer Protection.* Indianapolis: Bobbs-Merrill, 1971.

Nader, Ralph, ed. *The Consumer and Corporate Accountability.* New York: Harcourt Brace Jovanovich, 1973.

——. *Unsafe at Any Speed: The Designed-in Dangers of the American Automobile.* New York: Grossman, 1965.

Narins, Craig R., Ann M. Dozier, Frederick S. Ling, and Wojciech Zareba. "The Influence of Public Reporting of Outcome Data on Medical Decision Making by Physicians." *Archives of Internal Medicine* 165 (January 2005): 83–87.

National Women's Health Network. *Hysterectomy: Resource Guide* 2. Washington, D.C.: National Women's Health Network, 1980.

"Nationalized Doctors?" *Time,* June 21, 1937, 26–30.

"Needless Surgery—Doctors, Good and Bad" (interview with Dr. Paul Hawley). *U.S. News and World Report,* February 20, 1953, 48–55.

Nelson, Alondra. *Body and Soul: The Black Panther Party and the Fight against Medical Discrimination.* Minneapolis: University of Minnesota Press, 2011.

Nolen, Herman C., and Harold H. Maynard. *Drug Store Management.* New York: McGraw-Hill, 1941.

"Norman Rockwell Visits a Family Doctor." *Saturday Evening Post,* April 12, 1947, 30–34.

Novitch, Mark. "Direct-to-Consumer Advertising of Prescription Drugs." *Food Drug Cosmetic Law Journal* 39 (1984): 306–11.

Numbers, Ronald L. *Almost Persuaded: American Physicians and Compulsory Health Insurance, 1912–1920.* Baltimore: Johns Hopkins University Press, 1978.

Oberlander, Jonathan. *The Political Life of Medicare.* Chicago: University of Chicago Press, 2003.

Okrent, Daniel. *Last Call: The Rise and Fall of Prohibition.* New York: Scribner, 2010.

Okun, Mitchell. *Fair Play in the Marketplace: The First Battle for Pure Food and Drugs.* Dekalb: Northern Illinois University Press, 1986.

Oliver, Thomas R., Philip R. Lee, and Helene L. Lipton. "A Political History of Medicare and Prescription Drug Coverage." *Milbank Quarterly* 82 (June 2004): 283–354.

Olson, Laura Katz. *The Politics of Medicaid.* New York: Columbia University Press, 2010.

Omran, Abdel. "A Century of Epidemiological Transition in the United States." *Preventive Medicine* 6 (March 1977): 30–51.

——. "The Epidemiologic Transition: A Theory of the Epidemiology of Population Change." *Milbank Memorial Fund Quarterly* 49 (October 1971): 509–38.

"The Once-Ubiquitous Peoples Drug Stores / Streets of Washington." http://www.streetsofwashington.com/2011/11/once-ubiquitous-peoples-drug-stores.html. Accessed July 1, 2015.

Oppenheimer, Gerald M. "Becoming the Framingham Study." *American Journal of Public Health* 95 (April 2005): 602–10.

"Our Name Is Mud." *Medical Economics* 27 (November 1950): 79.

Owens, Thomas. "Health Questionnaires Aid History-Taking." *Medical Economics* 32 (June 1955): 135–38.

Packard, Vance. *Hidden Persuaders*. New York: McKay, 1957.

———. *The Status Seekers*. New York: McKay, 1959.

———. *The Waste Makers*. New York: McKay, 1960.

Parker, Robert S., and Edmund Polubinski. "Professional Associations and Corporations: Tax Considerations." *William and Mary Law Review* 11, no. 3 (1970): 685–705.

Parson, Esther Jane. *In the Doctor's Office*. Philadelphia: Lippincott, 1945.

"'Patent Medicine' Business Grows More Subtle." *Hygeia*, November 9, 1931, 1018.

"Patient-Centered Medical Homes." *Health Affairs*, September 14, 2010. Health Policy Brief. http://www.healthaffairs.org/healthpolicybriefs/brief.php?brief_id=25. Accessed July 1, 2015.

Patient-Centered Primary Care Collaborative. *Defining the Medical Home*. 2013. https://www.pcpcc.org/about/medical-home. Accessed July 1, 2015.

Paytash, Catherine A. "The Learned Intermediary Doctrine and Patient Package Inserts: A Balanced Approach to Preventing Drug-Related Injury." *Stanford Law Review* 51 (May 1999): 1343–71.

Pease, Otis A. *The Responsibilities of American Advertising: Private Control and Public Influence, 1920–1940*. New Haven: Yale University Press, 1958.

Peebles, Allon. *A Survey of the Medical Facilities of Shelby County, Indiana: 1929*. Washington, D.C.: Committee on the Costs of Medical Care, 1930.

Peña, Carolyn Thomas de la. *The Body Electric: How Strange Machines Built the Modern American*. New York: New York University Press, 2003.

Pennock, Pamela E. *Advertising Sin and Sickness: The Politics of Alcohol and Tobacco Marketing, 1950–1990*. DeKalb: Northern Illinois University Press, 2007.

Pennsylvania Department of Insurance. *Shoppers' Guide to Hospitals in the Philadelphia Area*. Harrisburg: Department of Insurance, 1971.

Perkins, Barbara Bridgman. "Economic Organization of Medicine and the Committee on the Costs of Medical Care." *American Journal of Public Health* 88 (November 1998): 1721–26.

Pernick, Martin S. "The Patient's Role in Medical Decisionmaking: A Social History of Informed Consent in Medical Therapy." In United States, President's Commission for the Study of Ethical Problems in Medicine and Biomedical and Behavioral Research, *Making Health Care Decisions: The Ethical and Legal Implications of Informed Consent in the Patient-Practitioner Relationship*, 3:1–35. 3 vols. Washington, D.C.: U.S. Government Printing Office, 1982.

Perrin, E. N. "He Thinks You Mishandle Patients." *Medical Economics* 37 (December 5, 1960): 38–42, 45–46, 48, 53–54, 56, 58, 60.

Perry, Armstrong. "Weak Spots in the American System of Broadcasting." *Annals of the American Academy of Political and Social Science* 177 (January 1935): 22–28.

Perry, Linda. "Physician Referral Service Touts Quality, Not Quantity." *Modern Health Care*, July 2, 1990, 36.

Pertschuk, Michael. *Giant Killers*. New York: Norton, 1986.

Pescosolido, Bernice A., Steven A. Tuch, and Jack K. Martin. "The Profession of

Medicine and the Public." *Journal of Health and Social Behavior* 42 (March 2001): 1–16.

Peterson, Osler L., Leon P. Andrews, Robert S. Spain, and Bernard G. Greenberg. *An Analytical Study of North Carolina General Practice, 1953–1954*. Evanston, Ill.: Association of American Medical Colleges, 1956.

Pew Charitable Trusts. *Persuading the Prescribers: Pharmaceutical Industry Marketing and Its Influence on Physicians and Patients*. November 11, 2013. http://www .pewtrusts.org/en/research-and-analysis/fact-sheets/2013/11/11/persuading-the-prescribers-pharmaceutical-industry-marketing-and-its-influence-on-physicians-and-patients. Accessed July 1, 2015.

Pew Research Center. *Mobile Technology Fact Sheet*. N.d. http://www.pewinternet .org/fact-sheets/mobile-technology-fact-sheet/. Accessed July 1, 2015.

Philbrook, Marilyn McLean. *Medical Books for the Layperson: An Annotated Bibliography*. Boston: Boston Public Library, 1976.

Phillips, Lauren B. *In the Name of the Patient: Consumer Advocacy in Health Care*. Chicago: National Society for Patient Representation and Consumer Affairs, 1995.

Pielke, Roger. *The Honest Broker: Making Sense of Science in Policy and Politics*. New York: Cambridge University Press, 2007.

Pierce, Russell. *Gringo Gaucho: An Advertising Odyssey*. Ashland, Ore.: Southern Cross, 1991.

Pinckney, Cathey, and Edward R. Pinckney. *The Patient's Guide to Medical Tests*. New York: Facts on File, 1982.

Pines, Wayne L. "New Challenges for Medical Product Promotion and Its Regulation." *Food and Drug Law Journal* 52 (1997): 61–65.

Pitofsky, Robert. "Beyond Nader: Consumer Protection and the Regulation of Advertising." *Harvard Law Review* 90 (February 1977): 661–701.

Pittman, David. "Concierge Medicine Gains Ground." *MedPage Today*, September 28, 2013. http://www.medpagetoday.com/MeetingCoverage/ AAFP/41936. Accessed July 1, 2015.

Piven, Frances Fox, and Richard A. Cloward. *Poor People's Movements: Why They Succeed, How They Fail*. New York: Vintage, 1979.

Podolsky, Doug. "America's Best Hospitals." *U.S. News and World Report*, August 5, 1991, 36–39.

Poen, Monte M. *Harry S. Truman versus the Medical Lobby: The Genesis of Medicare*. Columbia: University of Missouri Press, 1979.

Pollack, Craig E., Courtney Gidengil, and Ateev Mehrotra. "The Growth of Retail Clinics and the Medical Home." *Health Affairs* 29 (May 2010): 998–1003.

Poltrack, David. *Television Marketing: Network, Local, and Cable*. New York: McGraw Hill, 1983.

Pope, Tom. "FDA Reorganizes amid Generic Drug Scandal." *Management Review* 79 (February 1990): 36–40.

Porter, Roy. "Diseases of Civilization." In *Companion Encyclopedia of the History of Medicine*, edited by W. F. Bynum and Roy Porter. London: Routledge, 1993.

————. *Health for Sale: Quackery in England, 1660–1850*. Manchester: Manchester University Press, 1989.

"Postwar Project for Chain Drugstores." *Architectural Forum* 81 (October 1944): 114–15.

Potter, Samuel O. L., and R. J. E. Scott. *Therapeutics, Materia Medica, and Pharmacy.* 15th ed. rev. Philadelphia: Blakiston's, 1931.

"Practice-Building Offices." *Medical Economics* 5 (October 1927): 59–60.

Pray, W. Steven. *A History of Nonprescription Product Regulation*. Binghamton, N.Y.: Pharmaceutical Products Press, 2003.

Prentice, Kathy. "Airing Your Message in Doctors' Offices." *Media Life*, May 28, 2002. http://www.medialifemagazine.com:8080/news2002/may02/may27/2_tues/news5tuesday.html. Accessed July 1, 2015.

President's Commission on the Health Needs of the Nation. *Building America's Health: A Report to the President.* 5 vols. Washington, D.C.: President's Commission, 1952–53.

Preston, Lee, and Paul N. Bloom. "Concerns of the Rich/Poor Consumer." In *The Future of Consumerism*, edited by Paul N. Bloom and Ruth Belk Smith. Lexington, Mass.: Lexington Books, 1986.

Pringle, Henry F. "Aesculapius in Manhattan." *American Mercury*, March 1927, 364–69.

————. "What Do the Women of America Think about Medicine?" *Ladies' Home Journal*, September 1938, 14–15, 42–43.

Public Citizen and the Health Research Group. *A Consumer's Directory of Prince George's County Doctors*. Washington, D.C.: Public Citizen, 1974.

Pusey, William A. "Medical Education and Medical Service: Some Further Facts and Considerations." *Journal of the American Medical Association* 86 (May 15, 1926): 1501–8.

————. "The Old Time Country Doctor." *Journal of the American Medical Association* 85 (August 22, 1925): 580–84.

"Pushing Drugs to Doctors." *Consumer Reports*, February 1992, 87–94.

Quirke, Viviane, and Jean-Paul Gaudillière. "The Era of Biomedicine: Science, Medicine, and Public Health in Britain and France after the Second World War." *Medical History* 52 (October 2008): 441–52.

Rados, Carol. "Medical Device and Radiological Health Regulations Come of Age." *FDA Consumer Magazine* January–February 2006. http://www.fda.gov/aboutfda/whatwedo/history/productregulation/medicaldeviceandradiological healthregulationscomeofage/default.htm. Accessed July 1, 2015.

Raloff, Janet. "Drugs That Don't Work." *Science News* 119 (February 7, 1981): 92–93.

Rasmussen, Nicolas. *On Speed: The Many Lives of Amphetamine*. New York: New York University Press, 2008.

Ratcliff, J. D. "Aspirin: King of Drugs." *Coronet* 28 (June 1950): 30–32.

Reade, J. M., and R. M. Ratzan. "Yellow Professionalism: Advertising by Physicians in the Yellow Pages." *New England Journal of Medicine* 316 (May 21, 1987): 1315–19.

Reed, Louis S. Review of *American Medicine: Expert Testimony Out of Court*. *American Economic Review* 27 (September 1937): 611–13.

Rees, Alan M. "Communication in the Physician-Patient Relationship." *Bulletin of the Medical Library Association* 81 (January 1993): 1–10.

Rees, Alan M., and Blanche A. Young. *Consumer Health Information Source Book.* New York: Bowker, 1981.

Regier, Hilda. "Drug Labeling for Laymen?" *Journal of Legal Medicine* 4 (January 1976): 15–16.

Reidelbach, Maria. *Completely Mad: A History of the Comic Book and Magazine.* Boston: Little, Brown, 1991.

Relman, Arnold. "The New Medical-Industrial Complex." *New England Journal of Medicine* 303 (October 23, 1980): 963–70.

Remington, Joseph P. *The Practice of Pharmacy.* 4th ed. Philadelphia: Lippincott, 1905.

Remington, Joseph P., and E. Fullerton Cook. *Practice of Pharmacy.* Easton, Pa.: Mack, 1948.

Remington, Joseph P., E. Fullerton Cook, and Eric Wentworth Martin. *Remington's Practice of Pharmacy.* Easton, Pa.: Mack, 1951.

———. *Practice of Pharmacy.* Easton, Pa.: Mack, 1956.

"A Restrained Suburban Drugstore." *Architectural Forum* 88 (May 1948): 140.

Reverby, Susan. *Examining Tuskegee: The Infamous Syphilis Study and Its Legacy.* Chapel Hill: University of North Carolina Press, 2009.

———. "Stealing the Golden Eggs: Ernest Amory Codman and the Science and Management of Medicine." *Bulletin of the History of Medicine* 55 (Summer 1981): 156–71.

Reynolds, James A. "What If You're Listed in a Nader-Style Doctor Directory?" *Medical Economics* 51 (November 11, 1974): 290–93.

Ricciardi, Lygeia, Farzad Mostashari, Judy Murphy, Jodi G. Daniel, and Erin P. Siminerio. "A National Action Plan to Support Consumer Engagement via E-Health." *Health Affairs* 32 (February 2013): 376–84.

Rinehart, Stanley M. "The High Cost of Keeping Alive." *Saturday Evening Post,* January 9, 1926, 38–39, 92, 94, 96.

Risse, Guenter B., Ronald L. Numbers, and Judith Walzer Leavitt. *Medicine without Doctors: Home Health Care in American History.* New York: Science History Publications/USA, 1977.

Robert Graham Center. *Medical School Production of Primary Care Physicians Falls Far Short of Nation's Needs, Study Shows.* June 12, 2013. http://www.graham-center .org/online/graham/home/news-releases/2013/gmemapper.html. Accessed July 1, 2015.

Robins, Natalie S. *Copeland's Cure: Homeopathy and the War between Conventional and Alternative Medicine.* New York: Knopf, 2005.

Robinson, Leonard. "Don't Be Your Own Doctor." *Coronet* 48 (June 1960): 154–58.

Rodale, J. J. *The Health Finder: An Encyclopedia of Health Information from the Preventive Point-of-View.* Emmaus, Pa.: Rodale, 1954.

Rodwin, Marc A. *Conflicts of Interest and the Future of Medicine: The United States, France, and Japan.* New York: Oxford University Press, 2011.

———. *Medicine, Money, and Morals: Physicians' Conflicts of Interest.* New York: Oxford University Press, 1993.

Rogers, Carl R. "Significant Aspects of Client-Centered Therapy." *American Psychologist* 1 (October 1946): 415–22.

Rogers, Naomi. *An Alternative Path: The Making and Remaking of Hahnemann Medical College and Hospital.* New Brunswick, N.J.: Rutgers University Press, 1998.

———. "Caution: The AMA May Be Dangerous to Your Health." *Radical History Review* 80 (Spring 2001): 5–34.

———. *Polio Wars: Sister Kenny and the Golden Age of American Medicine.* New York: Oxford University Press, 2013.

Rorem, C. Rufus, and Robert F. Fischelis. *The Costs of Medicines: The Manufacture and Distribution of Drugs and Medicines in the United States and the Services of Pharmacy in Medical Care.* Chicago: University of Chicago Press, 1932.

Rorty, James. *American Medicine Mobilizes.* New York: Norton, 1939.

———. *Our Master's Voice.* New York: Day, 1934.

Rose, Nikolas. *The Politics of Life Itself: Biomedicine, Power, and Subjectivity in the Twenty-First Century.* Princeton: Princeton University Press, 2006.

Rosen, George. *Fees and Fee Bills: Some Economic Aspects of Medical Practice in Nineteenth Century America.* Baltimore: Johns Hopkins University Press, 1946.

Rosen, George, and Charles E. Rosenberg. *The Structure of American Medical Practice, 1875–1941.* Philadelphia: University of Pennsylvania Press, 1983.

Rosenberg, Charles. "The Book in the Sickroom." In *"Every Man His Own Doctor": Popular Medicine in Early America.* Essays by Charles E. Rosenberg and William H. Hefland. Philadelphia: Library Company, 1998.

———. *The Care of Strangers: The Rise of America's Hospital System.* New York: Basic Books, 1987.

———. *The Cholera Years: The United States in 1832, 1849, and 1866.* Chicago: University of Chicago Press, 1962.

———. "Codes Visible and Invisible: The Twentieth-Century Fate of a Nineteenth-Century Code." In *The American Medical Ethics Revolution,* edited by Robert Baker. Baltimore: Johns Hopkins University Press, 1999.

———. *Explaining Epidemics and Other Studies in the History of Medicine.* New York: Cambridge University Press, 1992.

———. "Health in the Home." In *Right Living: An Anglo-American Tradition of Self-Help Medicine and Hygiene,* edited by Charles E. Rosenberg. Baltimore: Johns Hopkins University Press, 2003.

———. "John Gunn: Everyman's Physician." In Rosenberg, *Explaining Epidemics and Other Studies in the History of Medicine.* New York: Cambridge University Press, 1992.

———. "Medical Text and Social Context: Explaining William Buchan's Domestic Medicine." In Rosenberg, *Explaining Epidemics and Other Studies in the History of Medicine.* New York: Cambridge University Press, 1992.

———. *No Other Gods: On Science and American Social Thought.* Baltimore: Johns Hopkins University Press, 1976.

————. *Our Present Complaint: American Medicine, Past and Present.* Baltimore: Johns Hopkins University Press, 2007.

————. "The Practice of Medicine in New York City a Century Ago." In Rosenberg, *Explaining Epidemics and Other Studies in the History of Medicine.* New York: Cambridge University Press, 1992.

————. "The Therapeutic Revolution: Medicine, Meaning, and Social Change in Nineteenth-Century America." In *The Therapeutic Revolution,* edited by Morris Vogel and Charles Rosenberg. Philadelphia: University of Pennsylvania Press, 1979.

————. *The Trial of the Assassin, Guiteau: Psychiatry and Law in the Gilded Age.* Chicago: University of Chicago Press, 1968.

————, ed. *Healing and History: Essays for George Rosen.* New York: Science History and Dawson, 1979.

————, ed. *Right Living: An Anglo-American Tradition of Self-Help Medicine and Hygiene.* Baltimore: Johns Hopkins University Press, 2003.

Rosenberg, Charles, and Janet Golden. *Pictures of Health: A Photographic History of Health Care in Philadelphia, 1860–1945.* Philadelphia: University of Pennsylvania Press, 1991.

Ross, Mary. "The Issue of Health." *Survey Graphic,* December 1934, 581.

Rothman, David. *Beginnings Count: The Technological Imperative in American Health Care.* New York: Oxford University Press, 1997.

————. "The Public Presentation of Blue Cross, 1935–1965." *Journal of Health Politics, Policy, and Law* 16 (Winter 1991): 671–93.

————. *Strangers at the Bedside: A History of How Law and Bioethics Transformed Medical Decision Making.* New York: Basic Books, 1991.

Rothman, David, and Sheila M. Rothman. *The Willowbrook Wars.* New York: Harper and Row, 1984.

Rothman, Sheila M. *Living in the Shadow of Death: Tuberculosis and the Social Experience of Illness in American History.* New York: Basic Books, 1994.

Rothstein, William G. *American Physicians in the Nineteenth Century: From Sects to Science.* Baltimore: Johns Hopkins University Press, 1972.

————. *Public Health and the Risk Factor: A History of an Uneven Medical Revolution.* Rochester: University of Rochester Press, 2008.

————. "When Did a Random Patient Benefit from a Random Physician?" *Caduceus* 12 (Winter 1996): 2–8.

Roueché, Berton. "Ten Feet Tall." *New Yorker,* September 10, 1955, 47–48, 50–51, 54–56, 58–60, 62, 65–69, 71–72, 74–77.

Rowe, Frederick M. "The Decline of Antitrust and the Delusions of Models: The Faustian Pact of Law and Economics." *Georgetown Law Journal* 72 (June 1984): 1511–70.

Rowe, Howard M. "Patient Package Inserts: The Proper Prescription?" *Food and Drug Law Journal* 50 (1995): 95–124.

Rowell, Hugh Grant. "How to Get Your Money's Worth from Your Doctor." *American Magazine,* May 1931, 76–77, 100.

Rozovsky, Faye. *Consent to Treatment: A Practical Guide.* 2nd ed. Boston: Little, Brown, 1990.

Rubinow, I. M. "In Defense of Socialized Medicine." *The Nation,* May 2, 1928, 508–10.

Ruderman, Florence A. "A Placebo for the Doctor." *Commentary* 69 (May 1980): 54–60.

Ruzek, Sheryl Burt. *The Women's Health Movement: Feminist Alternatives to Medical Control.* New York: Praeger, 1978.

Saad, Lydia. *On Healthcare, Americans Trust Physicians over Politicians.* June 17, 2009. http://www.gallup.com/poll/120890/healthcare-americans-trust-physicians-politicians.aspx. Accessed July 1, 2015.

"Sale of Dangerous Drugs Restricted by New Law." *Public Health Reports* 67 (March 1952): 292.

Salsberg, Edward S., and Gaetano J. Forte. "Trends in the Physician Workforce, 1980–2000." *Health Affairs* 21 (September/October 2002): 165–73.

Saltzstein, Harry. "Cancer—Its Status Today." *Hygeia* 12 (March 1934): 218–20.

Sanders, Marion K., ed. *The Crisis in American Medicine.* New York: Harper, 1961.

Sandroff, Ronni. "Got Side Effects?" *Consumer Reports,* June 2008, 2.

Sanjek, Roger. *Gray Panthers.* Philadelphia: University of Pennsylvania Press, 2009.

Sardell, Alice. *The U.S. Experiment in Social Medicine: The Community Health Center Program, 1965–1986.* Pittsburgh: University of Pittsburgh Press, 1988.

Scalise, Dagmara. "Patient Satisfaction and the New Consumer." *Hospitals and Health Networks* 80 (December 2006): 57, 59–62.

Schacht, Wendy H., and John R. Thomas. "Patent Law and Its Application to the Pharmaceutical Industry." Congressional Research Service Report for Congress, January 10, 2005. http://www.law.umaryland.edu/marshall/crsreports/crsdocuments/rl3075601102005.pdf. Accessed July 1, 2015.

Schafer, James A., Jr. *The Business of Private Medical Practice: Doctors, Specialization, and Urban Change in Philadelphia, 1900–1940.* New Brunswick, N.J.: Rutgers University Press, 2013.

Schiedermayer, D. L. "The Hippocratic Oath—Corporate Version." *New England Journal of Medicine* 314 (January 2, 1986): 62.

Schlesinger, Mark. "The Dangers of the Market Panacea." In *Healthy, Wealthy, and Fair: Health Care and the Good Society,* edited by James A. Morone and Lawrence R. Jacobs. New York: Oxford University Press, 2005.

Schluster, Daniel H. "FDA's Experience with Patient Package Inserts: A Program That Just Won't Go Away." 1995. Unpublished paper in author's possession originally downloaded from http://leda.law.harvard.edu/leda/data/95/dschlust.html.

Schmidt, Alexander M. Interview by James Harvey Young and Robert G. Porter, March 8–9, 1985. http://www.fda.gov/downloads/AboutFDA/WhatWeDo/History/OralHistories/SelectedOralHistoryTranscripts/UCM264361.pdf. Accessed July 1, 2015.

Schnabel, Truman G. "Esther Everett Lape—The American Foundation, and American Medicine 50 Years Ago." *Transactions of the American Clinical and Climatological Association* 110 (1999): 62–72.

Schoenfeld, Eugene. *Advice Your Family Doctor Never Gave You.* New York: Grove, 1968.

Schorr, Daniel. *Don't Get Sick in America*. Nashville: Aurora, 1970.

———. *Staying Tuned: A Life in Journalism*. New York: Pocket Books, 2001.

Schudson, Michael. *Advertising: The Uneasy Persuasion*. New York: Basic Books, 1982.

———. *Watergate in American Memory: How We Remember, Forget, and Reconstruct the Past*. New York: Basic Books, 1992.

Schwartz, Barry. *The Paradox of Choice: Why More Is Less*. New York: HarperCollins, 2004.

Schwartz, Howard D., and Cary S. Kart. "The Changing Role of the Patient: The Patient as Consumer." In *Dominant Issues in Medical Sociology*, edited by Howard D. Schwartz and Cary S. Kart. Reading, Mass.: Addison-Wesley, 1978.

Scroop, Daniel. "A Faded Passion? Estes Kefauver and the Senate Subcommittee on Antitrust and Monopoly," *Business and Economic History* 5 (2007). http://www .thebhc.org/sites/default/files/scroop.pdf. Accessed July 1, 2015.

Seaman, Barbara. *The Doctors' Case against the Pill*. 25th anniv. ed. Alameda, Calif.: Hunter House, 1995.

Sehnert, Keith W. "A Course for Activated Patients." *Social Policy* 8, no. 3 (1980): 40–46.

Sehnert, Keith W., and Howard Eisenberg. *How to Be Your Own Doctor (Sometimes)*. New York: Grosset and Dunlap, 1975.

"Self Service Reaches the Drugstore." *Business Week*, March 7, 1953, 43–44.

Shapiro, Howard S. *How to Keep Them Honest: Herbert Denenberg on Spotting the Professional Phonies, Unscrewing Insurance, and Protecting Your Interests*. Emmaus, Pa.: Rodale, 1974.

Shapiro, Joseph P. *No Pity: People with Disabilities Forging a New Civil Rights Movement*. New York: Times Books, 1993.

Shepard, C. David, and Daniel Fell. "Marketing on the Internet." *Journal of Health Care Marketing* 15 (Winter 1995): 12–15.

"Should Prescription Drug Ads Be Reined In?" *Room for Debate: A New York Times Blog*, August 4, 2009. http://roomfordebate.blogs.nytimes.com/2009/08/04/ should-prescription-drug-ads-be-reined-in/?_r=0. Accessed July 1, 2015.

Shryock, Richard Harrison. *Medical Licensing in America, 1650–1965*. Baltimore: Johns Hopkins University Press, 1967.

———. *Medicine and Society in America, 1660–1860*. New York: New York University Press, 1960.

Shumsky, Neil Larry, James Bohland, and Paul Knox. "Separating Doctors' Homes and Doctors' Offices: San Francisco, 1881–1941." *Social Science and Medicine* 23, no. 10 (1986): 1051–57.

Silber, Norman. *Test and Protest: The Influence of Consumers Union*. New York: Holmes and Meier, 1983.

Silverman, Milton, and Philip R. Lee. *Pills, Profits, and Politics*. Berkeley: University of California Press, 1974.

Sinai, Nathan, Maurice Leven, Kathryn Robertson, and Elizabeth Sulloway. *A Survey of the Medical Facilities of San Joaquin County, California, 1929*. Chicago: University of Chicago Press, 1931.

Sivulka, Juliann. *Soap, Sex, and Cigarettes: A Cultural History of American Advertising*. 2nd ed. Boston: Wadsworth, Cengage Learning, 2012.

Sizemore, Lula, and Allison Sizemore. Interview by Claude V. Dunnagan, November 8, 1938. U.S. Work Projects Administration, Federal Writers' Project (Folklore Project, Life Histories, 1936–39), Manuscript Division, Library of Congress. http://hdl.loc.gov/loc.mss/wpalh2.27030109. Accessed July 1, 2015.

Sloan, Frank A. "Effects of Health Insurance on Physicians' Fees." *Journal of Human Resources* 17 (Fall 1982): 533–57.

Sloan, Frank A., and Lindsey M. Chepke. *Medical Malpractice.* Cambridge, Mass.: MIT Press, 2008.

Sloane, David, and Beverlee Sloane. *Medicine Moves to the Mall.* Baltimore: Johns Hopkins University Press, 2003.

Smith, Austin. "The Changing Health Care Scene." *Vital Speeches* 39 (December 1972): 98–103.

———. "Doctors Say . . ." *Hygeia* 22 (September 1944): 658–59, 696, 698.

———. "The Health of the Nation: The Stewardship of the Pharmaceutical Industry." *Vital Speeches* 26 (January 15, 1960): 210–15.

Smith, Dale. "Appendicitis, Appendectomy, and the Surgeon." *Bulletin of the History of Medicine* 70 (Fall 1996): 414–41.

Smith, Mark D., et al., eds. *Best Care at Lower Cost: The Path to Continuously Learning Health Care in America.* Washington, D.C.: National Academies Press, 2012.

Smith, Mickey C. *The Rexall Story: A History of Genius and Neglect.* New York: Pharmaceutical Products Press, 2004.

———. *Small Comfort: A History of the Minor Tranquilizers.* New York: Praeger, 1985.

Smith, W. Eugene. "The Country Doctor." *Life*, September 20, 1948, 115–26.

Snow, Margie. "Open for Business." *Health Facilities Management* 25 (July 2012): 29–32.

Somers, Anne Ramsay. *Promoting Health: Consumer Education and National Policy: Report of the Task Force on Consumer Health Education.* Germantown, Md.: Aspen, 1976.

Somers, Herman, and Anne Somers. *Doctors, Patients, and Health Insurance: The Organization and Financing of Medical Care.* Washington, D.C.: Brookings Institution, 1961.

Sommers, Roseanna, Susan Dorr Goold, Elizabeth A. McGlynn, Steven D. Pearson, and Marion Danis. "Focus Groups Highlight That Many Patients Object to Clinicians' Focusing on Costs." *Health Affairs* 32 (February 2013): 338–46.

Sonnedecker, Glenn. *Kremers and Urdang's History of Pharmacy.* 4th ed. Madison, Wis.: American Institute for the History of Pharmacy, 1986.

Sontag, Susan. *Illness as Metaphor.* New York: Farrar, Straus, and Giroux, 1978.

Speaker, Susan. "From 'Happiness Pills' to 'National Nightmare': Changing Cultural Assessment of Minor Tranquilizers." *Journal of the History of Medicine and Allied Sciences* 52 (July 1997): 338–76.

Spears, Jack. *Hollywood: The Golden Era.* New York: Castle, 1971.

"Special Procedure in Certain Types of Advertising Cases." In *Annual Report of the Federal Trade Commission, 1938.* Washington, D.C.: U.S. Government Printing Office, 1938.

Squires, David. *The U.S. Health System in Perspective: A Comparison of Twelve Industrialized Nations.* New York: Commonwealth Fund, 2011. http://www

.commonwealthfund.org/publications/issue-briefs/2011/jul/us-health-system-in-perspective. Accessed July 1, 2015.

Starr, Paul. *Remedy and Reaction: The Peculiar American Struggle over Health Care Reform*. Rev. ed. New Haven: Yale University Press, 2013.

———. *The Social Transformation of American Medicine*. New York: Basic Books, 1982.

"State Regulation of Drugs: Who May Sell 'Patent and Proprietary' Medicines." *Yale Law Journal* 63, no. 4 (February 1954): 550–59.

Steiner, Gary A. *The People Look at Television: A Study of Audience Attitudes*. New York: Knopf, 1963.

Steinhart, Yael, Ziv Carmon, and Yaacov Trope. "Warnings of Adverse Side Effects Can Backfire over Time." *Psychological Science* 24 (September 2013): 1842–47.

Stevens, M. L. Tina. *Bioethics in America: Origins and Cultural Politics*. Baltimore: Johns Hopkins University Press, 2000.

Stevens, Rosemary. *American Medicine and the Public Interest*. Updated ed. Berkeley: University of California Press, 1998.

———. *In Sickness and in Wealth: American Hospitals in the Twentieth Century*. New York: Basic Books, 1989.

Stevens, Rosemary, Charles E. Rosenberg, and Lawton R. Burns, eds. *History and Health Policy in the United States: Putting the Past Back In*. New Brunswick, N.J.: Rutgers University Press, 2006.

Stone, Brad. "Fast Tracking the First AIDS Drug." *FDA Consumer* 21 (October 1987): 13–15.

Stout, Wesley. "Alagazam, The Story of Pitchmen, High and Low." *Saturday Evening Post*, October 19, 1929, 26.

Strasser, Susan. "A Historical Herbal: Healing with Plants in a Developing Consumer Culture." Unpublished manuscript.

———. *Satisfaction Guaranteed: The Making of the American Mass Market*. Washington, D.C.: Smithsonian Institution Press, 1989.

———. "Sponsorship and Snake Oil: Medicine Shows and Contemporary Public Culture." In *Public Culture: Diversity, Democracy, and Community in the United States*, edited by Marguerite S. Shaffer. Philadelphia: University of Pennsylvania Press, 2008.

Strout, Richard Lee. "The Radio Nostrum Racket." *Nation*, July 17, 1935, 65–66.

"Study Reveals Too Few Grievance Committees." *Medical Economics* 30 (December 1953): 278, 280–81.

Sullivan, Mark. *The Education of an American*. New York: Doubleday, Doran, 1938.

Swackhamer, Gladys V. *Choice and Change of Doctors: A Study of the Consumer of Medical Services*. New York: Committee on Research in Medical Economics, 1939.

Swan, Carroll J. "New Packages Aid Shift to National Advertising." *Printers' Ink*, June 25, 1948, 32–33, 56, 61.

Swann, John. "The 1941 Sulfathiazole Disaster and the Birth of Good Manufacturing Practices." *Pharmacy in History* 40, no. 1 (1999): 16–25.

———. "FDA and the Practice of Pharmacy: Prescription Drug Regulation to 1951." *Pharmacy in History* 36, no. 2 (1994): 55–70.

Szasz, Thomas, and Marc Hollender. "A Contribution to the Philosophy of Medicine: The Basic Models of the Doctor-Patient Relationship." *Archives of Internal Medicine* 97 (May 1956): 585–92.

Tannenbaum, Samuel A., and Paul M. Branden. *The Patient's Dilemma: A Public Trial of the Medical Profession.* New York: Coward-McCann, 1935.

Taylor, Rosemary C. R. "Free Medicine." In *Co-Ops, Communes, and Collectives: Experiments in Social Change in the 1960s and 1970s,* edited by John Case and Rosemary C. R. Taylor. New York: Pantheon, 1979.

Temin, Peter. *Taking Your Medicine: Drug Regulation in the United States.* Cambridge, Mass.: Harvard University Press, 1980.

Temkin-Greener, Helen. "Medicaid Families under Managed Care." *Medical Care* 24 (August 1986): 721–32.

[Tennent, John]. *Every Man His Own Doctor; or, The Poor Planter's Physician.* 2nd ed. Williamsburg, Va.: Parks, 1734.

Thaler, Richard H., and Cass R. Sunstein. *Nudge: Improving Decisions about Health, Wealth, and Happiness.* New Haven: Yale University Press, 2008.

Theoharis, Athan, ed. *A Culture of Secrecy: The Government versus the People's Right to Know.* Lawrence: University Press of Kansas, 1998.

Thomas, Karen Kruse. *Deluxe Jim Crow: Civil Rights and American Health Policy, 1935–1954.* Athens: University of Georgia Press, 2011.

Thomasson, Melissa A. "From Sickness to Health: The Twentieth-Century Development of U.S. Health Insurance." *Explorations in Economic History* 39 (July 2002): 233–53.

———. "The Importance of Group Coverage: How Tax Policy Shaped U.S. Health Insurance." *American Economic Review* 93 (September 2003): 1373–84.

Thompson, Morton. *Not as a Stranger.* New York: Scribner, 1954.

"Time to Get That Step Fixed." *Medical Economics* 28 (August 1951): 63.

Tobbell, Dominique A. *Pills, Power, and Policy: The Struggle for Drug Reform in Cold War America and Its Consequences.* Berkeley: University of California Press, 2012.

Toffler, Alvin. *Future Shock.* New York: Bantam, 1970.

Tomes, Nancy. *The Gospel of Germs: Men, Women, and the Microbe in American Life.* Cambridge, Mass.: Harvard University Press, 1998.

———. "The Great American Medicine Show Revisited." *Bulletin of the History of Medicine* 79 (Winter 2005): 627–63.

———. "The Information RX: Historical Perspectives, Contemporary Challenges." In *Medical Professionalism in the New Information Age,* edited by David Blumenthal and David J. Rothman. New Brunswick, N.J.: Rutgers University Press, 2010.

———. "Merchants of Health: Medicine and Consumer Culture in the United States, 1900–1940." *Journal of American History* 88 (September 2001): 519–47.

———. "The Patient as a Policy Factor: A Historical Case Study of the Consumer-Survivor Movement in Mental Health." *Health Affairs* 25 (May–June 2006): 720–29.

———. "Patients or Health Care Consumers? Why the History of Contested Terms Matters." In *History and Health Policy in the United States: Putting the Past Back In,* edited by Rosemary Stevens, Charles E. Rosenberg, and Lawton R. Burns. New Brunswick, N.J.: Rutgers University Press, 2006.

———. "Reshuffling the Cards: Reflections on the New Disease Order in the Interwar United States." Unpublished manuscript.

———. "An Undesired Necessity: The Commodification of Medical Service in Interwar America." In *Commodifying Everything: Relations of the Market*, edited by Susan Strasser. New York: Routledge, 2003.

Tone, Andrea. *The Age of Anxiety: A History of America's Turbulent Affair with Tranquilizers*. New York: Basic Books, 2009.

———. *Devices and Desires: A History of Contraceptives in America*. New York: Hill and Wang, 2001.

"Too Many Wrong Ideas about Doctors" (interview with Dr. R. B. Robins). *U.S. News and World Report*, April 3, 1953, 44–51.

Toon, Elizabeth. "Managing the Conduct of the Individual Life: Public Health Education and American Public Health, 1910 to 1940." Ph.D. diss., University of Pennsylvania, 1998.

Trafford, Abigail. "As Controversy Mounts over Hospitals-for-Profit." *U.S. News and World Report*, December 10, 1984, 61–62.

Tu, Ha T., and Catherine Corey. "State Prescription Drug Price Websites: How Useful to Consumers?" *HSC Research Brief*, February 2008. http://www.hschange .com/CONTENT/966/. Accessed July 1, 2015.

Turner, Judith A. "Consumer Report/FDA Pursues Historic Role amid Public, Industry Pressures." *National Journal Reports* 7 (February 15, 1975): 250–59.

Turow, Joseph. *Playing Doctor: Television, Storytelling, and Medical Power*. Ann Arbor: University of Michigan Press, 2010.

Twerski, Aaron D. "Liability for Direct Advertising of Drugs to Consumers: An Idea Whose Time Has Not Come." *Hofstra Law Review* 33 (Summer 2005): 1149–54.

Ulrich, Laurel Thatcher. *A Midwife's Tale: The Life of Martha Ballard, Based on Her Diary, 1785–1812*. New York: Knopf, 1990.

Underground Newspaper Collection. Ann Arbor: University Microfilms International, 1963–85.

"Unique Survey." *Business Week*, November 25, 1944, 88.

U.S. Congress. House. Committee on Interstate and Foreign Commerce. Hearings on Federal Food, Drug, and Cosmetic Act. 82nd Cong., 1st sess., May 1–5, 1951.

U.S. Congress. Senate. Committee on the Judiciary. *Administered Prices: Drugs: Report of the Committee on the Judiciary, United States Senate, Made by Its Sub-committee on Antitrust and Monopoly, Pursuant to S. Res. 52*. 87th Cong., 1st sess., June 27, 1961.

U.S. Federal Trade Commission. *Drug Product Selection: Staff Report to the Federal Trade Commission*. Washington, D.C.: Bureau of Consumer Protection, 1979.

U.S. Food and Drug Administration. "Proposed Rule. Prescription Drugs Products: Patient Labeling Requirements." *Federal Register* 44, no. 131 (July 6, 1979), 40016–41.

"U.S. Medicine in Transition." *Fortune*, December 1944, 156–63, 184–93.

U.S. Office of Technology Assessment. *Defensive Medicine and Medical Malpractice*. Washington, D.C.: U.S. Government Printing Office, 1994.

U.S. Task Force on Prescription Drugs. *Final Report*. Washington, D.C.: Office of the Secretary, Department of Health, Education, and Welfare, 1969.

"Use of, and Satisfaction with, C.M.A. Relative Value Studies by Physicians in Active Practice in California." *California Medicine* 97 (November 1962): 323–25.

Vares, Tina. "Viagra and 'Getting It Up.'" *M/C: A Journal of Media and Culture* 5 (November 2003). http://journal.media-culture.org.au/0311/7-vares-viagra.php. Accessed July 1, 2015.

Vernon, John, Antonio Trujillo, Sara Rosenbaum, and Barbara DeBuono. *Low Health Literacy: Implications for National Health Policy*. October 2007. http://hsrc .himmelfarb.gwu.edu/sphhs_policy_facpubs/172. Accessed July 1, 2015.

Veteran Patient. "Some Dressing Rooms I've Seen." *Medical Economics* 5 (December 1927): 19, 21.

Vickery, Donald M., and James F. Fries. *Take Care of Yourself: A Consumer's Guide to Medical Care*. Reading, Mass.: Addison-Wesley, 1976.

———. *Take Care of Yourself: Your Personal Guide to Self-Care and Preventing Illness*. 4th ed. Reading, Mass.: Addison-Wesley, 1989.

Vincent, Terry S. "Patient Package Inserts—Like It or Not, Here They Come!" *Medical Times* 104 (December 1976): 133–38.

Vogl, A. J. "See Yourself as Ralph Nader Sees You." *Medical Economics* 51 (April 1, 1974): 141–46, 153–54, 159, 162–63, 166–67, 171–73, 176.

Wailoo, Keith. *How Cancer Crossed the Color Line*. Oxford: Oxford University Press, 2011.

———. *Pain: A Political History*. Baltimore: Johns Hopkins University Press, 2014.

Walker, Edward T. *Grassroots for Hire: Public Affairs Consultants in American Democracy*. New York: Cambridge University Press, 2014.

Wallace, C. R. "How Prosperous Should You Look?" *Medical Economics* 37 (November 1960): 282–88.

Walsh, Charles, and Alissa Pyrich. "FDA Regulation of Pharmaceutical Advertising." *Seton Hall Law Review* 24 (1994): 1325–35.

Walsh, James J. "Medicine Men." *Commonweal*, April 15, 1938, 685–86.

Walters, Orville S. "Show Them What They're Paying For." *Medical Economics* 28 (January 1951): 59, 203–5.

Ward, George Gray. "What You Should Know about Cancer." *Hygeia* 14 (September 1936): 822–24.

Ward, Patricia Spain. "In Recognition of Esther Everett Lape." *Women and Health* 5 (Summer 1980): 1–3.

———. "United States versus American Medical Association et al.: The Medical Antitrust Case of 1938–1943." *American Studies* 30 (Fall 1989): 123–53.

Warner, John Harley. "The Aesthetic Grounding of Modern Medicine." *Bulletin of the History of Medicine* 88 (Spring 2014): 1–47.

Watkins, Elizabeth Siegel. "'Doctor, Are You Trying to Kill Me?' Ambivalence about the Patient Package Insert for Estrogen." *Bulletin of the History of Medicine* 76 (Spring 2002): 84–104.

———. *The Estrogen Elixir: A History of Hormone Replacement Therapy in America*. Baltimore: Johns Hopkins University Press, 2007.

————. *On the Pill: A Social History of Contraceptives.* Baltimore: Johns Hopkins University Press, 1998.

"We Die Differently Now." *Literary Digest* 113 (June 18, 1932): 26.

Weems, Robert E., Jr. *Desegregating the Dollar: African American Consumerism in the Twentieth Century.* New York: New York University Press, 1998.

Weisman, Carol Sachs. *Women's Health Care: Activist Traditions and Institutional Change.* Baltimore: Johns Hopkins University Press, 1998.

Weiss, Edward H. "A New Slant on Buying." *Challenge* 1 (September 1953): 36–40.

Weisz, George. *Divide and Conquer: A Comparative History of Medical Specialization.* Oxford: Oxford University Press, 2006.

————. "Epidemiology and Health Care Reform: The National Health Survey of 1935–1936." *American Journal of Public Health* 101 (March 2011): 438–47.

————. *The Medical Mandarins: The French Academy of Medicine in the Nineteenth and Early Twentieth Centuries.* New York: Oxford University Press, 1995.

Welke, Barbara. "The Cowboy Suit Tragedy: Spreading Risk, Owning Hazard in the Modern American Consumer Economy." *Journal of American History* 101 (June 2014): 97–121.

"A Well-Equipped Office Is a Sound Investment." *Medical Economics* 5 (October 1927): 22.

Wendt, Diane, and Eric W. Jentsch. "The Pharmacy Collections." *Caduceus: A Museum Quarterly for the Health Sciences* 13 (Winter 1997): 33–42.

Werner, Rachel M., and D. A. Asch. "The Unintended Consequences of Publicly Reporting Quality Information." *Journal of the American Medical Association* 293 (March 9, 2005): 1239–44.

Wertheimer, Albert I. "A Prescription Is Not a Simple Matter Anymore." *American Journal of Public Health* 73 (August 1983): 844–45.

"What Americans Spend." *Medical Economics* 32 (June 1955): 102–3.

"When Patients Know What's Good for Them." *AEI Journal on Government and Society* 5 (Fall 1981): 6–10.

"Where Are All the Salesclerks? Look Again!" *American Magazine* 156 (September 1953): 119.

White, Paul D. "Heart Disease—Then and Now." *Hygeia* 11 (October 1933): 877–80, 950–52.

"Whoever Shouts the Loudest Still Sells the Most." Howard Fulcher, interview by Susan Levitas, August 17, 1994. Working in Patterson Project Collection, American Folklife Center, Library of Congress. http://hdl.loc.gov/loc.afc/afcwip .sla01506. Accessed July 1, 2015.

Whole Earth Catalog. Menlo Park, Calif.: Portola, 1968.

Whorton, James C. *Inner Hygiene: Constipation and the Pursuit of Health in Modern Society.* New York: Oxford University Press, 2001.

————. *Nature Cures: The History of Alternative Medicine in America.* Oxford: Oxford University Press, 2002.

"Why M.D.s Have a Tough Time Explaining Fees." *Medical Economics* 37 (July 18, 1960): 60–61.

"Why the Doc's Bills Aren't Paid." *Medical Economics* 5 (October 1927): 65.

Wilkes, M. S., R. A. Bell, and R. L. Kravitz. "Direct-to-Consumer Prescription Drug Advertising: Trends, Impact, and Implications." *Health Affairs* 19 (March–April 2000): 110–28.

Williams, Greer. "How to Choose Your Doctor." *Hygeia* 20 (June 1942): 430–32.

——. "Unjustified Surgery." *Harper's*, February 1954, 35–41.

Williams, Lawrence P. *How to Avoid Unnecessary Surgery.* Los Angeles: Nash, 1971.

Williams, Linsly R. "Your Doctor's Bill." *Collier's*, October 3, 1931, 21, 28.

Wilson, Natalia A., Eugene S. Schneller, Kathleen Montgomery, and Kevin J. Bozic. "Hip and Knee Implants: Current Trends and Policy Considerations." *Health Affairs* 27 (November 2008): 1587–98.

Wilson, Sloan. *The Man in the Gray Flannel Suit.* New York: Simon and Schuster, 1955.

Wolfe, Audra. *Competing with the Soviets: Science, Technology, and the State in Cold War America.* Baltimore: Johns Hopkins University Press, 2012.

Wolfe, Sidney M., Christopher M. Coley, and Public Citizen Health Research Group. *Pills That Don't Work: A Consumers' and Doctors' Guide to 610 Prescription Drugs That Lack Evidence of Effectiveness.* Washington, D.C.: Public Citizen's Health Research Group, 1980.

Wolfe, Sidney M., Lisa Fugate, Elizabeth P. Hulstrand, and Laurie E. Kamimoto. *Worst Pills, Best Pills: The Older Adult's Guide to Avoiding Drug-Induced Death or Illness.* Washington, D.C.: Public Citizen, 1988.

"Women Who." *off our backs* 1 (August 31, 1971): 8.

Woolley, Ernest S. *Physicians' Systems: A Short Course of Business Instructions for the Doctor and His Assistant.* Kansas City, Mo.: Physicians Pub. Co., 1928.

Wright, Harold N., and Mildred L. Montag. *A Textbook of Materia Medica, Pharmacology, and Therapeutics.* Philadelphia: W. B. Saunders Co., 1939.

Wylie, Philip. "The Doctors' Conspiracy of Silence." *Redbook*, March 1952, 24–25, 90–94.

Yegian, J. M., P. Dardess, M. Shannon, and K. L. Carman. "Engaged Patients Will Need Comparative Physician-Level Quality Data and Information about Their Out-of-Pocket Costs." *Health Affairs* 32 (February 2013): 328–37.

Young, James H. *The Medical Messiahs: A Social History of Health Quackery in Twentieth-Century America.* Princeton: Princeton University Press, 1967.

——. *Pure Food: Securing the Federal Food and Drugs Act of 1906.* Princeton: Princeton University Press, 1989.

——. *The Toadstool Millionaires: A Social History of Patent Medicines in America before Federal Regulation.* Princeton: Princeton University Press, 1961.

Younkin, Peter. "Making the Market: How the American Pharmaceutical Industry Transformed Itself during the 1940s." http://www.irle.berkeley.edu/culture/papers/Younkin-Mar08.pdf. Accessed July 1, 2015.

Zussman, Robert. *Intensive Care: Medical Ethics and the Medical Profession.* Chicago: University of Chicago Press, 1994.

INDEX

Numbers in italic refer to illustrations.

American Health Empire, The (Health Policy Advisory Center), 258
American Hospital Association (AHA), 179, 259, 271, 272, 332
American Medical Association (AMA): activism against, 258–60; advertising and, 93–94, 120–21; antitrust and, 130; Committee of Physicians for the Improvement of Medical Care and, 126; Committee on the Costs of Medical Care and, 75; consumer education by, 93–95; Council on Pharmacy and Chemistry, 231, 426 (n. 30); Cousins Affair and, 309–10; decline of, 330; formation of, 22–23; FTC and, 295–96, 331; Hawley Affair and, 183–84; Health in America documentary and, 269; health insurance and, 142–43; increasing influence of, 50; labeling legislation and, 115; Medicare/Medicaid and, 255, 256; National Welfare Rights Organization and, 270–71; public relations efforts of, 177, 187; Pure Food and Drugs Act and, 34–35; state medical societies and, 26–27
American Medicine: Expert Testimony Out of Court (American Foundation), 125–26
American Medicine Mobilizes (Rorty), 124
American Patient, 266
American Patients Association, 12, 144, 417, 424 (n. 14), 438 (n.15)
American Pharmaceutical Association, 32, 59, 96, 97, 153–54
American Pharmaceutical Manufacturers Association, 153–54
American Revolution, 20
"American way of life," 11
Amphetamines, 151, 155, 314
Anthony, Norman, 103
Antibiotics, 149, 150, 155, 166, 172, 185, 235, 244; marketing of, 150, 238, 240; price-fixing of, 241, 450 (n. 8)
Antipsychotics, 447 (n. 41)
Antitrust, 130, 142–43, 149

Appel, James, 197
Appendectomy, 59, 68, 180, 212
Apprenticeships, 21
Architecture, 169–70, 207, 222
Armstrong, Donald, 65, 70, 430 (n. 61)
Arnold, Denis G., 417
Arnold, Thurman, 130
Arrowsmith (Lewis), 70
Arsenic Act (United Kingdom), 25
Ask-A-Nurse, 332–33
Aspirin, 85, 224–25
Assembly line, 74
Authoritarian Personality, The (Adorno), 162
Automobile industry, 4, 242, 265, 420
Automobiles: as consumer good, 4, 38, 66, 163, 178, 209, 222; imagery of used in medicine, 1, 2, 41, 66, 71–72, 102, 157, 176, 180–81, 189, 238, 243, 251, 258, 306, 383, 389, 390, 417
Autonomy, 9, 10, 134, 162, 230, 242, 288, 312–13, 322, 329–30
Ayres, William H., 233

Baby boomers, 290–91, 417, 455 (n. 9)
Bailey, William J., 71
Baker, John Newton, 178
Baker, Norman, 65, 429 (n. 48)
Baketel, H. Sheridan, 54, 180
Baldwin, Louise, 117
Ballard, Martha, 21
Balliett, Gene, 338, 341
Banting, Frederick, 85
Barbiturates, 151, 152, 153, 155
Barclay, William, 316
Barker, Karlyn, 345
Barnes, Frederick, 320
Barnett, E. Dwight, 179
Bates v. State Bar of Arizona, 296
Baxter, Lenore, 143–44, 177
Baylor Hospital, 141
Bazell, Robert J., 287
Beals, Dick, 228
Bebinger, Martha, 414
Bedrosian, John, 323

CCMC. *See* Committee on the Costs of Medical Care
Celebrities, 88, 381
Center for Law and Social Policy, 314
Center for Science in the Public Interest, 264
Center for Study of Responsive Law, 265
Center for the Study of Civil Liberties and Civil Rights, 280
Centers for Medicare and Medicaid Services, 326–27
Ceriani, Ernest, 163
Chaney, Lon, 40
Chase, Stuart, 102, 108, 134
"Cherry picking," 353
Chiropractic, 27, 118, 160
Chisari, Francis, 300
Chloromycetin, 235, 237
Chlorpromazine, 236
Christian Science, 118, 160
Christy, Jack, 348
Cigarettes, 4, 14, 38, 42, 56, 76, 94, 104, 120, 160, 206, 238, 251, 257, 319
Ciphers, 99
Cities, doctors' offices in, 54–55
Citizens' Advisory Committee (FDA), 233–34
Clendenning, Logan, 44
Clinics: community, 260–62; retail, 394; walk-in, 321–22, 338
Clinton, Bill, 355–56, 382
Clinton, Hillary, 355–56
Cochrane, Archie, 357
Cochrane Collaboration, 357
Code of ethics, of AMA, 23, 331
Coding, 181
Codman, Ernest Armory, 311, 458 (n. 68)
Cohen, Wilbur, 255
Cohn, Victor, 345–46, 373
Cold War, 156–57, 163–64, 166–67
Collins, Joseph, 72
Commission on the Health Needs of the Nation, 156
Committee of Physicians for the Improvement of Medical Care, 126

Committee on Medical Practice, 184, 443 (n. 58)
Committee on the Costs of Medical Care (CCMC), 73–76, 110, 122, 129–30, *201*
Commonwealth Fund, 188
Community clinics, 260–62
Community Mental Health Centers Act, 260
Comparative effectiveness studies, 399
Competition: between drugstores, 364–65; between health insurance companies, 353–54; between hospitals, 332–34; between physicians, 336–37
Confidential Bulletin (Consumers' Research), 105, 108–9
Consent, 269, 270, 271, 274, 275–76, 276–80, 285, 318, 385, 394, 417, 453 (n. 69)
Console, Dale, 244
Consumer activism, 263–67, 280–81
Consumer culture, 163, 321, 390, 420; interwar, 38, 41, 44, 45; medicine and, xii, 5, 10, 19, 45, 68, 193
Consumer education. *See* Education, consumer
Consumer Federation of America, 264
Consumer Health Coalition, 263
Consumer Health Information Source Book, 303
Consumerism, 8; medical vs. health, 14; as term, 424 (n. 7). *See also* Critical consumerism; Medical consumerism
Consumerists, 424 (n. 7)
Consumer Price Index, 178, 237, 445 (n. 87)
Consumer Product Safety Commission, 264
Consumer Reports, 157, 284
Consumers' Bill of Rights, 253, 271
Consumers' Guide to Health Care (Chisari, Nakamura, and Thorup), 300
Consumer spending: doctor bills in spectrum of, 69–70; drugstores and, 81; in economy, 4, 8, 38; habits, *211*;

rising, in 1920s, 38; shifts in, 178, 221–22

Consumers' Research, 105, 108–10

Consumers Union, 109, 110, 157, 246–47, 264, 302, 361, 449 (nn. 69–70)

Continuing medical education, 61, 408

Contraceptives, 276, 293–94, 385. *See also* Birth control

Cooley, Charles, 42

Cooper, Donald L., 287

Cooper, Marian G., 338–39

Copeland, Royal, 44, 115, 117

Cornell Medical Index, 171

Corporations: health care, 323–24; physicians as, 324

Corticosteroids, 235–36; marketing of, 150, 238

Cosmetics: drugstores and, 78, 80, 82, 83, 92, 104, 364, 366; safety and, 102, 106, 110, 111, 113, 114, 117

Costs: advertising by, 332; as "bitter pill," 178–82; business considerations and, 65–67; Committee on the Costs of Medical Care and, 73–76; consumer concerns over, 68–69, 70, 76, 91, 100, 106, 120, 128–29, 134, 178–80, 192, 194, 271, 354; as consumer spending, 69–70; culture of, 179–80; discussion of before treatment, 180–81; drugs and, 99–100, 216, 220–21, 241–42, 254–55, 368; fee splitting and, 120–21, 182, 443 (n. 58); in "free trade" era, 23; health insurance and, 145–46, 198, 325, 400; itemized billing and, 48, 66–67, 180–81, 184, 209, 210, 271; life span and, 41–42; in media, 197; medical consumerism and, 120–21; of medical education, 48; Medicare and, 327; outcomes vs., 400–401; of over-the-counter drugs, 229–30; philanthropy and, 73; physicians' justifications for, 48, 65–68, 76, 179–80, 194, 398; rising, 48–49, 65–66, 69, 197, 323–24, 413–14; setting of, 179–81; of surgery, 68; variations in, 67–68

Costs, Risks and Benefits of Surgery (Bunker, Barnes, and Mosteller), 320

Council of Senior Citizens, 438 (n. 15)

Council on Pharmacy and Chemistry (AMA), 231, 426 (n. 30)

Country doctor, 48, 58, 64, 161, 165, 203, 438 (n. 15)

Cousins, Norman, 162, 308–10, 317

"Cousins Affair," 308–10

Cramp, Arthur, 86, 88, 97, 102, 120

Crawford, Charles, 233

"Creaming," 353

Crenner, Chris, 453 (n. 69)

Crile, George, 278, 303

Critical consumerism, 5. *See also* Consumerists; Medical consumerism

Cron, Theodore, 12, 266–67

"Cultural lag," 74, 191

Culture: autonomy in, 10; of billing, 179–80; individualism in, 10; of medicine, xi–xii

Curran, William, 278

Customer service, pharmacists and, 100–101

Cutler, David M., 398–99

CVS, 365

Dabes, Mrs. Joseph, 233

Dalkon Shield, 293–94

Dao, Thomas, 278

Dartmouth Atlas, 312

Davis, Adelle, 161

Davis, Edward, 113

Davis, Michael Marks, 58, 110, 173, 401

Dear Abby, 279

Decision aids, 410–11

"Defensive medicine," 401

Defibrillator, 404

Delacrote, George T., Jr., 103

"Delores ad," 378, 382

Democracy, 11, 140

Democratic National Convention (1968), 257

Democratic Party, 240–41, 257, 264, 267, 355

Food and Drugs Act and, 19, 32–37; safety with, 253–54; side effects of, 234–40, 275–76, 360, 386, 395, 405; testing of, 254; "wonder," 150, 241–42. *See also* Prescriptions

Drugstores, *204, 205, 215*; advertising and, 78, 225, 366; antiregulatory mood and, 360–61; aspirin and, 224–25; competition between, 364–65; consumer spending and, 221–22; counter service to self-service in, 221–30; criticism of, 102–3; customer service and, 100–101; dominance of, 81–82; drugs and, 81–83, 84–86; expansion of, 364; grocery stores and, 223–334; hygiene and, 83; medical consumerism and, 111–12; nonmedical merchandise at, 83–84; pharmaceutical industry and, 85–86; pharmacists and, 81; from pharmacy to, 79–84, 92; physicians and, 91–92; pine board, 99–100; prescriptions and, 82–83, 230–31, 386–87; products offered at, 365–66; reputation of early, 82; role of, 77–78; science and, 79, 84–85; self-medication and, 53, 92–93; shoplifting in, 226–27

Dubos, René, 196–97, 418–19
Due process, 279
Dunbar, Paul, 152–53
Dunham, Donald, 179
Durante, Jimmy, 227
Durham, Carl, 153
Durham-Humphrey Amendments, 154, 156, 231, 232, 233, 446 (n. 28)
Dyott, Thomas, 22

Eaton, George D., 133
Let's Eat Right to Keep Fit (Davis), 161
Eclectic medicine, 22
Economic Opportunity Act, 260
Economic transformation, 323–24
Economy, consumer spending in, 4, 8, 38. *See also* Consumer Price Index
Edstrom, Eve, 198

Education: 10, 11, 14, 72, 109, 163; consumer, 93–95, 226, 446 (n.14), 455 (n.9), 466 (n. 32); rising levels of, 134–35, 183, 226, 290–91; health and patient, 42, 44, 83, 297, 300, 302, 310–11; patient, 310–11
Education, medical. *See* Medical education
Ehrenreich, Barbara, 269
Ehrlich, Paul, 85
Elixir Sulfanilamide, 116, 447 (n. 35)
Emerson, Haven, 438 (n. 15)
Employee Retirement Income Security Act, 292–93, 460 (n. 17)
Endorsement, celebrity, 381
Engagement, patient, 391–92
Entrepreneurship, 20
Environmental Protection Agency, 264
Ephraim, Jerome W., 110, 135, 433 (n. 59)
Equipment, in doctors' offices, 57–58. *See also* Technology
Estrogen, 71, 244, 315
Ethnicity. *See* Race
Evans Rule, 99
Everett, Ann, 377
Evidence-based medicine, 312–13, 357, 358, 393, 393, 399, 400, 403, 406
Ewing, Oscar, 12, 144, 417, 424 (n. 14), 438 (n. 15)

Fad, 70, 71, 243, 245
Fagerlin, Angela, 403
Falk, I. S., 55, 62, 69–70, 74–75, 110, 123, 128
Family doctor, x, 31, 48, 63–64, 163, 169, 192, 196, 251, 298, 337, 385, 407. *See also* Country doctor; General practitioner; Primary care physician
Family Doctor, The (Rockwell), 163, *203*
Fanon, Frantz, 258
Fash, Robert, 222
Fashion, 70, 71, 243, 245
Fast-tracking, of drugs, 360, 370–71
FCC. *See* Federal Communications Commission

Health Left, 287, 326

Health maintenance organizations (HMOs), 292, 328–29, 330, 352

Health Policy Advisory Center, 258, 259

Health Research Group, 265, 266, 303, 347–48, 351, 384

Health Rights News, 262

Health Security Act, 292

Heart disease. *See* Cardiovascular disease

Heller, Jean, 277

Henderson, Lawrence H., 3, 424 (n. 4)

Henderson, Ruth Evelyn, 62

Heric, Thomas M., 336

Hertzler, Arthur, 24, 50, 54, 55

Hiebert, J. Mark, 230

Hill-Burton Act, 140–41

Hippocratic Oath, 330, 336, 343

"Hip-pocket" operations, 303, 414, 457 (n. 44)

Hip replacement, 325, 404

History, medical, in patient evaluation. *See* Medical history

HIV/AIDS, 370

Hoff, Lawrence C., 379

Hoffman, Felix, 85

Holmes, Oliver Wendell, 29, 36

Home, as locus of care, 21, 23, 53–54, 170. *See also* Domestic medicine

Home economics, 42, 107, 110, 114, 226, 233

Homeopathy, 13, 22, 27, 115, 118, 299

Hooper, Benjamin, 165–66, 341

Hopkins, Charles, 32

Hormone replacement therapy. *See* Estrogen

Hospital Corporation of America (HCA), 324, 328

Hospitals: in 1800s, 21–22; advertising and, 332–35, 408–9; competition between, 332–34; for-profit, 328–29; health insurance and, 141–42; influence of on medical billing culture, 179, 181–82; in medical training, 49–50; Medicare and, 327; mortality data of, 348; Patients' Bill of Rights and, 272–73; ranking of, 349–50; specialization and, 50–51; in *U.S. News and World Report*, 349–50

Hospitals and Health Network, 1

Hours, office, 338–39

House calls, ix, 48, 53–54, 170, 188, 213

House Committee on Un-American Activities, 154, 157, 449 (n. 68)

Household medicine, 21

How to Avoid Unnecessary Surgery (Williams), 302–3

How to Be Your Own Doctor (Sometimes) (Sehnert), 310

Hoyt, Daniel, 95

Humana, 321, 324, 328, 332, 334

Humphrey, Hubert, 153

Hygiene, drugstores and, 83

Hysterectomy, 180, 185, 194, 457 (n. 44)

Iacocca, Lee, 327

Ibuprofen, 375

"If" (Kipling), 47

If Disney Ran Your Hospital: 9 ½ Things You Would Do Differently (Lee), 389–90

Image, of physicians. *See* Physicians, image of

Imaging devices, 324–25

Incomes, of physicians, 52, 168, 194–95, 251–52

Index Medicus, 303

Individualism, 9, 10, 52, 134

Industrialization, 20

Infectious disease, decline in, 41–42

Inflation, 107, 363; and medical costs, 146, 147, 197

Information leaflet. *See* Patient information leaflet

Informed consent, 269, 270, 271, 274, 276–80, 285, 318, 385, 394, 417, 453 (n. 69)

Ingelfinger, Franz J., 308, 313

Innovation, 325

Institute of Medicine (IOM), 348, 392

Insulin, 85
Insurance. *See* Health insurance
Interactions, drug, 405
Interdepartmental Committee on
    Health and Welfare Activities, 130
Internet, x, xv, 1, 2, 3, 15, 19, 44, 333, 365,
    384, 387, 391, 394, 396, 410, 415
Internships, 49–50
Itemization, of bills, 180–81, *209*, *210*

Jarvis, D. C, 161
J. B. Williams Company, 229
Jehovah's Witnesses, 279
Jewish medical school applicants, 50
Jingles, 228
Johns Hopkins Medical School, 27
Johnson, Lyndon, 252, 255–56
Joint Council for the Accreditation of
    Hospitals, 270–71
Joubert, Pieter, 304
Journal of the American Medical Associa-
    tion, 34, 75, 120, 122, 126–27
Journals, medical, 168
"Judo politics," 273–74, 280–81
Jungle, The (Sinclair), 33–34
J. Walter Thompson (ad agency), 45, 89,
    90, 94

Kaiser Permanente, 142, 412
Kaiser Permanente Foundation, 418
Kallet, Arthur, 70, 106, 109, 111–13, 134,
    157, 246, 384, 430 (n. 61), 449 (n. 68)
Kamholtz, Theodore, *212*
Katz, Norman D., 449 (n. 68)
Kefauver, Estes, 220, 241–42, 253–54
Kefauver-Harris Amendment, 252, 254,
    257, 293
Keller, Reamer, *212*
Kellock, Katharine A., 121, 122, 183, 303,
    436 (n. 45)
Kennedy, John F., 5, 199, 252, 253–55, 257
Kennedy, Ted, 267, 292
Kent, James, 24
Kerlan, Irvin, 231
Kessler, David, 382

King, James, 388
King, Martin Luther, Jr., 257
Kingsbury, John, 123
Kingsley, Sidney, 70
Kipling, Rudyard, 47
Kirk, Paul Harden, 169
Kirlin, Florence, 117
Kisch, Arnold, 290
Klein, Herbert, 306
Klerman, Gerald, 244
Kmart, 363
Knauer, Virginia, 466 (n. 32)
Knee replacement, 325, 404
Knowles, John H., 318–19
Koch, Ed, 346
Koop, C. Everett, 373
Koos, Earl Lomon, 159, 188–89, 443
    (n. 66)
Kopetzky, Samuel J., 126
Krause, Arlene, 321
Kresge, S. S., 363
Kris, Joseph, 165–66, 341
Kroger, 223, 363, 464 (n. 6)
Kushner, Rose, 278, 344

Labels, 100, 114–17, 232, 274–76, 314–15.
    See also Packaging
Laboratory-based science, 26, 28–29
Lamb, Ruth deForest, 110, 114, 134, 153
Lander, Louise, 318
Langford, Elizabeth, 157
Language, in prescriptions, 98–99, 233
Lape, Esther Everett, 124
Lasagna, Louis, 244, 304
Latin, 98–99, 233
Lavin, John H., 313
Lazarsfeld, Paul, 189
Lear, Walter, 272
"Learned intermediary," 245, 268, 274–75,
    384–86, 403, 448 (n. 66), 452 (n. 47)
LeBlanc, Thomas, 77, 84
Lee, C. Marshall, Jr., 193–94
Lee, Fred, 389–90
Legal activism, 268
"Legend drugs," 220–21

Legitimacy, 4
Legler, William, 89–90, 90–91
Leno, Jay, 382
Lerner, Barron, 453 (n. 69)
Let the Seller Beware! (Hubbard and Bishop), 267–69
Leven, Maurice, 54
Lewis, Sinclair, 70
Liberty Mutual, 146
Librium, 236
Licensure: doctor-shopping and, 61; early, 23, 25; education and, 27–28; internships and, 50; in late 1800s, 26–27
Life span, 41–42, 43, 159–60
Lifestyle diseases, 43
Liggett, Louis, 77, 81
Lincoln Hospital, 260
Linde, Shirley, 301–2
Lipkin, Mack, 307
Literacy, 22, 100, 446 (n. 30)
Lobbyists, 12–13, 265
Loeb, Eleanor, 430 (n. 61)
Looking-glass self, 42, 84, 386
Loos, Earl Komon, 159
Lord, Audre, 424 (n. 12)
Loss leaders, 230
Luce, Henry, 126
Lucky Strike cigarettes, 94
Luxury, 71–73
Lynch, John, 336–37

Magaziner, Ira, 355
Magnuson, Warren G., 229, 267
Malpractice: activism and, 268; communication and, 310; consent and, 277, 278, 279; "free trade" era and, 24–25; "reasonable patient" standard and, 278; rise in suits for, 350; testing and, 401
Mammogram, 10, 342, 353, 406, 419
Mammon, MD (stock character), 70
Managerial medicine: advertising and, 331–36; decline of, 356–57; doctor-patient relationship and, 330–31; economic transformation and, 323–24;

emergence of, 322; health insurance and, 327–28, 352–53; health maintenance organizations and, 328–29; Medicaid and, 346–47; medical consumerism and, 357–58; Medicare and, 325–26; patients and, 322–23; physicians and, 329–30; private practice and, 336–43
Mantle, Mickey, 381
Marketing. *See* Advertising
Mason, Cleon, 63
Mason, James, 236
Masters, Dexter, 247, 449 (n. 68)
Maurer, Herrymon, 194–95
May, Charles, 245
Maynard, Harold H., 80, 101
McCarthy, Eugene G., 312
McCarthyism, 154, 157
McGarrah, Rob, 283–84
McKeown, Thomas, 440 (n. 57)
Means, J. H., 174
Meat Inspection Act, 35
Meatpacking industry, 33–34
Mechanic, David, 312
MedFirst, 321, 338
Media: in early 1800s, 22; health education and, 44–45; Kefauver hearings and, 242; "medical breakthrough" narrative in, 40; medical fiction in, 158; "red clause" and, 33
Medic (television program), 158
Medicaid, 252, 255–57, 292, 346–47, 402, 450 (n. 10), 462 (n. 65)
Medical Advisory Committee, 124, 126
Medical arms race, 167, 333–34, 339, 401, 403
Medical Assistant, The (Cooper and Bredow), 338–39
Medical assistants, 171, 181, 340, 341, 441 (n. 17)
"Medical breakthrough" narrative, 40
Medical Committee for Human Rights, 259, 262, 263, 265–66, 298
Medical consumerism: and accusations of communist sympathies, 5, 75, 154,

157, 246, 391; Consumers' Research and, 108–10; costs and, 120–21; critical, 105–7; drugstores and, 111–12; flaws of, 419; health consumerism vs., 14; individualism and, 134; labels and, 114–17; managed care and, 357–58; patient clout and, 134–35; Patients' Bill of Rights and, 272; physician reactions to, 304–5, 306–7; popularization of, 110–11; prescription drugs and, 247–48; professionalism and, 134; radicalism and, 252–53; skepticism and, 118–24

"Medical democracy," 140

Medical devices, 325, 334, 404–5

Medical Economics (magazine), 66, 68, 180–81, 195, *208–12*, 273, 283–84, 287, 305–6, 313, 457 (n. 50)

Medical education: cost of, 48; curriculum advancement in, 49; curriculum advancement in early, 26; discrimination in, 50; doctor-patient relationship and, 191–92; hospitals in, 49–50; in media, 44–45; rankings in, 27–28, 61; science in, 167; "whole patient" and, 307–8

Medical history: in patient evaluation, 58, 300, 308, 429 (n. 30), 457 (n. 56)

"Medical home," 393, 402–3

Medical-industrial complex, 8, 141, 252–53, 258, 320, 328–29, 450 (n. 17), 453 (n. 70)

Medical insurance. *See* Health insurance

Medical journals, 168

Medical Letter on Drugs and Therapeutics, 246, 449 (n. 69)

Medical reference materials, patient use of, 297–98

Medicare, 199, 252, 255–57, 292, 325–28, 341, 438 (n. 15), 450 (n. 10), 459 (n. 11)

Medicare Prescription Drug, Improvement, and Modernization Act, 396

Medicine (drugs). *See* Drugs

Medicine at the Crossroads (Bernheim), 130, 132

Medicine Show, The (Consumers Union), 247, 302, 384

MedWatch, 384, 395

Men in White (film), 40

Men in White (Kingsley), 70

Mental health, 260, 279

Meprobamate, 236. *See also* Miltown

Merck, 149–50

Merck Manual of Diagnosis and Therapy, 168, 297, 456 (n. 27)

Mercurochrome, 430 (n. 61)

Merton, Robert, 444 (n. 68)

Middle class, 11, 14, 38, 162–63

Midwifery, 21

Milbank Fund, 123

"Milk Bottle Wars," 123–24

Milk of Magnesia, 96

Miller, Charles, 194

Miller, James C., III, 361

Miller, K. E., 92–93

Miller, Leslie J., 278

Miller, Roger, 377

Miller-Tydings Act, 100

Mills, C. Wright, 11, 162

Mills, Wilbur, 255

Milstein, Lloyd, 376

Miltown, 236, 244

Minot, George, 126

Mintz, Morton, 243, 254

"Miracle drugs," 157, 172, 221, 224, 234, 237

Mitchell, George, 356

Mitchell, Wesley C., 74

Modern Man Is Obsolete (Cousins), 162

Mondale, Walter, 277

Monetarization, 67, 324

Montgomery Ward Catalog, 39

Moore, Harry H., 54, 72, 436 (n. 46)

Morris, Lloyd, 63

Moss, Frank, 312

Moss, John E., 267

Mosteller, Frank, 320

Motherhood, 21

Movies, 40

Mrs. Winslow's Soothing Syrup, 37

Parke, Davis (pharmaceutical firm), 85, 86, *216*, 235, 240, 289, 291

Parking, 169–70, 173, 337, 338

Parsons, Talcott, 189, 444 (n. 68)

Pasteur, Louis, 40

Patent law, 149–50, 220, 254, 368–70

Patent medicines, 30

Paternalism: activism and, 258; informed consent and, 385; *Our Bodies, Our Selves* and, 299; and "patient" as term, 263; Patients' Bill of Rights and, 272; prescriptions and, 98; rejection of, 106; socioeconomic status and, 69

Patient(s): baby boomer, 290–91, 417, 455 (n. 9); defined, 14; as "doctor-shoppers," 1, 60–65, 119–20, 173–78, 337–38, 344–46, 462 (n. 65); drugs as expected by, 59, 244–45; education of, 310–11; engagement and, 391–92; first visit of, to physician, 62; "good," 132–33; health insurance and, 340–43, 354; as not passive, 297–304; privacy of, 170; as riled-up, 288–91; "safe," 383–86; skepticism of, 118–24; specializations and, 50–51; stakeholders and, 12–13; as term, 13, 263; trust in physicians by, 289; as watchdogs, 121, 344–45; "whole," 307–8. *See also* Doctor-patient relationship; Medical consumerism

Patient Care Partnership, The (American Hospital Association), 394

Patient information leaflet, 274–76, 314–17, 371–72, 373, 466 (nn. 32, 37)

Patient Prescription Drug Labeling Project, 314

Patient Protection and Affordable Care Act, 1, 397–98, 400

Patients' Bill of Rights, 269–74, 276, 318, 391

Patient's Guide to Successful Surgery, The (Galton), 303

Patients' Rights Digest, 280

Patten, Simon, 107

Peabody, Francis, 307

Peebles, Allon, 59

Penalty, The (film), 40

Penicillin, 148, 149, 150, 235, 237, 277

People's Drug Store, *204*, *205*, 375

People's Free Clinic of Austin, *218*

People's Handbook of Medical Care (Frank and Frank), 298

People's Pharmacy, The (Graedon), 302

Perez v. Wyeth Laboratories, 385–86

Pertschuk, Michael, 267, 296

Peters, John P., 124, 126

Pfizer, 240, 450 (n. 8)

Pfizer doctrine, 294

Pharmaceutical industry: drugstores and, 85–86; patent law and, 149–50; prescription drugs and, 147–56; Red Scare and, 154; regulation of, 240–44, 360, 370–71; as "sunrise industry," 367–68

Pharmaceuticals. *See* Drugs; Prescriptions

Pharmacists: ciphers used by, 99; drugstores and, 81; physicians vs., 100–101; price setting by, 99; responsibilities of, with prescription drugs, 231–33. *See also* Drugstores; Prescriptions

Pharmacy: from drugstore to, 79–84, 92; open floor plan of, 97. *See also* Drugstores

Philanthropy, 73

Phillips, Pauline, 279

Phillips' Milk of Magnesia, 96

Physical examination, 58, 429 (n. 30)

Physicians: advertising and, 93–95, 96–97, 331–36; apprenticeships of, 21; autonomy of, 9, 242, 288, 312–13, 322, 329–30; "best of" lists of, 350–51; as businesspeople, 48, 65–67, 178–79; competition between, 336–37; as corporations, 324; drug advertising and, 378–79; drugstores and, 91–92; in early 1800s, 21; education of (*See* Education); fees of (*See* Costs); first visit to, 62; general practice (*See* General Practitioner); house calls by, ix,

48, 53–54, 170, 188, 213; image of, 40, 65, 143, 165, 178, 186–96, 198, 213, 251, 256, 257, 322, 336–37, 385; improvements in, 49–52; incomes of, 52, 168, 194–95, 251–52; individualism of, 9, 52; insurance and, 339–43; internships of, 49–50; as "learned intermediaries," 245, 268, 274–75, 384–86, 403, 448 (n. 66), 452 (n. 47); licensure of (*See* Licensure); malpractice by (*See* Malpractice); managerial care and, 329–30, 336–43; medical consumerism and, 304–5, 306–7; Medicare and, 327; offices of, 52–60, 168–73, 202, *207, 208,* 337–38; patient information leaflets and, 316–17; patient views of, 190–91; personal service and, 74, 100, 176–77, 307, 325, 441 (n. 17); pharmacists vs., 100–101; professionalism of, 4, 28–29, 70–71, 134, 337; ranking of, 350–51, 388–89; in rural areas, 54; selection of, 60–61, 173–78; "shopping" for, 1, 60–65; specialization of, 50–52, 60, 64, 167–68; trust in, 289. *See also* Country doctor; Doctor-patient relationship; Primary care physician
Physician's Desk Reference (*PDR*), 297
Piggly Wiggly, 223
Pine board stores, 99–100
Pinkham, Lydia, 31, 33
Plant-based drugs, 21
Pneumovax, 375
Pogue, Alan, *218*
Poisons, 25
Polypharmacy, 362, 405
POP Radio, 366
Postal service, 22, 31
Potter, Samuel O., 98
Poverty: doctor shopping and, 346–47, 462 (n. 65); doctor's office locations and, 55; health care access and, 158–59; health care activism and, 257–58. *See also* Medicaid
Prescription Drug Law, 154–56
Prescription Drug User Fee Act, 395

Prescriptions: Consumers Union and, 246–47; defined, 231; drugstores and, 82–83, 230–31, 386–87; Durham-Humphrey Amendments and, 154, 156, 231, 232, 233; labels for, 232; language in, 98–99, 233; as loss leaders, 230; market expansion of, 231; medical consumerism and, 247–48; pharmaceutical industry and, 147–56; pharmacist responsibilities with, 231–33. *See also* Drugs
Press Ganey Associates, 1
Prevention, 161, 299
Preventive medicine, 12, 160–61
Prices. *See* Costs
Primary care physician, 175, 343, 389, 393, 402–3, 462 (n. 65), 470 (n. 36); as term, 337
Prince George's County Medical Society, 282–85
Pringle, Henry F., 128
Print revolution, 22
Privacy, 170, 279–80
Private practice, 52, 75, 141, 336–43
Product liability, 385–86
Product placement, 88
Professionalism, 4, 28–29, 70–71, 134, 337
Progressive era, 19, 20
Proprietary drugs, 29–31
Prozac, 370
Publications, 168
Public Citizen, 282, 283, 303, 306, 347–48, 351, 384
Public Citizen's Health Research Group, 265
Public relations, by AMA, 177–78, 187, 255
"Puffing," 90
Pure Food and Drugs Act, 19, 33–37, 95
Pusey, William Allen, 24, 67–68, 94, 433 (n. 51)

Quackery, 23, 28–29, 33, 62, 65, 71
Quality control, 399
Quinlan, Karen Ann, 279

Rabies vaccine, 40
Race: doctor's office locations and, 55;
    health care access and, 25, 158–59;
    health care activism and, 257–58;
    medical education and, 50
Radicals, 252–53. *See also* Activism
Radio, advertising on, 87–88, 103
Radium water, 71, 430 (n. 61)
Ramus, Michael, 217
Randolph, Gardner, 21
Ranking: of hospitals, 349–50;
    of medical schools, 27–28, 61;
    of physicians, 350–51, 388–89
Reader's Digest, 197–98
Reagan, Ronald, 292, 317, 322, 327, 360,
    361, 370
Real Folks (radio program), 88
"Red clause," 33
Red Scare, 154, 157, 246, 449 (n. 68)
Reeder, Leo, 290
Rees, Alan M., 302
Refilling of prescriptions, 37, 99,
    152–53, 154, 155, 231, 232–33
Reform, health care. *See* Health care
    system, reform of
Regulation: of drug advertising,
    88–89, 228–29; drugstores and,
    360–61; in late 1800s and early
    1900s, 32–37; of pharmaceutical
    industry, 240–44, 360, 370–71;
    rolling-back of, 360
Reinhardt, Uwe, 329
Religion, 279
Relman, Arnold, 328, 450 (n.17)
Remington, Joseph P., 98, 431 (n. 15)
Remuglia, Anthony, 146
Republican Party, 257, 267, 314
Resor, Stanley, 90
Resource-Based Relative-Value Scale,
    327, 341, 401
Retail. *See* Drugstores
Retail clinics, 394
Revolution, American, 20
Rexall Company, 81, 227
Reynolds, James, 284, 306

Rights of Hospital Patients, The (ACLU),
    318
Rinehart, Stanley M., 48, 53, 66
Ring, Martha D., 55, 62, 74–75
Robert Wood Johnson Foundation, 418
Robins, R. B., 184
Robinson, Leonard, 245–46
Rockefeller, Nelson, 292
Rockefeller Institute for Medical Re-
    search, 85
Rockwell, Norman, ix, 163, 203, 336, 385
Rodale, Jerome, 299
Rodale, J. J., 161
Rodale, Robert, 299
Roe, Jane, 285
Roessner, R. Gommel, 207
Roe v. Wade, 279–80
Rogers, Carl, 189, 444 (n. 68)
Rogers, Paul G., 372–73
Rollen Watterson Associates, 184,
    189–90
Romney, Mitt, 397
Roosevelt, Eleanor, 69, 113
Roosevelt, Franklin, Jr., 115
Roosevelt, Franklin D., 113, 115
Roosevelt, Theodore, 34, 35
Roper, Elmo, 128
Roper, Otis, 348
Roper, William, 348
Rorem, C. Rufus, 55, 62, 74–75, 85, 92
Rorty, James, 92, 103, 106, 110, 124, 128,
    131–32, 162, 258
Rothman, David, 453 (n. 69)
Roueché, Berton, 236
Rufen, 375
Rural areas, physicians in, 54
Russell, George A., 163, 203
Rutter, Richard, 176

"Safe patients," 383–86
Safety, drug, 34, 86, 116–17, 225, 251, 252,
    253–54, 384, 395
Sagwa (tonic), 31
Saltzstein, Harry, 43
Sartre, Jean-Paul, 258

STUDIES IN SOCIAL MEDICINE

Nancy M. P. King, Gail E. Henderson, and Jane Stein, eds., *Beyond Regulations: Ethics in Human Subjects Research* (1999).

Laurie Zoloth, *Health Care and the Ethics of Encounter: A Jewish Discussion of Social Justice* (1999).

Susan M. Reverby, ed., *Tuskegee's Truths: Rethinking the Tuskegee Syphilis Study* (2000).

Beatrix Hoffman, *The Wages of Sickness: The Politics of Health Insurance in Progressive America* (2000).

Margarete Sandelowski, *Devices and Desires: Gender, Technology, and American Nursing* (2000).

Keith Wailoo, *Dying in the City of the Blues: Sickle Cell Anemia and the Politics of Race and Health* (2001).

Judith Andre, *Bioethics as Practice* (2002).

Chris Feudtner, *Bittersweet: Diabetes, Insulin, and the Transformation of Illness* (2003).

Ann Folwell Stanford, *Bodies in a Broken World: Women Novelists of Color and the Politics of Medicine* (2003).

Lawrence O. Gostin, *The AIDS Pandemic: Complacency, Injustice, and Unfulfilled Expectations* (2004).

Arthur A. Daemmrich, *Pharmacopolitics: Drug Regulation in the United States and Germany* (2004).

Carl Elliott and Tod Chambers, eds., *Prozac as a Way of Life* (2004).

Steven M. Stowe, *Doctoring the South: Southern Physicians and Everyday Medicine in the Mid-Nineteenth Century* (2004).

Arleen Marcia Tuchman, *Science Has No Sex: The Life of Marie Zakrzewska, M.D.* (2006).

Michael H. Cohen, *Healing at the Borderland of Medicine and Religion* (2006).

Keith Wailoo, Julie Livingston, and Peter Guarnaccia, eds., *A Death Retold: Jesica Santillan, the Bungled Transplant, and Paradoxes of Medical Citizenship* (2006).

Michelle T. Moran, *Colonizing Leprosy: Imperialism and the Politics of Public Health in the United States* (2007).

Karey Harwood, *The Infertility Treadmill: Feminist Ethics, Personal Choice, and the Use of Reproductive Technologies* (2007).

Carla Bittel, *Mary Putnam Jacobi and the Politics of Medicine in Nineteenth-Century America* (2009).

Samuel Kelton Roberts Jr., *Infectious Fear: Politics, Disease, and the Health Effects of Segregation* (2009).

Lois Shepherd, *If That Ever Happens to Me: Making Life and Death Decisions after Terri Schiavo* (2009).

Mical Raz, *What's Wrong with the Poor?: Psychiatry, Race, and the War on Poverty* (2013).

Johanna Schoen, *Abortion after Roe* (2015).

Nancy Tomes, *Remaking the American Patient: How Madison Avenue and Modern Medicine Turned Patients into Consumers* (2016).

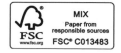